AF782861

Natural Immunity

NeuroImmune Biology, Volume 5

NeuroImmune Biology

Series Editors

I. Berczi, A. Szentivanyi

Advisory Board

B.G. Arnason, *Chicago, IL*
E. Artzt, *Buenos Aires, Argentina*
P.J. Bàrnes, *London, UK*
T. Bartfai, *La Jolla, CA*
L. Bertók, *Budapest, Hungary*
H.O. Besedovsky, *Marburg, Germany*
J. Bienenstock, *Hamilton, Canada*
C.M. Blatteis, *Memphis, TN*
J. Buckingham, *London, UK*
Ch. Chawnshang, *Rochester, NY*
R. Dantzer, *Bordeau, France*
M. Dardenne, *Paris, France*
N. Fabris, *Ancona, Italy*
R.C. Gaillard, *Lausanne, Switzerland*
Ch. George, *Bethesda, MD*
R. Good, *Tampa, FL*
R.M. Gorczynski, *Toronto, Canada*
C. Heijnen, *Utrecht, The Netherlands*
T. Hori, *Fukuoka, Japan*
H. Imura, *Kyoto, Japan*
M.D. Kendall, *Cambridge, UK*
E.A. Korneva, *St. Petersburg, Russia*
K. Kovacs, *Toronto, Canada*
G. Kunkel, *Berlin, Germany*
L.A. Laitinen, *Helsinki, Finland*
B. Marchetti, *Catania, Italy*
L. Matera, *Turin, Italy*
H. Ovadia, *Jerusalem, Israel*
C.P. Phelps, *Tampa, FL*
L.D. Prockop, *Tampa, FL*
R. Rapaport, *New York, NY*
S. Reichlin, *Tucson, AZ*
R. Schmidt, *Hannover, Germany*
A. Shmakov, *Novosibirsk, Russia*
K. Skwarlo-Sonta, *Warsaw, Poland*
E.M. Sternberg, *Bethesda, MD*
D.W. Talmage, *Denver, CO*
S. Walker, *Columbia, MO*
A.G. Zapata, *Madrid, Spain*

Natural Immunity

Volume Editors

Lóránd Bertók
Donna A. Chow

NRI for Radiobiology & Radiohygiene, Budapest, Hungary
and
University of Manitoba, Winnipeg, Manitoba, Canada

ELSEVIER

2005

AMSTERDAM – BOSTON – LONDON – NEW YORK – OXFORD – PARIS
SAN DIEGO – SAN FRANCISO – SINGAPORE – SYDNEY – TOKYO

ELSEVIER B.V.
Sara Burgerhartstraat 25
P.O. Box 211, 1000 AE
Amsterdam, The Netherlands

ELSEVIER Inc.
525 B Street
Suite 1900 San Diego
CA 92101-4495, USA

ELSEVIER Ltd.
The Boulevard
Langford Lane, Kidlington,
Oxford OX5 1GB, UK

ELSEVIER Ltd.
84 Theobalds Road
London WC1X 8RR
UK

© 2005 Elsevier B.V. All rights reserved.

This work is protected under copyright by Elsevier B.V., and the following terms and conditions apply to its use:

Photocopying
Single photocopies of single chapters may be made for personal use as allowed by national copyright laws. Permission of the Publisher and payment of a fee is required for all other photocopying, including multiple or systematic copying, copying for advertising or promotional purposes, resale, and all forms of document delivery. Special rates are available for educational institutions that wish to make photocopies for non-profit educational classroom use.

Permissions may be sought directly from Elsevier's Rights Department in Oxford, UK: phone (+44) 1865 843830, fax (+44) 1865 853333, e-mail: permissions@elsevier.com. Requests may also be completed on-line via the Elsevier homepage (http://www.elsevier.com/locate/permissions).

In the USA, users may clear permissions and make payments through the Copyright Clearance Center, Inc., 222 Rosewood Drive, Danvers, MA 01923, USA; phone: (+1) (978) 7508400, fax: (+1) (978) 7504744, and in the UK through the Copyright Licensing Agency Rapid Clearance Service (CLARCS), 90 Tottenham Court Road, London W1P 0LP, UK; phone: (+44) 20 7631 5555; fax: (+44) 20 7631 5500. Other countries may have a local reprographic rights agency for payments.

Derivative Works
Tables of contents may be reproduced for internal circulation, but permission of the Publisher is required for external resale or distribution of such material. Permission of the Publisher is required for all other derivative works, including compilations and translations.

Electronic Storage or Usage
Permission of the Publisher is required to store or use electronically any material contained in this work, including any chapter or part of a chapter.

Except as outlined above, no part of this work may be reproduced, stored in a retrieval system or transmitted in any form or by any means, electronic, mechanical, photocopying, recording or otherwise, without prior written permission of the Publisher.
Address permissions requests to: Elsevier's Rights Department, at the fax and e-mail addresses noted above.

Notice
No responsibility is assumed by the Publisher for any injury and/or damage to persons or property as a matter of products liability, negligence or otherwise, or from any use or operation of any methods, products, instructions or ideas contained in the material herein. Because of rapid advances in the medical sciences, in particular, independent verification of diagnoses and drug dosages should be made.

First edition 2005

Library of Congress Cataloging in Publication Data
A catalog record is available from the Library of Congress.

British Library Cataloguing in Publication Data
A catalogue record is available from the British Library.

ISBN: 0-444-51755-3
ISSN: 1567-7443 (Series)

∞ The paper used in this publication meets the requirements of ANSI/NISO Z39.48-1992 (Permanence of Paper).
Printed in The Netherlands.

Foreword

Susceptibility and resistance to disease have been known to people since prehistoric times. Catastrophic epidemic diseases in medieval times provided ample evidence for both of these concepts. Environmental effects were also identified as one of the factors that affect resistance to disease. The expression "catching a cold" refers to this association. Pasteur made observations between the relationship of chicken cholera (pasteurellosis) and the weather and Koch examined the effect of swimming in cold water on the susceptibility of chickens to anthrax [1]. Mediaeval shepherds knew that if they saved the scabs from pox lesions and inoculated young animals with this material, the disease could be prevented. Jenner and Ehrlich popularized this knowledge and the concept of *adaptive immunity* was born [2]. However, it was clear from numerous examples that adaptive immunity was not fully responsible for resistance to disease. With the advent of virology, it became apparent that there is *species specific resistance*. This means that a particular virus cannot cause disease in some host species but it could do it in other species. This is also true for bacteria, but the host-restrictions are often not as strict as for viruses. It was also obvious that healthy animals and human beings do demonstrate *nonspecific resistance* to infections and a number of other insults, which may be caused by diverse noxious agents. The term "nonspecific" was adopted in relation to adaptive immunity, which is antigen specific. Hans Selye described a syndrome elicited by diverse noxious agents [3], which he later named the *stress response* that resulted in elevated resistance to countless *stressors*. Physical, chemical, biological and in man even emotional agents could act as stressors. During the stress response the hypothalamus pituitary adrenal axis was activated, the thymus exhibited a profound shrinkage, atrophy of lymphoid organs and immunosuppression also occurred, except for gamma globulin, which was elevated. Stressed animals showed increased resistance to numerous noxious insults, and this was named by Selye the *general adaptation syndrome* [4]. Selye knew that in some way he was dealing with the immune system, but it was not possible to understand in those days the mechanisms involved. All that immunologists could see at the time was that the thymus was involuted and adaptive immunity was seriously suppressed or even eliminated by stress. This was in sharp contrast with Selye's conclusion that the stress response was an adaptive defence reaction.

In this book the natural immune system is presented. Its relationship to the adaptive immune system, the neuroendocrine system and to the entire host organism is discussed. This is the system we are born with and it will be with us for life. Most species of the animal kingdom rely on this immune system as the adaptive system is found only in vertebrates. The natural immune system protects us not only from infectious agents, but also from various noxious agents, and during acute danger, this system kicks into high gear, which manifests in febrile illness. In contrast with the commonly held perception, fever is a defence reaction, called the *acute phase response*. It is a very successful defence response as most people with febrile illness recover and become healthy again. The natural immune system also plays important *physiological roles* as presented in this volume. Clearly this is an incredibly effective system, which protects us practically from any kind of insult, and it is able to increase our resistance with unparalleled efficiency. Innate immune mechanisms are deeply embedded in our development and physiology.

This system provides the foundations for the adaptive immune system, which could not function or even exist without our innate system. There is little doubt that the recognition and appreciation of this system is a major milestone in Biology and is a perfect topic to be presented as volume 5 of Neuroimmune Biology.

Istvan Beczi, Lóránd Bertók, Donna Chow

REFERENCES

1. Metchnikoff E. Immunity in infective diseases. Cambridge: Cambridge Univ Press;1907.
2. Silverstein AM. The History of Immunology. In Fundamental Immunology, Third Ed. Paul WE. Ed. Raven Press, New York. 1993; pp. 21–41.
3. Selye H. A syndrome produced by diverse nocuous agents. Nature (Lond) 1936; 138: 32.
4. Selye H. The general adaptation syndrome and the diseases of adaptation. J Clin Endocrinol 1946; 6: 117–230.

Preface

Natural immunity is commonly considered to refer to the first line of host defence against microbial pathogens which provides protection before the development of the adaptive immune response. However the recent progressive explosion in molecular, cellular, animal and human research which has dramatically expanded our concept of the natural immune system and its functions, has been captured in this volume. Natural immunity is presented in its broadest terms focusing on the incredible richness in cellular and humoural mediators, their evolutionary origins in ancient times, their intimate interaction with the neuroendocrine system and their unquestionable ability to provide an interactive and multilayered defence against pathogenic invasion all of which must also be considered in the context of their less well acknowledged physiological roles in essential, complex biological processes. The aim of this volume is to mark the significant expansion in our understanding of the scope of natural immunity in order to strengthen the rational basis for both fundamental and applied research on the natural immune system.

Donna A. Chow

Acknowledgements

Donna A. Chow wishes to acknowledge the research support of The Bayer, Canadian Blood Services, Héma Québec Partnership Fund. We are grateful to Mrs. Susan Ness and Dr. Arthur Chow who assisted in the preparation of this volume and to Dr. Istvan Berczi who consistently provided excellent guidance, support and enthusiasm for the project.

Lóránd Bertók is grateful to Mrs. Éva Major-Foki, Mrs. Márta Horváth-Lovász and to Dr. András Székely for the preparation of this volume, and to Dr. István Berczi for his friendly help and cooperation.

List of Contributors

Alan Aderem
The Institute for Systems Biology, Seattle, Washington

Laura N. Arneson
Department of Immunology, Mayo Graduate School, Mayo Clinic Rochester, Rochester, Minnesota

Istvan Berczi
Department of Immunology, Faculty of Medicine, The University of Manitoba, Winnipeg, MB, Canada

Lóránd Bertók
"Fodor József" National Center of Public Health, "Frédéric Joliot-Curie" National Research Institute for Radiobiology and Radiohygiene, Budapest, Hungary

Steven E. Bosinger
Division of Experimental Therapeutics, University Health Network, Toronto General Research Institute, Toronto General Hospital, Toronto, ON, Canada
Department of Microbiology & Immunology, University of Western Ontario, London, ON, Canada

Cheryl M. Cameron
Department of Microbiology & Immunology, University of Western Ontario, London, ON, Canada

Mark J. Cameron
Division of Experimental Therapeutics, University Health Network, Toronto General Research Institute, Toronto General Hospital, Toronto, ON, Canada

Miriam Capri
Department of Experimental Pathology, University of Bologna, Bologna, Italy

Donna A. Chow
Department of Immunology, Faculty of Medicine, University of Manitoba, Winnipeg, MB, Canada

Jeff C. Coombs
Division of Experimental Therapeutics, University Health Network, Toronto General Research Institute, Toronto General Hospital, Toronto, ON, Canada

Edwin L. Cooper
Laboratory of Comparative Neuroimmunology, Department of Neurobiology, David Geffen School of Medicine at UCLA, University of California, Los Angeles, California

Mark E. Devries
Division of Experimental Therapeutics, University Health Network, Toronto General Research Institute, Toronto General Hospital, Toronto, ON, Canada
Department of Microbiology & Immunology, University of Western Ontario, London, ON, Canada

Adrian J. Dunn
Department of Pharmacology and Therapeutics, Louisiana State University Health Sciences Center, Shreveport, Louisiana

Trude H. Flo
The Institute for Systems Biology, Seattle, Washington

Christiana Fumelli
Department of Experimental Pathology, University of Bologna, Bologna, Italy

Claudio Franceschi
Department of Experimental Pathology, University of Bologna, Bologna, Italy

Ronald B. Herberman
University of Pittsburgh Cancer Institute, Department of Medicine and Pathology, University of Pittsburgh School of Medicine, Pittsburgh, Pennsylvania

Karoline A. Hoisawa
Division of Experimental Therapeutics, University Health Network, Toronto General Research Institute, Toronto General Hospital, Toronto, ON, Canada
Department of Microbiology & Immunology, University of Western Ontario, London, ON, Canada

Kenneth M. Huttner
Division of Neonatology, Department of Pediatrics, Harvard Medical School and the MassGeneral Hospital for Children, Boston, Massachussetts

Elizabeth Husztik
Institute of Pathophysiology, University of Szeged, Szeged, Hungary

David J. Kelvin
Division of Experimental Therapeutics, University Health Network, Toronto General Research Institute, Toronto General Hospital, Toronto, Canada

Susan J. Larson
Department of Psychology, Concordia College, Moorhead, Minnesota

Georege Lázár
Institute of Pathophysiology, University of Szeged, Szeged, Hungary

Georege Lázár Jr.
Department of Surgery, University of Szeged, Szeged, Hungary

Paul J. Leibson
Department of Immunology, Mayo Graduate School, Mayo Clinic Rochester, Rochester, Minnesota

Francesco Lescai
Department of Experimental Pathology, University of Bologna, Bologna, Italy

Daniela Monti
Department of Experimental Pathology and Oncology, University of Florence, Florence, Italy

Bente Klarlund Pedersen, MD
The Copenhagen Muscle Research Centre and The Department of Infectious Diseases, Righospitalet, University of Copenhagen, Copenhagen, Denmark

Stefano Salvioli
Department of Experimental Pathology, University of Bologna, Bologna, Italy

Hector R. Wong
Division of Critical Care Medicine, Cincinnati Children's Hospital Medical Centre, Children's Hospital Research Foundation, Cincinnati, Ohio

Contents

I. HOST DEFENSE MECHANISMS

Natural Immunity
Edited by L. Bertók and D.A. Chow
© 2005 Elsevier B.V. All rights reserved

Host Defence: An Interaction of Neuroendocrine-, Metabolic- and Immune Mechanisms in the Interest of Survival

ISTVAN BERCZI[1], LÓRAND BERTÓK[2] and DONNA A. CHOW[1]

[1]Department of Immunology, Faculty of Medicine, the University of Manitoba, Winnipeg, MB R3E 0W3, Canada; [2]"Fodor József" National Center of Public Health and "Frédéric Joliot-Curie" National Research Institute for Radiobiology and Radiohygiene, H-1221 Anna u. 5, Budapest, Hungary

ABSTRACT

The term natural resistance refers to the capacity of living organisms to withstand injury caused by physical, chemical and biological agents that may be present in the external or internal environment. This protection is mediated by the natural, or innate, immune system, a multi-factorial and polyspecific defence system. Evolutionarily preserved germ-line receptors mediate the activation of natural immune cells that recognize genetically preserved, cross-reactive homologous epitopes (homotopes) in micro-organisms, cancer cells, virus-infected cells and distressed cells. In general, protection is based on balancing the defence mechanisms of the organism with the damaging effects of harmful agents. This defence comprises epithelial, secretory and endogenous mechanisms in addition to the cellular and humoural components of the natural immune system. In recent years, a continuing surge of exploration and discussion has helped to crystallize our appreciation of the molecular mechanisms of this innate system, their basis in evolution, physiological, pathological and behavioural significance and their regulation, in particular their intimate connection with the neuroendocrine system. In higher animals natural immune mechanisms are boosted profoundly during acute febrile illness leading to the release of pro-inflammatory cytokines, IL-1, TNF-alpha and IL-6, which in turn activate the neuroimmune regulatory network. The HPA axis and the sympathetic nervous system is activated and catabolism prevails. IL-6, glucocorticoids and cathecolamines induce the production of acute phase proteins permitting a rapid activation of phagocytic and cytotoxic mechanisms under the command of natural antibodies and other recognition molecules (e.g. C-reactive protein, endotoxin binding and mannose binding proteins). The acute phase response is a highly co-ordinated emergency defence reaction, which relies on the interaction of neuroendocrine, immune and metabolic mechanisms in the interest of maximum host defence during emergency situations, such as sepsis. In most cases febrile illness leads to healing and recovery, which attests to the effectiveness of the natural immune system and excites the desire for the benefits which should accrue from mastering the manipulation of this system.

1. INTRODUCTION

Innate or natural immunity has had a long and exciting past of which we are increasingly being made aware. The origins of the natural immune system are clearly buried in the evolutionary struggle for life. All living organisms, whether eucariotic, procariotic, unicellular or multicellular, from the lowest evolutionary stage right to the top, must have adequate defences against infections and other environmental threats. There is rapidly increasing knowledge of the various invertebrate defence systems, all of which depend on genetically stable, hard-wired innate mechanisms, or "natural" immune mechanisms, as they most frequently are called. It is also becoming clear that many, if not all of the natural defence molecules, which are present in vertebrates are also represented in lower animals. Most of the mechanisms involved are redundant and mutipotent, aimed at highly conserved, cross-reactive homologous epitopes, or *homotopes* for short. Homotopes are present on the targets of the natural defence system which may be microbes, infected – and cancer cells, as well as on other external and internal targets, as presented in this volume [1–3].

The evolutionary connection of our natural immune system to that of lower animals is truly fascinating. For instance, bacteria are known to express heat shock proteins, which must serve their survival under difficult environmental circumstances. In higher animals and man, heat shock proteins have similar functions and are intimately associated with steroid hormone receptors. Steroid hormones play important roles in the stress response [4,5]. Fungi make antibiotic substances, which miraculously work well in higher animals and man to fight bacterial infections. Antibiotics may be regarded to be analogous to defensins, and other antimicrobial molecules in our natural immune arsenal. Ciliates, which are the most primitive unicellular animals, are phagocytic organisms. Do they eat, digest and, therefore, destroy their microbial enemies? We know little about this, but our own phagocytic cells are certainly capable of eating away our enemies and much more.

Multicellular plants, as well as animals, must possess an effective system for organization and adequate defence mechanisms in order to survive and withstand environmental challenges and infectious agents. We share adhesion molecules with plants as attested by the stimulatory effect of plant lectins, such as phytohemagglutinine and concanavalin-A, on lymphocytes [6]. The existence of plant derived hormones, contraceptives and many remedies testifies further for our physiological and pathophysiological ties with the *plant kingdom*.

One striking conclusion, which is apparent from this book, is that the natural immune system serves well and protects most species of the *animal kingdom* with its enormous variety of defence mechanisms, whereas adaptive immunity exists only in a small minority of animals. If most species rely on innate mechanisms and survive well and prosper, this must speak forcefully for the enormous potency and versatility of this system. It is also clear that cytokines predate the adaptive immune system and so do neuropeptides predate the development of the central nervous system (CNS). Neuroimmune interactions also existed prior to the development of the central nervous system [7]. It is also regarding the innate system, as it is for the adaptive system, that immune mechanisms play an important role in normal physiology and pathology [8–10].

Today immunological host defence may be categorised into three major constituents: (a) species-specific resistance, (b) natural immunity and (c) the adaptive immune response. Species-specific resistance depends on factors defined by evolution. For instance, pathogens are capable of causing disease in some species whereas others remain refractory [11]. In contrast, natural immunity is subject to changes according to the environment of the individual and represent a long-recognised, important but largely unresolved challenge in medicine. Much more is known about the adaptive immune response which exerts exquisite specificities towards antigenic determinants or epitopes of infectious agents and of other antigens. This has been the overwhelming subject of interest in modern immunology, with specificity the dominating concept in the study of immunity, so that we have learned much about the adaptive immune system [12]. Specific responses are detected more easily and the results may be presented in a quantitative form which offers to the scientist a more reasonable chance for success. It has been much more difficult to study natural immunity in spite of the fact that many of the cellular and immune factors that are involved in this system have long been recognised [13].

One may suggest without hesitation that the problem of natural immunity is one of the most important challenges in modern medicine. It is apparent that immune function, including natural immunity, is influenced by numerous medical interventions and other factors that include nutrition, surgical procedures, various forms of injury, ionizing radiation, chemotherapeutic and immunosuppressive drugs, environmental pollution and harmful lifestyle (incorrect nutrition, alcoholism, smoking, drug abuse, lack of exercise, etc.). These factors may decrease natural immunity, which could lead to disease or even death caused by facultative pathogenic organisms that are harmless to healthy individuals.

The AIDS epidemic has stimulated interest in natural immunity. It became apparent that AIDS patients died of secondary infections as a rule and these were due to the profound immunosuppression caused by HIV. Similar observations were made in cancer patients treated by chemotherapeutic agents and ionizing radiation, which suppress immune host defences. This fact emphasized the importance of natural immunity and the need for immunological rehabilitation and stimulation in such patients. It also became clear to immunologists that natural immunity was much more significant than previously recognised and that it deserved much more attention.

The phenomenon of natural resistance plays an important role in biology by allowing for the selection of individuals that are most resistant to disease. In our time, natural selection is curbed by human intervention. This demands further attention to the enhancement of immune mechanisms, which make it possible to save individuals who would have succumbed to disease in earlier times.

Clearly, we are just beginning to recognize the enormous complexity, efficiency and importance of this system in the Biology of animals and man and there is a lot to be clarified for a thorough understanding of natural immunity. The rationale for the evolution of this system is the focus of animated discussion and conjecture.

2. HISTORY: IMMUNE DEFENSE VERSUS SELF-ORGANIZATION

The concept of resistance to disease must have evolved simultaneously with the recognition of health and disease during prehistoric times. A decrease in resistance resulted in disease, which occurred in the weak and infirm as a rule. In spite of the common occurrence of disease throughout history, the underlying mechanisms remained unexplained for millennia. The scientists and physicians of ancient times were not able to define adequately the concept of resistance. Before the discovery of microbes, a number of factors (e.g. extreme cold or hot weather, starvation and environmental factors) were linked with the occurrence of certain infectious disease outbreaks or epidemics, often as a consequence of wars.

Experimentally *Pasteur* made the first observations with regard to the association of chicken cholera and abrupt changes in the weather. *Robert Koch* studied anthrax infection of chickens after forcing them to swim in cold water. These experiments indicated that environmental factors have an influence on resistance to disease. Nevertheless the exact definition of resistance was not put forward till our time. The situation is somewhat similar to the one described by János in the Book of "Phenomena": 'two people sat on the roof, one was taken, the other was left behind'. In other words, it was generally recognised that during epidemics in a human or animal population some individuals always remained healthy. This occurred even when the majority of the population succumbed to disease. The ability of certain individuals to face deadly diseases was defined as *resistance*. No further distinctions were made in this respect. The term *immunity* was also used to describe the resistance of an organism against infectious disease [13].

2.1. Inflammation and phagocytosis

While Cornelius Celsus (30BC-AD50) has been attributed with the first description of inflammation [14], in thinking about the development of our current understanding of natural immunity, the formative work of Metchnikoff is often cited, with thanks to Alfred Tauber for keeping the spotlight on Metchnikoff [15–18]. As described by Tauber, Chernyak and Podolsky [rev in 16,19], Metchnikoff's observation of the process of inflammation around thorns in starfish larvae led him to propose the "phagocyte as the amoeboid mediator of cellular immunity" in an expansion of the phagocyte aboriginal function of "eating to feed" to "eating to defend". This concept provided a basis for the investigation of cellular immunity and a counterpoint of debate for the subsequently developed (immunochemically focused) school of humoural immunity [17]. Further, according to his interpetation of Darwinism, Metchnikoff postulated a fundamentally disharmonious concept of the living organism, in contrast with the view of individual health at the time, a condition of harmony [19]. Metchnikoff considered that "embryological development proceeds with cell lineages that are potentially in competition", disharmonious and required "harmonizers", phagocytes, to decide which cells would survive [quoted as in 19]. Thus, phagocytes actively defined what would later be referred to as immune "self". One could imagine that the generation of spontaneous mutations could act as a 'disharmonizing' process. Metchnikoff also argued that phagocytes would continue to actively define an organism in the adult state and that phagocytes would also defend the host (all in the interest of survival !). The latter led to his *Bacillus bulgarus* therapy, to replace the toxic flora of the large intestine with exogenous "friendly" microbes, a for-runner of current-day probiotics and driver of the yogurt industry [19].

2.2. Self/non-self: early days and ancient times

In the history of the immune 'self' controversy outlined by Tauber [18], the idea that the immune system distinguished between self and non-self was implicit in Metchnikoff's phagocytosis theory, and was formally expressed when Burnet introduced the ideas of self, and self-non-self discrimination leading to his proposal of the clonal selection theory in 1959 [20]. This shifted the arbitration of self/non-self from phagocytes to the clonally selected T and B lymphocytes of the adaptive immune response. Jerne's (idiotypic) network theory of the immune system published in the early 1970's, proposed a highly integrated and self-sensing lymphocyte system [21]. The system knows only itself and perturbation of the system is required for activation. While in the Burnet model, defense of self was the foundation of immune reactivity, Jerne's self-sensing network challenged the concept of immune 'self' and expanded the role of the immune system to physiological functions.

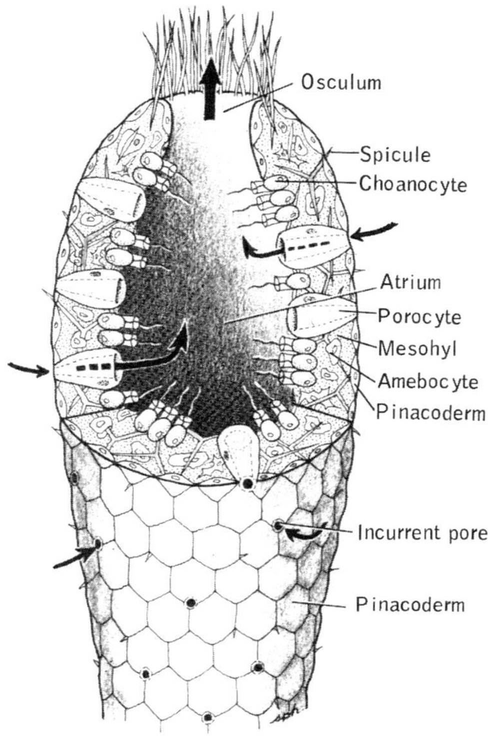

Figure 1. A partially cross-sectioned asconoid sponge [adapted from Ref. 22] .

As is obvious from the above overview, immunologists have thought for a long time that self-recognition was a feature exclusive to the immune system. However, zoologists have long established that self-recognition was easily demonstrable in the most primitive multi-cellular animals, sponges (Fig. 1). Sponges control their morphogenesis, cell proliferation and differentiation. They preserve their species characteristics and have immune defences as well. They are capable of rejecting grafts from other species of sponges. Phagocytic cells provide their immune defence. Sponges were disintegrated by passing them through a screen. When brought together under proper conditions, the cells re-aggregated with cells from the same species, but not with cells from other species, so as to form functional sponge units, which could vary in size but with the maintenance of function. Clearly, these seemingly loosely aggregated cells behave as a highly co-ordinated morphogenic regulatory system. Sponge cells will grow and differentiate into functional cells according to their topographical localization [22]. Similar observations were made in higher animals. Cells from different anlages of the amphibian embryo were mixed and they were able to sort out into a pattern that resembled the initial organisation of embryonic tissue. Such aggregation experiments were also performed with embryonic cells from birds or mammals. Cell adhesion molecules present in embryonic tissue mediate such re-aggregation and play a key role in morphogenesis [23,24].

Embryonic morphogenesis is regulated by cell-to-cell contact and by diffusible mediators. Adhesion molecules are non-diffusible, hence they are capable of signalling single cells very specifically. It is very clear from embryonic development and from antigen-induced lymphocyte proliferation that adhesion signals are dominant over growth factor signalling. This is an obligate requirement for morphogenesis, which is based on the positional relationship of cells/tissues to each other. Adherence signals determine, according to the local tissue/organ requirements, whether or not the cell is going to divide, differentiate and take up a function, or simply be on standby (survive), or perhaps be committed to the pathway of programmed cell death (apoptosis). Concentration gradients of tissue hormones and cytokines are important for morphogenesis during embryonic development [6]. This means that only certain cells will divide at any given time, while others will go into differentiation and take up the appropriate function according to their location in the body, or be on standby (stem cells, as well as differentiated cells) or may even be eliminated. Therefore, the systemic growth stimulus is modified according to the local needs, so that the morphological and functional integrity of the organism is maintained at all times. Growth hormone (GH) is well recognised as a hormone capable of stimulating the proportional growth of all tissues and organs. This dominance of local regulatory mechanisms over the systemic GH signal assures the development of a fully functional animal or human being.

Injured nerve cells in the CNS can be re-induced to grow axons and establish functional connections if exposed to non-neural elements of the peripheral nervous system [25]. This finding indicates that in adult tissues that lost their capacity to grow, stromal adherence signals are capable of inducing growth and regeneration.

Plants show a remarkable morphological and functional differentiation. Some proteins extracted from plants and collectively named lectins [26,27] activate animal cells, especially lymphoid cells for proliferation and function, including immunoglobulin secretion, cytotoxicity, helper or suppressor activity. Therefore, plant lectins function as regulatory molecules on animal cells and probably fulfil similar functions in the plants as well. Animal tissues also contain lectin-like adhesion molecules [27].

The restrictive power of cell-to-cell signalling is also fundamental to the adaptive immune response. Clearly, an antigen specific T lymphocyte clone must not proliferate unless it is triggered by the specific antigenic epitope in the context of self-MHC molecules. Without this restriction antigen-specific adaptive immune reactions would not be possible. Furthermore, MHC recognition by suppressor T lymphocytes and inhibitory receptors in natural killer and other cells serve as safeguards against the killing of normal non-infected and non-cancerous cells [28].

These facts indicate that adhesion molecules and locally active soluble mediators (cytokines) are required for organogenesis. It is likely that the same mediators are needed for the re-assembly of sponge cells after disintegration. Sponges exhibit a definite axis as vertebrates do, and it is also possible to define an imaginary head-tail orientation. There is no nervous system or endocrine system present in these primitive animals. On this basis, the principal regulatory circuits that are anticipated to operate in sponges and in similar primitive animals are shown in Fig. 2. During evolution the neuroendocrine system has been superimposed on this basic regulatory circuit, which reached its highest organization in man. So the situation has changed to the extent that the neuroendocrine system regulates the potential for growth and function (competence) in higher animals, whereas adhesion molecules and cytokines have the power to regulate competence locally according to the requirements in the various tissues and organs. Immune reactions, including natural immunity, are regulated according to this principle (Fig. 3). It is remarkable that in emergency situations (e.g. sepsis) the neuroimmune regulatory netwok is capable of selectively enhancing natural immune mechanisms, which provide instantaneous protection to the host, and at the same time to suppress the adaptive arm of the immune response, which is not capable of effective host defence under these conditions. This phenomenon has been coined as *immunoconversion* [1–3].

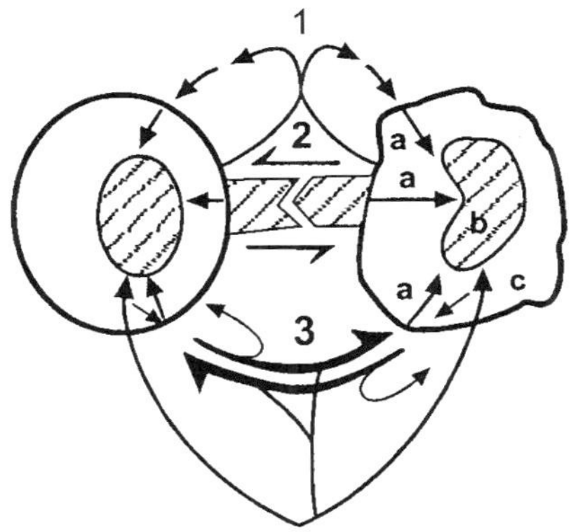

Figure 2. Hypothetical regulatory circuits of primitive animals without the presence of the neuroendocrine system.
1. Autocrine/paracrine secretion of competence (growth) factor. Competence is proposed to be a prerequisite of regulation by adhesion molecules and cytokines.
2. Adhesion molecules regulate the growth stimulatory signal according to the local requirements.
3. Cytokines complete the cell cycle. Some cytokines are of distant origin, which create gradients that are essential for axial and "head-tail" differentiation. Sponges already show such morphological differentiation.

Clearly, self recognition and self-non-self discrimination has been a prerequisite of the evolution for multi-cellular organisms and thus its development predates the development of the immune system in higher animals. The acceptance of self and rejection of non- self has been the rule right from the beginning for the phylogenesis of the multi-cellular animals and plants.

2.3. More mediators: the nude mutation

Beyond the abundant evidence for phagocytic cells, our understanding of the large number and variety of mediators contributing to the natural immune response was dramatically advanced by the discovery of nude mice. Mice bearing the nude mutation have a poorly developed thymus and lack of an effective T cell-mediated immune system. Yet, such mice did not develop an increased incidence of spontaneous tumours. This provided a strong impetus for the investigation of immune responses other than the thymus-dependent adaptive immunity [rev in 29]. This lead to a surge in research by many laboratories on the newly identified natural killer (NK) cells, which did not require previous exposure of the host to antigen, and exhibited instantaneous cytotoxicity towards tumour cells [30–32]. To a lesser extent observations of 'natural antibody' activity against tumours and apparently multi-specific, autoreactive antibodies from normal individuals also received (some) attention. The nature of immune 'self' became more complicated with the identification of such polyspecific and autoreactive NAb and with the demonstration of NK sensing MHC class I as "self" that delivers inhibitory signals and that 'missing self' leads to activation [33].

More recently, advances in cytokine research have allowed the study of dendritic cells, the major antigen presenting cell (APC) for naive T cell activation. This supported the search for the mechanism of the adjuvant effect, Janeway's 'immunologist's dirty little secret', needed to produce a vigorous adaptive immune response against a peptide antigen presented by MHC to TCRs. Investigations initiated by Janeway and Medzhitov [34], led to the pivotal finding that an array of Toll-like receptors on APC's could recognize different components on bacteria activat-

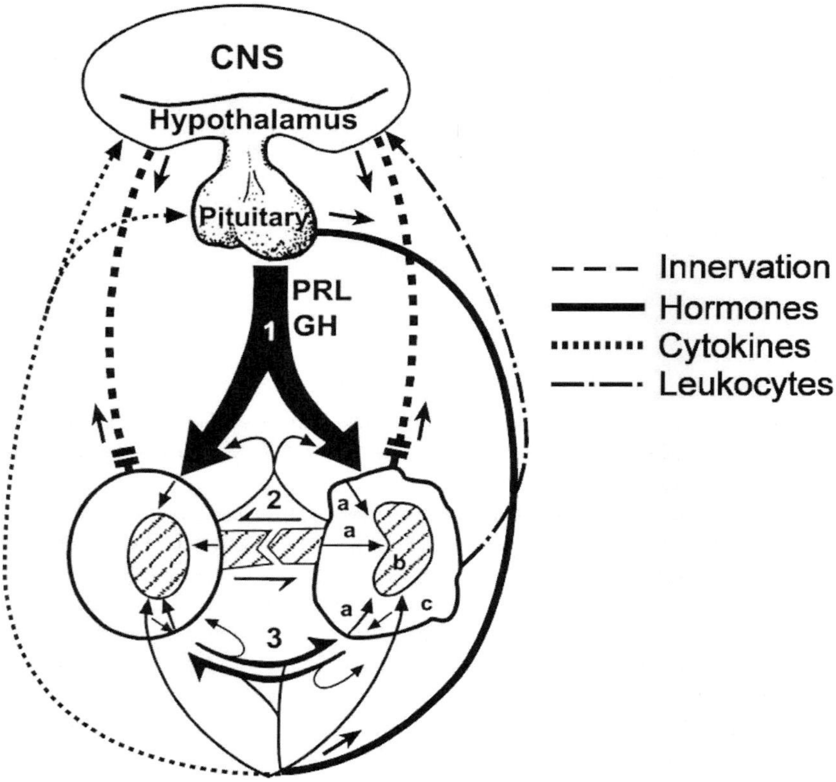

Figure 3. The neuroimmune regulatory circuit.
During evolution the neuroendocrine system has been super-imposed onto the basic regulatory circuit outlined above. The CNS, via the pituitary gland now controls systemically the competence signal for all organs and tissues that amounts to effective growth control of the organism. Adhesion molecules and cytokines remain in control of the local (e.g. positional) regulation of the systemic competence signal. The target organs/tissues provide feedback signals to the neuroendocrine system via innervation and by soluble mediators, such as hormones and cytokines. The neuroimmune regulatory circuitry is fundamental for the development and function of higher animals for their entire life cycle. It exerts physiological regulation and also fundamental to host defence, including regeneration and healing.

ing DC's to provide the needed costimulatory second signals for T lymphocyte activation. These discoveries brought the innate immune system attention, but it was chiefly framed as a supporter for the adaptive immune response.

2.4. An integrated system with expanded functions

Increasingly, investigators have viewed the immune system as a highly complex and integrated system, which communicates with the body in which it resides and self, non-self discrimination is less the issue, rather action is determined by the context of the interaction. Tauber [18], considers that the question of 'context' has been interpreted narrowly by some as being established at birth or shortly after, while for others (including Cohen, Coutinho, Grossman and Matzinger) the context is ever changing. The search to understand activation has focussed increasingly on, 1) the nature of signals, which are ancillary to antigen recognition in the adaptive immune response, 2) the functional structure of the immune system in which they operate and 3) the relationships between the clonally selected T and B lymphocytes of the adaptive response and the mediators of the evolutionarily ancient innate immune response. Recognition of phylogenetic and functional relationships between the innate and adaptive immune systems has led to the concept of a more integrated immune system with a wider scope of function. Matzinger in particular, in defining the context of activation as "danger" rather than the discrimination between self and non-self, assigned the decision-making role for activation to the phagocytic APC. This proposal was supported by her observation that necrotic but not healthy or apoptotic cells released factors which could activate dendritic cells in vitro [35].

2.5. LPS at the core of innate immune research

The recently reviewed [36] long history of endotoxin study, provides a continuous thread (a fuse really) that starts before Metchnikoff with Hippocrates and informs our current concept of innate immunity. Beutler's and Rietschel's story of innate immune sensing focussing on microbial 'endotoxin' which in time became synonymous with lipopolysaccharide (LPS) a protein-free product from Gram-negative bacteria, cites three major milestones in the quest to understand how microbes create disease: the identification of endotoxin as a definable chemical species, the identification of soluble, host-derived mediators of toxicity (e.g., tumour necrosis factor, TNF) coupled with the idea that toxicity and protection were not readily separable, and recently the identification of the LPS receptor itself, providing evidence that many microbial toxins share mechanisms of action similar to endotoxin.

Additional bacterial components including some from Gram-positive bacteria exhibit endotoxin-like biological effects in mammals among them lipopeptides, lipoteichoic acid double-stranded RNA and unmethylated DNA with CpG motifs, and all are recognized by paralogous receptors [36,37].

3. EPITHELIAL, SECRETORY AND ENDOGENOUS HOST DEFENSE

3.1. Antimicrobial peptides

Epithelial tissues and granulocytes express numerous antimicrobial peptides called defensins and cathelicidins. These molecules were recognised initially for their broad-spectrum antimicrobial properties. However, now they are known to play a role in both the regulatory and effector arms of the innate immune system. These peptides modulate bacterial adherence ; complement activation ; fibrinolysis; steroid synthesis; mast cell activation; monocyte, neutrophil, mast cell, T cell and immature dendritic cell chemoattraction; cytokine expression; cytotoxicity; cell proliferation; angiogenesis; protease inhibitor synthesis; keratinocyte differentiation; proteoglycan synthesis; phagocytosis and Ca^{+2} mobilisation. Genes of the adaptive immune system encoding immunoglobulins and T cell receptors undergo a series of genetic amplifications and rearrangements. Homologous events involving genes of the innate immune system can be seen as generating a protective diversity promoting survival of a population or species. The mechanisms for this "genome instability" in innate immunity genes remain to be elucidated [38].

3.2. Endogenous cytoprotective mechanisms

Endogenous cytoprotective mechanisms protect the mammalian host against various forms of injury and noxious stimuli. Since these mechanisms are activated upon encountering potentially cytotoxic conditions, *Haem-oxygenase* and the heat shock response confer protection against a broad array of cytotoxic stimuli. The activation of the *anti-oxidant pathways* is critical to survival in an aerobic environment. *Hypoxia inducible factor* is a key transcription factor that directs the expression of genes necessary for adaptation to hypoxia and/or ischemia. *Nitric oxide* is a ubiquitous molecule that impacts a number of biological, physiological and pathophysiological processes [39].

3.3. Bile acids and natural resistance

Bacterial endotoxin is toxic, when given parenterally but is harmless upon oral administration. In naturally occurring *entero-endotoxaemic diseases* (e.g. shock due to sepsis or to other causes), endotoxin is known to absorb from the intestinal tract. If the common bile duct of rats was chronically cannulated (bile deprived animals) orally administered endotoxin was absorbed from the intestinal tract and provoked shock. This absorption was prevented by sodium deoxycholate or by natural bile. Bile acids split the endotoxin macromolecule into non-toxic fragments. This detoxifying detergent action of bile plays a significant role in host defence against infectious agents with a lipoprotein outer structure (e.g. "big" viruses). This represents a *physico-chemical defence system.* Bile deficiency and the consequent endotoxaemia are important components in the pathogenesis of certain diseases, such as sepsis, intestinal syndrome of radiation disease, hepato-renal syndrome, parvovirus infection, herpes, psoriasis, atherosclerosis, etc. Finally, bile acids may be used for the prevention and/or therapy of some clinical conditions such as the hepato-renal syndrome and psoriasis [40].

4. THE NATURAL IMMUNE SYSTEM

4.1. Natural killer cells: history and current status

Natural killer (NK) cells are a major component of the immune system, which play important roles in host defences against cancer and microbial infections. NK cells are distinct from T or B lymphocytes, with a characteristic morphology of large granular cells, and can be readily identified by characteristic cell surface molecules. They have the ability to recognise and rapidly kill a wide array of tumour cells and also virus-infected normal cells. NK cytotoxic activity can be strongly augmented by interferon, interleukin-2, and other cytokines. NK cells are major producers of some cytokines, especially interferon gamma [41]; they produce a neutrophil-activating factor and upregulate polymorphonuclear leukocytes to kill *Candida albicans* [42].

4.2. The reticuloendothelial system

During the nineteenth century varied cell types, which acted in host defence by phagocytosing foreign invaders were grouped collectively into the reticuloendothelial system (RES). The depression or blockage of the granulopoetic activity of this system has attracted considerable attention. Gadolinium chloride ($GdCl_3$), depresses RES activity and selectively suppresses or eliminates the large Kupffer cells. Kupffer cell blockade modifies the immune response, exerts protective effects on anaphylactic and endotoxic/septic shock, and decreases the liver-damaging effects of several hepatotoxins and ischaemic reperfusion. Recent studies have elucidated the mechanisms by which $GdCl_3$-induced Kupffer cell blockade protects against a variety of hepatotoxic processes [43].

4.3. Effector mechanisms of natural immunity

Evolutionary approaches to the investigation of innate immune mechanisms has shown that monoclonal antibodies to human adhesion molecules react with earthworm, leech and sipunculan leukocytes. Many CD markers common to vertebrate leukocytes, especially to macrophages and natural killer cells are expressed. In earthworms, only those leukocytes which are positive are active as killers in cytotoxic responses, whereas larger, primarily phagocytic leukocytes are negative. The evolution of complement can be traced from sea urchins to the teleosts and tetrapods, exhibiting at each level a corresponding increase in the numbers of complement components and duplications in complement pathways. Invertebrates and vertebrates seem to possess common signalling molecules e.g. neuropeptides. These signalling molecules are immunomodulators in circulating blood. In vertebrates, release occurs during stress that triggers the hypothalamo-hypophyseal-adrenal (HPA) axis. Neuropeptides are conserved messengers that regulate innate immune responses in invertebrates and in humans. The evidence suggests that the cross talk between nervous and immune systems has an ancient evolutionary origin, which is essential to homeostasis [7].

4.4. Natural immune activation

Multiple recognition molecules are involved representing numerous structural families including, several lectin families, pentraxins, leucine-rich repeats, many members of the IgSF, integrins, scavenger receptors and the seven transmembrane receptor family. Invading pathogens exhibit a range of different repeating epitopes. Host molecules express a variety of receptors capable of recognising these epitopes and act in a combinatorial manner which confers specificity to the host response. The large number, diversity, and ancient evolutionary origin of these receptors argues for the essential nature of their functions. While providing a first line of defence against invading pathogens is clearly crucial for organism survival, evidence is accumulating that these same receptors also participate in essential physiological functions [44].

4.5. Signaling in natural killer cells

NK cells have the ability to recognize tumour- and virus-associated ligands. These cells express CD16, the low-affinity Fc receptor (FcR) for IgG. NK cells do not have a single type of receptor through which they recognize antigens. Rather, clonal subpopulations of NK cells differ in their expression of receptors that recognize a variety of ligands on target cells throughout the body. NK cell binding of these ligands initiates signalling cascades within the NK cell that control its response to the target [45].

4.6. Toll-like receptors

Macrophages are central in orchestrating the innate immune response to infection, which is not a trivial task: they must be able to discriminate microbes from self, and then initiate a proper response. The discovery of the Toll-like receptor (TLR) family of pattern-recognition receptors has provided insight into this kind of recognition. TLRs are expressed on macrophages and other innate immune cells, where they collaborate to read the molecular fingerprint of different microbes and initiate inflammatory signalling pathways. The TLR family is important in infectious diseases, and there is also evidence that they may play a role in autoimmunity and degenerative diseases in the central nervous system [46].

5. REGULATION OF NATURAL IMMUNITY

5.1. Leukocyte migration

Leukocyte migration is essential for reactions to inflammatory stimuli at various locations in the body. However, leukocyte movement is also crucial during non-inflammatory processes such as haematopoietic development and routine passage through secondary lymphoid organs, which is also required for effective antigen presentation. Immune defects occur in chemokine receptor deficient mice. Chemokines, their receptors and adhesion molecules play a key role in the regulation of the immune response during inflammatory and under homeostatic conditions. Leukocyte trafficking plays a role during developmental processes, for example in haematopoiesis and thymic maturation of T cells and in regulatory circuits that ensure immune surveillance and communication between the innate and adaptive components of immunity [47].

Leukocytes utilize an active process to halt chemotaxis and switch to effector activity, with the aid of the arrestin protein, which blocks chemotactic signalling from chemokine receptors and converts it to a signal for degranulation [48, 49]. The discovery of chemorepulsive activity mediated by CXCR4 provides a mechanism by which mature T cells may exit the thymus [50, 51].

5.2. Neuroendocrine regulation of natural immunity

Natural killer (NK) cells, $\gamma\delta$ T lymphocytes and CD5+ B lymphocytes are key effector cells in the natural immune system. These cells utilize germ-line coded receptors that recognize highly conserved, homologous epitopes (homotopes). Under physiological conditions the natural immune system is regulated similarly to the adaptive immune system: growth and lactogenic hormones (GLH), insulin-like growth factor-I (IGF-I), insulin, leptin, some steroid (glucocorticoid at physiological concentrations, dehydroepiandrosterone and some of its derivatives) and thyroid hormones are stimulatory. The peptides of the hypothalamus-pituitary-adrenal axis (CRF, AVP, ACTH, αMSH, βEND) exert an immunosuppressive, anti-inflammatory and anti-pyretic effect. Opioid peptides and estradiol are immunomodulators that promote some immune activities while inhibiting others. High (pathophysiological) levels of glucocorticoids, progesterone and testosterone act as immunosuppressive hormones. Beta-adrenergic agents are immunosuppressive and anti-inflammatory, whereas cholinergic agents promote immunity and inflammation. Substance P and calcitonin-gene related peptide are pro-inflammatory and promote immunity, whereas somatostatin is an antagonist of these neuropeptides [52].

Mild infection or a sublethal dose of endotoxin elicits a brief elevation of GH and PRL in the serum. Severe trauma, sepsis and shock results in the elevation of TNFα, IL-1 and IL-6 in the blood stream, the GLH-IGF-I axis is suppressed, whereas the hypothalamus-pituitary-adrenal axis is activated. LH, FSH, estrogens, androgens, progesterone, and thyroid hormones all decline during infection and endotoxin shock, as a rule. Leptin, insulin, glucagon, α-MSH, endorphin, and arginine vasopressin are increased during endotoxemia. A "sympathetic outflow" leads to elevated blood levels of catecholamines. Fever and catabolism prevails, whereas acute phase proteins in the liver, cell proliferation in the bone marrow, and protein synthesis by leukocytes are increased. This is an acute emergency reaction to save the organism after the adaptive immune system has failed to contain and eliminate the pathogenic agent. During sepsis and endotoxin shock, glucocorticoids potentiate the production of acute phase proteins and regulate pro-inflammatory cytokine production. Catecholamines also inhibit inflammatory responses and promote, even initiate, the acute phase response. Leptin regulates energy metabolism and it is a major stimulator of the immune system. If the acute phase reaction fails to protect the host, shock will develop and death will follow [52].

The acute phase response leads to *immunoconversion*, which involves the suppression of the T-cell regulated adaptive immune system and the amplification of natural immunity. Natural antibodies, C-reactive -, endotoxin binding- and mannose binding proteins are boosted and serve as polyspecific recognition molecules for leukocytes. The natural immune system provides the first and the last line of host defence and its functional integrity and massive activation is largely dependent on the neuroendocrine system [52].

5.3. Natural immunity – Effect of exercise

Natural immunity is influenced by pharmacological agents, the environment, exercise and diet. Exercise induces increased circulating levels of a number of cytokines, especially IL-6, which is produced locally in contracting skeletal muscles and accounts for the arterial IL-6 concentration. In turn, IL-6 stimulates the production of a number of anti-inflammatory cytokines such as IL-1ra and IL-10 and also works in a hormone-like fashion. IL-6 also stimulates cortisol production and in the recovery phase of heavy exertion, a cortisol-induced shift in leukocyte subsets is seen. The dominant features in the post-exercise period are lymphopenia, neutrophilia and a markedly suppressed natural killer cell activity. In addition secretory IgA is inhibited [53].

Many clinical physical stressors (e.g., surgery, trauma, burn, sepsis) and environmental factors such as hyperthermia and hypoxia induce hormonal and immunological responses that have similarities to the cellular response to exercise [54]. Training at an intense level over many years can result in a chronic suppression of salivary immunoglobulin levels. The degree of immune suppression and the recovery rates after exercise are associated with the intensity of exercise and the duration or volume of the training [55]. The effect of acute hypoxia on lymphocytes resembles the effect of exercise [56].

The production of IL-6 from working muscles is further enhanced if muscle glycogen content is low. Carbohydrate intake during exercise attenuates the IL-6 production and consequently exercise-induced cortisol production and fluctuations in NK cells and neutrophils. A major new finding is that exercise-induced immune changes are not a secondary phenomenon to exercise-induced hormonal changes. Rather, muscle contractions induce the release of IL-6. By producing IL-6, muscle fibres are directly involved in exercise-induced immune changes, and exercise-induced cortisol changes can be viewed as a secondary phenomenon, which in turn leads to altered leukocyte subset composition. As IL-6 works as an energy sensor, it is also clear that dietary factors such as carbohydrate, may influence the immune response to exercise. It is noteworthy, that a cytokine, previously known as a component of the natural immune defence, should now also be considered as an important player in metabolism [53].

5.4. Enhancement of natural immunity

Endotoxin injections produce endotoxin tolerance and elevate natural resistance. However, such injections may have serious side effects, such as high fever, hypotension and abortion. For this reason LPS injections are not suitable for the enhancement of natural immune mechanisms in endotoxin-sensitive mammalian species. Various techniques have been used (physical, chemical, etc.) for the detoxification of endotoxins while the beneficial effects were maintained. One of the best detoxification techniques is treatment with ionizing radiation. The irradiation of LPS with ^{60}Co (100–200 kGy) decreased its toxicity. Such radiodetoxified endotoxin (RD-LPS) preparations showed decreased toxicity, whereas the beneficial effects were preserved (150 kGy:TOLERIN®). Irradiation causes marked chemical alteration in LPS, such as the decrease of glucosamine, KDO and fatty acids. A single parenteral injection of TOLERIN® is capable of preventing various shock syndromes in experimental animals. Unlike endotoxin, TOLERIN has barely any hypotensive effect and pretreatment with this preparation can prevent practically all the haemodynamic changes induced by LPS. LPS plays an important role in the pathogenesis of the intestinal syndrome of radiation disease, which may be prevented by up to 70% in rats with RD-LPS pretreatment. TOLERIN retains the adjuvant activity of LPS and it is a good adjuvant for inactivated virus vaccines. TOLERIN can also evoke the regeneration of the immune system in irradiated animals. The decrease of natural immunity in immunodeficient or immunosuppressed patients is the most important cause of opportunistic infections that may lead to sepsis, endotoxaemia, pneumonia and so on. Boosting of natural resistance and the induction of endotoxin tolerance are important in such patients. RD-LPS could produce significant proliferation of lymphoid cells in germ-free animals, which are immunodeficient. Many other beneficial effects are exerted by RD-LPS preparations, such as the activation of macrophages and of the reticuloendothelial system, antitumour activity, etc. On the basis of these favourable experimental results, TOLERIN was tested on 350 surgical patients suffering from gastrointestinal tumours, on patients suffering from AIDS and on cancer patients treated with CYSPLATIN©. TOLERIN treatment prevented sepsis and activated bone marrow function in these patients [57].

6. PHYSIOLOGICAL, PATHOLOGICAL AND BEHAVIORAL SIGNIFICANCE

6.1. Physiological activities of the natural immune system

Recent research has revealed the extensive underlying physiological role of the innate immune system in the development and homeostasis of the organism. The impact on development is evident during embryogenesis and also during normal cyclical changes in reproductive tissues in the adult. Mediators of the innate immune system are essential for normal tissue renewal and healing, regeneration, air breathing, cell signalling and cancer control. Natural immunity contributes to the normal physiology of the organism in many and diverse ways arguing for an evolutionary selection centred on self-organization for survival [8].

6.2. Pathophysiological relevance

The natural immune response is a pre-programmed, poly-specific first line of defence that is primarily responsible for eliminating or containing pathogens at the site of entrance into the host. This evolutionary conserved system was described first in cells of the immune system. However, it became apparent this form of immune potential exists in various tissues, where its activation plays a significant role in host defence, autoimmunity, inflammatory disease and pathogenesis of sepsis-induced multiorgan dysfunction. It is possible that natural immunity plays a role in the aging process, and in tumour immunosurveillance [9].

6.3 Behavioural mechanisms in host defence

Behavioural strategies assist organisms to defend themselves against pathogens. Reflexive behaviours, like coughing and vomiting, can be instrumental in expelling pathogens from the body. The avoidance of excrement is an important strategy for minimizing contact with pathogens. Learned food aversions and the avoidance of stimuli previously associated with illness minimize contact with pathogens. Behavioural changes can be induced by immune activation, and it has been argued that this "sickness behaviour" may assist the organism to recover from infection. Immune activation is associated with the production of cytokines, some of which (most notably, interleukin-1, IL-1) have potent behavioural activities. IL-1 decreases several behavioural activities, such as food intake, and sexual activity in females, but not in males. Certain kinds of behavioural experiences, most notably stressful ones, may induce immune activation and cytokine production. Environmental stressors and immune activation produce some similar physiological responses: increased body temperature, and activation of the sympathetic nervous system, the adrenal medulla, and the hypothalamo-pituitary-adrenal axis, as well as brain catecholamines and indoleamines. These observations have led to the concept that pathogen invasion induces "immune stress". The physiological responses induced can assist the defence of the organism against infections, at least in part by changing behaviour. It is argued that learned and reflexive behavioural strategies, and physiological and behavioural responses to illness, are all important components of host defence against pathogens [58].

7. 'MISSING SELF' AS A KEY TO INNATE IMMUNE ACTIVATION

The concept of 'missing self' first was coined with respect to the failure of activating NK cells due to the recognition of self-MHC [33]. This now appears as an emerging common principle in innate immunity. Sponges have phagocytic cells for defence. Another form of this strategy relies on cell expression of terminal sialic acid on cell surface molecules versus the lack of sialic acid on most microorganisms [59]. Sialic acid binding siglecs are inhibitory receptors bearing tyrosine-based inhibitory motifs (ITIMs). The lack of, or reductions in sialic acid on pathogens, some virally infected or transformed cells and apoptotic cells may act as missing self, allowing phagocytosis to proceed.

Complement, the major noncellular system of innate immunity in humans, exhibits wide ranging and potent biological activities which are under heavy regulation employing several different strategies. Since complement can react ubiquitously by binding covalently to self and non-self, regulator recognition of self can provide one strategy for preventing attack on the host. In this regard inhibition based on terminal sialic acid again contributes in the form of sialic acid-binding factor H of the alternate complement activation pathway, which promotes the inactivation of C3b and spares self cells [30,60]. Furthermore, additional complement inhibitors, which are broadly expressed and important in the control of complement activation on self cells are membrane expressed CD46 and CD55 (decay-accelerating factor, DAF) and the soluble and secreted C1 inhibitor and clusterin [61, 62]. All of these molecules are considered to constitute "don't eat me" signaling markers (SAMPs) [61]. These contrast with "eat me" markers in the form of soluble or secreted bridging molecules of the innate immune system binding to pathogen-associated molecular patterns (PAMPs) on pathogens and from apoptotic cell-associated molecular patters (ACAMP). Additional "don't eat me" signals result from normal host cell expression of CD200, CD47 and CD31, all of which engage inhibitory pattern recognition receptors (PRRs) and down-regulate phagocyte activities [61]. While complex, this form of control is well adapted for attack on pathogens not previously encountered. Furthermore, the lack of complement-receptor 1-related gene/protein y (Crry), a membrane-bound complement-regulatory protein structurally similar to decay accelerating factor (DAF/CD55) and membrane cofactor protein (MCP/CD46), resulted in complement deposition at the fetomaternal interface and fetal loss in mice [63], clearly supporting the essential nature of such 'self' expression in normal reproductive physiological processes. Thus, normal self must also include complement regulatory molecules.

8. APOPTOTIC CELLS AND THEIR PHAGOCYTOSIS

Our increasing understanding of cellular "corpse" generation and elimination [64] has contributed immensely to our appreciation of the scope of innate immune function. The concept of physiological cell death emerged from studies of animal development during the latter half of the 19th century [65]. However, the idea that a cell can activate a suicidal program of self-destruction (programmed cell death), which can be modified by external signals has only been developed during the last half of the 20th century, and this was considered essential for the development, homeostasis and integrity of multicellular organisms [65]. The description of cell death by apoptosis in the early 1970's provided a phenotype which became a focus for the investigation of homeostatic, 'physiological' cell death (cellular homeostasis) in normal and pathological tissues (e.g. cancer regression) [66]. Apoptosis was viewed as a prelude to the orderly removal of the non-viable cells by phagocytosis in the absence of inflammation. The molecular processes of apoptosis was investigated as an active mechanism of cell death induced by steroids, antibody-dependent cytolysis by lymphocyte killer (K) cells, NK cells and cytotoxic CD8$^+$ T cells consistent with its generalized utility in biology [67, 68].

The science of phagocytosis has undergone a revolution in the last few years from a descriptive to an analytical approach [71], and combined with advances in cytokine and chemokine research so has our appreciation of innate imunity. The demonstration that while phagocytosis of necrotic cells, clearly a danger signal, produces an inflammatory response, phagocytosis of apoptotic cells does not, provided further support for Matzinger's "danger'" hypothesis. Phagocytosis of apoptotic cells which have undergone a process of programmed cell death is at the core of many biological processes, pathological or physiological, which depend on the innate immune system.

9. NATURAL IMMUNITY AND THE NATURAL IMMUNE SYSTEM

While the innate immune system has traditionally been considered by many to have evolved to defend against microbial pathogens [59,70–72], others have proposed that the immune system did not evolve to fight infection [73,74]. Analysis of allorecognition challenged the paradigm that vertebrate immunity is pathogenetically focussed and directed support toward the idea that preserving individuality against the threat of invading conspecific cells (based on polymorphic compatibility molecules) was probably the driving force for all innate and adaptive immune systems and the defence function developed later [74]. Key molecules of the mammalian innate and adaptive immune systems were identified in sponges (Porifera) and some were considered likely to have acquired dual functions during evolution, acting first in adhesion and growth control and later in immune self/self- and self/non-self-recognition [75]. The bountiful evidence for the role of innate immunity in cell modulatory pathways of normal development reminds us of the limitations, folly even, of taking a narrow reductionist approach to understanding and investigating innate immunity. Investigation increasingly exposes the critical contributions of components of the innate immune system in normal physiological functions including, embryological development, reproduction, organ regeneration, and wound healing [8]. Antimicrobial peptides contribute as growth factors to wound healing and tissue repair. Phagocytes regulate angiogenesis by secreting growth factors [76] and by remodelling vasculature through macrophage-induced apoptosis of vascular endothelial cells [77,78]. Complement participates in crucial processes of normal development and organ regeneration [69]. NK cells and macrophages are considered important for a successful pregnancy contributing to implantation, vascularization, growth factor production for the placenta and trophoblast differentiation and parturition [79,80].

Several investigators have refuted the idea that the innate immune system is non-specific [14,74], rather it is extremely selective [61] and polyspecific, which is due to the multiple specificity of receptors (e.g. natural antibodies), and the crossreactivity of homotopes recognized by them.

Thus, a broad definition of the innate immune system which allows for extensive interpretation, would be an evolutionarily ancient, germline gene-dependent, self-organizing system (implying self-recognition) acting in the interest of survival. This would encompass all components of the immune system which fit this description (including T and B cells activated other than through specific clonaly-selected antigen recognition) participating in defence and self-organizing functions.

10. LINKS BETWEEN INNATE AND ADAPTIVE IMMUNITY

There are many examples illustrating that the natural immune system serves as a foundation, on which the adaptive immune system has evolved. Briefly, the macrophage, which is a principal co-ordinator of natural immunity, is also fundamental to adaptive immunity as an antigen presenting cell. Moreover, macrophages initiate the acute phase response, which leads to the inactivation of the thymus and the inhibition of adaptive immunity. B lymphocytes secreting natural antibodies may have an effect on any lymphocyte of the adaptive system that expresses Fc-receptors. Natural killer cells produce IFN-gamma and other cytokones that affect cells of the adaptive system. Defensins also affect adaptive immunity. Complement has been established as a vital link between natural and acquired immunity, profoundly augmenting the antibody response to T-dependent antigens [79]. In turn, activated T cells produce INF-gamma, the major cytokine activator of macrophages.

11. CURRENT APPLICATIONS AND CHALLENGES

The scope of natural immunity is vast and complicated by extraordinary diversity, redundancy, cooperation and amplification. Research to date has established the legitimacy of the field but the surge in exploration must continue if we harbour any desire to live in harmony with our immune system. Nevertheless, our increasing understanding of the mechanisms of the natural immune system and its importance for the development of a strong adaptive response has provided a strong incentive to better understand the dynamic interplay between infectious agents and host defence in man [34] and to develop *new adjuvants* as a component of improved vaccines. Current approaches to immune potentiation and adjuvant design combined with vaccine delivery are rapidly moving the field forward [81]. Toll-like receptors, in particular, are being targeted in vaccine development and in cancer therapy [82].

The use of the innate immune system by itself has been proposed as a *biodefence strategy* for protection against a broad and largely unforseen range of microbial pathogens which may be employed in bioweaponry [83,84]. This could employ synthetic, conserved components of microbes recognized by the Toll-like receptors and other receptors of the innate immune system. Both prophylactic and post-exposure approaches appear to be working in animals to prevent or reduce infections.

The early suggestion of Metchnikoff to eat live bacteria to promote health has seen a dramatic rise in popularity and has developed into the field of *probiotics*, (eating live 'good' microbiota) and the related field, *prebiotics* (eating non-digestible oligosaccharides that target pathological microbiota) both with the idea of modifying the activity or composition of the endogenous microbiota [85–87]. While the gut has been the main focus of this probiotic research, endogenous microbiota found in other parts of the body, (e.g. urogenital tract, skin and nasopharynx) have also attracted attention and can be expected to yield success [87].

Clearly, our understanding of the *immunology of aging is of present and future economic and political importance* [88] considering the current large population of aging 'baby boomers' and future increases in the proportion of older people and in the age of old people that are generally predicted to happen. Since natural immunity seems to be less affected by age than the adaptive response (Salvioli et al, this volume), the ability to manipulate the natural immune system will be needed to maintain a good quality of life in old age. With regard to natural immunity, which is heavily regulated by the environment, both external and internal, probably the most important decision an individual can make is to choose a healthy life style in order to maintain the natural and adaptive immune systems for a long, high quality life.

REFERENCES

1. Berczi I. Neuroendocrine response to endotoxin. Ann NY Acad Sci 1998;851:411–415.
2. Berczi I, Bertok L, Chow DA. Natural immunity and neuroimmune host defence. Ann NY Acad Sci 2001;917:248–257.
3. Haeryfar SMM, Berczi I. The thymus and the acute phase response. Cell Mol Biol 2001;47:145–156.
4. Berczi I, Nagy E, Baral E, Szentivanyi, A. Sterid Hormones. In "Neuroimmmune Biology,

Volume 3: The Immune-Neuroendocrine Circuitry. History and Progress". Berczi I, Szentivanyi A, Editors, Elsevier, Amsterdam, 2003; pp. 221–270.

5. Gabry KE, Chrousos G, Gold PW. The hypothalamus – Pituitary – Adrenal (HPA) Axis: Mediator of the adaptive response to stress. In "Neuroimmmune Biology, Volume 3: The Immune-Neuroendocrine Circuitry. History and Progress". Berczi I, Szentivanyi A, Editors, Elsevier, Amsterdam, 2003; pp. 379–414.
6. Berczi I. The role of the growth and lactogenic hormone family in immune function. Neuroimmunomodulation 1994;1:201–216.
7. Cooper EL. Effector mechanisms of Natural Immunity: an invertebrate perspective. In Neuroimmmune Biology, volume 5. Chow DA and Bertok L. Eds; Berczi I and Szentivanyi A. Series Eds; Amsterdam: Elsevier, 2004; pp. 103–121.
8. Chow D. Physiological Activities of the Natural Immune System. In Neuroimmmune Biology, volume 5. Chow DA and Bertok L. Eds; Berczi I and Szentivanyi A. Series Eds; Amsterdam: Elsevier, 2004; pp. 311–329.
9. Salvioli S, Capri M, Fumelli M, Lescal F, Monti D, Franceschi C. Pathological relevance of the natural immune system. In Neuroimmmune Biology, volume 5. Chow DA and Bertok L. Eds; Berczi I and Szentivanyi A. Series Eds; Amsterdam: Elsevier, 2004; pp. 331–350.
10. Berczi I, Szentivanyi A. Immune reactions. In: The immune-neuroendocrine circuitry. History and progress. Neuroimmune Biology, Volume 3. Berczi I, Szentivanyi A. Eds, Series Eds. Amsterdam: Elsevier, 2003; pp 315–377.
11. Bertók L. Experiments for the alteration of the species specific resistance by inhibition of protein-synthesis (Hungarian). Budapest: PhD Thesis;1964.
12. Gergely J. Phylogenesis and ontogenesis of immune response. In: Csaba Gy, editor. Actual problems of biology. (Hungarian). Budapest: Medicina, 1974;9–53.
13. Metchnikoff E. Immunity in infective diseases. Cambridge: Camridge Univ Press;1907
14. Revillard JP. Innate immunology. Eur J Dermatol 2002; 12: 224–7.
15. Tauber AI. Metchnikoff and phagocytosis theory. Nature Reviews Molecular cell Biology 2003; 4: 897–901.
16. Tauber AI, Chernyak L. Metchnikoff and the Origins of Immunology: From Metaphor to Theory. Oxford University Press 1991: 25–67.
17. Tauber AI, Chernyak L. The birth of immunology. II. Metchnikoff and his critics. Cell Immunol 1989 Jul; 121(2): 447–73.
18. Tauber AI. Moving beyond the immune self. Immunology 2000; 12: 241–8.
19. Podolsky S. Cultural divergence: Elie Metchnikoff's *Bacillus bulgaricus* therapy and his underlying concept of health. Bull History Med 1998; 72.1:1–27.
20. Burnet FM. The clonal selection theory of acquired immunity. Vanderbilt University Press 1959.
21. Jerne NK. Toward a network theory of the immune system. Ann Inst Pasteur Immunol (Paris) 1974; 125C: 373–89.
22. Barnes RD. Invertebrate Zoology. Third Edition. Philadelphia: WB Saunders, 1974.
23. Hood L, Huang HV, Dreyer WJ. The area code hypothesis. The immune system provides clues to understanding the genetic and molecular basis of cell recognition during development. J Systamol Struct 1987;7:531–559.
24. Thiery JP. Cell adhesion molecules as morphoregulators. A short survey. In: Burger MM, Sordat B, Zinkernagel RM, editors. Cell to Cell Interaction. Basel: Karger, 1990;242–246.
25. Aguayo AJ, Villegas-Perez MP, Vidal-Sanz M, Carter D, Bray GM. Influences of non-

neuronal tissues on the regeneration of injured nerve cells in the central nervous system of adult mammals. In Burger MM, Sordat B, Zinkernagel RM, editors. Cell to Cell Interaction. Basel: Karger, 1990; 40–61.
26. Sharon N. Lectin-carbohydrate complexes of plants and animals: An atomic view. Trends Biochem Sci 1993;18:221–226.
27. Berczi I, Szentivanyi A. Adhesion molecules. In "Neuroimmmune Biology", Volume 3: The Immune-Neuroendocrine Circuitry. History and Progress. Berczi I, Szentivanyi A, Editors, Elsevier, Amsterdam, 2003; pp. 99–115.
28. Murphy WJ, Reynolds CW, Tiberghien P, Longo DL. Natural killer cells and bone marrow transplantation J Natl Cancer Inst 1993;85:1475–82.
29. Haller O, Örn A. In vivo activity of murine NK cells. Editor Herberman RB. in Natural Cell-Mediated immunity Against Tumors, 1980; 1105–15.
30. Crocker PR, Varki A. Siglecs in the immune system. Immunology 2001;103(2):137.
31. Keissling R, Klein E, Wigzell H. "Natural" killer cells in the mouse. I. Cytotoxic cells with specificity for mouse Moloney leukaemia cells. Specificity and distribution according to genotype. Eur J Immunol 1975;5:112–7.
32. Herberman RB, Nunn ME. Lavrin DH. Natural cytotoxic reactivity of mouse lymphoid cells against syngeneic and allogeneic tumours. I. Distribution of reactivity and specificity. Int J Cancer 1975;16:216–29.
33. Kärre K. How to recognize a foreign submarine. Immunol Rev. 1997;155:5–9.
34. Ezekowitz RAB, Hoffman JA. Innate Immunity. Totowa, NJ: Humana Press; 2003.
35. Gallucci S, Lolkema M, Matzinger P. Natural adjuvants: Endogenous activators of dendritic cells. Nat Med 1999; 5:1249–55.
36. Beutler B, Rietschel ET. Innate immune sensing and its roots: the story of endotoxin. Nature Reviews Immunology 2003; 3: 169–76.
37. Weber JR, Moreillon P, Tuomanen EI. Innate sensors for Gram-positive bacteria. Current Opin Immunol 2003; 15: 408–15.
38. Huttner, KM. Antimicrobial Peptides - The Defence Never Rests. In Neuroimmmune Biology, volume 5. Chow DA and Bertok L. Eds; Berczi I and Szentivanyi A. Series Eds; Amsterdam: Elsevier, 2004; pp. 29–48.
39. Wong HR. Endogenous cytoprotective mechanisms. In Neuroimmmune Biology, volume 5. Chow DA and Bertok L. Eds; Berczi I and Szentivanyi A. Series Eds; Amsterdam: Elsevier, 2004; pp. 49–65.
40. Bertok L, The Role of Bile Acids in Natural Resistance: physico-chemical host defence In Neuroimmmune Biology, volume 5. Chow DA and Bertok L. Eds; Berczi I and Szentivanyi A. Series Eds; Amsterdam: Elsevier, 2004; pp. 67–78.
41. Herberman RB. A Historical Introduction of Natural Killer (NK) Cells and Current Status of Their Role in Host Defences In Neuroimmmune Biology, volume 5. Chow DA and Bertok L. Eds; Berczi I and Szentivanyi A. Series Eds; Amsterdam: Elsevier, 2004; pp. 81–94.
42. Djeu JY, Blanchard DK. Regulation of human polymorphonuclear neutriphil (PMN) activity against Candida albicans by large granular lymphocytes via release of a PMN-activating factor J Immunol 1987;139:2761–2.
43. Lázár G, Husztik E, Lázár G, Jr. The Role of the Reticuloendothelial System in Natural Immunity In Neuroimmmune Biology, volume 5. Chow DA and Bertok L. Eds; Berczi I and Szentivanyi A. Series Eds; Amsterdam: Elsevier, 2004; pp. 95–101.
44. Chow DA. Natural immune activation: stimulators/receptors. In Neuroimmmune

Biology, volume 5. Chow DA and Bertok L. Eds; Berczi I and Szentivanyi A. Series Eds; Amsterdam: Elsevier, 2004; pp. 123–150.
45. Arneson LN, Leibson PJ. Signalling in Natural Immunity: Natural Killer Cells In Neuroimmmune Biology, volume 5. Chow DA and Bertok L. Eds; Berczi I and Szentivanyi A. Series Eds; Amsterdam: Elsevier, 2004; pp. 151–166.
46. Flo, TH, Aderem A. Pathogen recognition by Toll-like receptors In Neuroimmmune Biology, volume 5. Chow DA and Bertok L. Eds; Berczi I and Szentivanyi A. Series Eds; Amsterdam: Elsevier, 2004; pp. 185–214.
47. Bosinger SE, Hoisawa KA, Cameron CM, Devries ME, Coombs JC. Cameron MJ, Kelvin DJ. Molecular control of leukocyte trafficking - Internal regulatory circuits of the immune system: Leukocyte circulation and homing In Neuroimmmune Biology, volume 5. Chow DA and Bertok L. Eds; Berczi I and Szentivanyi A. Series Eds; Amsterdam: Elsevier, 2004 (this volume).
48. Barlic J, Khandaker MH, Mahon E, Andrews J, DeVries ME, Mitchell GB et al. beta-arrestins regulate interleukin-8-induced CXCR1 internalization. J Biol Chem 1999;274(23):16287–94.
49. Barlic J, Andrews JD, Kelvin AA, Bosinger SE, DeVries ME, Xu L et al. Regulation of tyrosine kinase activation and granule release through beta-arrestin by CXCRI. Nat Immunol 2000;1(3):227–33.
50. Zou YR, Kottmann AH, Kuroda M, Taniuchi I, Littman DR. Function of the chemokine receptor CXCR4 in haematopoiesis and in cerebellar development. Nature 1998;393(6685): 595–9.
51. Poznansky MC, Olszak IT, Evans RH, Wang Z, Foxall RB, Olson DP et al. Thymocyte emigration is mediated by active movement away from stroma-derived factors. J Clin Invest 2002;109(8):1101–10.
52. Berczi I. Neuroendocrine Regulation of Natural Immunity. In Neuroimmmune Biology, volume 5. Chow DA and Bertok L. Eds; Berczi I and Szentivanyi A. Series Eds; Amsterdam: Elsevier, 2004; pp. 215–262.
53. Pedersen BK. Natural immunity – Effect of exercise. In Neuroimmmune Biology, volume 5. Chow DA and Bertok L. Eds; Berczi I and Szentivanyi A. Series Eds; Amsterdam: Elsevier, 2004; pp. 263–288.
54. Pedersen BK, Kappel M, Klokker M, Nielsen HB, Secher NH. The immune system during exposure to extreme physiologic conditions. Int J Sports Med 1994;15 Suppl 3:S116–21.
55. Droller MJ, Perlmann P, Schneider MU. Enhancement of natural and antibody-dependent lymphocyte cytotoxicity by drugs which inhibit prostaglandin production by tumor target cells. Cell Immunol 1978;39(1):154–64.
56. Hoffman-Goetz L, Simpson JR, Cipp N, Arumugam Y, Houston ME. Lymphocyte subset responses to repeated submaximal exercise in men. J Appl Physiol 1990;68(3):1069–74.
57. Bertok L. A new prospect for the enhancement of natural immunity. In Neuroimmmune Biology, volume 5. Chow DA and Bertok L. Eds; Berczi I and Szentivanyi A. Series Eds; Amsterdam: Elsevier, 2004; pp. 289–307.
58. Larson SJ, Dunn A. Behavioral Mechanisms for Defense Against Pathogens In Neuroimmmune Biology, volume 5. Chow DA and Bertok L. Eds; Berczi I and Szentivanyi A. Series Eds; Amsterdam: Elsevier, 2004; pp. 351–368.
59. Medzhitov R, Janeway Jr CA. Decoding the patterns of self and nonself by the innate immune system. Science 2002; 296: 298–300.
60. Pilatte Y, Bignon J, Lambre CR. Sialic acids as important molecules in the regulation of the

immune system: pathophysiological implications of sialidases in immunity. Glycobiology 1993:3(3):201–18.
61. Elward K, Gasque P. Molecular Immunol. 2003; 40: 85–94.
62. Pangburn MK, Pangburn KL, Koistinen V, Meri S, Sharma AK. Molecular mechanisms of target recognition in an innate immune system: interactions among factor H, C3b, and target in the alternative pathway of human complement. J Immunol. 2000 May 1; 164(9): 4742–51.
63. Caucheteux SM, Kanellopoulos-Langevin C, Ojcius DM. At the innate frontiers between mother and fetus: linking abortion with complement activation. Immunity 2003; 18: 169–72.
64. Savill J, Fadok V. Corpse clearance defines the meaning of cell death. Nature 2000; 407: 784–8.
65. Ameisen JC. On the origin, evolution and nature of programmed cell death: a timeline of four billion years. Cell Death and Differentiation 2002; 9: 367–93.
66. Kerr JFR, Wylie AH, Currie AR. Apoptosis: a basic biological phenomenon with widespread implications in tissue kinetics. Brit J Cancer 1972; 26: 239–57.
67. Alenzi FQ, Warrens AN. Cellular and molecular themes in apoptosis. Wien Klin Wochenschr. 2003 Sep 15; 115(15–16): 563–74.
68. Lawen A. Apoptosis-an introduction. BioEssays 2003; 25: 888–96.
69. Sansonetti PJ. Phagocytosis, a cell biology view. J Cell Sci 2000;111(pt 19):3355–6.
70. Janeway CA Jr. The immune system evolved to discriminate infectious nonself from noninfectious self. Immunol Today 1992; 13(1):11–6.
71. Medzhitov R, Janeway CA Jr. Innate immunity: impact on the adaptive immune response. Curr Opin Immunol 1997;147(1):4–9.
72. Mushegian A, Medzhitov R. Evolutionary perspective on innate immune recognition. J Cell Biology 2001; 155: 705–10.
73. Stewart J. Immunoglobulins did not arise in evolution to fight infection. Immunol Today 1992; 13: 396–9.
74. Rinkevich B. Invertebrates versus vertebrates innate immunity: in the light of evolution. Scand J Immunol 1999; 50: 456–60.
75. Müller WEG, Blumbach B, Müller IM. Evolution of the innate and adaptive immune systems: relationships between potential immune molecules in the lowest metazoan phylum (porifera) and those in vertebrates. Transplantation 1999; 68(9): 1215–27.
76. Sunderkotter C, Steinbrink K, Goebeler M, Bhasdwaj R, Sorg C. Macrophages and angiogenesis. J Leuk Biol 1994; 55: 410–22.
77. Diez-Roux G, Lang RA. A macrophage induced apoptosis in normal cells *in vivo*. Development 1997; 124: 3633–38.
78. Diez-Roux G, Argilla M, Makarenkova H, Ko K, Lang R. Macrophages kill capillary cells in G phase of the cell cycle during programmed vascular regression. Development 1999; 126: 2141–7.
79. Veenstra van Nieuwenhovten AL, Heineman MJ, Faas MM. The immunology of successful pregnancy. Human Reproduction Update 2003; 9: 347–57.
80. Hunt JS, Petroff MG, Burnett TG. Uterine leukocytes: key players in pregnancy. Cell & Developmental Biology 2000; 11: 127–37.
81. O'Hagen DT, Valiente NM. Recent advances in the discovery and delivery of vaccine adjuvants. Nat Rev Drug Discov 2003;2:727–35.
82. Rogatsky I. Drug discovery for inflammatory diseases. Expert Opin Biol Ther 2003

Sep;3(6):1001–4.
83. Hackett CJ. Innate immune activation as a broad-spectrum biodefense strategy: Prospects and research challenges. J Allerg Clin Immunol 2003 ;112(4):686–94.
84. Hilleman MR. Overview: cause and prevention in biowarfare and bioterrorism. Vaccine 2002;20:3055–67.
85. Mercenier A, Pavan S, Pot B. Probiotics as biotherapeutic agents:present knowledge and future prospects. Curr Pharm Res 2003;9(2):175–91.
86. Tuohy KM, Probert HM, Smejkal CW, Gibson GR. Using probiotics to improve gut health. Drug Discov Today 2003;8:692–700.
87. Ouwehand AC. Probiotics: time to move beyond Metchnikoff? Drug Discov Today 2003 Dec;8(23):1063.
88. Butler RN. Economic and political implications of immunology and aging on tomorrow's society. Mech Ageing Dev 1997 Feb; 93(1–3):7–13.

II. EPITHELIAL, SECRETORY AND ENDOGENOUS HOST DEFENSE

Natural Immunity
Edited by L. Bertók and D.A. Chow
© 2005 Elsevier B.V. All rights reserved

Antimicrobial Peptides – The Defence Never Rests

KENNETH M. HUTTNER

Division of Neonatology, Department of Pediatrics, Harvard Medical School and the Mass-General Hospital for Children, Boston, MA 02114 U.S.

ABSTRACT

The era of genomics has arrived bringing with it the promise of novel insights into the molecular basis of human health and disease. True to this promise, the field of innate immunity has seen extraordinary advances in the identification of key molecules for pathogen recognition, cellular signalling and microbicidal activity. Prominent among them in both epithelial tissues and granulocytes are the abundant and evolutionary-ancient defensins and cathelicidins. These molecules, recognized initially for their broad-spectrum antimicrobial properties, are now shown to occupy critical junctions in both the regulatory and effector arms of the innate immune system. This review will focus on these unique peptides, highlighting their structure, function and regulation in epithelial host defence, with an emphasis on clinical implications and a role as therapeutic targets.

1. ANTIMICROBIAL PEPTIDES

1.1. Structures

The two salient features that identify an antimicrobial peptide are an ability to inactivate microorganisms, tested either *in vitro* or *in vivo*, and a size less than 100 amino acids. Given these rather broad definitions, over 500 molecules derived from either plant or animal species are now categorised as antimicrobial peptides [1–3]. As a general rule, they are derived from propeptides following constitutive or inducible processing. The active peptides vary in structure from disulfide-bridged circular peptides to amphipathic α-helical sequences enriched for a single amino acid (Fig. 1). A common feature is the formation of a tertiary structure permissive for interaction with the predominantly anionic, cholesterol-poor microbial membrane [4].

Many excellent reviews are available on the numerous classes of antimicrobial peptides, describing in a wealth of detail their gene, mRNA and peptide structures [5,6]. Here we will outline briefly the principle classes of antimicrobial peptides isolated from mammalian tissues, with particular emphasis on those from *H. sapiens*.

In the 1980's, investigators at UCLA published seminal work characterising neutrophil defensins, the most abundant class of mammalian antimicrobial peptides [5]. As a general rule, mammalian defensins are cationic, arginine-rich, cysteine-containing peptides 29–47 amino acids in length that are derived from larger, precursor molecules. Most commonly, these pre-

- **Linear Helix** LLGDFFRKSKEKIGKEFKRIVQRIKDFLRNLVPRTES

  LL-37

  ISRLAGLLRLGGEKIGEKLKKIGQKIKNFFQKLVPQPE

  CRAMP

- **Disulfide Containing**

  α- and β-defensins ACYCRIPACIAGERRYGTCIYQGRLWAFCC

  HNP-1

  DHYNCVSSGGQCLYSACPIFTKIQGTCYRGKAKCCK

  HBD-1

- **Rich in Specific Amino Acid Residues**

  proline RRRPRPPYLPRPRPPPFFPPRLPPRIPPGFPPRFPPRF

  PR-39

  tryptophan: ILPWKWPWWPWRRNH2

  Indolicidin

  aspartic acid: DDDDDDD, GDDDDDD

  Anionic Peptides

Figure 1. Chemical structural classification of some well-studied mammalian antimicrobial peptides (modified from [3] with permission).

cursor molecules are prepropeptides containing a signalling pre- sequence, a neutralizing propeptide and the carboxy-terminal defensin that is liberated following multiple processing steps. Nearly all mammalian defensins contain six cysteine molecules participating in three disulfide bonds. They can be sorted broadly into three groups based on cysteine spacing and disulfide-bond alignment (Fig. 1).

The α-defensins are generally shorter in length and contain disulfide bridges in a {C1-C6, C2-C4, C3-C5} pattern, while the β-defensins are more variable in length at both termini and contain disulfide bridges in a {C1-C5, C2-C4, C3-C6} pattern. The core tertiary structure of α- and β-defensins is considered to be a triple-stranded antiparallel β-sheet [7]. The third group of defensins, θ-defensins, has been identified only in rhesus macaques [8], and is unique both in structure (circular) and in mechanism of post-translational assembly (intermolecular disulfide bridging).

As an interesting aside, it was recognised recently that the CXC motif present in the N-terminal of defensins is analogous to the CXC motif present in a class of chemokines [9]. Specific CXC chemokines demonstrate a pattern of broad-spectrum antimicrobial activity similar to that of the defensins [9], perhaps blurring the distinction between antimicrobial and signalling molecules.

The second main class of mammalian antimicrobial peptides is the cathelicidins, all of which are cleaved from precursor proteins containing the highly conserved propeptide sequence termed cathelin [6]. Interestingly, the cathelin propeptide was discovered independently as a porcine inhibitor of cathepsin L [10,11]. Cathelicidin genes consist of 4 exons, with exons 1-3 encoding the tissue-targeting cathelin portion of the molecule, and exon 4 encoding the active peptide. The active cathelicidin peptides vary widely in their primary sequence, and the cathelicidin gene family varies markedly in size among species. To date, only a single human cathelicidin gene has been identified, hCAP18. hCAP18 refers to the 18 kd cathelicidin prepropeptide, while the processed, active moiety is termed LL-37 (N-terminal leu-leu with length 37 a.a.) (Fig. 1).

Peptides of the defensin and cathelicidin families follow the dual paradigm of being processed from a precursor propeptide and having an antimicrobial activity linked to their net cationic charge. However, nature in its abundant diversity is likely to have evolved multiple paradigms for providing molecular protection of the epithelial barrier. The search for additional, novel classes of antimicrobial peptides has required novel insights and novel laboratory approaches. Among the unique peptide classes under investigation are anionic peptides and histone fragments.

The former are zinc-binding small molecules detected in pulmonary tissues of both sheep and humans [12]. In both species, these molecules and their precursors are constitutively expressed in airway tissues [13]. It is interesting to speculate whether they contribute to the proven effectiveness of zinc supplements in ameliorating pulmonary infections.

Many investigators have reported the HPLC purification of histone fragments with antimicrobial activity, and for years this was thought to be of no real consequence. However, it is now better appreciated that cellular apoptosis may be a defence response to microbial invasion. Therefore, it is a reasonable hypothesis that the release of histone fragments from the apoptotic cell chromatin is a highly effective strategy for augmenting host defence [14,15].

1.2. Cellular origin

Each species examined has a unique pattern of antimicrobial peptide expression, perhaps reflective of its unique life cycle and environment. However, a feature common to all species is the presence of abundant antimicrobial peptides in circulating granulocytes (e.g., neutrophils [5] and eosinophils [16]). It has been estimated that the antimicrobial α-defensins stored in human neutrophil granules (termed HNP's) may constitute up to 50% of the total neutrophil protein [5]. A subset of these granule antimicrobial peptides can be detected in epithelial tissues, with the most prominent examples being the epidermal expression of human cathelicidin LL-37 and the orthologous mouse cathelicidin CRAMP [11,17]. Additionally, cells of both the T and B cell lineages, capable of infiltrating epithelial tissues, demonstrate transcription, translation and release of both defensins and cathelicidins [15].

Defensins and cathelicidins are the principle antimicrobial peptides expressed in the epithelium of every major organ system examined. In human tissues this includes the skin, ear canal, salivary glands, conjunctiva, breast tissue, GI tract from oesophagus to colon, pulmonary tract, and genitourinary tract [6,11,18–20]. In addition to their expression in the epithelial lining cells, antimicrobial peptides may be released locally from tissue monocytes encountering microbes or their products [21]. Their presence in circulating phagocytic cells as well as at sites of host-environment interface has lead investigators to hypothesise that they are the microbicidal effector molecules of the innate immune system. Recent evidence described below (section 1.8–1.10, and section 2) not only is supportive of this role in innate immunity, but also is suggestive of a more central role in regulating host immunity.

1.3. Mechanisms of microbicidal action

In general, defensins and cathelicidins are bactericidal *in vitro* against both Gram-positive and Gram-negative bacteria in assays using simplified, low ionic strength media. Subsets of these peptides demonstrate antiviral, antifungal and antiprotozoal activity as well. A working model for their mechanism of activity includes an initial interaction of the cationic moiety with the anionic bacterial membrane phospholipids, subsequent weakening of the microbial membrane integrity and a terminal disruption of membrane function [4,22,23]. This model is consistent with the repeated observations that: (1) elevation of salt or divalent cation concentration in the media may shield the charges on the microbial surface and reduce antimicrobial peptide activity; and (2) bacteria may acquire resistance to microbial activity through alterations in their surface lipid properties.

As we attempt to develop a unifying model for the antimicrobial peptide mechanism of action, we should recognise that a number of independent observations suggest a significant diversity to the microbicidal activity. For example, a novel approach to this question is the use of transcriptional profiling to investigate the bacterial response to treatment with an antimicrobial peptide. *E. coli* treated with a sublethal dose of an insect antimicrobial peptide, Cecropin A, demonstrated significant changes in transcript levels for 26 different bacterial genes, half of which are yet to be assigned a function [24]. These changes differed from those seen in response to thermal, osmotic or nutritional stress.

Other data that need to be considered are the following: (1) several cationic peptides demonstrate cidal activity independent of local salt-concentration, most notably the cathelicidins [7]; (2) transmission EM of *S. aureus* killed by human β-defensin-3 (hBD-3) demonstrated a cellular morphology similar to that produced by penicillin, suggesting that primary disruption of cell wall integrity had occurred [25]; (3) neutrophil α-defensins HNP1-3 may bind to viral co-receptors inhibiting HIV replication [26]; and (4) HNP-1 added to rat or mouse lung explants augmented killing of *E. coli* and *P. aeruginosa* via enhanced production of reactive oxygen intermediates [27]. The take-home message is that *in vivo*, antimicrobial activity may be a synergy of independent innate immune mechanisms not easily demonstrated in simplified culture conditions.

1.4. Constitutive expression at epithelial surfaces

Constitutive epithelial expression is a feature common to the α-defensins expressed in Paneth cells, but in general is rare for β-defensins with the exception of hBD-1/mBD-1 [3]. The Paneth cell defensins of mouse (cryptdins) and humans (HD5 and HD6) are stored as propeptides in intracellular granules. Their release, either spontaneous or induced, is accompanied by co-release of a processing enzyme that cleaves the propeptide internally, releasing the active moiety. In the mouse, the processing enzyme is a matrix metalloproteinase MMP-7 [matrilysin] [28], and in humans, the analogous activity has been ascribed to an intestinal-specific trypsin isoform [29]. Paneth cell propeptide synthesis and storage appears to be a constitutive process, although release can be regulated at least partially by bacterial exposure through stimulation of Ca^{2+}-activated K^+ channels [30].

While most studies of adult animals demonstrate a constitutive level of Paneth cell α-defensin expression, during development there is a well-documented progression in expression levels [31,32] as well as a progression from diffuse epithelial expression to Paneth cell localisation [33]. The discovery of this maturation process may shed light on the increased risk of premature individuals for infectious enterocolitis [32]. While the abundance of evidence supports the constitutive nature of Paneth cell α-defensin expression, a study in rats has demonstrated that following haemorrhagic shock, mRNA for rat α-defensin RD-5 was up-regulated 10-fold [34]. While this result may be unique to the rat defensins, our current use of the term "constitutive" may reflect more the lack of an inducible response to traditional proinflammatory mediators. Modulation of high level basal activity in the case of Paneth cell α-defensins may be a characteristic of infectious, inflammatory and hormonal conditions.

Expression of the cathelicidin LL-37 is considered to be constitutive in the human gastrointestinal tract, with highest levels detected in epithelial cells at the surface and upper crypts of the colon. Both *in vitro* and *in vivo*, LL-37 expression levels parallel the state of differentiation and are not induced by bacterial exposure nor by treatment with proinflammatory cytokines [35].

hBD-1 and its mouse ortholog mBD-1 are unique among the β-defensins discovered to date in that they are expressed constitutively in epithelia and detected generally at low levels in surface lining fluids. The lack of inducibility correlates with an absence of NF-kB and AP-1 binding sites in their promoter regions [7]. In the best studied examples, hBD-1 and mBD-1 mRNAs were detected at their highest levels in the lung and in the kidney (both proximal and distal tubular epithelial cells) [36], and hBD-1 peptide isoforms were detectable in human urine [37]. While the usual mediators of inflammation do not induce these gene products, hormonal influences and the state of cellular differentiation may influence their level of transcription/translation. As examples, concentrations of the hBD-1 peptide increase in urine and breast tissue during pregnancy [7,37], and hBD-1 expression in keratinocytes increased with keratinocytes differentiation [38].

There have been several reports of bacteria or inflammatory mediators down-regulating hBD-1 expression as they induce hBD-2/hBD-3 expression [38]. The virulence of organisms causing colonic infections, for example *Shigella*, appears to be linked to the ability of bacteria or bacterial DNA to down-regulate the "constitutive" expression of both LL-37 and hBD-1 [39]. Much remains to be discovered regarding the mechanisms underlying this shift in transcriptional programming and its consequence for host immunity.

The unique pattern of hBD-1/mBD-1 expression may suggest a unique role for this molecule in innate immunity. In sections to follow, we will highlight reported differences in the properties of β-defensin-1 vs. inducible β-defensins, and hypothesise how those properties might provide insights into the general framework of constitutive vs. inducible host defence. Clearly, whatever framework is proposed, recent advances in this field are likely to lead to future paradigm revisions.

First, and perhaps most importantly, computer analysis of the human and mouse genomes has revealed that the β-defensin gene family is far larger than had been predicted. Sophisticated searches have uncovered 5 chromosomal regions that contain clusters of β-defensin-related genes and are conserved between species [40]. With the knowledge that at least 30 human β-defensin family genes and >40 mouse β-defensin family genes may be contributing to the innate immune system, it may be premature to consider hBD-1/mBD-1 as the sole β-defensin expressed constitutively. Furthermore, with these large gene families, one might surmise that the classic approach to proving gene function via single gene knockout would be unlikely to lead to a detectable change in phenotype. Fortunately, the mBD-1 gene knockout mice were constructed prior to the genomic information being available, and they demonstrate a phenotypic change both in lung [41] and urinary tract immunity [42].

Second, a series of five hBD-1 isoforms have been detected that differ only in their N-termini, and may differ functionally [37]. N-terminal processing may be a regulatory step, and a tissue-specific or individual-specific variation in isoform distribution may underlie a variation in hBD-1 activity. As an example, there are distinct patterns of hBD-1 isoforms present in individual urine samples [37].

Third and perhaps most importantly, most of the investigations into β-defensin regulation have been carried out in culture and may not reproduce *in vivo* conditions. An example is the detection of both hBD-1 and hBD-2 expression in human renal tubular epithelial cells, while biopsy material showed only hBD-1 expression [36]. Included in this category may be the demonstration that *H. pylori* induces hBD-1 expression in some but not all gastric epithelial cell lines [43,44].

1.5. Mechanisms of induction and secretion at epithelial surfaces

Barrier invasion, tissue injury and inflammation all lead to activation of innate immune defence mechanisms. Prominent among the first molecules to be detected are β-defensins and cathelicidins. The most detailed knowledge of this process has come from *in vitro* and *in vivo* studies of the bovine tracheal antimicrobial peptide (TAP), a β-defensin [45,46]. *E. coli* LPS has been shown to be a potent inducer of TAP *in vivo* and in tracheal epithelial cells *in vitro*. The LPS molecule binds to a cell surface CD14/TLR4 receptor (likely to require MD-2 as well) initiating an intracellular signalling pathway whose end result is NF-kB activation. The TAP gene contains consensus NF-kB binding sites leading to enhanced transcription, translation, post-translational processing and active peptide release.

Further investigation into the inducible expression of hBD-2 suggests that epithelial cells undergo dual regulation of β-defensin genes [19,21,47]. High level bacterial and/or LPS exposure activates epithelial cell NF-kB directly via the TLR (Toll-like receptor) pathway. Alternatively, low level microbial stimulation of tissue monocytes results in proinflammatory cytokine release (IL-1α, IL-1β and TNF-α). These molecules bind to specific receptors on epithelial cells and at low concentrations are potent activators of NF-kB. In fact, in human epidermis, hBD-2 is among the most highly induced mRNAs following IL-1α exposure [47]. Theoretically, having these alternate mechanisms of hBD-2 induction allows for: (1) a direct epithelial cell response to high level bacterial exposure; and (2) in the sub-epithelial space, pathogen-macrophage contact leading to proinflammatory cytokine release that provokes a regional upregulation of antimicrobial peptide synthesis in order to limit bacterial spread.

As more and more defensin genes are sequenced, analysis of their promoter regions has uncovered a marked variation in the presence of consensus response elements for the proinflammatory transcriptional enhancers NF-κB, AP-1, NF-IL-6 and STAT [7]. For example, the hBD-2 gene contains response elements for NF-κB, NF-IL-6 and AP-1, while the hBD-3 gene has numerous AP-1 but no NF-κB response elements. hBD-2 and 3 expression can be detected in many of the same tissues, however their differential regulation and differential antimicrobial spectra (hBD-2 active primarily against Gm-negatives while hBD-3 active against Gm-negative and Gm-positive organisms including *S. aureus*) allows for flexibility in the nature of the epithelial innate response. As a corollary, pharmacologic regulation of defensin gene expression may vary based on the presence or absence of gene-specific response elements. Dexamethasone inhibits hBD-3 but not hBD-2 (nor constitutive hBD-1) expression in airway epithelial cells [7].

As we strive to formulate an induction paradigm that focuses on classical pathways, an unusual set of experiments may have identified a novel pathway to NF-κB activation. In an artificial system utilising transfected bovine kidney cells, investigators reported that micromolar levels of L-isoleucine specifically induced expression of a β-defensin/luciferase reporter construct through NF-kB activation [48]. The authors speculate that since this essential amino acid is normally in low abundance, elevated levels of isoleucine or a related compound, possibly secreted by bacteria, could be interpreted by epithelial cells as a sign of infection.

1.6. Mechanisms of recruitment and activation

Recruitment of antimicrobial peptide-containing cells to epithelial sites of injury, infection or inflammation involves both circulating granulocytes and monocytes. The recruiting signals include chemokines released from compromised epithelium at tissue surfaces, from exposed tissue macrophages and from injured vascular endothelium [49]. Many of these same signals are known to promote haemostasis and wound repair [6], hence it is not surprising that the recruited antimicrobial elements would be direct participants in the healing process as well.

Antimicrobial peptides can be cytotoxic to the synthesising eukaryotic cells at high concentrations, and it is a challenge for granulocytes/monocytes to avoid cell injury during peptide packaging into granules and long-term peptide storage. Two alternative strategies have evolved to protect host cells from their own antimicrobial peptides until recruited from the circulation into the tissues. The first is best demonstrated in human neutrophils [4]. Initial processing of neutrophil α-defensins cleaves prepropeptides into propeptides. Within the propeptide, the anionic, N-terminal pro segment balances the charge and toxicity of the cationic, C-terminal defensin peptide. Secondary cleavage separates propiece from mature peptide, but their co-storage in the azurophilic granules leads to trans-inactivation until released into the phagolysosome or the external milieu.

The second strategy is best exemplified by the cathelicidins [50,51]. It is well documented in both pig and human neutrophils that the cathelicidins are stored as unprocessed, propeptides in peroxidase-negative granules, while their processing enzymes are stored in a distinct set of granules in the same cell. No active peptides are present as the cell circulates, however cell activation leads to fusion of both sets of granules with the phagolysosome or release of both sets of granules into the tissues. Either results in activation of this binary antimicrobial weapon.

While the pig neutrophils utilise neutrophil elastase to activate their protegrin cathelicidins, human neutrophils cleave hCAP-18 to LL-37 via proteinase 3, a serine proteinase from azurophilic granules [51]. This activation pathway provides an opportunity for the host to dampen an exuberant inflammatory response through proteinase inhibitors present in tissues, e.g., elafin in human skin [52], or co-released by the neutrophil, e.g., alpha 1-antiprotease [53]. In addition, pharmacologic modulation of host inflammation may be accomplished through the use of small molecule proteinase inhibitors, e.g., the elastase inhibitor NX21909 [54]. Finally, it is likely that among the diversity of mechanisms used by microbial pathogens to escape host defences will be a molecular mimic of host proteinase inhibitors.

1.7. Mechanisms of peptide inactivation

Three mechanisms have been proposed for antimicrobial peptide inactivation: protein binding, proteinase degradation and post-translational modification. As examples of the first mechanism, defensin binding to serum albumin, α-1-antiprotease (also known as α-1-antitrypsin) and α-1-chymotrypsin inhibits its proinflammatory and cytotoxic effects [55]. As further evidence for the importance of this protective mechanism, a selected oligonucleotide inhibitor of elastase, NX21909, protects against lung inflammatory injury in an *in vivo* model of acute disease [54].

Bacterial proteinases from human pathogens including *P. aeruginosa* and *S. pyogenes* have been shown to inactivate the human cathelicidin LL-37, possibly revealing a common microbial virulence mechanism [56]. Molecules that block this degradation, e.g., the metalloproteinase inhibitor GM6001, may have significant therapeutic potential in combination with traditional antibiotic treatment.

Finally, ADP ribosyltransferase, present on or secreted from epithelial cells, lymphocytes and neutrophils, can ribosylate the arg-14 of HNP-1 [57]. Ribosylated-HNP-1 is detected at increased levels in the BAL from smokers, and the ribosylated product has decreased antimicrobial and cytotoxic effects. Interestingly, arg-14 HNP-1 ribosylation did not affect T cell chemotactic and IL-8-releasing activities, suggesting that this mode of peptide modification may provide new insights into HNP-1 structure-function relationships.

1.8. Non-antimicrobial effects

A current area of great interest in the study of antimicrobial peptides is the search for dual roles in host immunity. Most if not all antimicrobial peptides are multi-functional, potentiating the innate immune response via mechanisms as diverse as promotion of wound healing, chemokine activity and initiating an adaptive immune response [6]. Indeed, it remains an open question whether antimicrobial activity is their most prominent role *in vivo*. A note of caution here relates to the fact that molecules like defensins and cathelicidins are membrane active, may have non-specific effects on membrane functions such as maintenance of ion gradients, and hence may demonstrate activities in specialised assay systems that are of unclear significance to *in vivo* conditions.

That caveat aside, antimicrobial peptides demonstrate a remarkable spectrum of host defence-related, non-antimicrobial functions including modulation of: bacterial adherence [55,58]; complement activation [55]; fibrinolysis [55]; steroid synthesis [59]; mast cell activation [60]; monocyte, neutrophil, mast cell, T cell and immature dendritic cell chemoattraction [11,61,62]; cytokine expression [63]; cytotoxicity [64]; cell proliferation [7,65]; angiogenesis [66]; protease inhibitor synthesis [67]; keratinocyte differentiation [38]; proteoglycan synthesis [11]; phagocytosis [68] and Ca^{+2} mobilisation [59]. The breadth of potential functions has led some to consider these molecules as the key regulators of innate immunity. While many recent reviews can be found containing complete descriptions of these activities, here we will highlight four unique aspects.

1. A variety of activities ascribed to these peptides involve binding to specific, high-affinity cell surface receptors. Among the best characterised examples are: β-defensin binding to the chemokine receptor CCR6 inducing chemotaxis of T-cells and immature dendritic cells [69]; LL-37 binding to the formyl peptide receptor-like 1 (FPRL1) inducing monocyte chemotaxis and Ca^{+2} mobilisation [17]; and HNP1-3 binding to the chemoreceptor CXCR4 on CD8 T lymphocytes, effectively blocking the replication of HIV-1 virus type X4 and stabilising patients' immunologic status [26]. In general, this type of receptor-peptide ligand interaction has enormous potential for drug targeting through development of receptor antagonists, anti-receptor antibodies or soluble receptors [70].
2. Constitutive and inducible antimicrobial peptides differ significantly in their activities. The inducible hBD-2 and LL-37 peptides degranulate mast cells via a G protein –phospholipase C-dependent mechanism, while the constitutive hBD-1 lacks this activity [60]. Additionally, hBD-2 is a mast cell chemotaxin while hBD-1 is not [17]. As a third example, in immortalised human keratinocytes the state of differentiation regulates hBD-1 mRNA levels while hBD-2 mRNA levels are unchanged [38].
3. Dose-response curves for non-antimicrobial activities often are bell-shaped, with peak activity near the concentration at which peak antimicrobial activity is reached. HNP1-3 enhance proliferation of human lung tumour epithelial cell lines at 4–10 μg/ml, but are cytotoxic at concentrations $\geq$ 20 μg/ml [65]. LL-37 is chemotactic for mast cells at 5 μg/ml but not at 1 or 20 μg/ml [17]. Finally, pig protegrins, members of the cathelicidin family, trigger the cleavage and export of IL-1β from LPS-primed monocytes with a peak at 12.5 μg/ml but are inactive at 1 and 100 μg/ml [63]. Possible implications of this consistent dose-response pattern are discussed in Section 3.2.
4. The non-antimicrobial activities of these peptides can amplify the innate response via positive feedback loops. IL-8, a CXC chemokine, is one of several signals that attract neutrophils to the lungs in patients with chronic inflammatory diseases, e.g., chronic bronchitis or COPD

[71]. Subsequent neutrophil degranulation then releases α-defensins that induce airway epithelial cells to synthesise additional IL-8.

1.9. Interactions with components of the innate immune system

One should not underestimate the challenge faced by the innate immune system in protecting the delicate epithelial tissues, e.g., those of the pulmonary and gastrointestinal tracts that provide vital physiologic functions in the presence of recurrent and/or continuous pathogen exposure. In many situations, a brisk immune and inflammatory response to low level pathogen exposure is less than ideal, as it may damage and disrupt key tissue elements. Mechanisms to promote a *prompt* and *appropriate response* to microbial challenge must be in place, it is our challenge to delineate them.

Evidence is accumulating that polarisation of epithelial cells is a key element in regulation of epithelial innate immunity. The apical cell surface is the primary site of microbial exposure, and analysis of its surface molecules as well as the composition of its secreted surface fluid will continue to provide insights into how host tissues control their adjacent milieu. As a baseline, the apical secretory components include (but are not limited to) organics (e.g., HCl), lysozyme, lactoferrin, SLPI, PLA2 and constitutive antimicrobial peptides (e.g., hBD-1) [72,73]. In airway surface fluid there is ample evidence for synergistic interactions between these components, although the β-defensin component, hBD-1 is more additive in its effects. An analogous system is present in the crypts of the small intestine, where the primary antimicrobial peptides are α-defensins [74], and in vaginal fluid [75]. It is a recurring theme in these studies that individual and synergistic activities are reduced as ionic strength increases.

On the apical surface of epithelial cells can be found bactericidal-permeability inducing protein (BPI), a molecule with both antibacterial and LPS-binding properties [76]. It is hypothesised that surface BPI interacts with constitutive β-defensins in promoting antimicrobial activity against bacteria adhering to the host cell surface. β-defensin and BPI-binding of released Gm-negative bacteria LPS would prevent the initiation of potentially injurious inflammatory responses.

A more dramatic and complex host response is activated in the setting of barrier compromise and epithelial injury [21]. Microorganisms and their cellular constituents now will come into contact with the epithelial cell basolateral surface where the Toll-like receptors (TLR) are localised and can be activated. TLR activation leads to NF-kB stimulation of β-defensin synthesis, predominantly the hBD-2 and hBD-3 molecules in the human pulmonary and gastrointestinal tissues. Additionally, tissue monocytes/macrophages will be activated by the microbial stimuli leading to proinflammatory cytokine (TNF-α, IL-1α, IL-1β) and antimicrobial peptide release. These molecules will then recruit circulating granulocytes and monocytes to an area at risk for significant infection spread.

Surprisingly, while degranulation of the recruited neutrophils leads to release of α-defensins that enhance monocyte TNF-α and IL-1β expression in response to *S. aureus* or phorbol myristate acetate (positive feedback), the same molecules down-regulate endothelial cell VCAM-1 expression reducing cellular recruitment from the circulation (negative feedback) [5]. The released α-defensins also bind C1Q and may activate the classical complement pathway [77], another component of the innate immune system preserved in organisms from *Drosophila* to humans.

1.10. Liaison with the adaptive immune system

It has been a long time coming, but finally a model is evolving that includes the innate immune system in alerting, stimulating and regulating the adaptive immune response. This can be viewed not merely as a step-wise escalation of the host response, but in reality a commitment of the host to a long term expenditure of resources for combating what is perceived as a significant pathogenic organism.

Following this line of reasoning, the most convincing evidence for regulation of adaptive immunity revolves around chemoattraction. While both defensin and cathelicidin peptides are antimicrobial at micromolar concentrations, they are chemotactic for dendritic and memory T cells at nanomolar concentrations [5]. hBD-1 and 2 act through binding to the CCR6 chemokine receptor, LL-37 via formyl peptide receptor-like 1 (FPRL1) and the α-defensins through a receptor not yet identified.

The primary adaptive immune response plays out in draining regional lymph nodes somewhat distant from the infected/injured tissue. Initially, immature dendritic cells are recruited to the site of inflammation, they process foreign antigens for presentation, migrate to the regional nodes and finally activate unprimed T and B cells. These activated cells then migrate to the original site of infection/injury to deliver the first effective response of the adaptive immune system. These are key steps where the antimicrobial peptides function in co-ordination with cytokine and chemokine elements of the innate immune system. Four examples are outlined below.

First, hBD-1, hBD-2 and α-defensins are chemotactic for immature dendritic cells (iDC) eliciting their migration to the site of antimicrobial peptide synthesis (epithelial cells) or release (from recruited granulocytes) [49]. Second, upon iDC arrival, both mBD-2 and human α-defensins have been shown to induce iDC maturation including the upregulation of surface costimulatory molecules and the enhanced expression of proinflammatory cytokines including IL-12, IL-1α and IL-1β [62]. Third, antimicrobial peptides recruit memory T cells to sites of inflammation [78]. And fourth, α-defensins have been shown to increase the mouse IgG response in a model of immunoglobulin stimulation [79].

2. *IN VIVO* MODELS OF ANTIMICROBIAL PEPTIDE FUNCTION

2.1. Skin

The ready availability of epidermal tissues for *in vivo* and *in vitro* studies has lead to rapid advances in our knowledge of skin antimicrobial peptide biology. Intact and uninflammed, keratinocytes do not express significant amounts of either cathelicidin or defensin peptides. However, both in human and mouse tissues, injured/inflamed skin expresses high levels of one or more antimicrobial peptides [6]. Two lines of evidence support the relevance of antimicrobial peptide expression to skin defence.

First, it is well known from clinical experience that psoriatic lesions are less prone to infection than atopic dermatitis lesions. In a recently published study, immunoblotting and Western blot analysis were used to analyse epidermal expression of both the human cathelicidin peptide LL-37 and the human β-defensin hBD-2 [80]. These peptides have been shown to be synergistic in activity against *S. aureus*, a major skin pathogen. In psoriatic surface epidermis, there is *abundant expression* of both peptides correlating with a decreased risk for bacterial infection [80]. In contrast, in atopic dermatitis lesions there is a significant *suppression of expression* for both peptides correlating with an increased risk of bacterial infection. Additionally, IL-4 and IL-13, cytokines known to be increased in atopic dermatitis lesions but not in psoriatic lesions, block antimicrobial peptide induction by TNF-α in cultured keratinocytes.

Direct evidence for the role of antimicrobial peptides in skin was provided through use of mouse knockout technology. Mice in which the LL-37 ortholog, CRAMP, was inactivated (CR-/-), demonstrated increased susceptibility to necrotic skin infection by group A Streptococcus (GAS) compared to their wild type littermates (CR+/+) [81]. Heterozygous animals (CR+/-) were intermediate in susceptibility supporting a gene dosage effect. In complementary studies, mutating the GAS bacterium to make it resistant to killing by CRAMP, lead to equal infectivity in CR-/- and CR +/+ animals. This combination of mouse and bacterial genetics provides the most convincing evidence to date that a single antimicrobial peptide provides a critical role in host defence.

2.2. Pulmonary tract

An area of great interest, and of significant controversy, is the role of antimicrobial peptides in lung protection in general, and specifically in patients with cystic fibrosis [82]. The leap into studying antimicrobial peptides in cystic fibrosis derives from observations that: (1) CF patients are prone to airway colonisation by bacterial pathogens; (2) CF patients are prone to recurrent lung infections as a source of morbidity and mortality; (3) the airway secretions of CF patients have been reported to contain an increased salt concentration; and (4) airway antimicrobial peptides are salt-sensitive, losing protective activity in the presence of salt concentrations seen in CF airway fluid.

Several well-publicised research reports used both *in vitro* assays and bronchial xenografts to demonstrate that the activity of the constitutively-expressed lung hBD-1 against common CF pathogens was reduced in the presence of CF airway fluid. Additionally, antisense suppression of xenograft hBD-1 expression abolished airway surface fluid microbicidal activity, and over-expression of the less salt-sensitive LL-37 restored antimicrobial activity in CF xenograft tissue [83–85].

As tantalising as it is to have CF lung disease explained by salt-sensitive antimicrobial activity, this hypothesis is highly controversial, based on the following observations. First, recent data suggests that the purported high salt concentration in CF airway surface fluid may not exist *in vivo* [86]. Second, multiple β-defensin peptides are expressed in airway epithelial cells [7] so that the hypothesis that hBD-1 suppression alone could change the microbicidal activity has not been accepted readily. Third, there is a great deal of phenotypic variation in infection susceptibility within the CF population, even in patients with the same CFTR genotype, with some patients having little in the way of pulmonary complications and others infected frequently from their early childhood [87].

As an alternative approach to address some of the questions, two laboratories derived mouse lines in which the mBD-1 gene was inactivated. In one report, there was no change in pulmonary susceptibility to a nebulized *S. aureus* challenge [42], while in the other there was a reproducible, delayed clearance of *H. influenza* inoculated intranasally [41]. Differences in strain background, pathogen choice and CFU level of inoculation make it difficult to resolve this discrepancy. Additionally, it is a challenge to relate this to CF in humans, as the mouse CF model does not mimic the human condition in pulmonary pathology.

2.3. Gastrointestinal tract

Multiple antimicrobial peptides are expressed in mammalian gastrointestinal tissues, with the greatest abundance in Paneth cells of the distal ileal crypts [74]. Initial thoughts were that use of single gene knockouts would be unlikely to produce a detectable phenotype. A successful alternative approach was to inactivate processing pathways common to all mouse intestinal α-defensins. The matrix metalloproteinase matrilysin (MMP-7) co-localises with α-defensins in Paneth cell granules, and its inactivation leads to a deficiency of mature defensins in the Paneth cells, an accumulation of the inactive precursors (implying a block in processing) and an increased susceptibility to an oral challenge with the bacterial pathogen *Salmonella* [28]. While this is very convincing evidence for the role of α-defensins in intestinal immunity, it remains a possibility that the loss of other intestinal activities regulated by MMP-7 contributed to the change in host susceptibility.

In a complementary series of experiments, Bevins CL, Huttner KM, et al. (submitted for publication [96]) have produced and analysed transgenic mouse strains carrying the human Paneth cell defensin gene HD-5. In two independently-derived lines, Paneth cell expression of HD-5 is co-ordinated with that of the endogenous mouse defensins both in spatial orientation and in developmental time-frame. More surprisingly, the addition of this single peptide to the mouse Paneth cell expression of up to 20 different α-defensins led to a reproducible augmentation of host defence.

There are a growing number of published studies related to antimicrobial peptide function in the tongue, ocular mucosa, genitourinary tract and in breast milk. The reader is directed to recent reviews for specific papers in these areas [4,5,7]. Clearly this area of research is poised to grow in the next decade.

3. BRIEF EVOLUTIONARY PERSPECTIVES

3.1. Antimicrobial synergy

A myriad of reports on peptide antimicrobial properties has demonstrated that each peptide has its own pattern of microbial specificity and dose-response curve. Even minor differences in amino acid sequence may change properties significantly. It is likely that we under-appreciate how these molecules synergize, perhaps not being as creative in our laboratory studies as nature has been during evolution. Peptides may be weakly microbicidal, but may unmask bacterial structures that lead to increased vulnerability to other molecules of innate immunity. For example, in the horseshoe crab, the peptide tachycitin has low antimicrobial activity but synergistically enhances the activity of a defensin-like peptide fifty-fold [88].

Experience in antimicrobial drug therapy has taught us that multi-drug treatment is the most effective approach to minimising the selection of resistant organisms. Apparently, through expression of large families of active peptides at each site of pathogen exposure, nature has been following this approach for thousands of years in optimising the innate immune response.

3.2. Checks and balances

In a number of examples from the inflammatory, clotting and immune cascades, pathway activation also lays the groundwork for limiting the response. Examples in the field of antimicrobial peptides are present as well, with several described below.

In the first case, proinflammatory cytokines IFN- and IL-6 were shown to stimulate synergistically the *release* of LL-37 from human PBMC, T and NK cells [15]. Simultaneously, these same cytokines down-regulated *transcription* of the LL-37 gene leading to a net decrease in peptide release 24 hours later.

Second, LL-37 administration to mice protects against endotoxemia yet inhibits macrophage stimulation by bacterial LPS and lipoteichoic acid [89]. These results suggest that this potent antimicrobial peptide can modulate the host response through limiting release of proinflammatory cytokines. This was confirmed by expression profiling of LL-37-treated human and mouse monocytes/macrophages. In both cases, chemokines but not TNF-α were up-regulated, consistent with the recruitment of immune cells even while limiting the damaging effects of inflammation.

As a third example, neutrophil activation results in the release of antimicrobial propeptides and their activating proteases including elastase and proteinase 3. Coincidentally these cells release antiproteases that function to limit activation [53]. At the same site where these proteases are crucial for promoting inflammation through antimicrobial peptide release, there is speculative evidence that they dampen the inflammatory response via entry into endothelial cells and cleavage of NF-kB [90].

Lastly, we had outlined in an earlier section three examples of antimicrobial peptide affects with bell-shaped dose-response curves, i.e., HNP1-3 enhancing cell proliferation, LL-37 promoting mast cell chemotaxis and protegrins catalysing release of active IL-1β. This response profile implies that as peptide concentrations move off of their optimum in either direction, e.g., as a response builds or subsides, their effectiveness will diminish and the system will trend back to baseline equilibrium.

3.3. Gene amplification, rearrangement and mutation

From a broad perspective, genes of the adaptive immune system encoding immunoglobulins and T cell receptors are known to undergo a series of genetic amplifications, rearrangements and mutations that generate a protective diversity promoting survival of the individual. Homologous events involving genes of the innate immune system can be seen as generating a protective diversity promoting survival of a population or species. Specific examples are presented below. The mechanisms for this "genome instability" in innate immunity genes remain to be elucidated, but may represent a precursor for the more familiar examples described in the adaptive immune system.

3.3.1 Amplification

Whole genome sequencing in both humans and mice demonstrated a large collection of closely related α- and β-defensin genes, presumably derived from duplication events that cluster at a single locus on human chromosome 8p23 [91] and its mouse equivalent. The number of genes varies significantly both between species and even between individuals in the case of HNP1-3 [92]. Similar results are found in the cathelicidin family with humans and mice having one classic cathelicidin, while sheep, cows and pigs have variably large cathelicidin gene families, again clustered at a single chromosomal site [11]. The genetic relationship among the multiple genes of these families, hypothesised based on sequence comparisons of the signal and propiece regions, is consistent with gene duplications occurring both before and after speciation [7].

In addition to the gene duplication events expanding the defensins family at the 8p23 locus, sophisticated computational analysis of genome sequence data points to expansion of the β-defensin gene family to at least 4 additional sites in the genome and subsequent duplication at each of these sites [40].

3.3.2 Rearrangement

One well-documented example of genetic rearrangement altering tissue-specific expression of innate immune peptides is in the human α-defensins [93]. The Paneth cell-specific α-defensins HD-5 and 6 are encoded by two exon genes, while the neutrophil α-defensins are encoded by three exon genes. A detailed comparison revealed a specific recombination event that juxtaposed a new 5' exon onto a 2 exon Paneth cell defensin gene, retargeting expression from the GI tract to neutrophils and creating the first 3 exon neutrophil defensin gene.

3.3.3 Mutation

Genetic mutation has led to a family of mouse Paneth cell α-defensins, numbering perhaps 20 or more, that differ at a limited number of amino acid positions and have significant differences in peptide properties [94]. The importance of mutations in the β-defensin gene family can be demonstrated as well with the association between single nucleotide polymorphisms in the hBD-1 gene and COPD in Japanese populations, most specifically with an increased risk of chronic bronchitis (OR 6.1, (2-18.3)) [95].

4. CONCLUSIONS

As we further our understanding of host defence regulation at the organismal level, we can appreciate the complexity of pathways within the innate immune system and the central position held by antimicrobial peptides. Unravelling their molecular structure has provided investigators with novel insights into mechanisms for regulating their biosynthesis, processing and release. With many surprises still to come, it is likely that future generations of epithelial biologists will view the innate and adaptive immune systems as a continuum, with antimicrobial peptides playing key roles both as regulatory and effector elements.

ACKNOWLEDGEMENTS

The author would like to thank Dr. Charles Bevins for his thoughtful review of the manuscript and Ms. Wendy Calderon for all her assistance in manuscript and reference preparation.

REFERENCES

1. Zasloff M. Antimicrobial peptides in health and disease. N Engl J Med 2002;347:1199–200.
2. Ganz T. Antimicrobial proteins and peptides in host defense. Semin Respir Infect 2001;16: 4–10.

3. Huttner KM, Bevins CL. Antimicrobial peptides as mediators of epithelial host defense. Pediatr Res 1999;45:785–94.
4. Bevins CL. Antimicrobial peptides as effector molecules in mammalian host defense. In: Herwald H, editor. Host response mechanisms in infectious disease. Basel: Karger AG, 2003;106–48. (Contributions to Microbiology; vol 10).
5. Lehrer RI, Ganz T. Defensins of vertebrate animals. Curr Opin Immun 2002;14:96–102.
6. Gallo RL, Murakami M, Ohtake T, Zaiou M. Biology and clinical relevance of naturally occurring antimicrobial peptides. J Allergy Clin Immunol 2002;110:823–31.
7. Schutte BC, McCray PB Jr. β-defensins in lung host defense. Annu Rev Physiol 2002;64: 709–48.
8. Tran D, Tran PA, Tang YQ, Yuan J, Cole T, Selsted ME. Homodimeric theta-defensins from rhesus macaque leukocytes: isolation, synthesis, antimicrobial activities, and bacterial binding properties of the cyclic peptides. J Biol Chem 2002;277:3079–84.
9. Cole AM, Ganz T, Liese AM, Burdick MD, Liu L, Strieter RM. IFN-inducible ELR$^-$ CXC chemokines display defensin-like antimicrobial activity. J Immunol 2001;167:623–7.
10. Ritonja A, Kopitar M, Jerala R, Turk V. Primary structure of a new cysteine proteinase inhibitor from pig leukocytes. FEBS Lett 1989;255:211–4.
11. Zaiou M, Gallo RL. Cathelicidins, essential gene-encoded mammalian antibiotics. J Mol Med 2002;80:549–61.
12. Brogden KA, Ackermann M, Huttner KM. Detection of anionic antimicrobial peptides in ovine bronchoalveolar lavage fluid and respiratory epithelium. Infect Immun 1998;66: 5948–54.
13. Fales-Williams AJ, Brogden KA, Huffman E, Gallup JM, Ackermann MR. Cellular distribution of anionic antimicrobial peptide in normal lung and during acute pulmonary inflammation. Vet Pathol 2002;39:706–11.
14. Rose FRAJ, Bailey K, Keyte YW, Chan WC, Greenwood D, Mahida YR. Potential role of epithelial cell-derived histone H1 proteins in innate antimicrobial defense in the human gastrointestinal tract. Infect Immun 1998;66:3255–63.
15. Agerberth B, Charo J, Werr J, Olsson B, Idali F, Lindbom L, et al. The human antimicrobial and chemotactic peptides LL-37 and α-defensins are expressed by specific lymphocyte and monocyte populations. Blood 2000;96:3086–93.
16. Marchini G, Lonne-Rahm S, Agerberth B, Gudmundsson GH. The newborn infant is protected by an innate antimicrobial barrier: peptide antibiotic are present in the skin and vernix. Br J Dermatol 2002;147:1127–34.
17. Niyonsaba F, Iwabuchi K, Someya A, Hirata M, Matsuda H, Ogawa H, et al. A cathelicidin family of human antibacterial peptide LL-37 induces mast cell chemotaxis. Immunology 2002;106:20–6.
18. Quayle AJ, Porter EM, Nussbaum AA, Wang YM, Brabec C, Yip KP, et al. Gene expression, immunolocalization, and secretion of human defensin-5 in the human female reproductive tract. Am J Pathol 1998;152:1247–58.
19. Ganz T. Epithelia: not just physical barriers. PNAS 2002;99:3357–8.
20. Murakami M, Ohtake T, Dorschner RA, Gallo RL. Cathelicidin antimicrobial peptides are expressed in salivary glands and saliva. J Dent Res 2002;81:845–50.
21. Ganz T. Antimicrobial polypeptides in host defense of the respiratory tract. J Clin Invest 2002;109:693–7.
22. Zhang L, Rozek A, Hancock RE. Interaction of cationic antimicrobial peptides with model membranes. J Biol Chem 2001;276:35714–22.

23. Hoover DM, Rajasjankar KR, Blumenthal R, Puri A, Oppenheim JJ, Chertov O, et al. The structure of human beta-defensin-2 shows evidence of higher order oligomerization. J Biol Chem 2000;275:32911–8.
24. Hong RW, Shchepetov M, Weiser JN, Axelsen PH. Transcriptional profile of the *Escherichia coli* response to the antimicrobial insect peptide Cecropin A. Antimicrob Agents Chemother 2003;47:1–6.
25. Harder J, Bartels J, Christophers E, Schroder JM. Isolation and characterization of human β-defensin-3 a novel human inducible peptide antibiotic. J Bio Chem 2001;276:5707–13.
26. Zhang L, Yu W, He T, Yu J, Caffrey RE, Dalmasso EA, et al. Contribution of human α-defensin 1,2, and 3 to the anti-HIV-1 activity of CD8 antiviral factor. Science 2002;298: 995–1000.
27. Porro GA, Lee JH, de Azavedo J, Crandall I, Whitehead T, Tullis E, et al. Direct and indirect bacterial killing functions of neutrophil defensins in lung explants. Am J Physiol Lung Cell Mol Physiol 2001;281:L1240–7.
28. Wilson CL, Ouellette AJ, Satchell DP, Ayabe T, Lopez-Boado YS, Stratman JL, et al. Regulation of intestinal α-defensin activation by metalloproteinase matrilysin in innate host defense. Science 1999;286:113–7.
29. Ghosh D, Porter E, Shen B, Lee SK, Wilk D, Drazba J, et al. Paneth Cell trypsin is the processing enzyme for human defensin-5. Nat Immunol 2002;3:583–90.
30. Ayabe T, Wulff H, Darmoul D, Cahalan MD, Chandy KG, Ouellette AJ. Modulation of mouse Paneth cell alpha-defensin secretion by mIKCa1, a Ca2+-activated, intermediate conductance potassium channel. J Biol Chem 2002;277:3793–800.
31. Ouellette AJ, Lualdi JC. A novel mouse gene family coding for cationic, cysteine-rich peptides. Regulation in small intestine and cells of myeloid origin. J Biol Chem 1990;265: 9831–7.
32. Salzman NH, Polin RA, Harris MC, Ruchelli E, Hebra A, Zirin-Butler S, et al. Enteric defensin expression in necrotizing enterocolitis. Pediatr Res 1998;44:20–6.
33. Darmoul D, Brown D, Selsted ME, Ouellette AJ. Cryptdin gene expression in developing mouse small intestine. Am J Physiol 1997;272:G197–206.
34. Condon MR, Viera A, D'Alessio M, Diamond G. Induction of a rat enteric defensin gene by hemorrhagic shock. Infect Immun 1999;67:4787–93.
35. Hase K, Eckmann L, Leopard JD, Varki N, Kagnoff MF. Cell differentiation is a key determinant of cathelicidin LL-37/human cationic antimicrobial protein 18 expression by human colon epithelium. Infect Immun 2002;70:953–63.
36. Nitschke M, Wiehl S, Baer PC, Kreft B. Bactericidal activity of renal tubular cells: the putative role of human beta defensins. Exp Nephrol 2002;10:332–7.
37. Valore EV, Park CH, Quayle AJ, Wiles KR, McCray PB Jr, Ganz T. Human beta-Defensin-1: an antimicrobial peptide of urogenital tissues. J Clin Invest 1998;101:1633–42.
38. Frye M, Bargon J, Gropp R. Expression of human β-defensin-1 promotes differentiation of keratinocytes. J Mol Med 2001;79:275–82.
39. Islam D, Bandholtz L, Nilsson J, Wigzell H, Christensson B, Agerberth B, et al. Downregulation of bactericidal peptides in enteric infections: a novel immune escape mechanism with bacterial DNA as potential regulator. Nat Med 2001;7:180–5.
40. Schutte BC, Mitros JP, Bartlett JA, Walters JD, Jia HP, Welsh MJ, et al. Discovery of five conserved β-defensin gene clusters using a computational search strategy. PNAS 2002;99: 2129–33.
41. Moser C, Weiner DJ, Lysenko E, Bals R, Weiser JN, Wilson JM. β-defensin 1 contributes

to pulmonary innate immunity in mice. Infection Immun 2002;70:3068–72.
42. Morrison GM, Kilanowski F, Davidson D, Dorin J. Characterization of the mouse beta defensin 1, *Dfb*1, mutant mouse model. Infection Immun 2002;70:3053–60.
43. Bajaj-Elliott M, Fedeli P, Smith GV, Domizio P, Maher L, Ali RS, et al. Modulation of host antimicrobial peptide (beta-defensins 1 and 2) expression during gastritis. Gut 2002;51: 356–61.
44. O'Neil DA, Cole SP, Martin-Porter E, Housley MP, Liu L, Ganz T, et al. Regulation of human β-defensins by gastric epithelial cells in response to infection with *Helicobacter pylori* or stimulation with interleukin-1. Infection Immun 2002;68:5412–15.
45. Diamond G, Russell JP, Bevins CL. Inducible expression of an antibiotic peptide gene in lipopolysaccharide-challenged tracheal epithelial cells. PNAS 1996;93:5156–60.
46. Diamond G, Legarda D, Ryan LK. The innate immune response of the respiratory epithelium. Immunol Rev 2000;173:27–38.
47. Liu AY, Destoumieux D, Wong AV, Park CH, Valore EV, Liu L, et al. Human β-defensin-2 production in keratinocytes is regulated by interleukin-1, bacteria, and state of differentiation. J Invest Dermatol 2002;118:275–81.
48. Fehlbaum P, Rao M, Zasloff M, Anderson GM. An essential amino acid induces epithelial β-defensin expression. PNAS 2000;97:12723–8.
49. Luster AD. The role of chemokines in linking innate and adaptive immunity. Curr Opin Immunol 2002;14:129–35.
50. Cole AM, Shi J, Ceccarelli A, Kim Y, Park A, Ganz T. Inhibition of neutrophil elastase prevents cathelicidin activation and impairs clearance of bacteria from wounds. Blood 2001;97:297–304.
51. Sørensen OE, Follin P, Johnsen AH, Calafat J, Tjabringa GS, Hiemstra PS, et al. Human cathelicidin, hCAP-18, is processed to the antimicrobial peptide LL-37 by extracellular cleavage with proteinase 3. Blood 2001;97:3951–9.
52. Ying QL, Simon SR. Kinetics of the inhibition of human leukocyte elastase by elafin, a 6-kilodalton elastase-specific inhibitor from human skin. Biochemistry 1993;32:1866–74.
53. DuBois RM, Bernaudin JF, Paakko P, Hubbard R, Takahashi H, Ferrans V, et al. Human neutrophils express the alpha 1-antitrypsin gene and produce alpha 1-antitrypsin. Blood 1991;77:2724–30.
54. Bless NM, Smith D, Charlton J, Czermak BJ, Schmal H, Friedl HP, et al. Protective effects of an aptamer inhibitor of neutrophil elastase in lung inflammatory injury. Curr Biol 1997;7:877–80.
55. Aarbiou J, Rabe KF, Hiemstra PS. Role of defensins in inflammatory lung disease. Ann Med 2002;34:96–101.
56. Schmidtchen A, Frick IM, Andersson E, Tapper H, Bjorck L. Proteinases of common pathogenic bacteria degrade and inactivate the antibacterial peptide LL-37. Mol Microbiol 2002;46:157–68.
57. Paone G, Wada A, Stevens LA, Matin A, Hirayama T, Levine RL, et al. ADP ribosylation of human neutrophil peptide-1 regulates its biological properties. PNAS 2002;99:8231–5.
58. Gorter AD, Hiemstra PS, de Bentzmann S, van Wetering S, Dankert J, van Alphen L. Stimulation of bacterial adherence by neutrophil defensins varies among bacterial species but not among host cell types. FEMS Immun Med Microbiol 2000;28:105–11.
59. Yang D, Chen Q, Schmidt AP, Anderson GM, Wang JM, Wooters J, et al. LL-37, the neutrophil granule- and epithelial cell-derived cathelicidin, utilizes formyl peptide receptor-like 1(FPRL1) as a receptor to chemoattract human peripheral blood neutrophils,

monocytes, and T cells. J Exp Med 2000;192:1069–74.

60. Niyonsaba F, Someya A, Hirata M, Ogawa H, Nagaoka I. Evaluation of the effects of peptide antibiotics human beta defensins-1/-2 and LL-37 on histamine release and prostaglandin D(2) production from mast cells. Eur J Immunol 2002;31:1066–75.
61. Niyonsaba F, Iwabuchi K, Matsuda H, Ogawa H, Nagaoka I. Epithelial cell derived human b-defensin-2 acts as a chemotaxin for mast cells through a pertussis toxin-sensitive and phospholipase C-dependent pathway. Internat Immunol 2002;14:421–6.
62. Biragyn A, Rufini, PA, Leifer CA, Klyushnenkova E, Shakhov A, Chertov O, et al. Toll-like receptor 4-dependent activation of dendritic cells by β-defensin 2. Science 2002;298: 1025–30.
63. Perregaux DG, Bhavsar K, Contillo L, Shi J, Gabel CA. Antimicrobial peptides initiate IL-1ß posttranslational processing: a novel role beyond innate immunity. J Immunol 2002;168:3024–32.
64. van Wetering S, Mannesse-Lazeroms SP, Dijkman JH, Hiemstra PS. Effect of neutrophil serine proteinases and defensins on lung epithelial cells: modulation of cytotoxicity and IL-8 production. J Leukoc Biol 1997;62:217–26.
65. Aarbiou J, Ertmann M, van Wetering S, van Noort P, Rook D, Rabe K, et al. Human neutrophil defensins induce lung epithelial cell proliferation in vitro. J Leukoc Biol 2002;72:167–74.
66. Li J, Post M, Volk R, Gao Y, Li M, Metais C, et al. PR39, a peptide regulator of angiogenesis. Nat Med 2000;6:49–55.
67. van Wetering S, van der Linden AC, van Sterkenburg MA, de Boer WI, Kuijpers AL, Schwalkwijk J, et al. Regulation of SLPI and elafin release from bronchial epithelial cells by neutrophil defensins. Am J Physiol Lung Cell Mol Physiol 2000;278:L51–8.
68. Ichinose M, Asai M, Imai K, Sawada M. Enhancement of phagocytosis by corticostatin I (CSI) in cultured mouse peritoneal macrophages. Immunopharmacology 1996;35:103–9.
69. Yang D, Chertov O, Bykovskaia SN, Chen Q, Buffo MJ, Shogan J, et al. Beta-defensins: linking innate and adaptive immunity through dendritic and T cell CCR6. Science 1999;286:525–8.
70. Le Y, Yang Y, Cui Y, Yazawa H, Gong W, Qui C, et al. Receptors for chemotactic formyl peptides as pharmacological targets. Int Immunopharmacol 2002;2:1–13.
71. van Wetering S, Mannesse-Lazeroms SPG, van Strekenburg MA, Hiemstra PS. Neutrophil defensins stimulate the release of cytokines by airway epithelial cells: modulation by dexamethasone. Inflamm Res 2002;51:8–15.
72. Travis SM, Conway BD, Zabner J, Smith JJ, Anderson NN, Singh PK, et al. Activity of abundant antimicrobials of the human airway. Am J Respir Cell Mol Biol 1999;20: 872–9.
73. Singh PK, Tack BF, McCray PB Jr., Welsh MJ. Synergistic and additive killing by antimicrobial factors found in human airway surface liquid. Am J Physiol Lung Cell Mol Physiol 2000;279:L799–805.
74. Ouellette AJ, Bevins, CL. Paneth cell defensins and innate immunity of the small bowel. Inflamm Bowel Dis 2001;7:43–50.
75. Valore EV, Park CH, Igreti SL, Ganz T. Antimicrobial components of vaginal fluid. Am J Obstet Gynecol 2002;187:561–568.
76. Canny G, Levy O, Furuta GT, Narravula-Alipati S, Sisson RB, Serhan CN, et al. Lipid mediator induced expression of bactericidal/permeability increasing protein (BPI) in human mucosal epithelia. PNAS 2002;99:3902–7.

77. Prohaszka Z, Nemet K, Csermely P, Hudecz F, Mezo G, Fust G. Defensins purified from human granulocytes bind C1q and activate the classical complement pathway like the transmembrane glycoprotein gp41 of HIV-1. Mol Immunol 1997;34:809–16.
78. Chertov P, Michiel DF, Xu L, Wang JM, Tani K, Murphy WJ, et al. Identification of defensin-1, defensin-2, and CAP37/azurocidin as T-cell chemoattractant proteins released from interleukin 8-stimulated neutrophils. J Bio Chem 1996;271:2935–40.
79. Tani K, Murphy WJ, Chertov O, Salcedo R, Koh CY, Utsunomiya I, et al. Defensins act as potent adjuvants that promote cellular and humoral immune responses in mice to a lymphoma idiotype and carrier antigens. Int Immunol 2000;12:691–700.
80. Ong PY, Ohtake T, Brandt C, Strickland I, Boguniewicz M, Ganz T, et al. Endogenous antimicrobial peptides and skin infections in atopic dermatitis. N Engl Med 2002;347: 1151–60.
81. Nizet V, Ohtake T, Lauth X, Trowbridge J, Rudisill J, Dorschner RA, et al. Innate antimicrobial peptide protects the skin from invasive bacterial infection. Nature 2001;414: 454–7.
82. Bals R, Weiner DJ, Wilson JM. The innate immune system in cystic fibrosis lung disease. J Clin Invest 1999;103:303–7.
83. Goldman MJ, Anderson GM, Stolzenberg ED, Kari UP, Zasloff M, Wilson JM. Human beta-defensin-1 is a salt-sensitive antibiotic in lung that is inactivated in cystic fibrosis. Cell 1997;88:553–60.
84. Bals R, Weiner DJ, Moscioni AD, Meegalla RL, Wilson JM. Augmentation of innate host defense by expression of a cathelicidin antimicrobial peptide. Infect Immun 1999;67: 6084–9.
85. Bals R, Weiner DJ, Meegalla RL, Wilson JM. Transfer of a cathelicidin peptide antibiotic gene restores bacterial killing in a cystic fibrosis xenograft model. J Clin Invest 1999;103: 1113–7.
86. Boucher RC. An overview of the pathogenesis of cystic fibrosis lung disease. Adv Drug Deliv Rev 2002;54:1359–71.
87. Pier GB. CFTR mutations and host susceptibility to *Pseudomonas aeruginosa* lung infection. Curr Opin Microbiol 2002;5:81–6.
88. Iwanaga S. The molecular basis of innate immunity in the horseshoe crab. Curr Opin Immunol 2002;14:87–95.
89. Scott MG, Davidson DJ, Gold MR, Bowdish D, Hancock RE. The human antimicrobial peptide LL-37 is a multifunctional modulator of innate immune responses. J Immunol 2002;169:3883–91.
90. Preston GA, Zarella CS, Pendergraft WF 3rd, Rudolph EH, Yang JJ, Sekura SB, et al. Novel effects of neutrophil-derived proteinase 3 and elastase on the vascular endothelium involve in vivo cleavage of NF-kappaB and proapoptotic changes in JNK, ERK, and p38 MAPK signaling pathways. J Am Soc Nephrol 2002;13:2840–9.
91. Linzmeier R, Ho CH, Hoang BV, Ganz T. A 450-kb contig of defensin genes on human chromosome 8p23. Gene 1999;233:205–11.
92. Mars WM, Patmasiriwat P, Maity T, Huff V, Weil MM, Saunders GF. Inheritance of unequal numbers of the genes encoding the human neutrophil defensins HP-1 and HP-3. J Biol Chem 1995;270:30371–6.
93. Bevins CL, Jones DE, Dutra A, Schaffzin J, Muenke M. Human enteric defensin genes: chromosomal map position and a model for possible evolutionary relationships. Genomics 1996;31:95–106.

94. Ouellette AJ, Hsieh MM, Nosek MT, Cano-gauci DF, Huttner KM, Buick RN, et al. Mouse Paneth cell defensins: primary structures and antibacterial activities of numerous cryptdin isoforms. Infect Immun 1994;62:5040–7.
95. Matsushita I, Hasegawa K, Nakata K, Yasuda K, Tokunaga K, Keicho N. Genetic variants of human β-defensin-1 and chronic obstructive pulmonary disease. Biochem Biophys Res Commun 2001;291:17–22.
96. Salzman NH, Ghosh D, Huttner KM, Paterson Y, Bevins CL. Protection against enteric salmonellosis in transgenic mice expressing a human intestinal defensin. Nature 2003;422;522–6.

Natural Immunity
Edited by L. Bertók and D.A. Chow
© 2005 Elsevier B.V. All rights reserved

Endogenous Cytoprotective Mechanisms

HECTOR R. WONG

Associate Professor of Pediatrics, Director, Division of Critical Care Medicine, Cincinnati Children's Hospital Medical Center, Children's Hospital Research Foundation, 3333 Burnet Avenue, Cincinnati, OH 45229-3039, USA

ABSTRACT

A number of fundamental mechanisms have evolved to protect the mammalian host against various forms of injury and noxious stimuli. Since these mechanisms are harnessed upon encountering potentially cytotoxic conditions, and are distinct from classical immune responses, they are referred to as endogenous cytoprotective mechanisms. Induction of haem-oxygenase and induction of the heat shock response confer protection against a broad array of cytotoxic stimuli. Activation of anti-oxidant pathways is critical to survival in an aerobic environment, which is both permissive to life as we know it, but at the same time carries the ever present risk of generating toxic oxygen free radicals and their derivatives. Hypoxia inducible factor is a key transcription factor that directs the expression of genes necessary for adaptation to hypoxia and/or ischemia. Finally, nitric oxide is a ubiquitous molecule that appears to impact an ever increasing number of biological, physiological, pathophysiological processes. In keeping with this complexity, nitric oxide appears to have important cytoprotective properties that are dependent on both the context in which it is produced and the amount that is produced.

1. INTRODUCTION

Apart from technological, cultural, and social factors, the human species has thus far managed to survive because of fundamental endogenous cytoprotective mechanisms that allow for adaptation and survival in adverse conditions. This chapter will focus on some selected, major endogenous cytoprotective mechanisms. Realizing that other mechanisms could be included, this chapter will focus on haem oxygenase, anti-oxidant systems, the heat shock response, hypoxia inducible factor, and nitric oxide.

2. HAEM OXYGENASE

Haem oxygenase (HO) is responsible for catalyzing the first and rate-limiting step in the degradation of haem to bilirubin [1,2]. It exists as three isoforms: HO-1, -2, and -3. HO-1 is a 32 kDa protein that is highly inducible by a variety of cellular stressors and stimuli, including haem, nitric oxide, cytokines, heavy metals, hyperoxia, hypoxia, endotoxin, and heat shock [3–5]. HO-1 activity is present in virtually all organs and is thought to primarily account for the cytoprotective properties of HO. HO-2 is a 36 kDa protein that is constitutively active and localized primarily to the brain and testes. HO-3 is a recently cloned isoform of 33 kDa and the exact role of this isoform remains to be defined.

The observation that HO-1 is induced by a variety of potentially cytotoxic stimuli, its relative high level of conservation throughout evolution, and its wide tissue distribution have logically led to numerous investigations to determine if HO-1 can serve a cytoprotective role. Numerous *in vitro* and *in vivo* studies have clearly established the cytoprotective properties of HO-1. The more definitive *in vitro* studies ascribing a cytoprotective role for HO-1 have involved gene transfection/transfer studies in which HO-1 was genetically overexpressed in cultured cells. For example, overexpression of HO-1 in hamster fibroblasts [6], rat foetal lung cells [7], or a human respiratory epithelial cell line [8] conferred protection against oxygen toxicity. In cultured rabbit coronary endothelial cells, overexpression of HO-1 conferred protection against haem and haemoglobin toxicity [9]. Finally, in cultured murine fibroblasts, regulated overexpression of HO-1 conferred protection against tumour necrosis factor-α-mediated apoptosis [10].

Experiments in animal models have confirmed that the *in vitro* cytoprotective properties of HO-1 are also operative *in vivo*. For example, induction of HO-1 by intravenous haemoglobin, protected rats against the lethal effects of endotoxemia, as well as ameliorating endotoxin-mediated hypotension, renal dysfunction, hepatic dysfunction, and inflammation [11,12]. Co-administration of tin protoporphyrin, a competitive inhibitor of HO, substantially reduced these protective effects, thus providing further evidence that HO-1 can play an important protective role against endotoxemia. Increased expression of HO-1 in the bronchiolar epithelium, via an adenovirus vector, conferred *in vivo* protection against hyperoxic lung injury in rats [13]. Finally, increased expression of HO-1 was demonstrated to enhance cardiac xenograft (mouse to rat) survival in a model of heart transplantation [14] and to induce tolerance to cardiac ischemia in a murine model [15].

Further evidence of the cytoprotective properties of HO-1 comes from gene knockout studies. HO-1 null mice generally do not survive to term. When HO-1 null mice do survive to term, they die within one year of age, and have growth retardation, anaemia, iron deposition in the kidneys and liver, and evidence of chronic inflammation in many organs [16]. Interestingly, complete HO-1 deficiency was recently described in a child that exhibited many of the same abnormalities seen in HO-1 null mice [17]. In other investigations HO-1 null mice have been demonstrated to be more susceptible to: 1) renovascular-related hypertension, renal failure, and cardiac hypertrophy [18], 2) endotoxin-mediated lethality [19], and 3) right ventricular dilation and infarction secondary to chronic hypoxia [20]. Collectively, the *in vitro*, *in vivo*, and gene deletion studies outlined above provide compelling evidence regarding the broad cytoprotective role of HO-1. What remains relatively elusive, however, is the mechanism(s) by which HO-1 confers this broad level of protection.

The byproducts of HO enzymatic activity include carbon monoxide (CO), bilirubin, and ferritin [3–5]. Each of these byproducts has been postulated to play a role in cytoprotection (e.g., ferritin can protect cells during oxidant stress and bilirubin is well known as a potent antioxidant) and it is likely that the three byproducts synergize in some way to confer cytoprotection. The most recent work in the field, however, points to direct CO-related cell signalling as the key component of HO-1-dependent cytoprotection [3,21,22]. Apart from its gaseous nature, CO also shares a variety of properties with nitric oxide, including neurotransmission, regulation of vascular tone, and activation of soluble guanylate cyclase. In addition, CO appears to have potent anti-

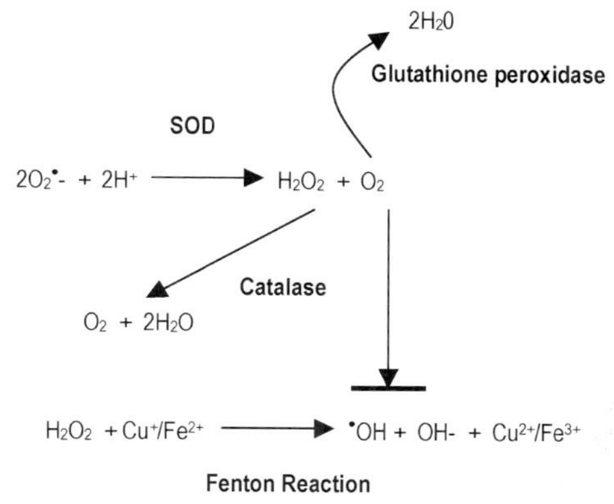

Figure 1. Schematic depicting the activities of superoxide dismutase (SOD), catalase, and glutathione peroxidase. SOD converts two molecules of superoxide anion to form hydrogen peroxide and water. The hydrogen peroxide produced from this reaction can be further reduced by either catalase or glutathione peroxidase. Catalase converts two molecules of hydrogen peroxide to oxygen and water. Glutathione peroxidase converts hydrogen peroxide to two molecules of water using glutathione as a substrate. In addition, the reduction of hydrogen peroxide by catalase and glutathione peroxidase decreases the participation of hydrogen peroxide in the Fenton reaction, which can lead to the formation of hydroxyl radicals.

inflammatory (via the MAP kinase pathway), anti-apoptotic, and antioxidant properties [23–30]. The rapidly evolving data strongly suggest that HO-1-derived CO is the key mechanism by which HO-1 confers cytoprotection, and further work in this area holds tremendous potential for therapeutic strategies involving HO-1 and/or CO.

3. ANTIOXIDANT SYSTEMS

Normal biological processes that make use of oxygen inevitably lead to the production of reactive oxygen species (ROS), including hydrogen peroxide, superoxide, hydroxyl radicals, nitric oxide, and peroxynitrite. While a limited amount of ROS production can serve important cell signalling and anti-microbial functions [31], when produced in larger amounts, ROS can cause oxidant stress to the host leading to cellular and tissue injury. The mechanisms by which oxidant stress causes cellular and tissue injury include damage to genomic and mitochondrial DNA, lipid peroxidation, and protein modification [32–34]. Cell death secondary to oxidant stress can be from either necrosis or apoptosis [34]. In keeping with many biological processes that have counter-acting or counter-regulatory mechanisms, all aerobic organisms have well-developed antioxidant systems to protect cells and tissues against high levels of ROS production.

Superoxide dismutases (SOD) exist in several forms including Mn-SOD, Cu/Zn-SOD, and Fe-SOD [35]. In addition, SOD exists within the cytoplasmic and mitochondrial cellular compartments and in the extracellular compartment. SOD efficiently (diffusion limited) converts two superoxide molecules to hydrogen peroxide and oxygen (Fig. 1). The importance of SOD in host defence against oxidant stress is illustrated by gene knock-out studies and by numerous studies demonstrating that genetic overexpression of SOD confers protection against oxidant stress [36–39]. In addition, mutations of human SOD can cause amyotrophic lateral sclerosis [40–41].

Catalases convert hydrogen peroxide to water and oxygen (Fig. 1) [42,43]. Thus, they can operate in conjunction with SOD to defend against oxidant stress (i.e., the hydrogen peroxide formed by SOD catalysis can be converted by catalases). In addition, by lowering intracellular levels of hydrogen peroxide, catalase can prevent formation of hydroxyl radicals that could occur via the Fenton reaction (Fig. 1). Glutathione (GSH) peroxidases consist of at least four isoforms in mammals and are widely distributed [43]. Similar to catalase, all members of the GSH peroxidases can convert hydrogen peroxide to water by using glutathione as a substrate.

Haemoglobin is a known scavenger of nitric oxide in mammalian systems and given the abundance of haemoglobin in all mammals, this mechanism is likely to be a central component for mammalian detoxification of nitric oxide [44]. Gardner et al., however, have recently discovered enzymatic systems within both aerobic and anaerobic bacteria that can efficiently detoxify/scavenge nitric oxide [45–49]. It is anticipated that homologous nitric oxide reducing systems will be described in mammalian cells in the near future [50].

Another major antioxidant mechanism in mammals is the thioredoxin system, which is composed of the oxidoreductase enzymes thioredoxin and thioredoxin reductase [51]. In conjunction with NADPH, thioredoxin reductase leads to the reduction of the active disulfide site of thioredoxin. Thioredoxin, in turn, can broadly function as a protein disulfide reductant. Another mechanism by which the thioredoxin system serves as an antioxidant is by the regeneration of various low molecular weight antioxidants such as vitamin E, vitamin C, selenium-related compounds, lipoic acid, and ubiquinones [51].

In summary, potent antioxidant systems have evolved to counter balance the normal production of ROS that occurs during many cellular processes, as well as the excessive amounts of ROS that can occur during pathological states. Despite this elegant counter-regulatory system, ROS can lead to cellular injury when either a component of the antioxidant system is defective, or when the high level production of ROS overwhelms an otherwise intact antioxidant system. Recognition of this critical balance and the mechanisms involved in defending against ROS holds tremendous potential for the design of therapeutic strategies directed toward restoring the balance between ROS production and endogenous antioxidant systems.

4. THE HEAT SHOCK RESPONSE

The heat shock response is another fundamental endogenous cytoprotective mechanism found in virtually all organisms [52–55]. Originally described in *Drosophila* [56], it is now known to occur throughout the animal kingdom from prokaryotes through humans. The heat shock response is defined by the rapid expression of a class of proteins known as heat shock proteins, when a cell, tissue, or intact organism is exposed to elevated temperatures. In addition, heat shock proteins can be induced by a wide variety of non-thermal stressors and pharmacological agents (Table I).

One functional significance of the heat shock response, whether induced by thermal or non-thermal stress, is that it confers protection against subsequent and otherwise lethal hyperthermia; a phenomenon referred to as thermotolerance [57,58]. Perhaps more interesting from a clinical standpoint is the phenomenon of cross-tolerance, whereby induction of the heat shock response confers protection against non-thermal cytotoxic stimuli. For example, *in vitro* experiments have demonstrated that induction of the heat shock response protects endothelial cells against endotoxin-mediated apoptosis [59]. Other examples include heat shock response-dependent protection against nitric oxide [60], peroxynitrite [61], and hydrogen peroxide [62]. *In vivo*, induction of the heat shock response protects animals against endotoxemia/sepsis [63,64], acute

Table I Non-thermal inducers of the heat shock response.

Inducer	Comments
Sodium Arsenite	Used extensively *in vitro* and *in vivo*
Prostaglandin-A_1	Other prostaglandins also active
Dexamethasone	Variable effect
Bimoclomol	Hydroxylamine derivative, non-toxic
Herbimycin A	Tyrosine kinase inhibitor
Geldanamycin	Tyrosine kinase inhibitor and HSP 90 inhibitor
Aspirin	Lowers temperature threshold for HSP induction
Non-steroidal antiinflammatory drugs	Lowers temperature threshold for HSP induction
Serine Protease Inhibitors	Concomitant inhibition of NF-κB.
Pyrrolidine Dithiocarbamate	Antioxidant; inhibitor of NF-κB
Diethyldithiocarbamate	Similar to PDTC
Glutamine	May be specific for intestinal epithelium
Heavy Metal Ions	Cadmium, Zinc
Phosphatase Inhibitors	Tyrosine and Ser/Thr phosphatases
Curcumin	Major constituent of turmeric; antiinflammatory
Geranylgeranlyacetone	Anti-ulcer drug

lung injury [65], and ischemia-reperfusion injury [66].

The mechanisms by which the heat shock response confers such broad cytoprotection are not fully understood. Several lines of evidence, however, indicate that heat shock protein 70 (HSP70) plays a central role in cytoprotection. For example, HSP70 is the most highly induced heat shock protein in cells and tissues undergoing the heat shock response [52–55], and is known to be induced in patients with a variety of critical illnesses or injuries [67,68]. Microinjection of anti-HSP70 antibody into cells impairs their ability to achieve thermotolerance [69]. Increased expression of HSP70 by gene transfer/transfection has been demonstrated to confer protection against *in vitro* toxicity secondary to lethal hyperthermia [70], endotoxin [59], nitric oxide [60], and hyperoxia [71], and *in vivo* ischemia-reperfusion injury [72–74]. Mice deficient in heat shock factor-1, the transcription factor responsible for high level expression of HSP70, have a drastically reduced ability to express HSP70, and cells from these animals can not be made thermotolerant and are more susceptible to oxidant stress [75–77]. In addition, heat shock factor-1 deficient mice demonstrate an increase in mortality when challenged with systemic endotoxin [76]. Collectively, these data strongly suggest that HSP70 is central to the cytoprotective properties of the heat shock response. The mechanisms by which HSP70 confers protection are not fully understood, but most likely relate to the ability of HSP70, and other heat shock proteins, to serve as molecular chaperones by binding, re-folding, transporting, and stabilizing damaged intracellular proteins [52–55].

Another potential mechanism by which the heat shock response may confer cytoprotection is by modulating inflammatory responses. The heat shock response has been demonstrated to inhibit a number of genes related to inflammation, including tumour necrosis factor-α, interleukin-1β, inducible nitric oxide synthase, interleukin-8, RANTES, C3, macrophage chemotactic protein-1, and intracellular adhesion molecule-1 [78–85]. In addition, it has been postulated that the inhibitory effects of the heat shock response are relatively selective for inflammation-associated genes [86]. The mechanisms by which the heat shock response inhibits proinflammatory gene expression involves inhibition of NF-κB. Several *in vitro* and *in vivo* studies have demonstrated that induction of the heat shock response inhibits activation of NF-κB, a pluripotent transcription factor that regulates the expression of many genes associated with inflammation [87–91]. The latest work in the area has identified IκB kinase (IKK) as the most upstream target through

Table II Genes regulated by HIF-1 (adapted from Ref. [97]).

Adrenomedullin	Aldolase A and C
Endothelin-1	Enolase 1
Erythropoietin	Glucose transporter 1 and 3
Heme oxygenase-1	Glyceraldehyde phosphate dehydrogenase
Hexokinase 1 and 2	Insulin-like growth factor-II
Lactate dehydrogenase A	Insulin-like growth factor binding protein 1 and 3
Nitric oxide synthase 2	p21
P35srj	Phosphofructokinase L
Phosphoglycerate kinase 1	Pyruvate kinase M
Transferrin	Transferrin receptor
Vascular endothelial growth factor	Vascular endothelial growth factor receptor

which the heat shock response modulates NF-κB activity. IKK is the rate limiting step in the activation of NF-κB in that it phosphorylates the endogenous NF-κB inhibitor, IκBα. Phosphorylation of IκBα leads to its rapid degradation by a ubiquitin/proteasome-dependent mechanism, thus releasing NF-κB to enter the nucleus. Induction of the heat shock response inhibits activation of IKK, in part by an intracellular phosphatase-dependent mechanism [85,92–94]. Inhibition of IKK subsequently inhibits phosphorylation and degradation of IκBα [95], thus keeping NF-κB in an inactive state. Finally, the heat shock response also leads to *de novo* expression of IκBα, thus providing another potential mechanism for inhibiting NF-κB activity [81,89,96].

In summary, the heat shock response serves a very broad cytoprotective role in virtually all organisms. HSP70 and heat shock factor-1 play key roles in cytoprotection and it would appear that anti-inflammatory effects of the heat shock response also play a prominent role in cytoprotection. The challenge remains to devise an effective and safe method (i.e., gene therapy or pharmacology) for inducing the heat shock response as a therapeutic strategy in the clinical setting.

5. HYPOXIA INDUCIBLE FACTOR

There are several proteins that belong to the hypoxia inducible factor (HIF) family. In addition, HIF is thought to function in both cytoprotection and the pathophysiology of several diseases [97,98]. This section will focus specifically on HIF-1 and its role in cytoprotection. HIF-1 is a heterodimeric transcription factor containing the subunits HIF-1α and HIF-1β [97,98]. In the context of this chapter, HIF-1 can be thought of as a major regulator of genes necessary for adaptation to hypoxia. The list of genes thought to be dependent on HIF-1 include genes for vascularization [99], energy metabolism [100], vascular tone [101], and erythropoiesis [102] (Table II). In addition, haem oxygenase-1 expression is, in part, dependent on HIF-1 activity [103].

The transcriptional activity of HIF-1 is primarily dependent on the intracellular level of the HIF-1α subunit, which is in turn highly dependent on the rate of HIF-1α protein degradation [97,98]. Under conditions of normal oxygen tension, the HIF-1α protein subunit undergoes ubiquitination and subsequent degradation by proteasome activity, thereby preventing formation of the HIF-1α/HIF-1β heterodimer [104,105]. In response to hypoxia, the HIF-1α protein subunit is no longer degraded, thereby increasing intracellular levels of HIF-1α protein and allowing formation of the HIF-1α/HIF-1β heterodimer, which is then transcriptionally active and allows for the expression of HIF-1-dependent genes. The exact mechanism by which cells "sense" hypoxia and curtail the degradation of the HIF-1α protein subunit is not fully understood, but likely involves inhibition of ubiquitination and is related to the von Hipple-Lindau tumour suppressor protein [97,106,107].

The cytoprotective properties of HIF-1 relate primarily to the HIF-1-dependent genes that allow for adaptation to hypoxia. For example, induction of the HIF-1-dependent gene, erythropoietin, leads to increased production of red blood cells, thereby increasing the oxygen carrying capacity of blood in the setting of hypoxia. This type of cytoprotective response is particularly important, for example, in children with cyanotic heart disease. Another example involves the HIF-1-dependent gene, vascular endothelial growth factor (VEGF), which is a critical growth factor for the development of blood vessels. In tissues subjected to ischemia, such as the myocardium, expression of VEGF promotes the development of neovascularization as a potential means of increasing blood flow to the ischemic tissue [108]. Yet another role for HIF-1 involves HIF-1-dependent expression of inducible nitric oxide synthase (see below) and ischemic preconditioning of the myocardium [109,110].

The biological importance of HIF-1 has been further established in transgenic mice having targeted deletions of the HIF-1α or HIF-1β subunit. Mice homozygous for deletion of either subunit (HIF-1α -/- or HIF-1β -/-) die during embryogenesis secondary to insufficient vascular development [100,111]. In contrast, heterozygote animals (HIF-1α +/-) seem to develop normally compared to wild-type animals. When exposed to hypoxia, however, heterozygote animals have an impairment in the classical responses and adaptations to hypoxia (e.g., blunted increase of haematocrit, blunted increase of right ventricular mass [112]).

In summary, HIF-1-dependent gene expression warrants classification as an endogenous cytoprotective mechanism by allowing for adaptation to cellular hypoxia, whether it be secondary to low oxygen tension *per se* or due to decreased blood flow (ischemia). While some of the aforementioned cytoprotective mechanisms (e.g., the heat shock response) allow for more immediate forms of cytoprotection, the cytoprotective responses and adaptations associated with HIF-1 activation are comparatively slower to develop. In addition, some of the responses induced by HIF-1 activation can be maladaptive/pathologic depending on duration of activation (e.g., the development of pulmonary hypertension in the setting of chronic hypoxia). Thus a greater understanding of HIF-1 regulation and activity will be necessary in order to manipulate HIF-1 activity as a therapeutic option. These options will include, depending on the therapeutic goals and clinical scenario, either augmenting HIF-1 activity (e.g., in ischemic tissues as a means of increasing vascularity) or blunting HIF-1 activity (e.g., as a means of preventing pulmonary hypertension in the setting of chronic hypoxia).

6. NITRIC OXIDE

Nitric oxide (NO) is produced by the enzyme nitric oxide synthase (NOS), which converts L-arginine to citrulline and NO [113]. Three known isoforms of NOS exist: endothelial NOS (eNOS), neuronal NOS (nNOS) and inducible NOS (iNOS). The terms "eNOS" and "nNOS" reflect the original tissues from which these isoforms were cloned; however, both isoforms are widely distributed beyond the endothelium and central nervous system, respectively. Generally speaking, both eNOS and nNOS are constitutively active, dependent on intracellular calcium for activity, and produce relatively small amounts of NO. iNOS derives its name from the observation that it requires *de novo* gene expression for maximal activity. In addition, iNOS is calcium independent and is responsible for high level production of NO following proinflammatory and other forms of stimuli. Although historically these isoforms have been classified as being "constitutive" and "inducible," it is now recognized that the eNOS and nNOS genes can undergo regulation (i.e., induction) under certain conditions, and that iNOS can also be constitutively active [113,114]. Finally, the human genes for the NOS isoforms are now categorized based on the order in which they were cloned; thus human nNOS, iNOS, and eNOS are termed NOS1, NOS2, and NOS3, respectively [115].

One of the primary mechanisms by which NO affects cellular function is through the activation of soluble guanylate cyclase leading to increased intracellular levels of cGMP. Since NO is a free radical gas, other important NO mechanisms that affect cellular function include reactions with metal complexes, nitrosation, nitration, and oxidation reactions [116]. The degree to which any one of these mechanisms is operative in a given biological process is, in turn, highly dependent on the amount of NO produced and the biological milieu.

An abundance of quality data indicate that NO can function as a cytoprotective molecule. Assigning biological significance to these data, however, is difficult given that the literature suggests that a very broad spectrum of biological processes are affected by NO and that equally abundant and quality data indicate that NO can be either directly cytotoxic or mediate cytotoxic/pathologic processes. Thus, NO appears to have dual properties as both a cytoprotective and a cytotoxic molecule. Unscrambling this controversy is not feasible within the context of this chapter. Examples of NO-dependent cytoprotection will be provided below, but the reader is reminded that for virtually each example of cytoprotection, there is an example of NO functioning in an opposite manner (i.e., cytotoxicity).

Apoptosis, or programmed cell death, can be modulated by NO and is perhaps the most prominent and well studied example of NO-mediated cytoprotection [117,118]. Various examples exist demonstrating that NO can either inhibit apoptosis or promote apoptosis. The anti-apoptotic effects of NO have been demonstrated in various cultured cells such as human B lymphocytes [119], endothelial cells [120], splenocytes [121], and hepatocytes [122,123], and in whole animal models [124,125]. In addition, NO has been demonstrated to prevent apoptosis secondary to diverse signals such as tumour necrosis factor, growth factor withdrawal, and Fas [117,118]. The mechanisms by which NO inhibits apoptosis are also quite diverse. For example, NO can induce expression of the aforementioned cytoprotective proteins, haem oxygenase-1 and heat shock protein 70, and thereby prevent apoptosis [122,126]. Since cGMP can also prevent apoptosis, NO-mediated activation of cGMP is another mechanism by which NO can prevent apoptosis, possibly by lowering intracellular calcium levels [121]. NO has also been shown to inhibit caspase activity [123] and inhibit cytochrome C release [127], two key events in the pro-apoptotic pathway. Finally, NO has been demonstrated to maintain or preserve intracellular levels of Bcl-2, a key anti-apoptotic protein [121,127].

NO can also be protective to whole organs. Examples include the liver [128], kidney [129], brain [130], heart [131], and intestine [132]. The mechanisms by which NO protects these organs involve many of the known physiologic and biologic functions of NO, such as vascular dilation, prevention of platelet and neutrophil adherence, antioxidant effects by reactions with reactive oxygen species, anti-apoptotic effects, and induction of other cytoprotective mechanisms (e.g., heat shock protein 70 and haem oxygenase-1). Thus, NO can protect organs during various forms of injury or stress by maintaining blood flow, preventing thrombosis, limiting inflammation, decreasing oxidant stress, and/or preventing apoptosis [128–132]. Again, the degree to which any one of these mechanisms is operative, or predominant, is dependent on the type of injury/stress, the amount of NO produced, and the biological context in which the NO is produced.

The cytoprotective properties of NO are indisputable and many biologically plausible mechanisms account for the observed cytoprotective effects. The availability of commonly used NO-donors (e.g., sodium nitroprusside and nitroglycerin) and novel NO-donors allows for the direct application of these principles in the clinical setting as a means of affording organ and tissue protection during a variety of disease states [125,131]. Enthusiasm for this approach must be tempered, however, by the known dual nature of NO as both a cytoprotective and cytotoxic molecule.

7. CONCLUSION

This chapter has attempted to describe some of the more powerful and ubiquitous endogenous mechanisms that exist to counter-act the multitude of cytotoxic stimuli that can adversely affect the human host. Certainly, other mechanisms exist that have not been described in this particular chapter. The next formidable challenge is to devise therapeutic strategies (either through pharmacology or gene therapy) that will allow for the safe and efficacious manipulation of these endogenous mechanisms of cytoprotection.

REFERENCES

1. Tenhunen R, Marver HS, Schmid R. The enzymatic conversion of heme to bilirubin by microsomal heme oxygenase. Proc Natl Acad Sci USA 1968;61:748–55.
2. Tenhunen R, Marver HS, Schmid R. Microsomal heme oxygenase. Characterization of the enzyme. J Biol Chem 1969;244:6388–94.
3. Ryter SW, Otterbein LE, Morse D, Choi AM. Heme oxygenase/carbon monoxide signaling pathways: regulation and functional significance. Mol Cell Biochem 2002 May-Jun;234–235(1-2):249–63.
4. Morse D, Choi AM. Heme Oxygenase-1. The "emerging molecule" has arrived. Am J Respir Cell Mol Biol 2002;27:8–16.
5. Otterbein LE, Choi AM. Heme oxygenase: colors of defense against cellular stress. Am J Physiol Lung Cell Mol Physiol 2000 Dec;279(6):L1029–37. Review.
6. Dennery PA, Sridhar KJ, Lee CS, Wong HE, Shokoohi V, Rodgers PA, Spitz DR. Heme oxygenase-mediated resistance to oxygen toxicity in hamster fibroblasts. J Biol Chem 1997 Jun 6;272(23):12937–42.
7. Suttner DM, Sridhar K, Lee CS, Tomura T, Hansen TN, Dennery PA. Protective effects of transient HO-1 overexpression on susceptibility to oxygen toxicity in lung cells. Am J Physiol 1999 Mar;276(3 Pt 1):L443–51.
8. Lee PJ, Alam J, Wiegand GW, Choi AMK. Overexpression of heme-oxygenase-1 in human pulmonary epithelial cells results in cell growth arrest and increased resistance to hyperoxia. Proc Natl Acad Sci USA 1996;93:10393–8.
9. Abraham NG, Lavrovsky Y, Schwartzman ML, Stoltz RA, Levere RD, Gerritsen ME, Shibahara S, Kappas A. Transfection of the human heme oxygenase gene into rabbit coronary microvessel endothelial cells: protective effect against heme and hemoglobin toxicity. Proc Natl Acad Sci USA 1995;92:6798–801.
10. Petrache I, Otterbein LE, Alam J, Wiegane GW, Choi AM. Heme oxygenase-1 inhibits TNF-α-induced apoptosis in cultured fibroblasts. Am J Physiol Lung Cell Mol Physiol 2000 Feb;278(2):L312–9.
11. Otterbein L, Sylvester S, Choi AMK. Hemoglobin provides protection against lethal

endotoxemia in rats: the role of heme oxygenase-1. Am J Respir Cell Mol Biol 1995;13: 595–601.
12. Otterbein L, Chin BY, Otterbein SL, Lowe VC, Fessler HE, Choi AM. Mechanism of hemoglobin-induced protection against endotoxemia in rats: a ferritin-independent pathway. Am J Physiol 1997 Feb;272(2 Pt 1):L268–75
13. Otterbein LE, Kolls JK, Mantell LL, Cook JL, Alam J, Choi AMK. Exogenous administration of heme oxygenase-1 by gene transfer provides protection against hyperoxia-induced injury. J Clin Invest 1999;103:1047–54.
14. Soares MP, Lin Y, Anrather J, Csizmadia E, Takigami K, Sato K, Grey ST, Colvin RB, Choi AM, Poss KD, Bach FH. Expression of heme oxygenase-1 can determine cardiac xenograft survival. Nat Med 1998;4:1073–7.
15. Yet SF, Tian R, Layne MD, Wang ZY, Maemura K, Solovyeva M, Ith B, Melo LG, Zhang L, Ingwall JS, Dzau VJ, Lee ME, Perrella MA. Cardiac-specific expression of heme oxygenase-1 protects against ischemia and reperfusion injury in transgenic mice. Circ Res 2001;89:168–73.
16. Poss KD, Tonegawa S. Heme oxygenase 1 is required for mammalian iron reutilization. Proc Natl Acad Sci USA 1997;94:10910–24.
17. Yachie A, Niida Y, Wada T, Igarashi N, Kaneda H. Oxidative stress causes enhanced endothelial cell injury in human heme oxygenase-1 deficiency. J Clin Invest 1999;103: 129–35.
18. Wiesel P, Patel AP, Carvajal IM, Wang ZY, Pellacani A, Maemura K, DiFonzo N, Rennke HG, Layne MD, Yet SF, Lee ME, Perrella MA. Exacerbation of chronic renovascular hypertension and acute renal failure in heme oxygenase-1-deficient mice. Circ Res 2001;88:1088–94.
19. Wiesel P, Patel AP, DiFonzo N, Marria PB, Sim CU, Pellacani A, Maemura K, LeBlanc BW, Marino K, Doerschuk CM, Yet SF, Lee ME, Perrella MA. Endotoxin-induced mortality is related to increased oxidative stress and end-organ dysfunction, not refractory hypotension, in heme oxygenase-1-deficient mice. Circulation 2000;102:3015–22.
20. Yet SF, Perrella MA, Layne MD, Hsieh CM, Maemura K, Kobzik L, Wiesel P, Christou H, Kourembanas S, Lee ME. Hypoxia induces severe right ventricular dilatation and infarction in heme oxygenase-1 null mice. J Clin Invest 1999;103:23–9.
21. Choi AM, Otterbein LE. Emerging role of carbon monoxide in physiologic and pathophysiologic states. Antioxid Redox Signal 2002;4:227–8.
22. Morse D, Sethi J, Choi AM. Carbon monoxide-dependent signaling. Crit Care Med 2001;30:S12–7.
23. Sethi JM, Otterbein LE, Choi AM. Differential modulation by exogenous carbon monoxide of TNF-alpha stimulated mitogen-activated protein kinases in rat pulmonary artery endothelial cells. Antioxid Redox Signal 2002;4:241–8.
24. Chapman JT, Otterbein LE, Elias JA, Choi AM. Carbon monoxide attenuates aeroallergen-induced inflammation in mice. Am J Physiol Lung Cell Mol Physiol 2001 Jul;281(1): L209–16.
25. Sato K, Balla J, Otterbein L, Smith RN, Brouard S, Lin Y, Csizmadia E, Sevigny J, Robson SC, Vercellotti G, Choi AM, Bach FH, Soares MP. Carbon monoxide generated by heme oxygenase-1 suppresses the rejection of mouse-to-rat cardiac transplants. J Immunol 2001;166:4185–94.
26. Otterbein LE, Bach FH, Alam J, Soares M, Tao Lu H, Wysk M, Davis RJ, Flavell RA, Choi AM. Carbon monoxide has anti-inflammatory effects involving the mitogen-activated

protein kinase pathway. Nat Med 2000;6:422–8.
27. Otterbein LE, Mantell LL, Choi AM. Carbon monoxide provides protection against hyperoxic lung injury. Am J Physiol 1999 Apr;276(4 Pt 1):L688–94.
28. Ke B, Buelow R, Shen XD, Melinek J, Amersi F, Gao F, Ritter T, Volk HD, Busuttil RW, Kupiec-Weglinski JW. Heme oxygenase 1 gene transfer prevents CD95/Fas ligand-mediated apoptosis and improves liver allograft survival via carbon monoxide signaling pathway. Hum Gene Ther 2002;13:1189–99.
29. Liu X, Chapman GB, Peyton KJ, Schafer AI, Durante W. Carbon monoxide inhibits apoptosis in vascular smooth muscle cells. Cardiovasc Res 2002;55:396–405.
30. Soares MP, Usheva A, Brouard S, Berberat PO, Gunther L, Tobiasch E, Bach FH. Modulation of endothelial cell apoptosis by heme oxygenase-1-derived carbon monoxide. Antioxid Redox Signal 2002;4:321–9.
31. Kamata H, Hirata H. Redox regulation of cellular signaling. Cell Signal 1999;11:1–14.
32. Yiä-Herttuala S. Oxidized LDL and atherogenesis. Ann NY Acad Sci 2000;899:191–208.
33. Marnett LJ. Oxyradicals and DNA damage. Carcinogenesis 2000;21:361–70.
34. Stadtman ER, Berlett BS. Reactive oxygen-mediated protein oxidation in aging and disease. Drug Metab Rev 1998;30:225–43.
35. McCord JM. Superoxide dismutase in aging and disease: an overview. Methods Enzymol 2002;349:331–41.
36. Tsan MF, White JE, Caska B, Epstein CJ, Lee CY. Susceptibility of heterozygous MnSOD gene-knockout mice to oxygen toxicity. Am J Respir Cell Mol Biol 1998;19:114–20.
37. Tsan MF. Superoxide dismutase and pulmonary oxygen toxicity: lessons from transgenic and knockout mice (Review). Int J Mol Med 2001;7:13–9.
38. Wispe JR, Warner BB, Clark JC, Dey CR, Neuman J, Glasser SW, Crapo JD, Chang LY, Whitsett JA. Human Mn-superoxide dismutase in pulmonary epithelial cells of transgenic mice confers protection from oxygen injury. J Biol Chem 1992;267:23937–41.
39. White CW, Avraham KB, Shanley PF, Groner Y. Transgenic mice with expression of elevated levels of copper-zinc superoxide dismutase in the lungs are resistant to pulmonary oxygen toxicity. J Clin Invest 1991;87:2162–8.
40. Garcia-Redondo A, Bustos F, Juan Y Seva B, Del Hoyo P, Jimenez S, Campos Y, Martin MA, Rubio JC, Canadillas F, Arenas J, Esteban J. Molecular analysis of the superoxide dismutase 1 gene in Spanish patients with sporadic or familial amyotrophic lateral sclerosis. Muscle Nerve 2002;26:274–8.
41. Hosler BA, Nicholson GA, Sapp PC, Chin W, Orrell RW, de Belleroche JS, Esteban J, Hayward LJ, Mckenna-Yasek D, Yeung L, Cherryson AK, Dench JE, Wilton SD, Laing NG, Horvitz RH, Brown RH Jr. Three novel mutations and two variants in the gene for Cu/Zn superoxide dismutase in familial amyotrophic lateral sclerosis. Neuromuscul Disord 1996;6:361–6.
42. Bai J, Cederbaum AI. Mitochondrial catalase and oxidative injury. Biol Signals Recept 2001;10:189–99.
43. Mates JM, Perez-Gomez C, Nunez de Castro I. Antioxidant enzymes and human diseases. Clin Biochem 1999;32:595–603.
44. Joshi MS, Ferguson TB Jr, Han TH, Hyduke DR, Liao JC, Rassaf T, Bryan N, Feelisch M, Lancaster JR Jr. Nitric oxide is consumed, rather than conserved, by reaction with oxyhemoglobin under physiological conditions. Proc Natl Acad Sci U S A 2002;99: 10341–6.
45. Gardner AM, Helmick RA, Gardner PR. Flavorubredoxin, an inducible catalyst for nitric

oxide reduction and detoxification in Escherichia coli. J Biol Chem 2002;277:8172–7.
46. Gardner AM, Gardner PR. Flavohemoglobin detoxifies nitric oxide in aerobic, but not anaerobic, Escherichia coli. Evidence for a novel inducible anaerobic nitric oxide-scavenging activity. J Biol Chem 2002;277:8166–71.
47. Gardner PR, Gardner AM, Martin LA, Dou Y, Li T, Olson JS, Zhu H, Riggs AF. Nitric-oxide dioxygenase activity and function of flavohemoglobins. sensitivity to nitric oxide and carbon monoxide inhibition. J Biol Chem 2000 Oct 13;275(41):31581–7.
48. Gardner PR, Costantino G, Salzman AL. Constitutive and adaptive detoxification of nitric oxide in Escherichia coli. Role of nitric-oxide dioxygenase in the protection of aconitase. J Biol Chem 1998;273:26528–33.
49. Gardner PR, Gardner AM, Martin LA, Salzman AL. Nitric oxide dioxygenase: an enzymic function for flavohemoglobin. Proc Natl Acad Sci U S A 1998;95:10378–83.
50. Gardner PR, Martin LA, Hall D, Gardner AM. Dioxygen-dependent metabolism of nitric oxide in mammalian cells. Free Radic Biol Med 2001;31:191–204.
51. Nordberg J, Arnér ESJ. Reactive oxygen species, antioxidants, and the mammalian thioredoxin system. Free Radic Biol Med 2001;31:1287–312.
52. Wong HR, Wispe JR. The stress response and the lung. Am J Physiol 1997 Jul;273(1 Pt 1): L1–9. Review.
53. Wong HR. Potential protective role of the heat shock response against sepsis. New Horiz 1998;6:194–200.
54. Kregel KC. Heat shock proteins: modifying factors in physiological stress responses and acquired thermotolerance. J Appl Physiol 2002;92:2177–86.
55. Hasday JD, Singh IS. Fever and the heat shock response: distinct, partially overlapping processes. Cell Stress Chaperones 2000;5:471–80.
56. Ritossa FM. A new puffing pattern induced by a temperature shock and DNP in Drosophila. Experientia 1962;18:571–3.
57. Gerner EW, Schneider MJ. Induced thermal resistance in HeLa cells. Nature 1975 Aug 7;256(5517):500–2.
58. Li GC, Werb Z. Correlation between synthesis of heat shock proteins and development of thermotolerance in Chinese hamster fibroblasts. Proc Natl Acad Sci USA 1982;89: 3218–22.
59. Wong HR, Mannix RJ, Rusnak JM, Boota A, Zar H, Watkins SC, Lazo JS, Pitt BR. The heat shock response attenuates lipopolysaccharide-mediated apoptosis in cultured sheep pulmonary artery endothelial cells. Am J Respir Cell Mol Biol 1996;15:745–51.
60. Wong HR, Ryan M, Menendez IY, Denenberg A, Wispe JR. Heat shock protein induction protects human respiratory epithelium against nitric oxide-mediated cytotoxicity. Shock 1997;8:213–8.
61. Szabo C, Wong HR, Salzman AL. Heat shock phenotype inhibits peroxynitrite-induced activation of poly (ADP) ribosyl synthetase and protects against peroxynitrite cytotoxicity in J774 macrophages. Br J Pharmacol 1996;315:221–6.
62. Wang JR, Xiao XZ, Huang SN, Luo FJ, You JL, Luo H, Luo ZY. Heat shock pretreatment prevents hydrogen peroxide injury of pulmonary endothelial cells and macrophages in culture. Shock 1996;6:134–41.
63. Ryan AJ, Flanagan SW, Moseley PL, Gisolfi CV. Acute heat stress protects rats against endotoxin shock. J Appl Physiol 1992;73:1517–22.
64. Hauser GJ, Dayao EK, Wasserloos K, Pitt BR, Wong HR. HSP induction inhibits iNOS mRNA expression and attenuates hypotension in endotoxin-challenged rats. Am J Physiol

1996 Dec;271(6 Pt 2):H2529–35.
65. Villar J, Edelson JD, Post M, Mullen JB, Slutsky AS. Induction of heat stress proteins is associated with decreased mortality in an animal model of acute lung injury. Am Rev Respir Dis 1993;147:177–81.
66. Hiratsuka M, Yano M, Mora BN, Nagahiro I, Cooper JD, Patterson GA. Heat shock pretreatment protects pulmonary isografts from subsequent ischemia-reperfusion injury. J Heart Lung Transplant 1998;17:1238–46.
67. Kindas-Mugge I, Hammerle AH, Frohlich I, Oismuller C, Micksche M, Trautinger F. Granulocytes of critically ill patients spontaneously express the 72 kD heat shock protein. Circ Shock 1993;39:247–52.
68. Pittet JF, Lee H, Morabito D, Howard MB, Welch WJ, Mackersie RC. Serum levels of Hsp 72 measured early after trauma correlate with survival. J Trauma 2002;52:611–7.
69. Riabolow, KT, Mizzen LA, Welch WJ. Heat shock is lethal to fibroblasts microinjected with antibodies against hsp70. Science 1989;242:433–6.
70. Li GC, Li L, Liu Y-K, Mak JY, Chen L, Lee WMF. Thermal response of rat fibroblasts stably transfected with human 70-kD heat shock protein-encoding gene. Proc Natl Acad Sci USA 1992;89:2036–40.
71. Wong HR, Menendez IY, Ryan MA, Denenberg A, Wispe JR. Increased expression of heat shock protein-70 protects human respiratory epithelium against hyperoxia. Am J Physiol 1998;275:L836–41.
72. Hiratsuka M, Mora BN, Yano M, Mohanakumar T, Patterson GA. Gene transfer of heat shock protein 70 protects lung grafts from ischemia-reperfusion injury. Ann Thorac Surg 1999;67:1421–7.
73. Marber MS, Mestril R, Chi SH, Sayen MR, Yellon DM, Dillman WH. Overexpression of the rat inducible 70-kD heat stress protein in a transgenic mouse increases the resistance of the heart to ischemic injury. J Clin Invest 1995;95:1446–56.
74. Plumier J-CL, Ross BM, Currie RW, Angelidis CE, Kazlaris H, Kollias G, Pagoulatos GN. Transgenic mice expressing the human heat shock protein 70 have improved post-ischemic myocardial recovery. J Clin Invest 1995;95:1854–60.
75. McMillan DR, Xiao X, Shao L, Graves K, Benjamin IJ. Targeted disruption of heat shock transcription factor 1 abolishes thermotolerance and protection against heat-inducible apoptosis. J Biol Chem 1998;273:7523–8.
76. Xiao XZ, Zuo XX, Davis AA, McMillan DR, Curry BB, Richardson JA, Benjamin IJ. HSF1 is required for extra-embryonic development, postnatal growth and protection during inflammatory responses in mice. EMBO J 1999;18:5943–52.
77. Malhotra V, Kooy NW, Denenberg AG, Dunsmore KE, Wong HR. Genetic ablation of heat shock factor-1 increases susceptibility to hyperoxia-mediated cellular injury. Exp Lung Res 2002;28:1–14.
78. Snyder YL, Guthrie L, Evans GF, Zuckerman S. Transcriptional inhibition of endotoxin-induced monokine synthesis following heat shock in murine peritoneal macrophages. J Leuko Biol 1992;51:181–7.
79. Schmidt JA, Abdulla E. Down-regulation of IL-1β biosynthesis by inducers of the heat-shock response. J Immunol 1988;141:2027–34.
80. Wong HR, Finder JD, Wasserloos K, Pitt BR. Expression of inducible nitric oxide synthase in cultured rat pulmonary artery smooth muscle cells is inhibited by the heat shock response. Am J Physiol 1995;269:L843–8.
81. Thomas SC, Ryan MA, Shanley TP, Wong HR. Induction of the stress response with

prostaglandin-A, increases I-κBα gene expression. FASEB J 1998;12:1371–8.
82. Ayad O, Stark JM, Fiedler MA, Menendez IY, Ryan MA, Wong HR. The heat shock response inhibits RANTES gene expression in cultured human lung epithelium. J Immunol 1998;161:2594–9.
83. Moon R, Pritts TA, Parikh AA, Fischer JE, Salzman AL, Ryan M, Wong HR, Hasselgren PO. Stress response decreases the interleukin-1beta-induced production of complement component C3 in human intestinal epithelial cells. Clin Sci (London) 1999 Sept;97(3): 331–7.
84. Malhotra V, Eaves-Pyles T, Odoms K, Quaid G, Shanley TP, Wong HR. Heat shock inhibits activation of NF-κB in the absence of heat shock factor-1. Biochem Biophys Res Comm 2002;291:453–7.
85. Kohn G, Wong HR, Bshesh K, Zhao B, Vasi N, Denenberg A, Morris C, Stark J, Shanley TP. Heat shock inhibits TNF-induced ICAM-1 expression in human endothelial cells via Iκ kinase (IKK) inhibition. Shock 2002;17:91–7.
86. Wong HR, Ryan M, Gebb S, Wispe JR. Selective and transient *in vitro* effects of heat shock on alveolar type II cell gene expression. Am J Physiol 1997 Jan;272(1 Pt 1):L132–8.
87. Wong HR, Ryan M, Wispe JR. The heat shock response inhibits inducible nitric oxide synthase gene expression by blocking Iκ-B degradation and NF-κB nuclear translocation. Biochem Biophys Res Comm 1997;231:257–63.
88. Pritts TA, Want Q, Sun X, Moon MR, Fischer DR, Fischer JE, Wong HR, Hasselgren PO. Induction of the stress response in vivo decreases NF-κB activity in jejunal mucosa of endotoxemic mice. Arch Surg 2000;135:860.
89. Wong HR, Ryan M, Wispe JR. Stress response decreases NF-κB nuclear translocation and increases I-κBα and expression in A549 cells. J Clin Invest 1997;99:2423–8.
90. Pritts TA, Wang Q, Sun X, Fischer DR, Hungness ES, Fischer JE, Wong HR, Hasselgren P.O. The stress response decreases NF-κB activation in liver of endotoxemic mice. Shock 2002;18:33–7.
91. Malhotra V, Wong HR. Interactions between the heat shock response and the nuclear factor-kappaB signaling pathway. Crit Care Med 2002 Jan;30(1 Supp):S89–95.
92. Curry HA, Clemens RA, Shah S, Bradbury CM, Botero A, Goswami P, Gius D. Heat shock inhibits radiation-induced activation of NF-κB via inhibition of I-κB kinase. J Biol Chem 1999;274:23061–7.
93. Yoo CG, Lee S, Lee CT, Kim YW, Han SK, Shim YS. Anti-inflammatory effect of heat shock protein induction is related to stabilization of IκBα through preventing IκB kinase activation in respiratory epithelial cells. J Immunol 2000;164:5416–23.
94. Grossman BJ, Shanley TP, Odoms K, Dunsmore KE, Denenberg AG, Wong HR. Temporal and mechanistic effects of heat shock on LPS-mediated degradation of IκBα in macrophages. Inflammation 2002;26:129–37.
95. Shanley TP, Ryan MA, Eaves-Pyles T, Wong H. Heat shock inhibits phosphorylation of I-kappaBalpha. Shock 2000;14:447–50.
96. Wong HR, Ryan MA, Menendez IY, Wispe JR. Heat shock activates the I-κBα promoter and increases I-κBα mRNA expression in BEAS-2B cells. Cell Stress Chaperones 1999;4: 1–7.
97. Smenenza GL. HIF-1: mediator of physiological and pathophysiological responses to hypoxia. J Appl Physiol 2000;88:1474–80.
98. Semenza GL. Signal transduction to hypoxia-inducible factor 1. Biochem Pharmacol 2002;64:993–8.

99. Carmeliet P, Dor Y, Herbert JM, Fukumura D, Brusselmans K, Dewerchin M, Neeman M, Bono F, Abramovitch R, Maxwell P, Koch CJ, Ratcliffe P, Moons L, Jain RK, Collen D, Keshert E, Keshet E. Role of HIF-1alpha in hypoxia-mediated apoptosis, cell proliferation and tumour angiogenesis. Nature 1998 Jul;394(6692):485–90.
100. Iyer NV, Kotch LE, Agani F, Leung SW, Laughner E, Wenger RH, Gassmann M, Gearhart JD, Lawler AM, Yu AY, Semenza GL. Cellular and developmental control of O2 homeostasis by hypoxia-inducible factor 1 alpha. Genes Dev 1998;12:149–62.
101. Hu J, Discher DJ, Bishopric NH, Webster KA. Hypoxia regulates expression of the endothelin-1 gene through a proximal hypoxia-inducible factor-1 binding site on the antisense strand. Biochem Biophys Res Commun 1998;245:894–9.
102. Jiang BH, Rue E, Wang GL, Roe R, Semenza GL. Dimerization, DNA binding, and transactivation properties of hypoxia-inducible factor 1. J Biol Chem 1996;271:17771–8.
103. Lee PJ, Jiang BH, Chin BY, Iyer NV, Alam J, Semenza GL, Choi AM. Hypoxia-inducible factor-1 mediates transcriptional activation of the heme oxygenase-1 gene in response to hypoxia. J Biol Chem 1997;272:5375–81.
104. Huang LE, Gu J, Schau M, Bunn HF. Regulation of hypoxia-inducible factor 1alpha is mediated by an O2-dependent degradation domain via the ubiquitin-proteasome pathway. Proc Natl Acad Sci U S A 1998;95:7987–92.
105. Huang LE, Arany Z, Livingston DM, Bunn HF. Activation of hypoxia-inducible transcription factor depends primarily upon redox-sensitive stabilization of its alpha subunit. J Biol Chem 1996;271:32253–9.
106. Jaakkola P, Mole DR, Tian YM, Wilson MI, Gielbert J, Gaskell SJ, Kriegsheim Av, Hebestreit HF, Mukherji M, Schofield CJ, Maxwell PH, Pugh CW, Ratcliffe PJ. Targeting of HIF-alpha to the von Hippel-Lindau ubiquitylation complex by O2-regulated prolyl hydroxylation. Science 2001 Apr 20;292(5516):468–72.
107. Mole DR, Maxwell PH, Pugh CW, Ratcliffe PJ. Regulation of HIF by the von Hippel-Lindau tumour suppressor: implications for cellular oxygen sensing. IUBMB Life 2001;52:43–7.
108. Lee SH, Wolf PL, Escudero R, Deutsch R, Jamieson SW, Thistlethwaite PA. Early expression of angiogenesis factors in acute myocardial ischemia and infarction. N Engl J Med 2000;342:626–33.
109. Melillo G, Musso T, Sica A, Taylor LS, Cox GW, Varesio L. A hypoxia-responsive element mediates a novel pathway of activation of the inducible nitric oxide synthase promoter. J Exp Med 1995;182:1683–93.
110. Bolli R, Dawn B, Tang XL, Qiu Y, Ping P, Xuan YT, Jones WK, Takano H, Guo Y, Zhang J. The nitric oxide hypothesis of late preconditioning. Basic Res Cardiol 1998;93:325–38.
111. Maltepe E, Schmidt JV, Baunoch D, Bradfield CA, Simon MC. Abnormal angiogenesis and responses to glucose and oxygen deprivation in mice lacking the protein ARNT. Nature 1997;386:403–7.
112. Yu AY, Shimoda LA, Iyer NV, Huso DL, Sun X, McWilliams R, Beaty T, Sham JS, Wiener CM, Sylvester JT, Semenza GL. Impaired physiological responses to chronic hypoxia in mice partially deficient for hypoxia-inducible factor 1alpha. J Clin Invest 1999;103:691–6.
113. Michel T, Feron O. Nitric oxide synthases: which, where, how, and why? J Clin Invest 1997;100:2146–52.
114. Guo FH, De Raeve HR, Rice TW, Stuehr DJ, Thunnissen FB, Erzurum SC. Continuous nitric oxide synthesis by inducible nitric oxide synthase in normal human airway

epithelium in vivo. Proc Natl Acad Sci U S A 1995;92:7809–13.
115. Moncada S, Higgs A, Furchgott R. International Union of Pharmacology nomenclature in nitric oxide research. Pharmaol Rev 1997;49:137–43.
116. Wink DA, Mitchell JB. Chemical biology of nitric oxide: insights into regulatory, cytotoxic, and cytoprotective mechanisms of nitric oxide. Free Radic Biol Med 1998;25: 434–56.
117. Kim YM, Bombeck CA, Billiar TR. Nitric oxide as a bifunctional regulator of apoptosis. Circ Res 1999;84:253–6.
118. Dimmeler S, Zeiher AM. Nitric oxide and apoptosis: another paradigm for the double-edged role of nitric oxide. Nitric Oxide 1997;1:275–81.
119. Mannick JB, Asano K, Izumi K, Kieff E, Stamler JS. Nitric oxide produced by human B lymphocytes inhibits apoptosis and Epstein-Barr virus reactivation. Cell 1994;79:1137–46.
120. Dimmeler S, Haendeler J, Nehls M, Zeiher AM. Suppression of apoptosis by nitric oxide via inhibition of interleukin-1beta-converting enzyme (ICE)-like and cysteine protease protein (CPP)-32-like proteases. J Exp Med 1997;185:601–7.
121. Genaro AM, Hortelano S, Alvarez A, Martinez C, Bosca L. Splenic B lymphocyte programmed cell death is prevented by nitric oxide release through mechanisms involving sustained Bcl-2 levels. J Clin Invest 1995;95:1884–90.
122. Kim YM, de Vera ME, Watkins SC, Billiar TR. Nitric oxide protects cultured rat hepatocytes from tumor necrosis factor-alpha-induced apoptosis by inducing heat shock protein 70 expression. J Biol Chem 1997;272:1402–11.
123. Li J, Bombeck CA, Yang S, Kim YM, Billiar TR. Nitric oxide suppresses apoptosis via interrupting caspase activation and mitochondrial dysfunction in cultured hepatocytes. J Biol Chem 1999;274:17325–33.
124. Ou J, Carlos TM, Watkins SC, Saavedra JE, Keefer LK, Kim YM, Harbrecht BG, Billiar TR. Differential effects of nonselective nitric oxide synthase (NOS) and selective inducible NOS inhibition on hepatic necrosis, apoptosis, ICAM-1 expression, and neutrophil accumulation during endotoxemia. Nitric Oxide 1997;1:404–16.
125. Saavedra JE, Billiar TR, Williams DL, Kim YM, Watkins SC, Keefer LK. Targeting nitric oxide (NO) delivery in vivo. Design of a liver-selective NO donor prodrug that blocks tumor necrosis factor-alpha-induced apoptosis and toxicity in the liver. J Med Chem 1997;40:1947–54.
126. Kim YM, Bergonia H, Lancaster JR Jr. Nitrogen oxide-induced autoprotection in isolated rat hepatocytes. FEBS Lett 1995;374:228–32.
127. Kim YM, Kim TH, Seol DW, Talanian RV, Billiar TR. Nitric oxide suppression of apoptosis occurs in association with an inhibition of Bcl-2 cleavage and cytochrome c release. J Biol Chem 1998;273:31437–41.
128. Wang Y, Vodovotz Y, Kim PK, Zamora R, Billiar TR. Mechanisms of hepatoprotection by nitric oxide. Ann N Y Acad Sci 2002;962:415–22.
129. Heeringa P, Steenbergen E, van Goor H. A protective role for endothelial nitric oxide synthase in glomerulonephritis. Kidney Int 2002;61:822–5.
130. Lipton SA. Neuronal protection and destruction by NO. Cell Death Differ 1999;6:943–51.
131. Dawn B, Bolli R. Role of nitric oxide in myocardial preconditioning. Ann N Y Acad Sci 2002;962:18–41.
132. Lefer AM, Lefer DJ. Nitric oxide II. Nitric oxide protects in intestinal inflammation. Am J

Physiol 1999;276:G572–5.

Natural Immunity
Edited by L. Bertók and D.A. Chow

© 2005 Elsevier B.V. All rights reserved

The Role of Bile Acids in Natural Resistance: Physico-Chemical Host Defence

LÓRÁND BERTÓK

"Fodor József" National Center of Public Health, "Frédéric Joliot-Curie" National Research Institute for Radiobiology and Radiohygiene, H-1221 Anna u. 5, Budapest, Hungary

ABSTRACT

The toxic effects of endotoxin, the cell wall component of Gram negative intestinal bacteria, under experimental conditions, can be induced only when they are administered parenterally. However, in naturally occurring *entero-endotoxaemic diseases* (e.g., septic and various shocks, etc.), the endotoxin is absorbed from the intestinal tract. The cause and mode of translocation was unknown. The generally used experimental shock models differ from natural diseases only in the mode by which endotoxin enter the blood circulation. If the common bile duct of rats was chronically cannulated (bile deprived animals) orally administered endotoxin was absorbed from the intestinal tract into the blood circulation and provoked endotoxin shock. This *translocation of endotoxins* and the consequent shock can be prevented by sodium deoxycholate or natural biles. The bile acids split the endotoxin macromolecule into atoxic fragments. A similar detoxifying detergent action plays a significant role in host defence against infectious agents with a lipoprotein outer structure (e.g., so-called "big" viruses). This defence mechanism of macroorganisms based on the *detergent activity of bile acids* is called *physico-chemical defence system.* Since bile deficiency and the consequent endotoxaemia are important components in the pathogenesis of certain diseases (e.g., sepsis, intestinal syndrome of radiation disease, hepato-renal syndrome, parvovirus infection, herpes, psoriasis, atherosclerosis, etc.), bile acids may be used for the prevention and/or therapy of some clinical conditions such as the hepato-renal syndrome and psoriasis.

1. INTRODUCTION

In addition to immunological reactions, numerous other mechanisms contribute to host defence. One such mechanism is the *detergent action* exerted in the gut by bile acids produced in the liver. This was discovered during our studies on the absorption of endotoxins from the gastrointestinal tract. It is well known that endotoxins are capable of inducing a syndrome similar to septic shock when applied parenterally [1–4]. Experimentally induced endotoxin shock is based on an artificial situation, which differs from the natural disease with regard to the entry of endotoxin into the host organism. Under natural conditions, during the so-called entero-endotoxaemic syndrome (e.g., various forms of shock) endotoxin will enter the circulation invariably from the gastrointestinal tract. It is known that endotoxin impairs the movement of intestinal villi [5], but the mechanism of its absorption was not known. In spite of this lack of knowledge, intravenously or intraperitoneally injected endotoxin induced a shock syndrome in mammals, which is similar to the natural disease (entero-endotoxaemia) that occurs prior to death (diarrhoea, inactivity, circulatory disturbances). The pathological findings in animals that succumbed to endotoxin shock are similar to those seen in animals that died of natural disease (intestinal oedema, haemorrhages). There are major differences in the sensitivity of various species to parenterally given endotoxin, which shows a correlation with phylogenetic development [6–7]. However, when given orally endotoxin is not able to exert toxicity even in the most sensitive animal species [1]. The reason for this remained unknown for some time, because intestinal enzymes did not affect the endotoxin molecule.

In our initial experiments we observed that oral endotoxin was harmless when given to rats at doses that were 500 to 3000 times higher than the parenteral lethal dose. Moreover, such treatment was harmless even when the gut mucosa had been damaged by histamine release induced by compound 48/80 and the animals had been sensitised to lipopolysaccharide (LPS) toxicity by the intravenous application of lead acetate. It was also observed that endotoxin given orally to rats could be re-isolated from gut content by the method of phenol-water extraction. No endotoxin absorption could be demonstrated even when the animals were made extremely susceptible to endotoxin by the use of lead acetate [1]. Although the intestinal syndrome during radiation disease is due to *entero-endotoxaemia*, in irradiated animals endotoxin absorption can be demonstrated only on day 6 to 7 with sensitisation using lead acetate [8].

The above experiments did not shed light on the mechanism of endotoxin absorption from the gastrointestinal tract. The reason for the extreme tolerance of healthy animals to orally given endotoxin could not be explained. Research was restricted to the study of animals/individuals with natural disease or, alternatively, of animals parenterally injected with endotoxin. There was little interest in the problem of *endotoxin absorption,* which is the prerequisite for the biological effect of endotoxin.

The lack of knowledge stimulated our interest in the problem of endotoxin absorption. We have been inspired by the *in vitro* experiments of an American research group, which observed that the treatment of endotoxin with a bile acid, sodium deoxycholate, resulted in the production of small atoxic units, which did not exert toxicity, but it was possible to revert to the toxic form if sodium deoxycholate was removed by dialysis. If protein was present in the system, the process became irreversible because the endotoxin fractions were adsorbed to the protein molecules. In this case it was necessary to extract the endotoxin (e.g., with phenol-water) and then it was possible to restore the molecule with some loss [9]. On the basis of these findings we considered the possibility that bile acids may play an important role *in vivo* in the *detoxification of endotoxin.* If indeed this was the case, it was possible to recover orally given endotoxin from the gastrointestinal tract by extraction even though it was present there in the 'fragmented', atoxic form.

Our hypothesis was further supported by the pathological observation that faecal samples of calves and piglets suffering from Escherichia coli *(E. coli)* diarrhoea were deficient in bile acids and contained significant quantities of neutral fat [10]. We predicted that bile deficiency was present. This hypothesis was also supported by the pathological observation that in newborn animals that succumbed to *E. coli* diarrhoea, the *gallbladders* were fully loaded, indicating the lack of release into the intestinal lumen. This resulted in acholic faeces [11]. We observed oedema and a yellow colour in the small intestine in mice given endotoxin parenterally, which suggested infiltration with bile acids. Perhaps parenterally injected endotoxin triggered the release of bile acids into the small intestine as a defence reaction but in this case no protection

Table I Deaths due to chronic bile fistula and orally administered ^{3}H-endotoxin in rats.

Group	Treatment	Death ratio (dead/total)
1	^{3}H-endotoxin (5 mg per os at 0 hr) + lead acetate (5 mg iv at 3 hr)	0/5
2	Bile fistula + lead acetate (5 mg iv)	1*/5
3	Bile fistula + ^{3}H-endotoxin (5 mg per os after 0 Hr) + lead acetate (5 mg iv after 3 hr)	5/5

* Died of intercurrent bile peritonitis.

could be achieved [12,13]. It is known that bacterial endotoxin chemically is a lipopolysaccharide molecule, in which the toxic moiety has been identified as the lipid A portion rich in fatty acids [14,15]. On the basis of the above observations one may suggest that bile acids detoxify endotoxin within the gastrointestinal tract.

2. EXPERIMENTS ON BILE-DEPRIVED RATS

We designed experiments for the clarification of this question *in vivo*. Because rats do not have gallbladders, it was possible to produce bile deficiency by the *cannulation of the common bile duct*. With this technique we successfully produced a *chronic bile deficiency*, which was suitable for the study of endotoxin absorption from the gastrointestinal tract. We favoured the hypothesis that in healthy animals orally given endotoxin, or the endotoxin released from Gram-negative bacteria within the gastrointestinal tract, did not cause clinical symptoms because bile acids which are present in the gut on a permanent basis, will take apart the endotoxin molecule due to the detergent action. Non-toxic small fractions are produced which are adsorbed by protein molecules present in the gut. It was anticipated on this basis that bile deficiency was necessary for the development of entero-endotoxaemia. This hypothesis has been proven experimentally in rats [16,17]. Endotoxin labelled with tritium or radioactive chromium was not absorbed in normal animals after oral application [18]. No clinical symptoms were produced by such treatment. In contrast, if such endotoxin was given to rats having a bile fistula for 1–2 weeks, which led to bile acid deficiency, the animals succumbed to endotoxin shock (Table I). It was possible to detect radioactive endotoxin in the blood of these animals (by the measurement of ^{3}H and ^{51}Cr activity), and we could sensitise such animals further to endotoxin by treatment with lead acetate [19]. These experiments revealed that bile deficiency is required for the absorption of endotoxin from the gastrointestinal tract. In further experiments we treated the endotoxin with sodium deoxycholate prior to oral application to rats having bile fistulas. Complete protection was observed even when the rats had been sensitised to endotoxin by treatment with lead acetate (Table II). Identical results were obtained when bile was used from rats, pigs and cows for the restoration of missing bile acids. Such treatment prevented the development of endotoxin shock [6]. The ligation of the bile duct in rats increased the blood cholesterol, bile acid and bilirubin levels, as shown in Table III.

These experiments provided proof for the role of bile acids in host defence against endotoxin, and indicated that bile deficiency leads to the absorption of intestinal endotoxin, both of which have clinical significance. Other investigators confirmed our results in animal experiments and also in clinical situations (endotoxaemia of patients suffering from bile duct occlusion and

Table II Sodium deoxycholate prevents deaths due to endotoxin in rats with bile fistula and lead acetate sensitisation.

Group	Treatment	Death ratio (dead/total)
1	Bile fistula + lead acetate (5 mg iv)	1*/6
2	Bile fistula + LPS (10 mg per os 0 hr) + lead acetate (5 mg iv + 3 hr)	5/6
3	Bile fistula + sodium deoxycholate (40 mg per os) + LPS (10 mg per os) + lead acetate (5 mg iv + 3 hr)	2/6

* Died of intercurrent bile peritonitis.

Table III The effect of ligation of the common bile duct in rats on serum bile acid, cholesterol, lipoprotein and bilirubin levels.

	Intact	Ligated
Glycocholic acid (μmol/l) (n = 15)	1.4 ± 0.84	45.5 ± 43.45
Glycodeoxicholic acid (μmol/l) (n = 15)	2.1 ± 0.79	7.36 ± 5.68
Cholesterol (mmol/l) (n = 15)	2.26 ± 0.34	3.5 ± 0.30
HDL (mmol/l) (n = 15)	0.55 ± 0.16	0.58 ± 0.18
LDL (mmol/l) (n = 15)	.36 ± 0.42	2.69 ± 1.04
Bilirubin (μmol/l) (n = 15)	7.0 ± 1.22	115.00 ± 89.67
Bilirubin D (μmol/l) (n = 14)	4.4 ± 1.30	45.00 ± 34.41

icterus), see for example *Bailey* [20], *Cahill* [21] and later *Gaffin* [22]. It was found that the treatment of patients suffering from icterus with bile acids prior to surgery prevented the impairment of renal function and the development of renal deficiency [21–24]. Our experimental observations made it possible to prevent a severe clinical disease. It seems obvious that this beneficial effect of bile acids is based on the physico-chemical, surface-active, detergent action. Our results support the hypothesis that the inactivation of endotoxin in the gastrointestinal tract by bile acids is due to the detergent action [25]. For this reason we studied other detergents in addition to sodium deoxycholate that are present in the bile of various animal species. Our goal was to find out whether or not they are capable of detoxifying endotoxin by fractionation of the molecule.

3. THE EFFECT OF VARIOUS DETERGENTS

Studies were done also with some commonly used *detergents* (e.g., sodium lauryl sulphate, cetylammonium bromide, polyoxyethylene stearate, Tween 20, benzalkonium chloride). Two rapid methods were developed for the determination of their activity. One approach was to inject a mixture of a lethal dose of endotoxin and a tolerated concentration of the detergent intraperitoneally into animals. If the detergent applied could detoxify endotoxin, the mortality of the animals was decreased. According to the second procedure the animals were sensitised to endotoxin by lead acetate. In this case microgram quantities of endotoxin could be used, mixed with detergent and given intravenously. Here it was also necessary to titrate detergent toxicity prior to its use. Again, a decrease in mortality indicated the anti-endotoxic effect of the detergent investigated. These experiments indicated that *sodium deoxycholate* and *bile* obtained from various animals (e.g., cow, pig, rat, and rabbit) showed 100% efficacy in protection, whereas sodium lauryl sulphate gave 80%, cetylammonium bromide 60%, and benzalkonium chloride 20% protection against the lethal dose of endotoxin, and Tween 20 was ineffective. We concluded that the best results were obtained with bile acids or with natural bile [26].

Our experimental results made it possible to explain the pathomechanism of entero-endotoxaemia in new-born babies, which occurred frequently some time ago, but decreased in number lately because of improved hygienic conditions in hospitals. However, this disease still has veterinary significance because 10–15% of newborn calves and piglets will fall victim to entero-endotoxaemia. It is likely that in a proportion of newborn animals bile production (probably because of disturbed liver function) or bile secretion into the small intestine (probably because of the lack of cholecystokinin) does not coincide with parturition, which leads to bile deficiency. There is a rapid penetration of Gram-negative bacteria into the gastrointestinal tract of newborn animals, which release endotoxins that would absorb in bile-deficient animals and cause disease and death. The situation is analogous to rats having a bile fistula and receiving endotoxin by the oral route. It follows that such newborn animals would be protected if given after parturition detergent preparations, optimally bile acids, that would prevent disease. Such treatment would restore the bile content in the gut which would enter the enterohepatic circulation, stimulate the production of bile acids and their secretion into the gut, in other words initiate the function of this fundamental host defence mechanism.

4. PROTECTIVE EFFECT OF BILE ACIDS PREPARATIONS AGAINST ENDOTOXIN SHOCK

On the basis of the above experiments therapeutic preparations of bile acids (DETERTOXON-S and B) have been produced which seem to be beneficial for the treatment of entero-endotoxaemia in newborns [27]. Comparative pathological studies conducted during these therapeutic trials demonstrated that these preparations were able to decrease mortality due to *E. coli* diarrhoea. For instance, in a cattle herd 195 calves received conventional treatment and 23 of them died, whereas after the treatment of 234 calves with the bile acid preparation only 6 were lost because of *E. coli diarrhoea.* Essentially similar results were obtained during the trial in other herds. The results were similar though inferior in a pig farm where 120 piglets were lost out of 2027 untreated animals, whereas 68 died of 1803 bile acid treated animals due to *E. coli* diarrhoea [28].

These results are significant because of the experience gained during several decades that the treatment of entero-endotoxaemic newborn animals with drugs or vaccines is of limited value. Vaccines provide protection only against specific strains that have been used for its production and become useless against other strains that frequently occur in a given population. This is a serious limitation, as approximately 150 different *E. coli* strains are known simply on the basis of O serotypes. For this reason the induction of specific immunity seems impossible. Perhaps the new, so-called pilus antigen vaccines or the use of DNA vaccines will improve the situation [29,30]. The problem is similar when antibacterial agents (antibiotics, sulphonamides) are used for treatment. Resistance will occur within a short period of time, which renders these drugs ineffective. One may hope, on the basis of our results, that this disease could be prevented by the restoration of bile acid deficiency. Current evidence indicates that in *E. coli* diarrhoea the entero- and protein toxins [30] could facilitate the translocation of endotoxin by causing damage to the gut mucosa. Such damage would inhibit or prevent the secretion of *cholecystokinin,* which in turn would lead to bile retention and allow the absorption of endotoxin into the bloodstream, resulting in endotoxaemia and shock. This explanation is compatible with those views that emphasise the fundamental pathogenic role of endotoxin in these conditions.

The above examples of animal disease have comparative pathological significance and serve as models for human conditions. It is well known that a significant proportion of the human population suffers from problems of bile secretion and of gallbladder function (*Bertók Jr.* and *Bertók*, unpublished observations). It is possible that the use of bile acid preparations would be of advantage in such patients.

5. PHYSICO-CHEMICAL HOST DEFENCE

The pathophysiological significance of these findings may be summarised as follows: A unique host defence mechanism has been discovered the significance of which is likely to lie way beyond protection against bacterial endotoxins. We call this mechanism the *physico-chemical defence* of the organism. The basis of this defence mechanism is the detergent effect of bile acids [6,31,32]. One may pose the question whether or not the protection based on detergent action provides defence against enterotoxaemia only or perhaps there are other situations in which endotoxin plays a role.

6. THE ROLE OF BILE ACIDS IN INTESTINAL ISCHAEMIA

We found in subsequent experiments that *intestinal ischaemia* is aggravated by bile deficiency [33,34]. Moreover, it was found that bile production is decreased under these conditions [35]. This was further supported by the observation that the administration of bile acids (500 mg pulverised and radiation-sterilised pig bile) to dogs with intestinal ischaemia prevented death in 60–70% of the animals [36]. The protective value of bile acids was also indicated in rats suffering from 'strangulated ileus', where endotoxin plays a fundamental role in the pathogenesis. Bile acids given into the intestinal lumen (20 mg pulverised and radiation-sterilised pig bile) prolonged the survival of the animals by 7 hours (50%) [37]. These results indicate that the use of proper bile acid preparations will provide new opportunities for the treatment of patients with acute abdominal conditions.

7. THE EFFECT OF BILE ACIDS ON VIRUSES

One may ask the question whether or not the protective effect of bile acid detergents is limited to bacterial endotoxins. *Theiler* observed that the virus of yellow fever and other 'arthropod-borne' viruses (belonging to the Toga group) are inactivated by bile or sodium deoxycholate. In contrast, the poliovirus, the virus of mouse encephalitis and endocarditis and Coxsackie viruses resist such treatment [38]. This observation served as a basic principle for the classification of viruses according to which two groups, sodium deoxycholate sensitive ('big viruses') and resistant ('small viruses') could be distinguished. It is interesting that nobody, including *Theiler*, recognized the pathological significance of these observations despite the fact that *Theiler* was actually working with the virus of yellow fever when he discovered the antiviral effect of bile. If we compare the bile acid sensitive and resistant viruses, it becomes clear that the viruses having lipoprotein capsule are sensitive and those that do not possess such a capsule are resistant. It follows that bile acids would affect *in vivo* all the viruses that possess lipoprotein 'capsule' (peplon). Those without capsules are all resistant. Therefore, it is logical to assume that the detergent effect of bile acids would act *in vivo* on all those viruses that have lipoprotein capsules and that this fact could be used for protection against such viruses. In an experimental model using Aujeszky's disease virus, a herpes virus, we demonstrated the protective effects of bile acids. It was found in rats that bile deficient animals contracted disease after the oral administration of Aujeszky's disease virus whereas intact rats were resistant [39]. It is possible that temporary or partial bile acid deficiency plays an important role in infections with herpes viruses that may occur after alimentary overloads (e.g., weddings and other feasts).

8. BILE ACIDS AND PSORIASIS

In our view, *psoriasis,* a condition considered to be inherited in a polygenic manner [40], is also associated with bile or bile acid deficiency, as in most cases supplementation of the usual treatment with bile acids will diminish the severity of the clinical signs within a short period. One of my co-workers (Klára Gyurcsovics) treated a total of 551 psoriasis patients with bile acids (Suprachol®; Acidum dehydrocholicum) given orally for 1–8 weeks. The clinical efficacy of the treatment was evaluated by means of the Psoriasis Area Severity Index (PASI score). During this treatment 434 patients (78.8%) became asymptomatic. Of 249 psoriatics receiving the conventional therapy, only 62 (24.9%) showed clinical recovery during the same period of time ($p<0.05$). The curative effect of bile acids was even more pronounced in the acute form of psoriasis (95.1% of the patients became asymptomatic). Two years later 319 out of the 551 acute and chronic psoriasis patients treated with bile acid (57.9%) were asymptomatic, compared to only 15 out of the 249 patients (6.0%) receiving the conventional treatment ($p<0.05$). At the end of the two-year follow-up, only 10 out of 139 acute psoriasis patients (7.2%) receiving the conventional therapy and 147 out of 184 such patients (79.9%) treated with bile acids were asymptomatic ($p<0.01$). On the basis of clinical observations (digestive disorders, ultrasonographically confirmed gallbladder changes, etc.) it may be assumed that the deficiency of bile acids can indeed play a role in the pathogenesis of psoriasis. In bile acid deficiency the absorption ('translocation') of endotoxins becomes possible [41], and this will trigger the release of inflammatory cytokines in the skin of individuals having a hereditary predisposition. If the absorption of endotoxins is prevented by bile acid supplementation, the release of inflammatory cytokines can be blocked [42]. Probably this is the mechanism that explains the success of our treatment approach. Thus, the effect that cytokines have been recognized to exert in the pathogenesis of psoriasis suggests the indirect role of bacterial endotoxins. However, this effect probably occurs only if bile production or excretion is deficient (cholecystokinin deficiency, disturbance of cholesterol metabolism and bile production). Thus, the treatment of psoriasis with bile acids should actually be regarded as supplementation of a physiological substance rather than a medicinal therapy. In our view, its effectiveness, safety, simplicity and low cost make this treatment modality suitable for a wider use in the *therapy of psoriasis* [42]. The successful treatment of psoriasis with bile acids is an example demonstrating that the recognition of physico-chemical defence has practical importance. Thus, recognition of the role of bile acids enables us to provide cause-based treatment to psoriatics who have mostly been given only symptomatic treatment so far.

9. BILE DEFICIENCY AND PARVOVIRUS INFECTION

The importance of bile acids is further emphasised by the observation that the symptoms of acute *parvovirus* infection, which causes severe intestinal haemorrhage in dogs, closely resemble experimental endotoxin shock. During autopsy the characteristic finding is a dilated, tightly filled gallbladder. Endotoxin could be detected in the serum of such dogs using lead acetate sensitised animals [43]. These observations suggest that parvovirus induced mucosal damage in the small intestine, which leads to haemorrhage, is likely to inhibit cholecystokinin (CCK) synthesis and CCK deficiency leads to bile retention. Partial bile acid deficiency occurs in the gut, which makes the absorption of endotoxin possible. It is likely that the sick dogs die of endotoxin shock [43].

10. BILE DEFICIENCY AND RADIATION-INDUCED INTESTINAL-SYNDROME

It is clear that the intestinal syndrome associated with radiation disease is caused by bacterial endotoxins. Because bile acids are capable of endotoxin detoxification and bile deficiency permits the absorption of endotoxins into the bloodstream ('translocation'), one may ask the question whether or not bile deficiency would play a role in radiation disease. For this reason we studied in rats the effect of experimental bile deficiency on the development of radiation-induced intestinal syndrome. It was observed that the rats having bile fistulas died of radiation disease within five days, whereas the control irradiated and sham-operated irradiated animals survived for 11 days. Apparently bile deficiency accelerated the development of endotoxaemia in this model [44].

11. BILE ACID COMPOSITION OF VARIOUS SPECIES

In relation to the importance of bile acids in host defence against endotoxins one may ask the question whether or not bile composition plays a role in the endotoxin sensitivity/resistance of various species [45]. We have observed earlier that there are major differences in bile acid composition of bile obtained from sensitive (e.g., man, cow, guinea pig) and resistant species (e.g., birds, fish) [39]. It is interesting to note that there is a direct correlation between endotoxin sensitivity and radiation sensitivity of various species. Perhaps the ontogeny of the production of bile acids in chickens bears relevance to the fact that chicken embryos show endotoxin sensitivity up to 11 days of age, which is the time of the initiation of bile acid synthesis in the liver. Older chicks or mature animals can only be made susceptible to endotoxin by lead acetate treatment. It is likely that bile acids function not only in the gut but also in the liver in addition to acyloxyacyl hydrolase enzyme discovered in 1989 to be active in the detoxification of bacterial endotoxins [46].

12. ENDOTOXIN INACTIVATION BY LIVER/BILE ACIDS

We have observed, as have others, that liver homogenates from healthy rats are capable of inactivating small (microgram) quantities of endotoxins. In contrast, if the rats received lead acetate intravenously prior to the preparation of liver homogenates, no endotoxin inactivation was

Table IV Proven and presumed roles of bile acids and endotoxins in certain pathological processes.

Intestinal infections
Surgical / septic shock
Intestinal ischemic shock
Tourniquet shock
Gastro-intestinal syndrome of radiation disease
Hepato-renal syndrome
Enteroviral infections (e.g., parvovirus)
Herpes viral infections
Psoriasis
Atherosclerosis
Endocrine disorders

observed [39]. Similar results were obtained if we incubated natural bile fluid with lead acetate. Such bile solutions lost their capacity to detoxify endotoxin. It is likely that lead acetate damages the side chains that play an important role in the detergent effect of bile acids, and for this reason the modified bile acids are unable to detoxify endotoxin. This phenomenon may play a role in the lead acetate induced endotoxin sensitivity *in vivo* [39].

We demonstrated that after the dissociation of endotoxin by bile acids to its basic units, the detoxified material maintains the capacity to induce endotoxin tolerance [31–32]. It is possible that this observation will lead to the isolation of non-toxic endotoxin subunits, which will be able to stimulate natural resistance without toxic side effects [39].

13. CONCLUSIONS

In conclusion, one may suggest that a physico-chemical defence mechanism, which is based on the detergent action of bile acids, provide the body with a general defence, which is not limited to bacterial endotoxins, but is also effective against other agents (e.g., viruses) that possess lipoprotein or lipid structures. This novel mechanism may be added to the known defence mechanisms, which are based on bile acids produced in the liver and present in the *enterohepatic circulation*. It is interesting to note in this respect that bile acids are the most important products of cholesterol metabolism, which are reusable end products that affect the production of steroid hormones (by the adrenal gland and gonads). It is possible that bile acids play a role also in the pathophysiology of endocrine and reproductive abnormalities, which remains to be elucidated [47] (Table IV).

It is possible that deficient bile production or secretion leads to the absorption of minute amounts of endotoxin, which may play a role in the induction of atherosclerosis. We showed in cholesterol-treated rabbits that endotoxin significantly increases the development of atherosclerosis [48]. Recently several authors recognized his fact [49–60]. Partial or temporary bile acid deficiency may occur for several reasons: CCK deficiency, disturbance of bile secretion and deficient bile production due to liver damage, leading to endotoxin absorption. In turn, the absorbed endotoxin will act on sessile phagocytes fixed to the wall of blood vessels according to known pathways (e.g., endotoxin-binding protein and CD14 endotoxin receptor), which leads to the production of cytokines and other biologically active materials. These mediators, in conjunction with elevated cholesterol levels, could precipitate and initiate plaque formation. On this basis one may suggest that the systematic investigation of bile production and secretion from a young age and correction of deficiencies would decrease the development of atherosclerosis and the development of related diseases.

It is clear from the facts presented here that bile acids and endotoxins play a significant role in many more pathological conditions than were reasonably anticipated. It is likely that further investigation of these questions and the application of experimental results to patients will lead to new approaches in clinical medicine.

REFERENCES

1. Berczi I, Bertók L, Baintner K, Veress B. Failure of oral E.coli endotoxin to induce either specific tolerance or toxic symptoms in rats. J Path Bact 1968;96:481–486.
2. Bertók L. Bacterial endotoxins and their effects (Hungarian). Orv Hetil 1998;139:1947–1953.
3. Gans H, Matsumoto K. Are enteric endotoxins able to escape from intestine? Proc Soc Exp Biol Med 1975;147:736–741.
4. Gans H, Matsumoto K. On the escape of endotoxin from the intestine. In: Urbaschek B, Urbaschek R, Neter E, editors. Gram-negative bacterial infections. Wien: Springer Verlag, 1975;429–436.
5. Ihász M, Karika Gy, Ludány Gy. Effect of endotoxin on motion of intestinal villi (Hungarian). Orv Hetil 1968;109:1381–1384.
6. Bertók L. Role of bile in detoxification of lipopolysaccharide. In: Schlessinger D editor. Microbiology. Washington: American Society for Microbiology,1980;91–3.
7. Berczi I, Bertók L, Bereznay T. Comparative studies on the toxicity of E.coli lipopolysaccharide endotoxin in various animal species. Can J Microbiol 1966;12:1070–1071.
8. Bertók L, Kocsár L. Die Rolle des Endotoxins beim intestinalen Syndrom der Strahlenkrankheit. Wiss Z Karl Marx Univ Math Naturwiss 1974;23:65–66.
9. Rudbach JA, Anacker RL, Haskins WT, Johnson AG, Milner KC, Ribi E. Physical aspects of reversible inactivation of endotoxin. Ann N Y Acad Sci 1966;133(8):629–635.
10. Mouwen JM, Schotman AJ, Wensing T, Kijkuit CJ. Some biochemical aspects of white scours in piglets. Tijdschr Diergeneeskd 1972;97(2):65–72.
11. Bertók L. Role of endotoxins in E.coli induced pathological processes. (Hungarian) Magy Állatorv Lapja 1998;120:668–672.
12. Bertók L. Role of endotoxins and bile acids in the pathogenesis of septic circulatory shock. Acta Chir Hung 1997;36:33–36.
13. Bertók L, Tóth B. Studies on the pathogenesis of the edema disease of swine. I. the effect of the purified lipopolysaccharide endotoxin of Escherichia coli on mice. Acta Vet Acad Sci Hung 1963;13:421–428.
14. Westphal O, Lüderitz O, Bister F. Über die Extraction von Bacterien mit Phenolwasser. Z Naturforsh 1952;7b:148–155.
15. Rietschel ET, Brade H, Holst O, Müller-Loennies S, Mamat U, Zähringer U, Beckmann F, Seydel U, Brandenburg K, Ulmer AJ, Mattern T, Heine H, Schletter J, Loppnow H, Schönbeck U, Flad HD, Hauschildt S, Schade UF, Padova FD, Kusumoto S, Schumann RR. Bacterial Endotoxin: Chemical constitution, biological recognition, host response, and immunological detoxification. In: Rietschel ET, Wagner H editors. Pathology of septic shock. Current Topics in Microbiology and Immunology, Berlin: Springer-Verlag, 1996;216:40–81.

16. Kocsár LT, Bertók L, Várterész V. Effect of bile acids on the intestinal absorption of endotoxin in rats. J Bacteriol 1969;100(1):220–223.
17. Kocsár L, Bertók L, Várterész V. Function of bile acids in the intestinal absorption of endotoxin in rats. Ann Immunol Hung 1974;17:49–52.
18. Kocsár L, Bertók L, Varga L. Double labeling of endotoxin with chromium and tritium. Ann Immunol Hung 1973;17:71–72.
19. Selye H, Tuchweber B, Bertók L. Effect of lead-acetate on the susceptibility of rats to bacterial endotoxins. J Bacteriol 1966;91:884–890.
20. Bailey ME. Endotoxin, bile salts and renal function in obstructive jaundice. Brit J Surg 1976;63:774–781.
21. Cahill CJ. Prevention of postoperative renal failure in patients with obstructive jaundice - role of bile salts. Brit J Surg 1983;70:590–595.
22. Gaffin SL. Control of septic shock - present day concept. S A J Hosp Med 1982;40: 118–124.
23. Dimond T, Parks W. Perioperative management of obstuctive jaundice. Br J Surg 1997;84: 147–149.
24. Kisida E, Hegedüs Z, Bertók L, et al. Prevention of the postoperative hepatorenal syndrome by means of bile acid (preliminary report) (Hungarian). Magy Seb 1996;49:1–7.
25. Bertok L. Effect of bile acids on endotoxin in vitro and in vivo (physico-chemical defense). Bile deficiency and endotoxin translocation. Ann N Y Acad Sci 1998;851:408–410.
26. Bertók L, Kocsár L. Studies on some biological properties of surfactant treated endotoxin in rats. Ann Immunol Hung 1972;16:77–81.
27. Kocsár L, Bertók L, Várterész V et al. Produce for the production of ionizing radiation-activated bile acid content preparation for the treatment of entero toxemias of newborns (Hungarian). Budapest: Hungarian Patent 162.789/A-61-k-27/02,17/00. 1973.
28. Bertók L. A new possibility for the increase of natural immunity (nonspecific resistance): the radiodetoxified endotoxin (Hungarian). Orv Hetil 1999;140:819–827.
29. Kohoe M, Sellwood R, Shipley P, et al. Genetic analysis of K88-mediated adhesion of enterotoxigenic Esherichia coli. Nature 1981;291:122–128.
30. Nagy B. Pathology and specific prevention of enteral infections of calves and piglets [Doct Thesis Hung Acad Sci]. (Hungarian). Budapest;1992.
31. Bertók L. Physico-chemical defense of vertebrate organisms: the role of bile acids in defense against bacterial endotoxins. Perspect Biol Med 1977;21:70–76.
32. Bertók L. Physico-chemical defense system (Hungarian). Biológia 1977;25:127–134.
33. Karika G, Bertók L, Kisida E. Effect of bile deficiency on the survival of rats in the shock induced by occlusion of arteria mesenterica cranialis (Hungarian). Magy Seb 1978;31: 164–166.
34. Karika G. Role of bile acids in the endotoxemia abdominal catastrophies [PhD Thesis Hung Acad Sci]. (Hungarian). Budapest;1981.
35. Karika G, Fehér T, Bertók L. Change of the bile production in the experimental mesenteric occlusion of rats (Hungarian). Kísérl Orvostud 1980;32:221–224.
36. Karika G, Bertók L, Kisida E, et al. Effect of bile acid treatment in the shock of dogs induced by the occlusion of arteria mesenterica superior (cranialis) (Hungarian). Kísérl Orvostud 1978;30:491–493.
37. Karika G, Bertók L, Kisida E. Effect of intraluminally given bile on the survival of rats in the strangulated ileus (Hungarian). Magy Seb 1978;31:355–357.
38. Theiler M. Action of sodium deoxycholate on arthropod borne viruses. Proc Soc Ex Biol

Med 1957; 96:380–388.
39. Bertók L. Role of endotoxins and bile acids in the pathogenesis of septic circulatory shock. Acta Chirurg Hung 1997;36:33–36.
40. Dobozy A, Horváth A, Hunyadi J, et al. Dermatology (Hungarian). Budapest: Eklektikon Kiadó; 1998.
41. Belew PW, Rosenberg EW, Skinner RB jr, et al. Endotoxemia in psoriasis. Arch Dermatol 1982;118:142–143.
42. Gyurcsovics K, Bertók L. Role of bile acids in the pathogenesis and therapy of psoriasis (Hungarian). Orv Hetil 2000;141:915–917.
43. Szaniszló F, Bertók L. Demonstration of endotoxaemia in case of hyperacute parvoviral enteritis in dogs (Hungarian). Magy Állatorv L 1990;45:109–112.
44. Bertók L Jr, Sztanyik LB, Bertók L. Possible role of bile deficiency in the development of intestinal syndrome of acute radiation disease. Acta Physiol Hung 1992;79:29–32.
45. Haslewood GAD. The biological importance of bile salts. Amsterdam: North-Holland Publishing Company; 1978.
46. Munford RS, Hall CL. Purification of acyloxyacyl hydrolase, a leukocyte enzyme that removes secondary acyl chains from bacterial lipopolysaccharides. J Biol Chem 1989;264(26):15613–15619.
47. Bertók L. Endotoxins and endocrine system. Domest Anim Endocrinol 1998;15:305–8.
48. Horváth A, Bertók L, Horváth I, Lapis K, Hortoványi E, Hársing J, Kocsis I, Bozóky Z, Greskovits D. Additional data on antigen use for immunisation against atherosclerosis (in press).
49. Havel RJ. Role of the liver in atherosclerosis. Arteriosclerosis 1985;5:569–580.
50. Liao W. Endotoxin: possible roles in initiation and development of arterosclerosis. J Lab Klin Med. 1996;128:452–460.
51. Liao W, Florén CH. Hyperlipidemic response to endotoxin. A part of the host-defense mechanism. Scand J Infect Dis 1993;25(6):675–682.
52. Chawla A, Saez E, Evans RM. Don't know much bile-ology. Cell 2000;103:1–4.
53. Cerwinka WH, Cheema MH, Granger DN. Hypercholesterolemia alters endotoxin-induced endothelial cell adhesion molecule expression. Shock 2001;16:44–50.
54. Charach G, Rabinovich PD, Konikoff FM, Grosskopf I, Weintraub MS, Gilat T. Decreased fecal bile acid output in patients with coronary atherosclerosis. J Med 1998;29:125–136.
55. Kalayoglu MV, Indrawati, Morrison RP, Morrison SG, Yuan Y, Byrne GI. Chlamydial virulence determinants in atherogenesis: the role of chlamydial lipopolysaccharide and heat shock protein 60 in macrophage-lipoprotein interactions. J Infect Dis 2000;181 Suppl 3: S483–489.
56. Moseley RH. Bile-ology. Gastroenterology 2001;121:218–220.
57. Saikku P. Chlamydia pneumoniae in atherosclerosis. J Intern Med 2000;247:391–396.
58. Wiedermann CJ, Kiechl S, Dunzendorfer S, Schratzberger P, Egger G, Oberhollenzer F, et al. Association of endotoxemia with carotid atherosclerosis and cardiovascular disease: prospective results from the Bruneck Study. J Am Coll Cardiol 1999;34:1975–1981.
59. Wiedermann CJ, Kiechl S, Schratzberger P, Dunzendorfer S, Weiss G, Willeit J. The role of immune activation in endotoxin-induced atherogenesis. J Endotoxin Res 2001;7: 322–326.
60. Wiedermann CJ, Kiechl S, Willeit J. Is endotoxemia a risk factor for atherosclerosis? Wien Klin Wochenschr 2001;113:77–79.

III. THE NATURAL IMMUNE SYSTEM

Natural Immunity
Edited by L. Bertók and D.A. Chow

© 2005 Elsevier B.V. All rights reserved

A Historical Introduction of Natural Killer (NK) Cells and Current Status of Their Role in Host Defences

RONALD B. HERBERMAN

University of Pittsburgh Cancer Institute, Department of Medicine and Pathology, University of Pittsburgh School of Medicine, Pittsburgh, PA 15232, USA

ABSTRACT

Natural killer (NK) cells are a major component of the immune system, which can play an important role in host defences against cancer and microbial infections. Their identification, characterization, elucidation of how they function and are regulated, exploration of their biological roles have all occurred during the past 30 years. NK cells have been found to be distinct from T or B lymphocytes, have a characteristic morphology of large granular lymphocytes, and can be readily identified by characteristic cell surface molecules. The hallmark of their function is the spontaneous ability to reorganize and rapidly kill a wide array of tumour cells and also virus-infected normal cells. In addition, their cytotoxic activity can be strongly augmented by interferon, interleukin-2, and other cytotkines. NK cells not only respond to various cytokines, but are also major producers of some cytokines, especially interferon gamma. NK cells have been found to play a major role in host resistance against tumour growth and to be particularly effective in resistance against metastatic spread of tumours. Their potential to inhibit tumour growth has led to an increasing interest in exploring the therapeutic effects of activated NK cells against various types of cancer.

1. INITIAL IDENTIFICATION AND CHARACTERIZATION OF NK CELLS

Natural killer (NK) cells are widely recognized as a major component of the immune system, which, in addition to specifically immune T cells, can play an important role in host defences against cancer and microbial infections. However, the recognition of the existence of NK cells and their extensive characterization has unfolded only during the past 30 years.

In the early 1970s, many tumour immunologists began to examine the ability of lymphocytes from tumour immune or tumour-bearing individuals to kill tumour cells *in vitro*. These studies were initially performed within the paradigm of expecting that specifically immune T cells, reactive against tumour associated antigens, would be detected. In parallel, studies were performed with lymphocytes of cancer patients, mainly in colony inhibition or microcytotoxicity assays, and with lymphocytes from tumour immunized mice or rats, mainly by the then recently developed assay of ^{51}Cr release. In most of these studies, lymphocytes from normal individuals were included as controls, presumed to set the baseline against which the levels of cytotoxic reactivity of specifically immune T cells might be quantitatively assessed. However, in a variety of instances, the ability of lymphocytes of normal individuals was found to be as high as or even higher than that of lymphocytes from tumour-immunized or tumour-bearing individuals [1–10]. For example, the very first report of such observations may have been in a study of anti-leukaemia reactivity of human twins [1], in which not only the normal twin but also some normal adults were found to be able to kill leukaemic blast cells. Since such results were unexpected and did not fit the existing paradigm, the killing of tumour cells by lymphocytes from some normal individuals was mainly attributed to technical problems in the assays and a workshop was even held by the National Cancer Institute in 1972 [11] to discuss the issue. However, over the next 3–4 years, it became increasingly clear that the ability of some lymphocytes from normal individuals to kill tumour cells was a valid aspect of the tumour immunobiology of a variety of mammalian species, including humans [1–4], rats [5,6] and mice [7–10].

Once the existence of natural cell-mediated immunity began to be appreciated, considerable efforts were expended to determine the characteristics of the reactive lymphocytes [reviewed in 12]. It was almost immediately clear that the normal lymphocytes responsible for the anti-tumour activity were not typical T cells, since nude, athymic mice had high levels of natural cell-medicated cytotoxic reactively. In fact, the initial characterization of the effector cells was one of exclusions, with the conclusion that they lacked the characteristic features of T cells, B cells, macrophages or polymorphonuclear neutrophils. Rather, the natural reactivity against tumours seemed attributable to a particular subpopulation of lymphoid cells that have been termed NK cells. The existence of NK cells rapidly attracted considerable attention by many immunologists and much of their early observations are summarized in two extensive books [13,14] and various reviews [e.g., 12,15].

2. CHARACTERISTICS OF NK CELLS

A major advance in the characterization of NK cells came from the observation that both human and rat NK activity was attributable to lymphocytes with a distinct morphology, termed large granular lymphocytes (LGL) [16,17]. LGL comprise about 5% of the peripheral blood or splenic leukocytes in man and other species and can be readily identified morphologically. They can be highly enriched by centrifugation on density gradients of Percoll [16,17]. The availability of such highly purified effector cell populations quickly led to the identification of distinct cell surface molecules on NK cells. Human NK cells can now be readily identified and quantitated among peripheral blood mononuclear cells, by flow cytometry, as $CD3^-CD56^+$ cells [18]. Similarly, rat NK cells are now mainly characterized by the presence of NKR.P1 [19] and mouse NK cells by the presence of NK1 [20], which is the mouse equivalent of NKR.P1.

The hallmark function of NK cells is their ability to spontaneously and rapidly kill a variety of tumour cells, especially leukaemia cells and certain tumour cell lines. Although most carcinomas and cell lines derived from solid tumours are resistant to ^{51}Cr release cytotoxicity, which has been related to perforin-mediated damage, Vujanovic et al. [21] have recently found that such tumour cells undergo apoptotic cell death upon interaction with human NK cells. The NK cell is a quite selective killer, which does not harm normal "self" but can eliminate a wide range of NK–susceptible target cells, which include virus-infected normal cells as well as other tumour cells, without the need for antigen processing or presentation by major histocompatibility complex (MHC) molecules as is the case for cytotoxic T cells [22].

The basis for the selective target cell repertoire of NK cells is not completely understood.

It has been thought that NK cell-mediated killing is not MHC-restricted, but this concept has been challenged recently [23]. Moretta and colleagues have provided evidence that NK cells show alloantigen specificity and that it is possible to define distinct alloantigen-reactive clones of NK cells [24]. Thus, receptors specific for alloantigens encoded by the HLA-C or a closely linked gene are thought to be present on NK cells [24]. The role of the MHC class I complex in the susceptibility of targets to NK-mediated lysis has been controversial. Transfection of MHC-deficient tumour cells with the MHC class I gene confers resistance to lysis by NK cells [25], and this resistance has been mapped to the α_1 and α_2 domains of HLA-A2 molecules [26]. It thus appears that expression of class I MHC molecules on target cells confers protection against NK cell lysis, while the absence of MHC molecules enhances susceptibility to lysis, as if NK cells were able to sense this absence ("missing-self hypothesis"). The possibility that a negative signal is delivered to NK cells by class 1 MHC molecules or MHC-associated ligands, inducing protection from NK-mediated lysis, provides an explanation of why NK cells are not harmful to self targets (i.e., normal tissue cells) and is consistent with the presence of alloantigen receptors on NK cells.

3. REGULATION OF NK ACTIVITY

In addition to the spontaneous cytotoxic activity of NK cells, NK cells have been found to be highly responsive to various upregulatory signals either *in vivo* or *in vitro* [27]. When recombinant cytokine molecules became available, it was possible to demonstrate that NK cells become rapidly activated by interferons, interleukin (IL)-2, IL-12, IL-15, and IL-18 [28,29]. Although IL-2 was initially thought to induce a novel category of highly active anti-tumour cytotoxic lymphocytes, termed lymphokine-activated killer (LAK) cells, it soon became clear that most LAK activity was attributable to IL-2-activiated NK cells [30]. Among lymphocytes, NK cells are the first to respond to activation by IL-2 and possibly other signals. In response to IL-2, a small subset of NK cells (10–30%) rapidly acquire the ability to adhere to plastic or other solid surfaces [31] and upregulate surface expression of IL-2R and other activation antigens as well as expression of mRNA for a variety of cytokines [32]. Vujanovic, et al. have named these cells A-NK cells, A for the adherence and activation that characterize this early response to IL-2 [31]. While all NK cells undergo activation and expansion in the presence of IL-2 and/or other cytokines, A-NK cells proliferate significantly better than nonadherent NK cells, perhaps because they receive a double stimulatory signal, i.e., IL-2 and adherence to plastic, and achieve very high levels of antitumour activity *in vitro* [31].

Activated NK cells produce a spectrum of cytokines [33]. This ability of NK cells to produce haematopoietic cell growth factors, interferons, interleukins, tumour necrosis factors α and β, transforming growth factor, and other growth factors coupled with their ability to respond rapidly to exogenous signals by upregulating mRNA production for various cytokines within minutes and increasing migration to tissue sites, is responsible for the importance of the NK cell as a mediator or effector of the intercellular communication network. Upon activation, NK cells also express and upregulate the receptors for a variety of chemotactic factors, cytokines, growth factors, and hormones, including neuropeptides, which allows them to remain responsive to signals generated not only within the immune system but also elsewhere in the body. NK cells are also capable of producing many enzymes, some of which are associated with the cellular membrane and are likely involved in cell-to-cell interactions; others, which are intracellular, may be released during NK cell-mediated lysis. Overall, the NK cell has the potential to register changes rapidly and respond spontaneously to signals generated in its immediate environment or at distant locations in the body without a need for antigen presensitization.

The interactions of NK cells with Ig, mediated by the FcR, probably play a crucial role in regulation of NK cell functions. Both stimulatory and inhibitory signals can be received and transduced via the FcγRIIIs [34,35], depending on whether monomeric, cross-linked or antigen-complexed IgG molecules are involved, and the intracellular pathways engaged in processing and directing these signals have been intensely investigated [36]. The possibility that different types of FcRs expressed on NK cells cooperate with each other as well as with other receptors on NK cells in the handling of exogenous signals has to be considered as one explanation for the cells ability to channel various stimuli into a response which best reflects the requirements imposed by its external microenvironment. The ability of NK cells to produce IFNγ in response to IL-2 or viral challenge [32] is important in host defence against infectious agents. In the presence of target-bound antibodies, especially those of the IgG3 isotype, expression of FcR on the NK cell surface provides it with an additional opportunity for binding to the target and initiating the lytic process, which is referred to as antibody-dependent cell-mediated cytotoxicity (ADCC).

The majority of circulating and tissue NK cells in healthy humans are in a resting state, i.e., they are not in cycle or proliferating. However, these resting NK cells are prepared to respond immediately to signals and thus are remarkably well suited to mediate the first line of defence against various pathogens [37,22]. While this swift responsiveness to antigen-independent stimuli is advantageous for the effector cell, it also requires a regulatory "check and balance" system. The functions of NK cells have to be carefully regulated because of the potential for inappropriate cytokine release or damage to normal cells or tissues. Both autocrine and paracrine types of regulatory mechanisms are probably involved, and the functions of NK cells may be controlled at the level of development, differentiation, activation, and availability of NK cells in the microenvironment as well as via the modulatory influences of other mononuclear cells [38].

The presence of NK cells at the site of tissue injury is a function of their availability, i.e., the number in the environment and the ability to proliferate and migrate. The latter is clearly determined by cytokines and chemotactic factors produced locally [reviewed in 39].

A number of cytokines and various subsets of mononuclear cells, as well as other cells present in a particular tissue environment modulate NK functions. *In vivo*, NK cell development, growth, activation, and proliferation may be orchestrated by events, which occur at a particular tissue site. The ability of NK cells to promptly and efficiently respond to such events qualifies them as excellent mediators of regulatory and defence mechanisms.

4. ROLE OF NK CELLS IN HOST DEFENSE AGAINST DISEASE

A particular, ongoing interest in NK cells, in addition to their intrinsic immunobiologic characteristics and functions, has been related to their potential roles in resistance to cancer and other diseases. As summarized below, and in large part reviewed previously [40], there has been mounting evidence that NK cells may be quite important in defence against disease.

4.1. Role in resistance against tumour cell lines

The initial focus of *in vivo* studies was to explore the role of NK cells in resistance against established cell lines of tumours *in vivo*, particularly those that show susceptibility to cytolysis by NK cells *in vitro*. A major approach has been to look for correlations between resistance to the growth of the tumour cell lines *in vivo* and the levels of NK activity in the recipients. In several different situations, a good correlation was observed. The various types of correlations between NK activity and antitumour resistance have only been observed with tumour lines with some susceptibility to lysis by NK cells. The growth of NK-resistant tumours has not been affected by the levels of NK activity in the recipients.

Beige mice have low NK activity, due to a recessive point mutation and have also provided a convenient model for examining the role of NK cells in resistance to growth of transplantable tumour lines. Several NK-susceptible syngeneic tumours have been shown to produce a higher incidence of tumours and particularly of metastases in beige than in normal heterozygous littermates.

Another approach to the role of NK cells *in vivo* in the growth of transplantable tumours has been the attempt to transfer increased resistance by NK cell-enriched populations. Mixture of such cells with an NK-sensitive tumour resulted in reduced tumour incidence after transplantation. Systemic adoptive transfer of cells with the characteristics of NK cells from normal or nude mice was also found, in an immunochemotherapy model system, to increase protection against a transplantable leukaemia.

In an alternative approach that used information about selective markers on mouse NK cells, nude mice treated with anti-asialo GM1 (an antibody against a glycolipid which has selective reactivity against NK cells) had almost no detectable NK activity and showed increased susceptibility to transplantation of syngeneic, allogeneic and human tumours. Similarly, treatment of mice with anti-NK 1.1, an alloantibody with some specificity for NK cells, resulted in increased growth of a transplanted syngeneic tumour cell line.

The transfer of increased antitumour resistance with cell populations enriched in NK cells, and the inhibition of antitumour resistance by antisera reactive with NK cells, are quite supportive to the contention that NK cells play a key role in the limitation of growth of transplanted NK-susceptible tumour cell lines.

To obtain more direct information about the role of NK cells in the direct and rapid elimination of tumour cells *in vivo*, [^{125}I]-deoxyuridine (^{125}IUdR)-labelled tumour cells were inoculated intravenously and clearance from the lungs and other organs was measured [41,42]. In mice with high NK activity, there was a greater clearance of radioactivity when measured at 2–4 hours after inoculation than seen in mice with low reactivity.

As further confirmation of the role of NK cells in resistance to growth of NK-susceptible transplantable tumours, transfer of NK cell-containing populations into mice with cyclophosphamide-induced depression of NK activity was shown to restore significantly both tumour clearance and NK reactivity [43]. The effectiveness of the transfer correlated with the levels of NK activity of donor cells in a variety of situations. As more conclusive evidence for the key role of NK cells, it was shown that highly purified populations of LGL could significantly restore clearance and NK activity in rats, which had been pretreated with anti-asialo GM1 [44]. Thus, it appears that NK cells alone, without the need for other accessory cells, can effectively transfer the ability to rapidly eliminate radiolabelled tumour cells.

A similar pattern of results was obtained when radiolabelled cells were inoculated subcutaneously into the footpads of mice [45]. Clearance correlated in several ways with the levels of NK activity in the recipients and cells with the characteristics of NK cells were effective in local adoptive transfer.

The results with the footpad assay and the various demonstrations of NK-related differences in outgrowth of subcutaneous tumours indicate that natural effector cells can enter and be active at sites of local tumour growth. Thus, NK cells have the potential to be involved in the primary line of defence against the local outgrowth of transplanted tumours. However, it appears that the effectiveness of this natural resistance mechanism is rather limited. Even with tumour cells that are highly susceptible to NK activity, development of progressively growing tumours can occur in animals with high NK activity.

4.2. Role in resistance against metastases

Effective control of tumour metastases is the central current issue in clinical oncology. There are increasing indications that NK cells may play a major role in host resistance against metastasis. The above-described ability of NK cells to rapidly eliminate intravenously-inoculated tumour cells might provide a very effective control of haematogenous spread of tumours. Experimental support for this possibility first came from the finding that cells from lung metastases of a transplantable tumour in mice were more resistant to NK activity than locally growing tumour cells [46]. Metastatic tumour cells might represent those, which evaded elimination by relative resistance to NK activity. This posibility was supported by the demonstration that selection of NK-resistant variant tumour cells *in vitro* was accompanied by an increase in the metastatic capability of such cells in syngeneic hosts [47].

An important role of NK cells in resistance against metastatic growth of transplantable tumours was further supported by observations that suppression or augmentation of NK activity of mice was associated with parallel alterations in resistance to artificial metastases produced by intravenous inoculation of tumour cells [48]. In addition, nude mice, which have elevated levels of NK activity, were found to have increased resistance to lung metastases, whereas beige mice, with deficient NK activity, developed increased numbers of lung metastases [49].

The ability to selectively depress NK activity by administration of anti-asialo GM1 *in vivo* has provided a good opportunity to evaluate in detail the role of NK cells in control of metastases. Gorelik, et al. [49] showed that mice treated with this antiserum developed increased numbers of pulmonary metastases after intravenous inoculation of either B16 melanoma or Lewis lung carcinoma cells. In addition, the treated mice also developed many metastases in the liver, an organ, which previously showed completely resistance to the metastatic spread of these tumour lines.

By varying the time of inoculation of anti-asialo GM1 in relation to tumour challenge, it has been possible to gain some insight into the period of effective NK cell-mediated resistance to metastases [49]. The most dramatic increases in metastases have been seen in mice treated with antiserum prior to tumour challenge. In contrast, administration of anti-asialo GM1 at one or three days following tumour challenge had little or no effect on the number of metastases that developed. Therefore, it appeared that NK cells primarily influence metastatic spread of tumours by acting during the phase of haematogenous dissemination, presumably by their ability to directly eliminate the tumour cells from the circulation or capillary beds. Once invasion of tumour cells into the parenchyma of the lungs or other organs has occurred, NK cells, at least without stimulation of their activity, would seem to have less or no influence on the growth of the tumour colonies.

A limitation to the conclusions to be drawn from experiments with anti-asialo GM1 was the possibility that the treatment also affected other effector mechanisms. Therefore, experiments were performed in rats treated with anti-asialo GM1, in which the depressed NK activity could be partially restored by adoptive transfer of highly purified LGL [50]. This selective restoration of NK activity was accompanied by increased resistance to pulmonary metastases from a transplantable tumour cell line [51].

In contrast to the rather extensive evidence in experimental animal tumour models for an important role of NK cells in resisting the metastatic spread of tumour cells, there is a paucity of analogous information in cancer patients. However, the few relevant reports have been in concert with the animal tumour data. Pross and Lotzova [52] summarized results of studies of levels of NK activity in the blood of treated cancer patients who were free of detectable disease, who were then followed for possible development of distant metastases. A significant correlation between low NK activity and subsequent recurrence of disease was observed in several studies. Similarly, Schantz and Goephart [53] found that low NK activity at the time of surgical removal of squamous cell carcinoma of the head or neck was significantly correlated with subsequent development of distant metastases.

Taken together, the available evidence strongly suggests that NK cells play a major role in resistance against metastatic spread of tumours. The presence of NK cells in the blood, with spontaneous cytotoxic reactivity which can be rapidly augmented, may allow them to be particularly effective in eliminating most, if not all, tumour cells which seed into the circulation. Therefore, development of agents and protocols, which can induce sustained augmentation of NK activity may be expected to lead to more effective prevention and control of metastatic dissemination of tumours.

4.3. Role in immune surveillance against tumours

Of paramount interest is whether NK cells may be involved in immune surveillance against the initial development of spontaneous or carcinogen-induced tumours. There are several pieces of circumstantial evidence that are consistent with, or suggestive of, a role for NK cells:

a) Patients with the genetically determined Chediak-Higashi syndrome have a high risk of development of lymphoproliferative disease [54]. In detailed studies on several patients with this disease, all were found to have profound deficits in NK and K-cell activities, whereas a variety of other immune functions, including cytotoxicity against tumour cells by T cells, monocytes and granulocytes, was essentially normal.
b) Similarly, beige mice, which have an analogous genetic defect, also have a substantial [55], but incomplete [56], selective deficiency in NK activity. Aged beige mice have been reported to have a high incidence of lymphomas and heterozygous mice without the beige phenotype had a lower incidence [57].
c) Another human genetic abnormality, X-linked lymphoproliferative disease, has been associated with a defect in the ability to control proliferation of B cells infected with Epstein-Barr virus (EBV). Low NK activity has been found in such individuals and this deficit has been suggested to be involved in the pathogenesis of the disease [58]. In support of this possibility, cells with the characteristics of NK cells have been found to inhibit the proliferation of autologous EBV-infected B cells *in vitro* [59].
d) Patients on immunosuppressive therapy after kidney allotransplants have a high risk of developing tumours, both haematologic malignancies and a variety of carcinomas. Patients on such treatment regimens have been found to have very low NK activity and this has been suggested as a contributing factor to the subsequent development of tumours [60].
e) Patients with paroxysmal nocturnal haemaglobinuria also have a high risk of developing leukaemia and have been reported to have deficient NK activity [61]
f) A large prospective study has recently been reported [62], in which the residents in a Japanese city were tested for their levels of NK activity. During the following 15 years, individuals with initially low NK activity were found to have a significantly increased incidence of cancer.

4.4. Role in natural resistance against microbial infections

There have been increasing numbers of suggestions that NK cells may play some role in resistance against microbial infections. Most of the studies have been related to viruses [63], with several investigators showing that cells infected by a variety of viruses become considerably more sensitive to lysis by NK cells [64,65] and persistently virus-infected tumour cells grow poorly in nude mice, apparently as a result of interferon induction and reactivity by NK cells [64]. Furthermore, resistance to infection by several types of viruses *in vivo* has been found to correlate with NK activity. There is considerable evidence for a role of NK cells in genetic resistance of mice to severe infection by herpes simplex virus type I [66]. A correlation has also been found between susceptibility to severe herpesvirus infections in patients and low NK activity against virus-infected target cells [67]. It also seems likely that NK cells play an important role in natural resistance to infection by mouse cytomegalovirus [68].

NK cells may also be involved in resistance against some other types of microbial infections. A correlation has been observed between NK activity and resistance of mice to the malarial parasite *Babesia microti* [69]. Beige mice were highly susceptible to infection whereas heterozygous normal mice were resistant. There has also been some suggestive evidence for a role of NK cells in infection by *Trypanosoma cruzi* and this parasite has been shown to be susceptible to cytotoxicity by NK cells *in vitro* [70]. There is evidence that NK cells participate in eliminating tissue cells infected by mycoplasma or bacteria [71]. NK cells also participate in regulatory interactions between immune cells and nonimmune cells. For example, NK cells are capable of directly upregulating polymorphonuclear leukocytes to kill *Candida albicans* [71]. NK cells produce neutrophil-activating factors, which allow polymorphonuclear leukocytes to more effectively kill *C. albicans* and possibly other infectious organisms [71]. NK cells may also play a role in natural resistance of mice to infection by the fungus *Cryptococcus neoformans* [72].

5. NK CELLS IN THERAPY OF CANCER

From the evidence reviewed above, indicating that chronically low levels of NK activity or numbers in patients with cancer or other diseases may be associated with more severe symptoms or increased risk of disease progression, one might infer that augmentation of NK activity in disease may be of benefit to the patient. Therapy aimed at augmenting NK activity could be particularly advantageous for patients with cancer or immunodeficiencies. Such therapy is available today, and it generally consists of attempts to increase NK activity *in vivo* by the administration of agents with known NK-potentiating activity or adoptive transfer of activated autologous NK cells either locally or systemically to patients deficient in NK activity.

A variety of agents, generally referred to as biologic response modifiers (BRMs), are known to increase the activation, proliferation, or cytotoxicity of existing NK cells; other BRMs promote NK cell extravasation and accumulation in tissues, e.g., lung and liver, resulting in higher local cytotoxic activity. A partial list of commonly used BRMs includes a spectrum of cytokines such as interferons, IL-2 and IL-12; bacterial products such as OK432 (picibanil); plant lectins such as lentinan; monoclonal antibodies (Mabs) that bind to triggering structures on NK cells (e.g., anti-CD16 Mab); and interferon inducers such as polyribonucleotides. The effects of BRMs, especially cytokines, on signal transduction in NK cells, their mobility in tissues or ECM, and their ability to lyse tumour cells or virally infected targets are under intense investigation at this time.

Among the best-known activators of NK cells are IL-2 and IFNα [28,73]. These two cytokines have been used extensively not only for patients with malignancies but also for those with viral infections. For example, IFNα has been therapeutically effective in a proportion of patients with chronic hepatitis B infection [74], and patients with human immunodeficiency virus have received systemic IL-2 therapy in combination with zidovudine [75]. For patients with advanced malignancies unresponsive to other treatments, both IL-2 and IFNα therapies have resulted in a low frequency of durable responses [76,77]. Systemic or locoregional therapy with IL-2, even at low or moderate doses, leads to well-documented increases in the number of circulating NK cells and NK activity [78]. Although the extent of this IL-2-induced stimulation of NK activity *in vivo* could not be directly linked to clinical response, it may be at least partly responsible for the antitumour effectiveness of cytokine-based immunotherapy.

Immunotherapy with adoptively transferred activated NK cells and cytokines has been used mainly for patients with advanced malignancies in the hope of capitalizing on the well-documented antimetastatic activity of NK cells. The earliest clinical trials were performed with LAK cells and high-dose IL-2 in patients with metastatic melanoma or renal cell carcinoma [79]. The results of these trials have been only mildly encouraging in that the rate of objective clinical responses achieved was about 20–30% [79]. However, it is important to note that these responses, some of long duration (>2 years), were achieved in patients with metastatic diseases unresponsive to conventional therapies. The LAK cells for the adoptive cellular therapy were autologous and mainly contained IL-2-activated NK cells [29]. More recently, clinical trials with purified NK cells, selected and expanded *in vitro* from patients' PBMNC, have been done on the hypothesis that transfer of a selected subset of highly activated antitumour effector cells may be therapeutically more effective and require fewer cells and possibly lower doses of cytokines to support their viability and *in vivo* activity. The results of two preliminary phase I trials with patients with metastatic melanoma or renal cell carcinoma demonstrated that immunotherapy with selected, highly purified, and *in vitro*-expanded subsets of NK cells is feasible, well tolerated and, in some cases, effective for metastatic disease [80,81].

Increasingly often, bone marrow transplantation or peripheral stem cell transfer has been used for the treatment of malignancies. The transfer of activated NK cells after transplantation is based on the rationale that NK cells have potent antitumour effects and thus can help eliminate minimal residual disease. Purified and activated human NK cells have been used for the therapy of patients with cancer after high-dose chemotherapy and peripheral blood stem cell transplantation [82]. Preliminary results from clinical trials evaluating this therapy suggest that systemic transfer of A-NK cells plus IL-2 within 2–3 days after peripheral blood stem cell transplantation may not only help eliminate minimal residual disease, but facilitate haematopoietic recovery [82].

While both *in vivo* augmentation of NK activity with BRMs and adoptive transfer of activated NK cells are promising new therapies, additional clinical and basic studies are needed to build on the progress achieved to date and to acquire a better understanding of the interactions between activated NK cells and their targets *in vivo*.

REFERENCES

1. Rosenberg EB, Herberman RB, Levine PH, Halterman RH, McCoy JL, Wunderlich, JR. Lymphocyte cytotoxicity reactions to leukemia-associated antigens in identical twins. Int J Cancer 1972;9:648–58.

2. Oldham RK, Siwarski D, McCoy JL, Plata EJ Herberman RB. Evaluation of a cell-mediated cytotoxicity assay utilizing ^{125}iododeoxyuridine labeled tissue culture target cells. Natl Cancer Inst Monogr 1973;37:49–58.
3. Takasugi M, Mickey JR, Terasaki PI. Reactivity of lymphocytes from normal persons on cultured tumor cells. Cancer Res 1973;33:2898–902.
4. Rosenberg EB, McCoy JL, Green SS, Donnelly FC, Siwarski DF, Levine PH, Herberman RB. Destruction of human lymphoid tissue culture cell lines by human peripheral lymphocytes in ^{51}Cr-release cellular cytotoxicity assays. J. Natl Cancer Inst 1974;52: 345–52.
5. Holtermann OA, Klein E, Casale GP. Selective cytotoxicity of peritoneal leucocytes for neoplastic cells. Cell Immunol 1973;9:339–52.
6. Nunn JE, Djeu JY, Glaser M, Lavrin DH, Herberman RB. Natural cytotoxic reactivity of rat lymphocytes against syngeneic Gross virus-induced lymphoma. J Natl Cancer Inst 1976;56:393–9.
7. Herberman RB, Nunn ME, Lavrin DH, Asofsky R. Effect of antibody to antigen on cell-mediated immunity induced in syngeneic mice by murine sarcoma virus. J Natl Cancer Inst 1973;51:1509–12.
8. Herberman RB, Ting CC, Kirchner H, Holden H, Glaser M, Bonnard GD, et al. Effector mechanisms in tumour immunity. In: Brent, L and Holorow, J , editors. Prog Immunol Int Congr Immunol, 2nd 1974 Vol. 3 Amsterdam:North-Holland Publishing Co. 1974;285–95.
9. Herberman, RB, Nunn, ME and Lavrin, DH. Natural cytotoxic reactivity of mouse lymphoid cells against syngeneic and allogeneic tumors I. Distribution of reactivity and specificity. Int J Cancer 1975;16:216–29.
10. Kiessling R, Klein E, Wigzell H. "Natural" killer cells in the mouse. II. Cytotoxic cells with specificity for mouse Moloney leukemia cells. Characteristics of the killer cell. Eur J Immunol 1975;5:112–7.
11. Herberman RB, Gaylord CE. Conference and workshop on cellular immune reactions to human tumor-associated antigens. Natl Cancer Inst Monogr 1973;37:1–221.
12. Herberman RB, Holden HT. Natural cell-mediated immunity. Adv Cancer Res 1978;27: 305–77.
13. Herberman RB. Natural Cell-Mediated Immunity Against Tumors New York:Academic Press 1980.
14. Herberman RB. Natural Killer Cells and Other Natural Effector Cells. New York:Academic Press, 1982.
15. Herberman RB, Ortaldo JR. Natural killer cells: their role in defenses against disease Science 1981;214:24–30.
16. Timonen T, Ortaldo JR, Herberman RB. Characteristics of human large granular lymphocytes and relationship to natural killer and K cells. J Exp Med 1981;153:569–82.
17. Reynolds CW, Timonen T, Herberman RB. Natural killer (NK) cell activity in the rat. I. Isolation and characterization of the effector cells. J Immunol 1981;127:292–87.
18. Lanier LL, Cwirla S, Federspiel N. Human natural killer cells isolated from peripheral blood do not rearrange T cell antigen receptor beta chain genes. J Exp Med 1986;163: 200–14.
19. Chambers WH, Vujanovic NL, DeLeo AB, Olszowy MW, Herberman RB, Hiserodt JC. Monoclonal antibody to a triggering structure expressed on rat natural killer cells and adherent lymphokine-activated killer cells. J Exp Med 1989;169:1373–89.

20. Sentman CL, Kumar V, Koo G, Bennett M. Effector cell expression of NK1.1, a murine natural killer cell-specific molecule, and ability of mice to reject bone marrow allografts. J Immunol 1989;142:1847–53.
21. Vujanovic NL, Nagashima S, Herberman RB, Whiteside TL. Non-secretory apoptotic killing by human natural killer cells. J Immunol 1966;157:1117–26.
22. Trinchieri G. Biology of natural killer cells Adv Immunol 1989;47:187–376.
23. Moretta L, Ciccone E, Pende D, Tripodi G, Bottino C, Moretta A. Human natural killer cells: clonally distributed specific functions and triggering surface molecules. Lab Invest 1992;66:138–42.
24. Moretta A, Vitle M, Bottino C, Orengo AM, Morelli L, Augugliaro R, et al. p58 molecules as putative receptors for major histocompatibility complex (MHC) class I molecules in human natural killer (NK) cells. Anti-p58 antibodies reconstitute lysis of MHC class I-protected cells in NK clones displaying different specificities. J Exp Med 1993;178: 597–604.
25. Storkus WJ, Alexander J, Payne JA, Cresswell P, Dawson JR. The alpha 1/alpha 2 domains of class I HLA molecules, confer resistance to natural killing. J Immunol 1989;143:3853–7.
26. Storkus WJ, Sulter RD, Alexander J, Ward FE, Ruiz RE, Cresswell P, et al. Class I induced resistance to natural killing: identification of nonpermissive residues in HLA-A2. Proc Natl Acad Sci USA 1991;88:5989–92.
27. Herberman RB. Immunoregulation and natural killer cells. Mol Immunol 1982;19:1313–21.
28. Herberman RB, Ortaldo JR, Bonnard GD. Augmentation by interferon of human natural and antibody-dependent cell-mediated cytotoxicity. Nature 1979;277:221–3.
29. Kuribayashhi K, Gillis S, Kern DE, Henney CS. Murine NK cell cultures: effects of interleukin-2 and interferon on cell growth and cytotoxic reactivity. J Immunol 1981;126: 2321–7.
30. Ortaldo JR, Mason A, Overton R. Lymphokine-activated killer cells: analysis of progenitors and effectors. J Exp Med 1986;164:1193–205.
31. Vujanovic NL, Rabinowich H, Lee YJ, Jost L, Herberman RB, Whiteside TL. Distinct phenotypic and functional characteristics of human natural killer cells obtained by rapid interleukin-2-induced adherence to plastic. Cell Immunol 1993;151:133–57
32. Vitolo D, Vujanovic N, Rabinowich H, Schlesinger M, Herberman RB, Whiteside, TL. Rapid interleukin-2-induced adherence of human natural killer (NK) cells. II Expression of mRNA for cytokines and IL-2 receptors in adherent NK cells. J Immunol 1993;151: 1926–37.
33. Whiteside TL, Herberman RB. Role of human natural killer cells in health and disease. Clin Diag Lab Immunol 1994;1:125–33.
34. Cassatella M, Anegon AI, Cuture MC, Griskey P, Trinchieri G, Perussia B. Fc gamma R (CD16) interaction with ligand induces Ca2+ mobilization and phosphoinositide turnover in human natural killer cells. Role of Ca2+ in Fc gamma R (CD16) induced transcription and expression of lymphokine genes J Exp Med 1980;169:549–67.
35. Sulica A, Galatiuc C, Manciulea M, Bancu C, DeLeo A, Whiteside TL, Herberman RB. Regulation of human natural cytotoxicity by IgG. IV. Association between binding of monomeric IgG to the Fc receptors on large granular lymphocytes and inhibition of natural killer (NK) cell activity. Cell Immunol 1993;147:397–410.
36. Robertson MJ, Caligiuri MA, Manley TJ, Levine H, Ritz J. Human natural killer cell

adhesion molecules: differential expression after activation and participation in cytolysis J Immunol 1990;145:3194–201.
37. Haller O, Kiessling R, Orn A, Wigzell H. Generation of natural killer cells: an autonomous function of the bone marrow. J Exp Med 1977:145:1411–6.
38. Whiteside TL, Herberman RB. Characteristics of natural killer cells and lymphokine-activated killer cells. Their role in the biology and treatment of human cancer. Immunol Allergy Clin North Am 1990;10:663–704.
39. Whiteside TL, Jost LM, Herberman RB. Extravasation of antitumor effector cells. Invasion Metastasis 1992:12:128–46.
40. Herberman RB. Possible role of natural killer cells in host resistance against tumours and other diseases. In: Herberman RB. editor Clinics in Immunology and Allergy Eastbourne: WB Saunders Co Ltd, 1983;479–94.
41. Riccardi C, Puccetti P. Santoni A, Herberman RB. Rapid *in vivo* assay of mouse NK cell activity. J Natl Can Inst. 1979;63:1041–5.
42. Riccardi C, Santoni A, Barlozzari T, Puccetti P, Herberman RB. *In vivo* natural reactivity of mice against tumor cells Int J Cancer 1980;25:475–86.
43. Riccardi C, Barlozzari T, Santoni A, Herberman RB, Cesarini, C. Transfer to cyclophosphamide-treated mice of natural killer (NK) cells and *in vivo* natural reactivity against tumors. J Immunol 1981;126:1284–9.
44. Barlozzari T, Reynolds CW, Herberman RB. *In vivo* role of natural killer cells: involvement of large granular lumphocytes in the clearance of tumor cells in anti-asialo GM_1-treated rats. J Immunol. 1983;131:1024–7.
45. Gorelik E, Herberman RB. Assay for evaluation of *in vivo* natural cell-mediated resistance of mice to local transplantation of tumour cells Int J Cancer 1981;27:709–20.
46. Gorelik E, Fogel M, Feldman M, Segal S. Differences in resistance of metastatic tumor cells and cells from local growth to cytotoxicity of natural killer cells J Natl Cancer Inst 1979;63:1397–404.
47. Gorelik E, Segal S, Feldman M. Selection of 3LL tumor subline resistant to natural effector cells concomitantly selected for increased metasatic potency. Cancer Immunol Immunother 1982;12:105–9.
48. Hanna N, Fidler I. Relationship between metastastic potential and resistance to natural killer cell-mediated cytotoxicity in these murine tumor systems J Natl Cancer Inst 1981;66: 1183–90.
49. Gorelik E, Wiltrout RH, Okumura K. Habu S, Herberman RB. Role of NK cells in the control of metastatic spread and growth of tumor cells in mice Int J Cancer 1982;30: 107–12.
50. Barlozzari T, Lenhardt J, Wiltrout R, Herberman RB, Reynolds CW. Direct evidence for the role of LGL in the inhibition of experimental tumor metastases. J Immunol 1985;134: 2783–9.
51. Barlozzari T, Reynolds CW, Herberman RB. *In vivo* role of natural killer cells; involvement of large granular lymphocytes in the clearance of tumor cells in anti-asialo GM1-treated rats J Immunol 1983;131:1024–7.
52. Pross HF, Lotzova E. Role of natural killer cells in cancer. Nat Immunity 1993;12:279–92.
53. Schantz SP, Goephert H. Multimodality therapy and distant metastases. The impact of natural killer cell activity. Arch Otolaryng – Head Neck Surg. 1987;113:1207–13.
54. Roder JC, Lohmann-Matthes M-L, Domzig W, Wigzell H. The beige mutation in the

mouse. II. Selectivity of the natural killer (NK) cell defect J Immunol 1979;123:2174–81.
55. Roder JC, Duwe A. The beige mutation in the mouse selectively impairs natural killer cell function Nature 1979;278:451–3.
56. Brunda MJ, Holden HT, Herberman RB. Augmentation of natural killer cell activity of beige mice by interferon and interferon inducers. In:Herberman RB editor. Natural Cell-Mediated Immunity Against Tumors. New York:Academic Press 1980;411–5.
57. Haliotis T, Roder J, Texter D. Evidence for *in vivo* NK reactivity against primary tumors. In: Herberman RB editor. NK Cells and Other Natural Effector Cells. New York: Academic Press, 1982;1399–404.
58. Sullivan JL, Byron KS, Brewster FE, Purtilo DT. Deficient natural killer cell activity in X-linked lymphoproliferative syndrome Science 1980;210:543–45.
59. Masucci MG, Bejarano MT, Vanky F, Klein E. Cytotoxic and cytostatic activity of human large granular lymphocytes against allogeneic tumor biopsy cells and autologous EBV infected B lymphocytes. In Herberman RB editor. NK Cells and Other Natural Effector Cells. New York:Academic Press, 1982;1047–54.
60. Lipinski M, Tursz T, Kreis H, Finale Y, Amiel JL. Dissociation of natural killer cell activity and antibody-dependent cell-mediated cytotoxicity in kidney allograft recipients receiving high-dose immunosuppressive therapy. Transplantation 1980;29:214–8.
61. Yoda Y, Abe T, Mitamura K Saito K, Kawada K, Onozawa Y, et al. Deficient natural killer (NK) cell activity in paroxysmal nocturnal haemoglobinuria (PNH) Br J Haemotol 1982;52:559–61.
62. Imai K, Matsuyama S, Miyake S, Suga K, Nakachi K. Natural cytotoxic activity of peripheral-blood lymphocytes and cancer incidence: an 11-year follow-up study of a general population. Lancet 2000;356:1795–9.
63. Welsh RM. Regulation of virus infections by natural killer cells Nat Immun Cell Growth Reg 1986;5:160–99.
64. Bloom BR, Minato N, Neighbour A, Reid L, Marcus D. Interferon and NK cells in resistance to virus persistently infected cells and tumors. In:Herberman, RB, editor. Natural Cell Mediated Immunity Against Tumors. New York:Academic Press, 1980;505–24
65. Santoli D, Perussia B, Trinchieri G. Natural killer cell activity against virus-infected cells. In:Herberman, RB, editor. Natural Cell-Mediated Immunity Against Tumors New York: Academic Press, 1980;pp1171–9.
66. Lopez C. Genetic resistance to herpesvirus infections: role of natural killer cells. In: Skamene E, Kongshav PAL, Landy M. editors. Genetic Control of Natural Resistance to Infection and Malignancy. New York:Academic Press, 1980;253–65.
67. Lopez C, Kirkpatrick D, Fitzgerald P. The role of NK(HSV-1) effector cells in resistance to herpesvirus infections in man. In:Herberman, RB, editor. NK Cells and Other Natural Effector Cells. New York:Academic Press, 1982;1445–50.
68. Shellam GR, Grundy JE, Allan JE. The role of natural killer cells and interferon in resistance to murine cytomegalovirus. In:Herberman, RB, editor. NK Cells and Other Natural Effector Cells. New York:Academic Press, 1982;1451–8.
69. Ruebush MJ, Burgess DE. Induction of natural killer cells and interferon production during infection of mice with *Babesia microti* of human origin. In: Herberman, RB, editor. NK Cells and Other Natural Effector Cells. New York:Academic Press, 1982;1483–9.
70. Hatcher FM, Kuhn RE. Natural killer (NK) cell activity against extracellular forms of *Trypanosoma cruzi*. In: Herberman, RB, editor. NK Cells and Other Natural Effector Cells. New York:Academic Press, 1982;1091–7.

71. Djeu JY, Blanchard DK. Regulation of human polymorphonuclear neutriphil (PMN) activity against Candida albicans by large granular lymphocytes via release of a PMN-activating factor J Immunol 1987;139:2761–2.
72. Murphy WJ, Reynolds CW, Tiberghien P, Longo DL. Natural killer cells and bone marrow transplantation J Natl Cancer Inst 1993;85:1475–82.
73. Henney CS, Kuribayashi K, Kern DE, Gillis S. Interleukin 2 augments natural killer cell activity. Nature 1981;291:335–8.
74. Hoofnagle JH, Peters M, Mullen KD et al. Randomized controlled trial of recombinant human alpha interferon in patients with chronic hepatitis B. Gastroenterology 1988;95: 1318–25.
75. McMahon DK, Armstrong JA, Huang XL, Rinaldo Jr. CA, Gupta P, Whiteside TL, et al. A phase I study of subcutaneous recombinant IL-2 in patients with advanced HIV disease while on zidovudine. AIDS 1994;8:58–66.
76. Kirkwood JM, Ernstoff MS. Interferons in the treatment of human cancer. J Clin Oncol 1984;2:336–52.
77. Rosenberg SA, Lotze MT, Yang JC, Aebersold PM, Linehan WM, Seipp CA, et al. Experience with the use of high-dose interleukin-2 in the treatment of 652 cancer patients. Ann Surg 1989;210:474–85.
78. Caligiuri MA, Murray C, Robertson MJ, Wang E, Cochran K, Cameron C, et al. Selective modulation of human natural killer cells *in vivo* after prolonged infusion of low dose recombinant interleukin-2. J Clin Invest 1993;91:123–32..
79. Rosenberg SA, Lotze MT, Muul LM, Chang AE, Avis FP, Leitman S, et al. A progress report on the treatment of 157 patients with advanced cancer using lymphokine-activated killer cells and interleukin-2 or high-dose interleukin-2 along. N Engl J Med 1987;316: 889–97.
80. Hercend T, Farace F, Baume D, Charpentier F, Droz JP, Triebel F, et al. Immunotherapy with lymphokine-activated natural killer cells and recombinant interleukin-2: a feasibility trial in metastatic renal cell carcinoma. J Biol Response Modif 1990;9:546–55.
81. Whiteside TL, Herberman RB. The biology of human natural killer cells. Ann Ital Inst Health 1990;26:335–48.
82. Lister J, Pincus SM, Elder EM, Whiteside TL, Rybka WB, Donnenberg AD. Adoptive immunotherapy during peripheral blood stem cell (PBSC) transplantation: amplification of natural killer cell function early after transplantation. J Immunol 1993;150:218A.

Natural Immunity
Edited by L. Berczók and D.A. Chow
© 2005 Elsevier B.V. All rights reserved

The Role of the Reticuloendothelial System in Natural Immunity

GEORGE LÁZÁR, ELIZABETH HUSZTIK and GEORGE LÁZÁR, JR.[1]

Institute of Pathophysiology, [1]Department of Surgery, University of Szeged, Szeged, Hungary

ABSTRACT

In the nineteenth century, it was realized that certain cells were intensely phagocytic. These varied cell types which acted in host defence by phagocytosing of foreign invaders such as microbes were grouped collectively into the reticuloendothelial system (RES). In studies of the physiological and pathophysiological roles of the RES, depression or blockade of the granulopectic activity of this system has attracted considerable attention. Authors describe their experiments demonstrating that rare earth metal salts, among them gadolinium chloride ($GdCl_3$), depress the reticuloendothelial activity, selectively depressing or eliminating the large Kupffer cells. Recent studies from many laboratories have shown that the Kupffer cell blockade induced by $GdCl_3$ modifies the immune response, exerts protective effects on anaphylactic and endotoxic/septic shock, and decreases the liver-damaging effects of several hepatotoxins and ischaemic reperfusion. Recent studies have elucidated the mechanisms by which $GdCl_3$-induced Kupffer cell blockade protects against a variety of hepatotoxic processes. $GdCl_3$ is most likely protective because it prevents the release of inflammatory cytokines and toxic oxygen radicals produced by activated Kupffer cells. The causal roles of these mechanisms have been shown to be important in the prevention of hepatotoxic injuries caused by hepatotoxins, such as carbon tetrachloride and alcohol, or liver injuries associated with ischaemia-reperfusion, liver transplantation and sepsis.

1. INTRODUCTION

In the 19th century, the Russian zoologist Metchnikoff discovered that certain white cells, which he termed phagocytes, were able to ingest microorganisms and other foreign materials. He recognized the biological significance of phagocytes in the defence of the organism [1]. In the early 20th century, morphologists observed that certain cells took up dyes injected intravenously (called "vital dyes", since they stained live cells). The German pathologist Aschoff identified these cells as macrophages in connective tissues, microglia in the central nervous system, endothelial cells lining vascular sinusoids, and reticular cells of lymphoid organs. He suggested that these varied cell types functioned in host defence by phagocytosing foreign invaders such as microbes, and he grouped them collectively into the reticuloendothelial system (RES) [2].

The RES obviously consists of a working complex of macrophages, dendritic reticular cells, lymphocytes, and plasma cells as arrayed in the lymph nodes, spleen, thymus, bone marrow, gut-associated lymphoid tissues, inflammatory lesions, and elsewhere [3].

It was recognized that the pinocytosis, of which the endothelial and reticular cells are capable, is fundamentally different from the active phagocytosis of macrophages. After development of the concept of mononuclear phagocytic system [4], therefore, it is now more appropriate to classify monocytes and macrophages as members of the mononuclear phagocyte system.

2. GENERAL ASPECTS AND DEVELOPMENT OF CELLS IN THE MONONUCLEAR PHAGOCYTE SYSTEM

The cells in the mononuclear phagocyte system include promonocytes and their precursors in the bone marrow, monocytes in the circulation, and macrophages in the tissues. The cell line originates in the bone marrow as a common committed progenitor cell for the granulocyte and monocyte-macrophage pathways, the granulocyte-monocyte colony forming unit (CFU-GM). Glycoprotein hormones termed colony-stimulating factors induce differentiation of this cell into a monoblast, which differentiates into a promonocyte, the first morphologically identifiable cell in the series. Migration of monocytes into the different tissues appears to be a random phenomenon in the absence of localized inflammation. Once in the tissues, monocytes probably do not reenter the circulation. Rather, they undergo transformation into tissue macrophages with morphologic and sometimes functional properties that are characteristic for the tissue in which they reside; such transformation is presumably a response to tissue-specific stimuli [5]. In confirmation of studies showing that tissue macrophages in animals originate in the bone marrow [5–7], humans receiving transplanted bone marrow were found to have alveolar macrophages [8] and Kupffer cells [9] that express the sex karyotype of the donor.

3. MEASUREMENTS OF RETICULOENDOTHELIAL ACTIVITY

Quantitative measurements of reticuloendothelial activity are usually made by injecting a suitable colloid intravenously and subsequently measuring the rate of its disappearance from the blood. In his pioneering experiments, Jancsó [10] proposed the blood clearance of colloidal carbon for the estimation of phagocytic activity. The development and wide use of the carbon clearance test [11] enabled investigators to determine the functional ability of the RES. In this way, the RES modifications in response to infection, metabolism, tumour growth, shock and many other functions were studied. At present, the carbon clearance test is one of the most common procedures in experimental animals, though several other methods have been developed, for example, the clearance of microaggregates of heat-denatured albumin labelled with I^{125} [12] or of foreign red blood cells labelled with Cr^{51} [13]. By means of radioactive substances, it is possible to measure the activity of macrophages in different organs.

4. THE PRINCIPAL FUNCTIONS OF MONONUCLEAR PHAGOCYTES

Macrophages play a significant role in host defence mechanisms. When activated, they inhibit the growth of a wide variety of tumour cells and microorganisms [14]. Macrophages phagocytose foreign particles, such as microbes, macromolecules, including antigens, and even self-tissues that are injured or dead, such as senescent erythrocytes.

Phagocytosis is an evolutionarily conserved process utilized by many cells to ingest microbial pathogens, and apoptotic and necrotic corpses. By ingesting microbial pathogens, phagocytes accomplish two essential immune functions. Firstly, they initiate a microbial death pathway, in part by routing ingested pathogens to lysosomes rich in hydrolytic enzymes, and by targeting the phagocyte to oxidize a complex in the phagolysosome. Second, phagocytes, in particular dendritic cells, utilize phagocytosis to direct antigens to both MHC I and II compartments. Thus, phagocytosis serves a dual role: as an innate immune effector, and as a bridge between the innate and acquired immune responses [15]. This phylogenetically conserved process is critical for innate immunity, and mononuclear phagocytes play important roles in the recognition, activation and effector phases of specific immunity. Mononuclear phagocytes also are important participants in the bidirectional interactions between innate and specific immunity. Macrophages that respond to microbes as a reaction of innate immunity also function to trigger microbe-specific lymphocyte responses. Conversely, effector lymphocytes and their products enhance the antimicrobial functions of macrophages.

The phagocytic capacity of the macrophage is determined by the action of a composite of cell surface receptors, which can be classified generally as opsonic-dependent and opsonic-independent [16]. Opsonized pathogens may be recognized and internalized by receptors of the Fc portion of immunoglobulin, iC3b, and/or fibronectin. In the absence of opsonization, the clearance of micro-organisms, including *Candida* sp., *Cryptococcus neoformans*, *Pseudomonas aeroginosa, Pneumococcus carnii, Neiseria* sp., *Leischmanisa* sp., *Histoplasma* sp., and *Mycobacterium* sp., has been shown to be accomplished by lectinophagocytosis through the action of macrophage mannan and c-glucan receptors.

Macrophages produce cytokines that recruit other inflammatory cells, especially neutrophils, and are responsible for many of the systemic effects of inflammation, such as fever. One of the most potent inducers of these macrophage responses is a bacterial cell wall component called endotoxin [17], which binds to a macrophage surface molecule called CD14. Macrophages also produce growth factors for fibroblasts and vascular endothelium that promote the repair of injured tissues. Activated macrophages secrete proteolytic enzymes, active metabolites of oxygen (including superoxide anion and other oxygen radicals), arachidonic acid metabolites, cyclic adenosine monophosphate (cAMP), and cytokines such as interleukin-1 (IL-1), IL-6, IL-8 and tumour necrosis factor-α (TNF-α), among others. Many tissue-specific cells are of macrophage lineage, and function to process and present antigen (e.g. Langerhans cells, oligodendrocytes, etc.).

Neutrophils, monocytes, and tissue-based macrophages are major cellular components of the innate immune system, which serve as the initial line of host defence against infections by pathogenic bacteria, fungi and parasites. Cytokines such as granulocyte colony-stimulating factor (G-CSF), granulocyte-macrophage colony-stimulating factor (GM-CSF), macrophage colony-stimulating factor (M-CSF), and interferon (IFN)-γ have received increasing attention as potential adjunctive immunomodulatory agents for the treatment of infectious diseases. *In vitro* and *in vivo* studies have shown that G-CSF, GM-CSF and IFN-γ can augment the functional antimicrobial activities of neutrophils [17,18].

5. RETICULOENDOTHELIAL BLOCKADE

In studies of the physiological and pathophysiological roles of the RES, depression or blockade of the granulopectic activity of this system has attracted considerable attention. Among substances effectively depressing the reticuloendothelial activity are materials with different physicochemical properties. For example, various colloids [19], steroids such as cortisone [20], esters of fatty acids such as methyl palmitate [21], and liposome-encapsulated clodronate [22]. Different theories have been suggested to explain the mechanisms of action of these materials.

Our experiments [23] have demonstrated that rare earth metal salts, among them gadolinium chloride ($GdCl_3$), depress the reticuloendothelial activity and inhibit or completely abolish the effects of some reticuloendothelial stimulants. Our histological studies showed that the reticuloendothelial blockade induced by $GdCl_3$ is primarily due to the depression of the phagocytic activity by Kupffer cells [24], selectively depressing [25] or eliminating [26] large Kupffer cells.

Several studies have revealed that not only is the bulk of the intravenously injected particulate matter, colloidal particles, or cellular antigen taken up by the Kupffer cells, but the functional state of these cells strongly influences their distribution among the organs of the RES, which may have functional consequences [25,27].

Macrophages are the body's "alarm" cells that synthesize and excrete highly reactive materials, such as the superoxide anion, hydrogen peroxide, nitric oxide, eicosanoids, peptide mediators and proteolytic enzymes. These biologically active materials are very important in killing bacteria and tumour cells. However, macrophages not only act as a first line of defence but also have pivotal roles in regulating the immune response. The "over"-activation of macrophages and the excessive release of macrophage-derived destructive and immunosuppressive products may contribute to organ damage and the development of "multiple organ failure" in severe stress and injuries such as shock states [28].

Recent studies from many laboratories, including our own, have shown that the Kupffer cell blockade induced by $GdCl_3$ modifies the immune response [29], exerts protective effects on anaphylactic [30], and endotoxic/septic shock [31,32], and decreases the liver-damaging effects of several hepatotoxins [33–35] and ischaemic-reperfusion [36.

Hepatic macrophages (Kupffer cells) account for approximately 15% of the total number of liver cells, and they account for 80–90% of the resident macrophages in the entire body [37]. Kupffer cells are located on the inside of the sinusoidal wall and they are found predominantly in the periportal region, which may represent the best location for these cells to exhibit their endocytic role for blood-borne materials entering the liver. Kupffer cells exhibit vigorous phagocytic activity and produce many kinds of soluble mediators such as cytokines, prostanoids, oxygen radicals, and proteases. In response to septic stimuli, hepatic macrophages are activated and release monokines, such as IL-1 and TNF-α. The secreted monokines then activate circulating leukocytes as well as sinusoidal endothelial cells and induce ICAM-1 expression. The resultant leukocyte adhesion to the endothelium disturbs the sinusoidal microcirculation and causes tissue damage by injurious mediators such as oxygen radicals, proteases, prostanoids, and other substances released from activated leukocytes [38].

Recent studies have elucidated the mechanisms by which $GdCl_3$-induced Kupffer cell blockade protects against a variety of hepatotoxic processes. $GdCl_3$ is most likely protective because it prevents the release of inflammatory cytokines and toxic oxygen radicals produced by activated Kupffer cells [39]. The causal roles of these mechanisms have been shown to be important in the prevention of hepatotoxic injuries caused by hepatotoxins, such as carbon tetrachloride and alcohol [40,41], or liver injuries associated with ischaemia reperfusion [42], liver transplantation [43] and sepsis [44].

ACKNOWLEDGEMENTS

This work was supported by the National Science Foundation (OTKA, grant No. TO 23638) and Higher Education Development and Modernisation Program 0659/1999.

REFERENCES

1. Metchnikoff E. Sur la lutte des cellules de l'organisme contre l'invasion des microbes. Ann Inst Pasteur 1887;1:321–36.
2. Aschoff L. Das reticulo-endotheliale System. Ergebn inn Med Kinderheilk 1924;26: 1–118.
3. Friedman H, Escobar MR, Reichard SM. Introduction. The Reticuloendothelial System. A Comprehensive Treatise. Morphology. Carr I, Daems WT (Editors);Plenum Press, New York: London, 1980;l:XI-XII.
4. van Furth R, Raeburn JA, van Zwet TL. Characteristic of human mononuclear phagocytes. Blood 1979;54:485–500.
5. Johnston RB Jr. J Current Concepts: immunology. Monocytes and macrophages, New Engl J Med 1988;318(12):747–52.
6. Lázár G. Influence of splenectomy, partial hepatectomy and bile duct ligation on the granulopectic activity of the reticuloendothelial system. Acta Physiol Ac Sci Hung 1972;42:287–91.
7. van Furth R, Diesselhoff-den Dulk MMC, Sluiter W, van Dissel JT. New perspectives on the kinetics of mononuclear phagocytes. In: van Furth R, ed. Mononuclear phagocytes: characteristics, physiology and function. Dorbrecht: Martinus Nijhoff 1985;201–10.
8. Thomas ED, Ramberg RE, Sale GE, Sparkes RS, Golde DW. Direct evidence for a bone marrow origin of the alveolar macrophage in man. Science 1976;192:1016–8.
9. Gale RP, Sparkes RS, Golde DW. Bone marrow origin of hepatic macrophages (Kupffer cells) in humans. Science 1978;201:937–8.
10. Jancsó M. Histamine as a physiological activator of the reticulo-endothelial system. Nature (Lond.) 1947;160:227–8.
11. Biozzi G, Benacerraf B, Halpern BN. Quantitative study of the granulopectic activity of the reticuloendothelial system. II. A study of the kinetics of the granulopectic activity of the R.E.S. in relation to the dose of carbon injected. Relation between the weight of the organs and their activity. Brit J Path 1953;34:441–57.
12. Wagner HN Jr., Iio M. Studies of reticuloendothelial system (RES). Blockade of the RES in man. J Clin Invest 1963;42:427–34.
13. Schildt BE. Disappearance of i.v. injected ^{51}Cr-RBC from circulation as a possible measure of RS function in mice. Acta Chir Scand 1970;136:351–7.
14. Choi CY, You HJ, Jeong HG. Nitric oxide and tumor necrosis factor-α production by oleanolic acid via nuclear factor-ϲB activation in macrophages. Biochem Biophys Res Comm 2001;288:49–55.
15. Greenberg S, Grinstein S. Phagocytosis and innate immunity. Current Opin Immunol 2002;14:135–45.
16. Reichner JS, Fitzpatrick PA, Wakshull E, Albina JE. Receptor-mediated phagocytosis of rat macrophages is regulated differentially for opsonized particles and non-opsonized particles containing ϲ-glucan. Immunology 2001;104:198–206.

17. Berczi I, Bertók L, Chow DA. Natural immunity and neuroimmune host defense. Ann NY Ac Sci 2000;917:249–57.
18. Liles WC. Immunomodulatory approaches to augment phagocyte-mediated host defence for treatment of infectious diseases. Semin Respir Infect 2001;16(1):11–7.
19. Jancsó N. Speicherung. Budapest. Akadémiai Kiadó; 1955: pp. 1–468.
20. Bilbey DLJ, Nicol T. Effect of various natural steroids on the phagocytic activity of the reticuloendothelial system. Nature 1958;182:674.
21. DiLuzio NR, Wooles WR. Depression of phagocytic activity and immune response by methylpalmitate. Am J Physiol 1964;206:939–43.
22. Van Rooijen N. The liposome mediated macrophage "suicide" technique. J Immunol Meth 1989;124:1–6.
23. Lázár G. The reticuloendothelial blocking effects of rare earth metals. J Leukocyte Biol 1973;13:231–7.
24. Husztik E, Lázár G, Párducz Á. Electron microscopic study of Kupffer cell phagocytosis blockade induced by gadolinium chloride. Br J Exp Path 1980;61:624–30.
25. Lázár G, van Galen M, Scherphof GL. Gadolinium chloride shift in intrahepatic distributions of liposomes. Biochim Biophys Acta 1989;1011:97–101.
26. Hardonk MJ, Dijkhuis FW, Hulstaert CE, Koudstaal J. Heterogeneity of liver and spleen macrophages in gadolinium chloride-induced elimination and repopulation. J Leukoc Biol 1992;52:296–302.
27. Lázár G, Husztik E, Lázár G. Jr, Kiss I, Oláh J, Szakács J. Immunomodulation by gadolinium chloride-induced Kupffer cell phagocytosis blockade. J Alloys and Compounds 1998;228:908–10.
28. Lázár G. Stress: from concept to modern immunology. Ann NY Acad Sci 1998;85:16–8.
29. Lázár G Jr, Farkas Gy, Csanádi J, Lázár G. Gadolinium chloride (GdCl3)-induced macrophage blockade prevents rejection of human insulinoma cell xenograft in rats. Transplantation 1997; 63(5): 729-31.
30. Lázár G. Jr., Lázár G, Kaszaki J, Oláh J, Kiss I, Husztik E. Inhibition of anaphylactic shock by gadolinium chloride-induced Kupffer cell blockade. Agents Actions 1994;41:C97-8.
31. Lázár G, Jr., Husztik E, Lázár G. Effects of endotoxin and gadolinium chloride on acute septic peritonitis and septic shock in rats. In:First Vienna Shock Forum. Part B.: Monitoring and Treatment of Shock Schlag G, Redl H.editors, Alan R.Liss, New York, Progr. Clin. Biol. Res.1987;323-8.
32. Vollmar B, Rüttinger D, Wanner GA, Leider R, Menger MD. Modulation of Kupffer cell activity by gadolinium chloride in endotoxemic rats. Shock 1996;6:434-41.
33. Lázár G. Effect of reticuloendothelial stimulation and depression on rare earth metal chloride-induced splenic calcification and fatty acid degeneration of the liver. Experientia 1973;29:818-9.
34. Lázár G., Serra D, Tuchweber B. Effect of cadmium toxicity of substances influencing reticuloendothelial activity. Toxicol Appl Pharmacol 1974;29:367-76.
35. Barriault C, Audet M, Yousef IM, Tuchweber B: Effect of agents which modify reticuloendothelial system function on acute phalloidin-induced lethality and hepatotoxicity in mice. Toxicol Appl Pharmacol 1995; 131:206-15.
36. Suzuki S, Toledo-Pereyra LH, Rodrigez F, Lopez F. Role of Kupffer cells in neutrophil activation and infiltration following total hepatic ischemia and reperfusion. Circ Shock 1994;42:204-9.
37. Morio LA, Chiu H, Sprowles KA, Laskin DL. Functional heterogeneity of rat hepatic

and alveolar macrophages: effects of chronic ethanol administration. J Leukoc Biol 2000; 68(5):614-20.

38. Arii S, Imamura M. Physiological role of sinusoidal endothelial cells and Kupffer cells and their implication in the pathogenesis of liver injury. J Hepatobiliary Pancreat Surg 2000; 7(1):40-8.
39. Rose ML, Bradford BU, Germolec DR, Lin M, Tsukamoto H, Thruman RG. Gadolinium chloride-induced hepatocyte proliferation is prevented by antibodies to tumor necrois factor-α. Toxicol Appl Pharmacol 2001;170:39-45.
40. Edwards MJ, Keller BJ, Kauffman FC, Thurman RG. The involvement of Kupffer cells in carbon tetrachloride toxicity. Toxicol Appl Pharmacol 1993;119:275-9.
41. Cederbaum AI. Introduction serial review: Alcohol, oxidative stress and cell injury. Free Radical Biol and Med 2001;31:1524-6.
42. Kukan M, Vajdova K, Horecky J, Nagyova A, Mehendale HM, Tronec T. Effects of blockade of Kupffer cells by gadolinium chloride on hepatobiliary function in cold ischemia-reperfusion injury of rat liver. Hepatology 1997;26:1250-7.
43. Schauer RJ, Bilzer M, Kalmuk S, Gerbes AL, Leiderer R, Schildberg FW, Messmer K. Microcirculatory failure after rat liver transplantation is related to Kupffer cell-derived oxidant stress but not involved in early graft dysfunction. Transplantation 2001;72:1692-9.
44. Lázár G Jr., Duda E, Szakács J, Oláh J, Balogh A, Lázár G. Effect of Kupffer cell phagocytosis blockade on endotoxin sensitivity, endotoxin induced cytokine production in obstructive jaundice. In Cells of the Hepatic Sinusoid. Wisse E, Knook DL, Zanger R, Fraser R, editors. Kupffer Cell Foundation, 1999;7:237-8.

Natural Immunity
Edited by L. Bertók and D.A. Chow
© 2005 Elsevier B.V. All rights reserved

Effector Mechanisms of Natural Immunity: an Invertebrate Perspective

EDWIN L. COOPER

Laboratory of Comparative Neuroimmunology, Department of Neurobiology, David Geffen School Of Medicine at UCLA, University of California, Los Angeles, California 90095-1763, USA

ABSTRACT

There is a resurgence of interest in the duality of the immune system: innate, natural, non-specific, non-anticipatory, non-clonal responses of invertebrates; adaptive, induced, specific, anticipatory, clonal responses of vertebrates. Natural immunity is considered the most primitive and found in both groups, although invertebrates do not possess the adaptive system. Using monoclonal antibodies to human adhesion molecules, earthworm, leech and sipunculan leukocytes are positive for many CD markers common to vertebrate leukocytes, especially macrophages and natural killer cells. In earthworms, only those leukocytes active as killers in cytotoxic responses are positive, whereas a larger primarily phagocytic leukocyte is negative. Growing functional evidence focuses on invertebrate cytokines but prevailing controversy concerns molecular structure and presumed homology. Most credible information has been derived from the tunicates especially with the appearance of the draft genome of *Ciona intestinalis*. The evolutionary history of complement can be traced from sea urchins to the teleosts and tetrapods, exhibiting at each level a corresponding increase in the numbers of complement components and duplications in complement pathways. Invertebrates and vertebrates seem to possess common signalling molecules e.g. neuropeptides. These signalling molecules act as immunomodulators in circulating blood. In vertebrates, release occurs during stress that triggers the hypothalamo-hypophyseal-adrenal (HPA) axis. Neuropeptides also act as conserved messengers that initiate and stimulate innate immune responses in invertebrates and in humans. This system probably evolved in "simple" animals. Cross talk between nervous and immune systems has an ancient evolutionary origin essential to homeostasis. Comparative analyses using simpler animal models have enriched these views.

1. INTRODUCTION: INNATE VS ADAPTIVE IMMUNITY

1.1 Early history and scope

The world of immunology was split when Metchnikoff discovered invertebrate phagocytosis. It was then that the monolithic field underwent a major change [1]. Before Metchnikoff, immune systems were believed to be wholly humoral with little or no emphasis relegated to the role of cellular effectors (leukocytes) and the molecular products that they synthesize and secrete (mediators). Metchnikoff's discovery, however, initiated an enduring schism that we accept as fact; i.e., we added cellular immunity to the prevailing humoral immunity. Now almost 100 years later, this cellular component, and the animal models from which it was derived is, once again, at the centre of immunology. As a result, immunobiologists are more willing now to accept data and emerging concepts derived from intense analyses using invertebrate models than from work done in the fifty previous years when modern immunology was establishing itself. Knowing his strength of conviction, Metchnikoff would have savoured this intellectual turn of events! Because of his prescient influence and the discovery of phagocytosis we are now considerably further along toward a more complete understanding of the natural immune response and some of the mechanisms at the molecular and cellular levels. Otherwise we might not have emerged from what could have been a 19th century one-way "dark alley".

The scope of this chapter alerts us to the utility of models that offer more clues to the nature of animal immune systems than is available from the utilization of vertebrate models alone. This chapter, will focus on two major themes: a) natural immunity emphasizing certain characteristics that seem to be common for invertebrates and vertebrates (e.g. CD markers, cytokines, and complement); b) neuroendocrine components; c) linkages between the immune and neuroendocrine systems. These proposed overlaps of the three regulatory systems can be seen in the simplified figure.

1.2. Organization of the immune system

We are witnessing a resurgence of interest in the dual functional and morphological division of the immune system: innate, natural, non-specific, non-anticipatory, non-clonal responses in contrast to the adaptive, induced, specific, anticipatory, clonal responses typical of vertebrates. This duality is realized at every level: molecules, cells, tissues, organs, and whole organisms. Metchnikoff's discovery of phagocytosis an invertebrate cellular immune mechanism in an echinoderm (sea stars) became applicable to vertebrates. Vertebrate adaptive immunity utilizes the macrophage, T/B lymphocyte system that depends upon rearranging genes (RAG), whereas invertebrate innate immunity depends upon activities of complex leukocytes and molecules (non-clonally derived) that they synthesize and secrete [2]. Vertebrates have innate immunity and adaptive immunity and the innate capacity may act independently but overlap as a continuum with adaptive immunity [3–5]. Fearon and Locksley proposed that vertebrate natural or innate immunity effects a rapid, non-specific, incomplete antimicrobial host defence, until the slower, more specific acquired immune response develops [6]. Innate immunity may effect a supplementary role in determining which antigens the adaptive immune system responds to and the nature of that response. Innate immunity has also been considered *vis a vis* its cell products, those ubiquitous antimicrobial peptides [7]. Yet another view classifies vertebrate immunity as a specialized inflammatory response against infections. Adaptive immunity of vertebrates is considered to have evolved in response to counter measures successfully used by intracel-

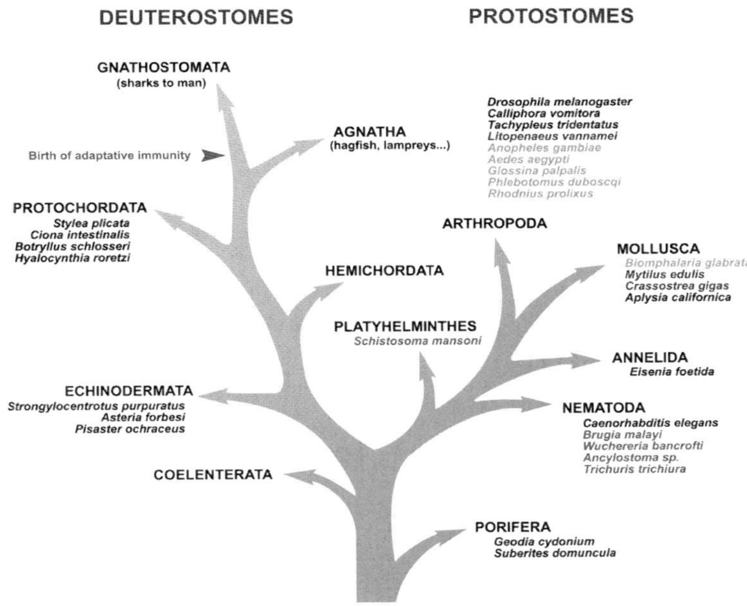

Figure 1. Simplified evolutionary tree showing the major divisions into the protostome and deuterostome invertebrates. Vertebrates are derived from the deuterostome line yet certain neuroendocrineimmune characteristics have been shown to be common among the members of these different groups. The protostome and deuterostome characterization is based upon the formation of the mouth. Modified from a version by Dr. Arnaud Lacoste, Post-Doctoral Fellow, Psychoneuroimmunology Program UCLA (Based upon: Giribet, G. 2002 Current advances in the phylogenetic reconstruction of metazoan evolution. A new paradigm for the Cambrian explosion? *Molecular Phylogenetics and Evolution*. 24: 343–357).

lular pathogens against non-specific immunodefence [8]. Analysing mammalian innate immune responses has revealed similarities with the invertebrate immune system. For example, insects possess an acute response that resembles human responses, implicating similar effectors, receptors and regulation of gene expression. Mussels that are mollusks and most other invertebrates evolved intracellular phagocytosis resembling that effected by vertebrate neutrophils, using cationic antibacterial peptides in phagolysosomes. Vertebrate innate immunity resembles a mosaic of invertebrate immune responses [9].

1.3. Bilaterians and the origins of chordates

A more precise taxonomy is essential at this point that shows the position of the invertebrates and vertebrates (Fig. 1). There are two major groups, the pre-bilaterians and the bilateria, that are sub-divided themselves into two other major groups, the protostomes and deuterostomes. Among protostomes there are two subgroups, the lophotrochozoa, which includes the annelids (e.g., segmented earthworms *Eisenia fetida* and leeches) and mollusks (e.g., oysters, snails, *Aplysia*) and the ecdysozoa to which the arthropods (e.g., flies, lobsters, shrimp, crabs) and nematodes (e.g., round worms *C. elegans*) belong. The deuterostomes consists of the echinoderms (e.g., starfish), hemichordates and chordates (urochordates [e.g., tunicates], cephalochordates and vertebrates [e.g., fish, amphibians, reptiles, birds and mammals]). Although not discussed

Table I General features of natural immunity in invertebrates.

Phagocytic cells; Encapsulation (granuloma/nodule formation see ERP)
Evidence of accelerated second set transplant rejection
Protease inhibitors; Lysozyme; Lysins
Agglutinins; C-Type lectins (Ca^{++}-dependent lectins)
S-Type lectins (Galectins); Prophenoloxidase System (proPO)
Metal-binding proteins (cysteine-rich metallothioneins)
Cytokines (functional homologues; no sequence data)
Transferrin and lactoferrin
Bacterial Permeability Increasing Protein (BPI)

in great detail here, the dominant evidence with respect to innate immunity and its relation to vertebrates (mammalian) and plants concern findings in *Drosophila* and *C. elegans*. Arthropods, especially insects, represent an important group of invertebrates because of their sheer numbers. Vertebrates, in particular mammals and including humans, are really insignificant. *Drosophila* as in times past with respect to genetics and development provides ample evidence that arthropods possess effective innate immune responses. Over-generalizing about the immune system of all invertebrates based upon this single species may in the long run be unwise since for example examining metazoan phylogeny based on small subunit rRNA, will yield certain interesting revelations, i.e., relationships that are perhaps closer than using other criteria. With more intense analysis as has been accomplished for fruit flies and round worms, it may be revealed that mollusks for example have solved problems of immunodefence in a special manner and so may have the annelids or even the urochordates the vertebrate's closest relatives [10].

Evolution of distinctive innate immunity genes concerns the urochordates where the very recent draft genome of *Ciona intestinalis*, a tunicate, focuses on chordate and vertebrate origins. This report finds no evidence of the pivotal genes implicated in adaptive immunity, such as immunoglobulin, T cell receptor, and major histocompatibility complex (MHC) class I and II genes. Evidence is still needed to confirm the possible existence of highly divergent orthologs of one or more of these genes. The numerous authors of this report found a large number of possible complement genes, including C1q-like and C6-like genes, three Toll-like receptor genes, and a variety of lectin genes. An interleukin-1 (IL-1) receptor and an IL-17 receptor gene were identified [11]. Genetic findings confirm a wealth of functional information performed long before defining genes became a prevailing technology in comparative immunology [2]. Invertebrates are endowed with natural immunity that is effected by cells and their humoral products, (Tables I + II). Cells synthesize and secrete molecular products, a survival strategy that protects invertebrates from microorganisms that they encounter in hostile, natural environments. These molecules lyse targets, naturally occurring microorganisms or experimentally introduced eukaryotic cells, including cancers providing a common effector mechanism in all invertebrates even one-cell protozoans [12–16]. Amoebapore, isolated from *Entamoeba histolytica*, a parasite that causes life-threatening disease in humans, is a polypeptide that forms ion channels in target cell membranes [17]. Amoebapore resembles NK-lysin, the novel lytic effector molecule from porcine cytotoxic lymphocytes [18].

1.4 Natural immunity in arthropods: Drosophila

Although evidence is mounting from the use of other invertebrate models, the most widely studied innate immune system is that of *Drosophila*. Aside from the fruit fly and its immune system for itself, we have learned an enormous amount about related immuno-defence systems in

Table II Invertebrate innate immune components.

Component/Characteristic	Metazoan Model
Encapsulating-Relating Factors (ERPs)	Insect (*Tenebrio molitor*)
Eicosanoids	Insects
Inducible inflammatory system (Toll, NF-κB)	Insects/arthropods *C elegans*
Acute phase proteins: Pentraxins, Ig superfamily, complement	Insects/Arthropods
α_2 macroblobulin family (protease inhibitor)	Nematodes, crustaceans, molluscs, echinoderms, tunicates; *Limulus polyphemus*
Lipoprotein-receptor related protein (LRP/$\__2$ M-R)	*C elegans*
Mannose Binding Lectin (MBL)	*C elegans*, tunicates
Antimicrobial peptides:	
Defensins e.g. Cecropins, Transferrin, Drosomycin Drosocin, Attacin, Metchnikowin	*Drosophila*
Defensins, eg: mytilins; myticins	*Mytilus galloprovincialis*
Lytic and Antimicrobial molecules:	Earthworms
Lysins (Fetidins, CCF-1, Lysenin, Eiseniapore)	
Antimicrobial peptide: (Non-lytic) Lumbricin I	
TNFα (Tumor necrosis factor alpha analogue)	
Reactive oxygen species (ROS)	Mollusks
Fibrinogen Related Proteins (FREPS)	Mollusks (planorbid snails)
NK-like cells with CD markers	Sipunculids, annelids, mollusks
Tachylectins	Horseshoe crab
Acute Phase Proteins: C-reactive protein, LPS-binding protein	Crustaceans/*Limulus*
C3 Homologue	Echinoderms; tunicates
Collectin (collagenous, carbohydrate binding protein lectin-mediated complement pathway)	Tunicates, Horseshoe crab
Mannose Binding Protein (MBP); Mannose Associated Serine Proteaseb (MASP)	Tunicates
Antimicrobial peptides: Clavanins, styelins	Tunicates

mammals and plants. Innate immune responses in *Drosophila* discriminate between pathogens and react by inducing the expression of specific antimicrobial peptide-encoding genes through distinct signalling cascades. Fungal infection activates NF-κB-like transcription factors via the Toll pathway, which also regulates innate immune responses in mammals. The pathways that mediate antibacterial defenses, in insects, however, are less well characterized. [19]· Nevertheless we can understand more by examining what has been done in *Drosophila* and the possible existence of parallels.

Natural immunity in insects depends upon multiple strategies as defense against microbial infection by: (a) activating proteolytic signaling cascades that lead to melanization and coagulation reactions at injury sites and around foreign objects; (b) utilizing blood cells to either phagocytose or encapsulate invading microbes; and (c) producing numerous antimicrobial peptides [20–22]. Antimicrobial peptides are synthesized in the fat body (an analog of the mammalian liver and the chlorogogen tissue in earthworms) in response to systemic infections of several epithelial tissues following local infections. Rel/Nuclear Factor (NF)-κB-like transcription factors are the major regulators relative to the expression of antimicrobial peptide genes in *Drosophila*, and their activity is modulated by signaling pathways that are similar to the interleukin-1 receptor (IL-1R) in mammals [23–25]. Similarities such as these strongly suggest an evolutionary link between the control of antimicrobial peptide gene expression and the control of mammalian innate immune responses [26,27]. The Toll signaling pathway, that was first identified as a regulator of embryonic dorsal-ventral patterning in *Drosophila*, is one regulator of antimicrobial peptide gene expression via the Rel/(NF)- κB system. [28]. The Toll and Imd pathways, however, do not share any components and each pathway regulates specific Rel proteins [19,24,29,30]. Although we understand more clearly concerning regulation of anti-microbial peptide gene expression in fruit flies, still various intermediates in the Toll and Imd pathways remain uncharacterized. This is also true for the earthworm where exploration is less, due to a dearth of international workers. Earthworms do have antimicrobial peptides and large lytic and agglutinating molecules.

2. CELL DIFFERENTIATION (CD) MARKERS AND INFLAMMATORY RESPONSES

2.1. Earthworms

According to Cooper, et al, (2002), earthworms, in particular, like other complex invertebrates, possess several leukocytes and the molecules that they synthesize and secrete [31]. Together they effect phagocytosis, encapsulation, agglutination, opsonization, clotting and lysis of foreign components. At least two major leukocytes: small coelomocytes, (SC) and large coelomocytes (LC) mediate lytic reactions against several targets. SC, the putative killer cells, are positive for CD11a, CD45RA, CD45R0, CDw49b, CD54 β_2-m, Thy-1 (CD90) and negative for CD1a, CD2, CD3, CD4, CD5, CD8, CD11b, CD14, CD16, CD18, CD19, CD25, CD34, CD36, CD44, CDw49d, CDw49e, CDw49f, CD56, CD57, CD69, CD71. LC the larger phagocytic cell that cleans up after cytotoxic responses is uniformly negative for these markers. Destruction of tumor cells in vitro reveals the dissociation of phagocytosis from natural killer cell responses. A third type, the chlorogogen cell (CC), synthesizes and sheds effector lytic molecules. Among the lytic molecules, three have been identified and sequenced (fetidins, CCF-1, lysenin) and another has been discovered (eiseniapore) three others H_1 H_2 H_3 share agglutinating and lysing functions and Lumbricin I is the only small antimicrobial but non-lytic molecule. Engelmann et al., (2002) identified conserved molecules (enzymes, peptides, cytokines) that might play a role in invertebrate innate immunity [32]. They detected the enzyme Cu-Zn-superoxide-dismutase (SOD), cytokines (tumor necrosis factor-α [TNFα], transforming growth factor-α [TGFα] and a peptide hormone (thyreotrope stimulating hormone, [TSH]) in earthworm coelomocytes with monoclonal antibodies developed originally against human and/or mouse antigens. Three coelomocyte subpopulations were identified according to their form, size and granularity by confocal microscopy and flow cytometric analysis. Two coelomocyte types showed cell surface positivity with anti-Thy-1, [CD90], CD24 and TNF-α antibodies. Strong cytoplasmic reactions were shown with anti-TNF-α and anti-SOD mAbs but a weaker but unambiguous reaction with thyroid stimulating hormone (TSH). The third population was negative for all of the monoclonal antibodies. Cellular and humoral components function to distinguish between *self and not self*, dispose of internal damaged components (cancer ?), and external antigens (microbes). Innate immunity evolved as an essential survival strategy in all living species.

2.2. Leeches

Leukocytes that mediate inflammatory responses in leeches have been characterized by immunohistochemistry. Macrophage-like cells, NK-like cells, and granulocytes migrate after pricking with bacterial lipopolysaccharide. Inflammatory responses increased progressively and provoked cell migration to the body wall and then to wound surfaces. Macrophages, NK cells, and granulocytes display similar features and behavior traits in invertebrates and vertebrates.

Table III CD and other markers identify invertebrate leukocyte types involved in natural immune responses.

Model and CD markers	Cell type function
Earthworms: *Eisenia foetida*	
CD11a, CD45RA, CD45RO CDw49b, CD54, β_2m, CD90	Small coelomocytes NK-like activity
Leeches: *Glossiphonia complanata*	
CD25, CD14, CD61, CD68, CD11b,CD11c	Macrophage-like
CD25, CD56, CD57 and CD16	NK-like
CD11b and CD11c	Granulocytes
Sipunculid worms: *Themiste petricola*	
CD44	Coelomocyte locomotion

Which leukocytes are involved in inflammation? [33]. Shortly after inflicting injury to the body wall in the presence of lipopolysaccharides, many cells resembling vertebrate macrophages, NK cells and granulocytes migrate to lesioned areas. Nuclei of migrating cells incorporated bromodeoxyuridine, suggesting replication. Using human monoclonal antibodies leech cells were positive: macrophage-like cells for CD25, CD14, CD61, CD68, CD11b and CD11c; NK-like cells for CD25, CD56, CD57 and CD16; granulocytes for CD11b and CD11c. In blots of leech extracts, the CD25 monoclonal antibody recognizes a band of about 55 kD; the CD56 monoclonal antibody, two bands of about 140 and 210 kD; the CD57 monoclonal antibody, two bands of about 106 and 70 kD; the CD14 monoclonal antibody, a band of about 50 kD; the CD16 monoclonal antibody, a band of about 60 kD. CD61 and CD68 both recognized a band of about 110 kD; CD11b recognized a band of 200 kD and CD11c, a band of 180 kD [34]. In other experiments, leeches were injected with bacterial lipopolysaccharide, fluoresceinated yeasts, sulfate spheres and ciliates (Protozoa). Shortly after injection, migrating cells appeared. Each injection first provokes cell migration towards non-self material followed by various responses (degranulation, phagocytosis, encapsulation, and melanization). In vertebrates, the structure and function of many CD are well known and strictly linked to specific cell types and functions. CD61 is an integrin belonging to the β3 family and found on migrating cells. CD14 is expressed on myelomonocytic cells including macrophages and Langerhans cells, and it is also a receptor for LPS. CD56 antigen is expressed on neuron, astrocytes, Schwann cells and NK cells. CD57 is associated with cells with natural killer activity. In leeches, all of these cells involved in the healing process are positive for CD61, CD14, CD56 and CD57 [35] (Table III).

2.3. Sipunculan worms

Cell migration is a key event in natural invertebrate and vertebrate immunity [36]. Microbial products like lipopolysaccharide (LPS) and formyl-methyl-leucyl-phenylalanine (fMLP) promote cell recruitment to infection sites. In mammals, complement activation by factors such as zymosan induces C5a production, and that in turn influences leukocyte migration. The endogenous factor hyaluronic acid (HA), an extracellular matrix component, also promotes cell migration through its receptor CD44. Using microchemotaxis chambers, leukocytes (coelomocytes) from the sipunculan worm *Themiste petricola* migrate towards exogenously and endogenously derived chemoattractants [LPS, fMLP, or zymosan treated plasma (ZTP)]. HA is a potent chemotactic signal and coelomocytes adhere strongly to plates coated with LMW-HA but not with HMW-HA. HA mediated effects are blocked by the monoclonal antibody IM7 directed to mouse CD44, suggesting that a CD44-like cross-reactive antigen might play a role in HA medi-

Table IV Presence of cytokine-like molecules (CLM) in invertebrates (from Ottaviani).

Animal Group	CLM
Mollusca	
Planorbarius corneus	
Viviparus ater	IL-1α, β, IL-2, IL-6, TNF-α, PDGF-AB, TGF-β1
Viviparus contectus	
Lymnaea stagnalis	PDGF-AB, TGF-β1
Mytilus galloprovincialis	IL-8, PDGF-AB, TGF-β1
Insecta	
Calliphora vomitoria	TNF-α, PDGF-AB, TGF-β1
Galleria mellonella	IL-1α, TNF-α
Estigmene acraea	IL-1α, TNF-α
Lymantria dispar	PDGF-AB, TGF-β1
Nematoda	
Caenorhabditis elegans	IL-1α, TNF-α, PDGF-AB
Annelida	
Eisenia foetida	IL-1α, TNF-α, PDGF-AB, TGF-β1
Tunicata	
Botryllus schlosserii	IL-1α, TNF-α
Ciona intestinalis	

Table V Effects of mammalian cytokines on different invertebrate functions (modified from Ottaviani).

Cytokine	Function
PDGF-AB, TGF-β1	Wound repair; apoptosis
PDGF-AB, TGF-β1, IL-8	Cell motility
PDGF-AB, TGF-β1, IL-1α, TNF-α, IL-8	Cell migration
IL-1α, TNF-α, IL-2	Phagocytosis; NOS production
IL-2	NK-like activity
PDGF-AB, TGF-β1, IL-1α,β, IL-2, IL-6, TNF-α,β	Stress response

ated coelomocyte locomotion.

3. CYTOKINE ACTIVITY

Since about 1986, there has been a growing literature focusing on cytokines in invertebrates [37,38] (Tables IV and V). Studies have yielded functional evidence but prevailing controversy concerns molecular structure. Several invertebrate species have been examined including arthropods, annelids, mollusks and echinoderms. However, the bulk of the more credible information has been derived from the tunicates. Within the last 10 years, this evidence is even more compelling especially when we view the noteworthy results recently published concerning the draft genome of *Ciona intestinalis* [11]. Thus the earlier functional evidence is corroborated by genetic data.

4. IMMUNE SYSTEM EVOLUTION

4.1. Invertebrate ancestors and the protostome line: the Japanese horseshoe crab

Because invertebrates lack an adaptive immune system, to survive they evolved effective intrinsic defence strategies against a variety of microbial pathogens. This ancient form of host defence, innate immunity, is present in all multicellular organisms including humans. The Japanese horseshoe crab *Tachypleus tridentatus*, is a model protostome organism. Its innate immune system includes a hemolymph coagulation system that participates both in immunity against microbes and in hemostasis. Early work on the evolution of vertebrate fibrinogen suggests a common origin of the arthropod hemolymph coagulation and the vertebrate blood coagulation systems. This assumption could not be verified by comparing the structures of coagulogen, the clotting protein of the horseshoe crab, and of mammalian fibrinogen. However, the crystal structure of tachylectin 5A (TL5A), a nonself-recognizing lectin from the hemolymph plasma of *Tachypleus tridentatus* provides new insights. TL5A shares not only a common fold but also related functional sites with the gamma fragment of mammalian fibrinogen. This is the first structural evidence of a common ancestor for innate immunity and the blood coagulation systems [39]. Both invertebrates and vertebrates are able to discriminate between self and non-self by lectins (carbohydrate-binding proteins). This is a strategy of innate immunity. Immune recognition in vertebrates is mediated by ficolins (lectins that consist of a fibrinogen-like and a collagen-like domain), as well as by mannose-binding lectins. These serve to trigger activation of the complement system and in turn the activation of novel serine proteases. The presence of a similar lectin-based complement system in ascidians, our closest invertebrate relatives, indicates that the complement system probably played a role in innate immunity before jawed vertebrates developed the adaptive immune system [40]

4.2. Invertebrate ancestors on the deuterostome line as revealed by echinoderms

Echinoderms share common ancestry with chordates within the deuterostome clade. Shared molecular features between their immune systems and that of mammals reveal the genetic framework on which these immune systems probably evolved. Coelomocytes are the immune effector cells of sea urchins in which their primary function is protection against invasive by marine pathogens. Six genes expressed in coelomocytes are homologues that are also expressed in leukocytes of the mammalian immune system. Three coelomocyte genes encode transcription factors: 1) NF–κB homologue (SpNFκB); 2) a GATA-2/3 homologue (SpGATAc); 3) a runt domain factor (SpRunt-1). All three coelomocyte genes respond in a pronounced manner to challenge by bacterial antigens. SpNFκB and SpRunt-1 genes are rapidly up regulated, but transcripts of SpGATAc factor disappear rapidly after injecting bacteria. Sham injection also activates more slowly SpNFκB and SpRunt. Bacterial injection does not affect SpGATAc levels. SpHS, another gene, encodes a protein related to the signal transduction intermediate HS1 of lymphocytes. SpSRCR1 and SpSRCR5, two other newly discovered genes, encode proteins featuring SRCR repeats. These genes are members of a complex family of SRCR genes all expressed specifically in coelomocytes. In vertebrates, the SRCR repeats most closely resemble those of mammalian macrophage scavenger receptors. Individuality is clearly present since each sea urchin expresses a specific pattern of SRCR genes. Shared immune functions and, more generally, a shared regulatory architecture are the most likely significance of these findings. The larger implication underlies immune system gene expression in all deuterostomes suggesting that the vertebrate immune system has evolved by inserting new genes into old gene regulatory networks that play a crucial role in immunity [41].

5. COMPLEMENT

5.1. Innate and adaptive immunity and the role of complement

Adaptive immunity in vertebrates can be traced to the appearance of ancestral RAG genes in ancestral jawed vertebrates. Innate immunity is more ancient and appeared about 450 million? years ago. The complement system a central subsystem within innate immunity has been identified throughout the animal groups but seems to be restricted to deuterostomes. The evolutionary history of complement can be traced from sea urchins (phylum Echinodermata), which have a simplified system homologous with the alternative pathway, through the agnathans (hagfish and lamprey) and the elasmobranchs (sharks and rays) to the teleosts (bony fish) and tetrapods, with increases in the numbers of complement components and duplications in complement pathways [42]. Complement in vertebrates comprises a complex enzyme system and non-enzymatic proteins essential for effecting innate and adaptive immune responses and for exerting immunoregulatory functions. Complement protein C3 is a central molecule in the complement system whose activation is essential for this system to function [43]. Complement activation can be induced through three pathways: 1) the classical initiated by antibody-antigen complexes; 2) the alternative initiated by certain structures on microbial surfaces; 3) an antibody-independent initiated by binding of mannan-binding lectin (MBL; first described as mannan-binding protein) to carbohydrates. MBL is structurally related to the complement C1 subcomponent, C1q, and seems to activate the complement system through an MBL associated serine protease known as MASP or p100, that is similar to C1r and C1s of the classical pathway. MBL binds to specific carbohydrate structures found on the surfaces of numerous microorganisms, including bacteria, yeasts, parasitic protozoa and viruses. Complement exhibits antibacterial activity effected through killing mediated by the terminal, lytic complement components or by promoting phagocytosis. MBL level in plasma is genetically determined, and deficiency is associated with frequent infections in childhood, and possibly also in adults. A new MBL-associated serine protease (MASP-2) has been identified. It shows a striking homology with MASP (MASP-1) and the two C1q-associated serine proteases C1r and C1s. Thus complement activation through MBL, like the classical pathway, involves two serine proteases and may have evolved before the development of the adaptive immune system of vertebrates [44].

5.2. How does complement work?

In lower vertebrates, the poikilotherms or ectotherms (fish, amphibians and reptiles), complement is activated by the alternative and lectin pathways and is primarily involved in the opsonization of foreign material. The Agnatha (the most primitive vertebrate-a jawless fish) possess the alternative and lectin pathways while cartilaginous fish are the first group in which the classical pathway appears following the emergence of immunoglobulins. All poikilotherms possess a well-developed complement system resembling that of the homeothermic (endothermic) vertebrates, i.e., birds and mammals. Most complement components seem to have evolved after the duplication of primordial genes encoding C3/C4/C5, fB/C2, C1s/C1r/MASP-1/MASP-2, and C6/C7/C8/C9 molecules, a process that may have led to the formation of distinct activation pathways. Unlike homeotherms, certain poikilotherms (e.g., trout) possess multiple forms of complement components (C3, factor B(fB)) that are structurally and functionally more diverse than those of higher vertebrates. Evidence strongly suggests that the complement system is present in all deuterostomes, and regulatory complement components have been identified in all species beyond the protochordates. Therefore, the mechanisms of complement activation and regulation probably developed in parallel [45].

5.3. Interaction of complement with other recognition factors

The recognition factor, MBL, is associated with a serine protease MASP which, upon MBL binding to the microbial ligand, activates the complement component C3, leading to either (a) phagocytosis of the opsonized target via the complement receptor, or (b) humoral cell killing via assembly of the membrane attack complex. Galectins (formerly S-type lectins) modulate activity of the complement receptor 3 (CR3), the macrophage membrane receptor for complement components C3b and iC3b, downstream products of the MBL pathway that are covalently bound to target cells. Galectins also mediate macrophage- and dendrocyte-adhesion to lymphocytes activated by signaling through another C-type lectin, the L-selectin, leading to immunoglobulin-mediated responses. The functional interplay of MBL, galectins and L-selectin in the acute phase response neutralizes the microbial challenge, and leads to adaptive immunity. Although the observation of various components of the lectin pathway in different invertebrate species demonstrates the high conservation and ancient roots of the components of innate immunity, there has previously been no evidence supporting the possibility that the integral lectin-mediated complement activation pathway is present in invertebrates. There is now evidence for the coexistence of homologs of all the pathway's key components (MBL, MASP, C3, and galectin) in the protochordate *Clavelina picta*. This suggests that the lectin-mediated pathway, an ancient pathway of complement activation preceded the immunoglobulin pathway and has been conserved intact throughout its evolution [46].

6. NATURAL IMMUNITY AND THE NEUROENDOCRINE SYSTEM

What are some of the general features of the neuroendocrineimmune system? The immune system has been referred to as the mobile brain because of shared molecules between the nervous, endocrine and immune systems, the three regulators that govern and control homeostasis--a balanced milieu. Opinions concerning the significance of these interrelations are divided. There are those who view the whole organism and therefore favor a unifying theme with respect to the three systems: central nervous system (CNS), endocrine system (ES), and immune system, (IS). Still others, the reductionists, prefer to retain a strict separation despite substantial evidence indicating enormous overlap. Within the CNS, neuropeptides are small molecules responsible for transmitting certain signals. In vertebrates the hypothalamus produces several of these transmitters, that cause pain (e.g., substance P) or suppress it (e.g., endorphins, enkephalins). In the ES the inner portion of the adrenal medulla, when stimulated by sympathetic nerves, releases adrenaline, causing effects similar to but more than that induced by prolonged noradrenaline (NA). The outer region of the adrenal cortex, when stimulated by adrenocorticotropic hormone (ACTH) from the anterior pituitary, secretes hydrocortisone (cortisol) whose synthetic derivatives have powerful anti-inflammatory effects. Cytokines are present and active within the IS. The most convincing immune-nervous-endocrine link is the induction of fever by TNF, IL-1,

IFNs. With respect to natural immunity, there are several characteristics, components or activities that are apparently shared by invertebrates and vertebrates. These include, complement, lysis, activities of leukocytes such as cytotoxicity and NK cell activity (Tables I and II). According to Ottaviani, there is evidence for ACTH and for cytokines throughout the animal kingdom [37,38].

According to Salzet et al., (2003), during evolution, invertebrates and vertebrates seem to possess common signaling molecules e.g., neuropeptides [47]. Complete hormonal-enzymatic systems for the biosynthesis of opioid peptides have been found in both the central nervous system (CNS) and immune systems (IS). These signaling molecules act as immunomodulators in circulating blood. In vertebrates, release occurs during stress (cognitive or pathogens), that triggers the hypothalamo-hypophysial-adrenal (HPA) axis. Neuropeptides are also employed as conserved messengers that initiate and stimulate innate immune responses in invertebrates and in humans. Given this new information concerning mammalian-like neuroendocrine processes found in invertebrates, in all probability, this system originated in "simple" animals suggesting a referral to the mammalian neuroendocrine system as invertebrate-like. Cross talk between nervous and immune systems has an ancient evolutionary origin essential to homeostasis [48–53].

7. STRESS-INDUCED IMMUNE CHANGES

7.1. The oyster is a model for understanding mechanisms of stress

The stress response comprises a series of coordinated physiological neuroendocrine responses increasing an organism's capacity to maintain homeostasis in the presence of threatening agents. Stress involves hormonal signaling to rapidly modulate strategic physiological functions in vertebrates but more precise evidence for invertebrates is lacking; yet there are some interesting results. Oysters *(Crassostrea gigas)* are permanently exposed to various microbes and their immune system is continuously challenged thus preventing infections by potentially pathogenic organisms. Impaired immune responses usually result in mass mortalities in cultured oyster stocks or increased bacterial loads in food products intended for humans. As indicated by NA and DA measurements, a 15-minute mechanical disturbance causes a transient state of stress. Blood cells (hemocytes) are a convenient indicator of activity measured before, during and after applying a stressor to analyze: 1) levels of circulating numbers; 2) migratory and phagocytic activities; 3) reactive oxygen species production. All immune functions are significantly down regulated during stress and a transient period of immuno-stimulation also occurs 30–240 min after the disturbance. Stress exerts a significant influence on immune functions that could explain why stress and the outbreak of disease are often linked in shellfish culture [54]. Oysters challenged with a low dose of the oyster pathogen *Vibrio splendidus* strain and subjected to a mechanical stress 3 days later showed variable responses. Mortality and *V. splendidus* loads increased in stressed but were low in unstressed oysters. Injection of NA or ACTH also caused higher mortality and increased accumulation of pathogens in challenged oysters. Physiological changes imposed by stress, or stress hormones, may influence host-pathogen interactions especially in immature immune systems [55].

7.2. The stress response in oysters and catecholamines (CA)

Mechanical disturbances (shaking) and temperature or salinity variations have been applied since oysters in aquaculture or in nature commonly encounter these stressors. Circulating NA and DA concentrations increased in response to stress. The catecholaminergic response to acute mechanical stressors was rapid (less than 5 min), transient (a return to basal CA levels after 60–90 min), and reflected the intensity and duration of the stressor. Responses to temperature and salinity variations were long lasting (up to 72 h). CA concentrations varied within the range, which induces physiological responses suggesting that stress-induced NA and DA changes exert a regulatory function in oysters [56].

7.3. Catecholamines and pro-opiomelanocortin (POMC) derived peptides

Both catecholamines such as NA and DA, and pro-opiomelanocortin- (POMC)-derived peptides such as ACTH, central regulators of the vertebrate stress-response, are also present in invertebrates. In oysters, NA and DA are released into the circulation in response to stress and their storage and release occurs in neurosecretory cells that are similar in morphology and biochemical responses to vertebrate chromaffin cells. The neurotransmitters, acetylcholine or carbachol, caused no significant release of NA or DA. The nicotinic antagonists hexamethonium and α-bungarotoxin and the muscarinic antagonist atropine caused no significant inhibition of CA release in stressed oysters. ACTH induced a significant release of NA but not DA. The oyster adrenergic stress-response, unlike the vertebrate responses, may not be controlled by acetylcholine but may be controlled by other factors, e.g., ACTH [57].

8. NORADRENALINE AND ADRENERGIC SIGNALING

8.1. Apoptosis and the invertebrate neuroimmune response

Apoptosis contributes to maintenance and preservation of a balanced immune system in vertebrates. With the exception of mollusks, information is scarce concerning apoptotic processes and regulation of immunity in other invertebrates. NA a catecholamine produced by the neuroendocrineimmune system induces apoptosis in oyster hemocytes. The apoptosis-inducing effect of NA can be mimicked by isoproterenol and blocked by propranolol, indicating that NA triggers apoptosis via a α-adrenergic signaling pathway. Exposure to the pan-caspase inhibitor Z-VAD-FMK or expression of the caspase inhibitor P35 under the transcriptional control of a mollusk heat shock protein 70 (hsp70) gene promoter reduces levels of apoptotic cells in hemocytes treated with isoproterenol. P35-sensitive caspases are probably involved in apoptosis and are triggered by α-adrenergic signaling. Moreover, mitogen-activated protein kinases and Rho, a member of the Ras GTPase family, may be involved in anti-apoptotic mechanisms that modulate the apoptotic effect of NA [58]

8.2. Heat shock proteins and neuroimmune responses

Expression of heat shock proteins is a homeostatic mechanism induced in prokaryotic and eukaryotic cells in response to metabolic and environmental insults. Increasing evidence suggests that in mammals, the hsp response is integrated with physiological responses through neuroendocrine signaling. Oyster and abalone hemocytes were transfected with a gene construct containing a gastropod hsp70 gene promoter linked to the luciferase reporter-gene. NA and α-adrenergic stimulations induced the expression of luciferase in these transfected mollusk immunocytes. Exposure of hemocytes to NA or to the α-adrenoceptor agonist phenylephrine (PE) causes expression of the inducible isoform of the hsp70 protein determined through immunoblotting. Pertussis toxin, the phospholipase C (PLC) inhibitor U73122, the protein kinase C (PKC) inhibitor calphostin C, the Ca^{++}-dependent PKC inhibitor Gö 6976 and the phosphatidylinositol 3-kinase (PI 3-kinase) inhibitor LY294002 blocked the PE-mediated induction of the hsp70 gene promoter. Thus, α-adrenergic signaling induces transcriptional upregulation of hsp70 in molluscan hemocytes through a PTX-sensitive G-protein, PLC, Ca^{++}-dependent PKC and PI 3-kinase. Neuroendocrine signaling and the hsp70 response share an apparent link in molluscan immune cells [59].

8.3. Catecholamines and neuroimmune regulation

Catecholamines regulate several physiological processes in mollusks. The β-adrenoceptor agonist isoproterenol mimics the inhibitory effects of NA on phagocytosis by oyster hemocytes, whereas the α-adrenoceptor agonist phenylephrine had no significant effect. The β-adrenoceptor antagonist propanolol, but not the α-adrenoceptor antagonist prazosin, prevented inhibition of phagocytosis by NA. The type IV phosphodiesterase inhibitor rolipram acted synergistically with a suboptimal concentration of isoproterenol to inhibit phagocytosis, and the protein kinase A inhibitor H-89, but not the protein kinase C inhibitor calphostin C, attenuated the effect of isoproterenol. NA modulates phagocytosis via a β-adrenergic receptor/cAMP/protein kinase A signaling pathway [60]. Catecholamines are present in the microenvironment of immunocytes. NA the principal CA circulating in bivalve hemolymph exerts a dose-dependent inhibitory effect on luminol-dependent chemiluminescence- (CL)-responses in oyster hemocytes. The α-adrenoceptor agonist phenylephrine exerts no significant effect whereas the β-adrenoceptor agonist isoproterenol mimicked the inhibitory effects of NA on the CL-response. The β-adrenoceptor antagonist propanolol, but not the α-adrenoceptor antagonist prazosin, prevents the negative effects of NA on the CL-response. β-adrenergic receptors are probably present on hemocyte surfaces thus allowing NA to down-regulate the CL-response [61]

9. PERSPECTIVES ON ORIGINS OF NATURAL IMMUNITY AND RELATION TO THE NEUROENDOCRINE SYSTEM

Interest in the dual functional and morphological division of the immune system is pervasive. Clearly access to the totality of immune capability is now balanced with all animals being considered. We now have innate, natural, non-specific, non-anticipatory, non-clonal responses of invertebrates in contrast to the adaptive, induced, specific, anticipatory, clonal responses typical of vertebrates. The innate is considered the most primitive and found in both animal groups; invertebrates do not possess the adaptive system. This duality is expressed at every level of biological organization: molecules, cells, tissues, organs, and organisms. Monolithic immunology, 19th century preoccupation with humoral mechanisms was split when Metchnikoff discovered phagocytosis in invertebrates. This discovery changed the face of immunology, creating a permanent schism and according equal importance to cellular effectors (leukocytes) obviously the sources of the molecular products that they synthesize and secrete (mediators), the mainstay of the humoral system. Now almost 100 years later, this essential cellular component, and the animal models from which it was derived are, once again, at the center of immunology. However, prevailing taxonomies are changing depending upon the amount and kind of molecular data that emerges. In fact, with discoveries of innate immunity and the Toll pathway, we witnessed a convergence of similar mechanisms between mammals, plants and invertebrates. Thus the strict lines of apparent separation are not at all blurred but are now in sharper focus revealing a pervasive uniformity.

Until technology is refined for the use of relevant invertebrate cells and their specific antibodies, the search for cell differentiation (CD) markers using reagents from mammals will rest as a plausible approach that edges us nearer to a better understanding of origins and possible homologies. With respect to cytokines, where must we go? Further proof and confirmation of the existing linkages invertebrate and vertebrate molecules will do more to explain the whole organism. Clearly we need to resolve relationships by performing more intense genetic analyses. Complement on the other hand is another matter with respect to the immune system where there is greater clarity. The complement cascades in higher vertebrates appear to have evolved from a few primordial genes through gene duplication and subsequent divergence of function. This view is based on similarities in protein sequence and function with complement protein families, the clustered organization of some complement genes, and parallels in organization and function of the lectin, alternative and classical pathways.

The most unique characteristics of natural immunity concern the relation with the immune and connection with the nervous and endocrine systems. This is an example of how linkages exist in the whole organism by means of the three regulatory systems. The stress response comprises a series of coordinated physiological neuroendocrine responses increasing an organism's capacity to maintain homeostasis in the presence of threatening agents. Stress involves hormonal signaling in order to rapidly modulate strategic physiological functions in vertebrates but this kind of more precise evidence for invertebrates is just beginning to emerge. What still needs to be resolved is the precise appearance of pro-opiomelanocortin-derived peptides (e.g., ACTH), as a unifying theme in the neuroendocrineimmune system and to eventually link this in more clearly with those characteristics that are closer to immune than those associated with the neuroendocrine system, [62–64].

ACKNOWLEDGEMENTS

A note of appreciation is extended to Dr. Arnaud Lacoste, Post doctoral Fellow, Program in Psychoneuroimmunology, UCLA for executing the original for Fig. 1.

REFERENCES

1. Besredka, A. Histoire d'une idee' de E. Metchnikoff: inflammation, immunitie, senescence, pathologie, philosophie. Masson, Paris. 1921.
2. Cooper EL, Rinkevich B, Uhlenbruck G, Valembois P. Invertebrate Immunity: another viewpoint. Scand. J. Immunol. 1992; 35:247–66.
3. Medzhitov R, Janeway C. Innate immunity. N Engl. J Med. 2000;343:338–44.
4. Medzhitov R, Janeway C. Innate immune recognition: mechanisms and pathways. Immunol Rev. 2000;173:89–97.

5. Hoffmann JA, Kafatos FC, Janeway CA, Ezekowitz RA. Phylogenetic perspectives in innate immunity. Science 1999;284:1313–8.
6. Fearon DT, Locksley RM. The instructive role of innate immunity in the acquired immune response. Science 1996;272:50–4.
7. Boman HG. Peptide antibiotics and their role in innate immunity. Ann. Rev. Immunol. 1995;67:1–92.
8. Quintans J. Immunity and inflammation: The cosmic view. Immunol. Cell Biol. 1994; 72: 262–6.
9. Salzet M. Vertebrate innate immunity resembles a mosaic of invertebrate immune responses. Trends in Immunology 2001;22:285–8.
10. Loker ES, Bayne CJ. Molecular studies of the molluscan response to digenean infection in Beck G, Sugumaran M, Cooper EL. Editors. Phylogenetic Perspectives on the Vertebrate Immune System. New York: Kluwer Academic /Plenum Publishers. 2001; 209–22.
11. Dehal, P, et al. The draft genome of *Ciona intestinalis*: insights into chordate and vertebrate origins. Science 2002;298:2157–67.
12. Cooper EL, Suzuki MM, Cossarizza A, Franceschi C. Cytotoxic reactions in invertebrates: the earthworm model. In: Söderhäll K, Iwanaga S, Vasta GR. Editors. New Directions In Invertebrate Immunology. Fair Haven, NJ: SOS Publications. 1996;23–42.
13. Cooper EL. Earthworm Immunity. In: Rinkevich B, Müller WEG. Editors; Invertebrate Immunology. Heidelberg: Springer Verlag. 1996;10–45.
14. Cooper EL, Cossarizza A, Kauschke E, Franceschi C. Cytotoxicity in earthworms. In: Maramorosch K, Loeb M, editors; Proc. World Cong In Vitro Biology. 1997;53–8.
15. Cooper, EL, Kauschke E, Cossarizza A, Franceschi C. Cell adhesion and the immune system: A case study using earthworms. Micros Res Tech. 1999;44:237–53.
16. Cooper EL, Kauschke E, Cossarizza A. Annelid humoral immunity: Cell lysis in earthworms. In Beck G, Cooper EL, Sugumaran M. editors; Phylogenetic Perspectives on the Vertebrate Immune system. New York: Plenum Publishing Co. 2001;169–84.
17. Andersson M, Gunne H, Agerberth B, Boman A, Bergman T, Sillard R, Jornvall H, Mutt V, Olsson B, Wigzell H, et al. NK-lysin, a novel effector peptide of cytotoxic T and NK cells. Structure and cDNA cloning of the porcine form, induction by interleukin 2, antibacterial and antitumour activity. EMBO. J. 1995;14:1615–25.
18. Leippe M, Müller-Eberhard HJ. The pore-forming peptide of *Entamoeba histolytica*, the protozoan parasite causing human amoebiasis. Toxicology 1994;87:5–18.
19. Leulier F, Rodriguez A, Khush, RS, Chen P, Abrams JM, Lemaitre B. The *Drosophila* caspase Dredd is required to resist Gram-negative bacterial infection. EMBO J. 2000; 1: 353–8.
20. Vidal S, Khush RS, Leulier F, Tzou P, Nakamura M, Lemaitre B. Mutations in the *Drosophila* dTAK1 gene reveal a conserved function for MAPKKKs in the control of rel/NF-B-dependent innate immune responses. Genes & Development 2001;15:1900–12.
21. Hoffmann J, Reichhart J. Drosophila immunity. Trends Cell. Biol. 1997;7:309–16.
22. Khush RS, Lemaitre B. Genes that fight infection: What the Drosophila genome says about animal immunity. Trends Genet. 2000;16: 442–9.
23. Engstrom Y. Induction and regulation of antimicrobial peptides in Drosophila. Dev. Comp. Immunol. 1999;23:345–58.
24. Anderson KV. Toll signaling pathways in the innate immune response. Curr. Opin. Immunol. 2000;12:13–9.
25. Khush RS, Leulier F, Lemaitre B. Drosophila immunity: Two paths to NF-κB. Trends

Immunol. 2001;22:260–4.
26. Hoffmann JA, Kafatos FC, Janeway CA, Ezekowitz RA. Phylogenetic perspectives in innate immunity. Science 1999;284:1313–8.
27. Aderem A, Ulevitch RJ. Toll-like receptors in the induction of the innate immune response. Nature 2000;406:782–7.
28. Lemaitre B, Nicolas E, Michaut L, Reichhart J, Hoffmann J. The dorsoventral regulatory gene cassette spätzle/Toll/cactus controls the potent antifungal response in *Drosophila* adults. Cell 1996;86:973–83.
29. Rutschmann S, Jung AC, Zhou R, Silverman N, Hoffmann JA, Ferrandon D. Role of Drosophila IKK in a Toll-independent antibacterial immune response. Nat. Immunol. 2000;1:342–7.
30. Lu Y, Wu LP, Anderson KV. The antibacterial arm of the Drosophila innate immune response requires an IB kinase Genes & Dev. 2001;15:104–10.
31. Cooper EL, Kauschke E, Cossarizza A. Digging for innate immunity since Darwin and Metchnikoff. Bioessays 2002;24:319–33.
32. Engelmann P, Pál J, Timea B, Cooper EL, Németh P. Earthworm leukocytes react with different mammalian antigen-specific monoclonal antibodies Zoology 2002;105:257–65.
33. de Eguileor M, Tettamanti G, Grimaldi A, Boselli A, Scari G, Valvassori R, Cooper EL, Lanzavecchia G. Histopathological changes after induced injury in leeches. J Invertebr Pathol 1999;74:14–28.
34. de Eguileor M, Grimaldi A, Tettamanti G, Valvassori R, Cooper EL, Lanzavecchia G. Lipopolysaccharide-dependent induction of leech leukocytes that cross-react with vertebrate cellular differentiation markers. Tissue and Cell 2000a;32:437–45.
35. de Eguileor M, Grimaldi A, Tettamanti G, Valvassori R, Cooper EL, Lanzavecchia G. Different types of response to foreign antigens by leech leukocytes Tissue and Cell 2000b 32:40–8.
36. Cabrera PV, Blanco G, Ernst G, Alvarez E, Cooper EL, Hajos S. Coelomocyte locomotion in the sipunculan *Themiste petricola* induced by exogenous and endogenous chemoattractants: role of a CD44-like antigen--HA interaction. J. Invertebr. Pathol. 2002; 79:111–9.
37. Ottaviani, E. The evolutionary paradox of invertebrate cytokines. Mod. Asp. Immunobiol 2002;1:253–5.
38. Ottaviani, E. Invertebrate ACTH Immuno-neuroendocrine regulation. Mod. Asp. Immunobiol. 2001;2:215–6.
39. Kairies, N., et al. The 2.0-A crystal structure of tachylectin 5A provides evidence for the common origin of the innate immunity and the blood coagulation systems. Proc Natl Acad Sci USA 2001;98:13519–24.
40. Fujita T. Evolution of the lectin-complement pathway and its role in innate immunity. Nat Rev Immunol 2002;2:346–53.
41. Pancer Z, Rast JP, Davidson EH. Origins of immunity: transcription factors and homologues of effector genes of the vertebrate immune system expressed in sea urchin coelomocytes. Immunogenetics 1999;49:773–86.
42. Smith LC, Clow LA, Terwilliger DP. The ancestral complement system in sea urchins. Immunol Rev 2001;180:16–34.
43. Sahu A, Lambris JD. Structure and biology of complement protein C3, a connecting link between innate and acquired immunity. Immunol Rev 2001;180:35–48.
44. Thiel S. et al, A second serine protease associated with mannan-binding lectin that

activates complement. Nature 1997;386:506–10.
45. Zarkadis IK, Mastellos D, Lambris JD. Phylogenetic aspects of the complement system. Dev Comp Immunol 2001;25:745–62.
46. Vasta GR, Quesenberry M, Ahmed H, O'Leary N. C-type lectins and galectins mediate innate and adaptive immune functions: their roles in the complement activation pathway. Dev Comp Immunol 1999;23:401–20.
47. Salzet M, Tasiemski A, Lefebvre Cooper EL. Comparison of molecular neuroimmune processes between leeches and human Proc. 18th Zoology Congress Athens 2003. Legakis, et al., Editors. Pensoft, Sofia-Moscow, 2003; 147–157.
48. Salzet M, Salzet B, Cocquerelle C, Verger-Bocquet M, Pryor S, Laurent V, Stefano GB. Biochemical and molecular characterization of ACTH, its precursor and receptor in the leech *Theromyzon tessulatum* : morphine increases ACTH levels. J. Immunol. 1997;159: 5400–11.
49. Salzet M, Vieau D, Stefano GB. Serpins: an evolutionarily conserved survival strategy. Immunol. Today 1999;20:541–4.
50. Salzet M. Molecular neuroimmune processes. Brain Res Rev. 2000;34:69–79.
51. Salzet M, Vieau D, Day R. Cross-talk between nervous and immune systems through the animal kingdom : focus on opioids. Trends in Neurosc. 2000a;23:500–5.
52. Salzet M, Capron A, Stefano GB. Molecular cross talk in host parasite relationships: schistosomes or leeches -host interactions. Parasitol. Today 2000b;12:536–40.
53. Salzet M, Breton C, Bisogno T, Di Marzo V. Comparative biology of endogenous endocannabinoids system : possible role in immune response. Eur. J. Biochem. 2000c; 267:4917–27.
54. Lacoste A, Malham SK, Gelebart F, Cueff A, Poulet SA. Stress-induced immune changes in the oyster *Crassostrea gigas*. Dev Comp Immunol 2002;26:1–9.
55. Lacoste A, Jalabert F, Malham SK, Cueff A, Poulet SA. Stress and stress-induced neuroendocrine changes increase the susceptibility of juvenile oysters (*Crassostrea gigas*) to *Vibrio splendidus*. Appl Environ Microbiol 2001;67:2304–9.
56. Lacoste A, Malham SK, Cueff A, Poulet SA. Stress-induced catecholamine changes in the hemolymph of the oyster *Crassostrea gigas*. Gen Comp Endocrinol 2001;122:181–8.
57. Lacoste A, Malham SK, Cueff A, Jalabert F, Gelebart F, Poulet SA. Evidence for a form of adrenergic response to stress in the mollusc *Crassostrea gigas*. J Exp Biol 2001; 204: 1247–55.
58. Lacoste A, Cueff A, Poulet SA. P35-sensitive caspases, MAP kinases and Rho modulate beta-adrenergic induction of apoptosis in mollusc immune cells. J Cell Sci 2002; 115: 761–8.
59. Lacoste A, De Cian MC, Cueff A, Poulet SA. Noradrenaline and alpha-adrenergic signaling induce the hsp70 gene promoter in mollusc immune cells. J Cell Sci 2001; 114: 3557–64.
60. Lacoste A, Malham SK, Cueff A, Poulet SA. Noradrenaline modulates oyster hemocyte phagocytosis via a beta-adrenergic receptor-cAMP signaling pathway. Gen Comp Endocrinol 2001;122:252–9.
61. Lacoste A, Malham SK, Cueff A, Poulet SA. Noradrenaline modulates hemocyte reactive oxygen species production via beta-adrenergic receptors in the oyster *Crassostrea gigas*. Dev Comp Immunol 2001;25:285–9.
62. Cooper EL. Evolutionary development of the neuroendocrineimmune system. Adv. Neuroimmunol. 1991;1:83–96.

63. Cooper EL. Overview of immunoevolution. Boll. Zool., 1992;59:119–28.
64. Cooper EL. Perspectives in neuroimmunomodulation: Lessons from the comparative approach. Anim. Biol. 1992;1:169–80.

Natural Immunity
Edited by L. Bertók and D.A. Chow
© 2005 Elsevier B.V. All rights reserved

Natural Immune Activation: Stimulators/Receptors

DONNA A. CHOW

Department of Immunology, University of Manitoba, Winnipeg, MB Canada, R3M 0P9

ABSTRACT

The activation of the natural immune response is initiated through multiple recognition molecules representing numerous structural families including, several lectin families, pentraxins, leucine-rich repeats, many members of the IgSF, integrins, scavenger receptors and the seven transmembrane receptor family, which have been maintained through evolution. Invading pathogens exhibit a range of different repeating epitopes. Host molecules, soluble or on cell surfaces, express a variety of receptors capable of recognising these epitopes and act in a combinatorial manner which confers specificity to the host response. The number, diversity and ancient evolutionary origin of these receptors argues for the essential nature of their functions. While providing a first line of defence against invading pathogens is clearly crucial for organism survival, evidence is accumulating that these same receptors participate in essential functions unrelated to defence against invaders.

1. INTRODUCTION

The increased attention focussed on the natural immune response over the past decade has markedly expanded our knowledge regarding the number of the mediators and range of their functions, and has renewed interest and discussion on issues associated with the natural immune system including the evolutionary pressure for the development of the system and its relationship with the adaptive response.

The natural immune system has long been considered a first line of defence against invading pathogens. The mediators are widely distributed in mammalian tissues and systemically in the circulation. They are preformed and ready to act or are rapidly inducible. Activation of the natural immune system implies a recognition event followed by a sequence of events aimed at destroying an invader or alternatively maintaining the integrity of the organism. Our awareness has increased regarding the multiplicity of receptors contributing to recognition, their structures, their redundancy, the use of facilitating or amplifying, intermediary molecules (opsonins, LBP) to reach the threshold of interaction for functional activation. The receptors which contribute to the innate response include secreted molecules in blood and lymph which act as bridging molecules between the effector cell and the target for phagocytosis, cell surface receptors for pathogens leading to phagocytosis and cell surface receptors which lead to signalling and induction of proinflammatory cytokines.

The dual concepts of pathogen-associated molecular patterns (PAMPs), invariant structures associated with essential microbial functions, which act as the main targets of the innate response against pathogens, and their non-clonal, germline-specified pattern-recognition receptors (PRRs), developed by Janeway and Medzhitov [1–4], have provided a productive framework for discussing the induction of natural immune responses, particularly against microbial pathogens. Their view of natural immune strategies for recognition encompassed recognition of "microbial nonself" and Kärre's 'recognition of missing self' [3,5]. This was extended with the addition of "induced or altered self"[6]. The first strategy distinguishes between "infectious non-self" and "non-infectious self" through recognition of conserved metabolic products unique to microbes leading to activation of the innate immune system. The second acknowledged the benefit of self-recognition and this was coupled to inhibitory signalling pathways, so that when "markers of normal self"are not recognized on an abnormal cell, activation would occur. The last strategy was considered to end in apoptosis through a " cell-autonomous mechanism" or as the result of a signal from another cell, following recognition of markers of infection or cell transformation [6]. In addition, markers on apoptotic cells can trigger clearance mechanisms of the innate immune response. An alternate view proposed by Matsinger suggests that pattern recognition receptors react in response to 'danger' recognized as self-antigens exposed upon cell destruction through necrotic cell death [7]. Berczi's concept of homotopes and their receptors [8,9], with homotopes being highly conserved homologous or cross-reactive epitopes which may also be expressed on self tissue, suggests an additional contribution from self-recognition in the evolutionary development and conservation of natural immune reactivity. This thinking is also evident in the description of antigen presenting cell (APC) dual-specific pattern recognition receptors which recognize both endogenous and exogenous ligands suggesting their participation in normal tissue functions and in defence mechanisms [10].

2. ACTIVATION RECEPTORS/ AND THEIR LIGANDS

Recognition molecules contributing to the initiation of activation of the natural immune system are widely distributed for pervasive surveillance of the organism, with their presence detected on cell surfaces, in cells (in granules or in cytoplasm, for example HSP), or on soluble mediators. In contrast with the receptors of the adaptive immune response, they are highly conserved in evolution, originate from the germline, do not require clonal expansion, do not tend toward somatic mutation and are generally of weak affinity. Proteins of many different structural gene families contribute to this function [11,12] suggesting the essential nature of natural immunity.

2.1. Lectins

Lectins have long been implicated in cell aggregation. Three molecular strategies contribute to cell adhesion in prokaryotic and eukaryotic systems. Cell surface molecules can bind through homophilic or heterophilic interactions, or through the linking action of a multivalent, soluble molecule. Our knowledge of the diversity of lectins participating in natural immune responses has increased markedly in the last 15 years [13]. However, x-ray crystallographic studies have also revealed surprising evidence of tertiary structure evolutionary convergence among some lectins [reviewed in 13].

2.1.1. *C-Type (Lectins)*

Collectins, are oligomers of a cysteine-rich region and a collagen-like domain joined through a neck region to a C-type lectin carbohydrate-recognition domain (CRD), present in plasma and on mucosa surfaces [14]. For example serum mannose-binding lectin (MBL) which binds mannose and N-acetyl-glucosamine [15] consists of three polypeptide chains with globular heads wound into triplets which oligomerize and exhibit structural and functional similarities with C1q and IgM [16]. MBL produced in the liver can activate complement through MBL-associated serine proteases, MASPs, splitting C4 and C2, and similar to the classical pathway, leading to the non-specific covalent binding of the intermediary molecule C3b which increases phagocytosis of the MBL target. MBL is opsonic for bacteria but can also bind an endogenous epitope on CD45RO of immature murine thymocytes [17]. This provides evidence for homotopes and links MBL-recognized PAMPs with carbohydrate expression on the leukocyte common antigen (LCA), CD45. Since this epitope was expressed on a lymphocyte subpopulation during a transient stage of maturation, mannose-binding lectins of the innate immune system, MBL or possibly the homologous cell surface DEC-205 of thymic DCs may contribute to a physiological process, the selective maturation of thymocytes [reviewed in 17]. Conversely, considering that CD45 has been identified in hagfish [18] and is a negative regulator of JAKs-dependent signalling by cytokines [19] which includes, the innate system cytokines, IL-6, Il-10 and IL-15, it has been argued that CD45 plays a crucial role in innate immunity [reviewed in 18]. Surfactant proteins S and D (SP-A and SP-D) are collectins found coating pulmonary epithelial cells and in the gastrointestinal tract [20]. They aggregate pathogens reducing their infectivity and increase their phagocytosis via SP-specific receptors on phagocytes [reviewed in 14,21].

Selectins are membrane glycoproteins, a subfamily of C-type lectins bearing a C-type domain, an epidermal growth factor receptor-like domain and variable numbers of complement regulatory protein-like domains [13]. They include the murine lymph node homing receptor (L-selectin), the endothelial-leukocyte adhesion molecule (E-selectin) and the platelet granule membrane protein-140 (P-selectin). They exhibit approximately 50% homology in their C-type lectin domains and possess fairly similar saccharide specificities and functions [13]. They participate in cell trafficking and contribute to the recruitment of neutrophils to inflammatory sites.

Macrophage mannose-binding receptors contribute to the phagocytosis of bacteria. They consist of twelve domains, eight of which are C-type lectins with the carbohydrate-binding activity detected between the fourth and the eighth domains [22]. The cysteine-rich (CR) domain has been identified as a lectin [23].

2.1.2. *Natural killer (NK) cell transmembrane receptors*

The Ly49 C-type lectins are a family of MHC-class I-specific receptors. The Ly49D and LY49H members are activating receptors for murine NK cells. LY49H binds m157 produced by murine cytomegalovirus (MCMV) which has ben shown by protein structural prediction studies to be similar to class I MHC with similarities to H-2M3, MICA and CD1d non-classical MHC class I molecules [24]. However, in another strain of mice, m157 binds the inhibitory MHC-specific Ly49I receptor arguing that m157 binding to Ly49H may have evolved as a defence against MCMV [24].

NKG2 C-type lectin-like family member NKG2D, is considered the most widely expressed NK receptor and a potent activator of natural immune responses [11]. In humans it is present on NK cells, $CD8^+$ T cells and intraepithelial lymphocyte (IEL) $\gamma\delta$ T cells, and recognizes, through protein-protein interactions, molecules distantly related in sequence to MHC-class I which are upregulated in response to stress, oncogenic transformation or virus infection. These include the non-classical MHC class I molecules MIC-A and MIC-B [25] , which exhibit a limited distribution on the surface of normal cells including, mainly epithelial cells, the epithelial lining of the gastrointestinal tract and the thymic cortex, and fibroblasts [24,26,27]. However, MICA is also induced on anti-CD3- or anti-CD28- plus PMA-activated T cells [28,29], and on IFN-α-stimulated dendritic cells [30], suggesting that MICA is a marker of activated cells. Expression of MICA on the epithelium of the gastrointestinal tract, cells which undergo continued rapid renewal during life [31], is consistent with this thinking. In addition, the demonstration of heat shock elements defined by HSP70 in the promoter regions of MICA and MICB [32], link expression of these nonclassical class I molecules to situations where HSPs are expressed. Heat shock proteins (HSPs) 27, 60, 70 and 90 are constitutively expressed inside all cells under normal physiological conditions [reviewed in 33]. They act as intracellular molecular chaperones for the proper assembly, folding, translocation and degradation of proteins. Their differential cellular and subcellular expression in human decidua and placenta during pregnancy [33] and the presence of HSP70 mRNA in human fetal membranes [34] raise questions regarding whether MICA or MICB, which exhibit heat shock elements defined by HSP70 in their promoter regions [32] may also be induced in this metabolically active tissue providing targets for cells bearing NKG2 receptors to participate in morphological development or control of the pregnancy. This is supported by the requirement for the major heat shock transcriptional factor HSF1 for extra-embryonic development beginning at mid-gestation and for postnatal growth in mice coupled with the failure to detect changes in basal HSP levels associated with extra-embryonic abnormalities in HFS1-deficient mice, suggesting the activation of non-HSP genes [35]. Could activation of these genes lead to expression of MICA and/or MICB ?

Murine NKG2D recognize molecules with weak homology to MHC class I including the retanoic acid early inducible 1 protein family Rae1 and the H60 family of dominant histocompatibility antigens of BALB/c mice. They are detected on tumour but not normal cells and interestingly, H60 is also expressed at low levels on activated lymphoblasts and at high levels on the thymocytes of BALB/c [24]. Human NKG2D also binds ULBPs or binding proteins for human cytomegalovirus UL16 glycoprotein [24]. The MHC-binding surfaces of NKG2D and other C-type lectin MHC-binding NK receptors to date appear to be relatively flat consistent with their protein-binding capacity and they are missing the Ca^{++} binding residues [25].

The NKR-P1 family of C-type lectin receptors in mice includes NK1.1 which is expressed on NK and T cells and is implicated in NK cell activation. However, some NKR-P1 bear ITIMs and are considered to exert an inhibitory function on NK cell activation [36].

2.1.3. *Galectins (S-Type Lectins)*

Galectins are a growing and widely distributed family of structurally-related lectins which bind β-galactoside and are considered master regulators of immune cell homeostasis [37]. Their specificity including that of the ubiquitously expressed N-acetyl-lactosamine-binding lectins, is conserved through evolution in their carbohydrate-recognition domains (CRDs) [38,39]. Genomic studies of galectin-like domains suggest that the galectin gene family may have originated at or before the development of multicellularity [39]. Galectins in the main, are soluble proteins, synthesized in the cytosol and are secreted through a non-classical mechanism. They are not endocytic receptors; however, their binding to cell surface molecules regulates the inflammatory response. Expression of the core 2β-1,6-N-acetylglucosaminyltransferase (C2GnT) which is developmentally regulated and increased after T cell activation, has been proposed as the basis of T cell susceptibility to galectin-1 induced cell-cycle arrest and/or apoptosis during development in the thymus and in the periphery after activation [38]. In contrast, galectin-3 is considered an amplifier of the inflammatory response. As an extracellular molecule galectin activated cells including monocytes, macrophages, neutrophils, mast cells and basophils [reviewed in 37,40], and as an intracellular molecule provided a critical role in phagocytosis by macrophages [40]. Galectin-3 was first identified as a cell surface antigen Mac-2 on thioglycolate-elicited macrophages and then as a glycoform-specific IgE-binding protein (epsilon bp/Mac-2), exhibits two independent sites for LPS, a C-terminal carbohydrate-binding site inhibitable by lactose and an N-terminal site which bound LPS from β-galactoside-negative bacterium [41]. Galectin-3 is also able to aggregate and cross-link ligands, extending its functional capacity. Thus, galectin-3 and its ligands appear to fulfil the definition of a homotope/homotope receptor system, binding both exogenous microbial epitopes and endogenous epitopes, through its carbohydrate-binding site.

2.1.4. *The Pentraxins*

C-reactive protein (CRP) and serum amyloid P component (SAP) are acute phase proteins (APP) which exhibit calcium-dependent binding to several different molecules and pathogens. They are members of the ancient family of pentraxins which are composed of five identical segments joined to form a five sided doughnut structure. CRP exhibits high affinity binding to phosphorylcholine expressed on microbes, oxidized phospholipids and apoptotic host cells [42,43]. Through a different site CRP binds galactans and galactose phosphates [44]. CRP acts as an opsonin indirectly through activation of complement. It has been reported to act directly as an opsonin by reacting with Fc receptors on phagocytic cells; however, recent experiments have not confirmed this [reviewed in 45]. SAP has a preference for binding phosphoethanolamine and activates complement.

2.1.5. *Ficolins*

Ficolins are oligomers, somewhat similar to collectins, of a cysteine-rich region, a collagen-like domain attached through a neck structure to a carbohydrate-binding fibrinogen-like domain found in plasma and on mucosa surfaces [14,15]. Serum ficolins bind N-acetyl-glucosamine (GlcNAc) with human serum L-ficolin/35 (ficolin L) and H-ficolin (Hakata antigen) reported to activate complement through MASPs.

2.1.6. *Scavenger receptors (SRs)*

SRs are transmembrane receptors detected on macrophages, dendritic cells and some epithelial cells [46] which internalize modified low-density lipoproteins and phagocytose apoptotic cells, microorganisms and their products [46]. These structurally heterogeneous receptors include molecules with C-type lectin, collagenous, cysteine-rich or other domains, arguing for diverse mechanisms in the binding of their diverse ligands including the polyanionic targets of the collagenous domains.

2.2. The Ig superfamily (IgSF)

IgSF genes encode the most common domain type in the human proteome [reviewed in 47], a clear indicator of its importance. The IgSF codes for a broad spectrum of molecules which exert diverse functions such as cell-cell recognition and adhesion, recognition of soluble molecules and specific antigen recognition. Most Fc receptors (FcRs) function as multichain receptors with the α chain, which recognizes the Fc portion of immunoglobulins being itself a member of the IgSF. Recent identification of Fc receptor homologs in humans [reviewed in 47], holds a promise of unveiling additional activating receptors of natural immunity.

2.2.1. *Fc Receptors*

FcγRI (CD64), bears three IgSF domains and is constitutively expressed on monocytes and macrophages [reviewed in 48,49]. The murine FcγRI is the high affinity receptor for T-dependent IgG_{2a} but also the low affinity receptor for complexed IgG_3 [50]. Since IgG_3 is the first IgG class produced in mice, is T-independent with the class switch from IgM promoted by INF-γ produced largely from NK cells, recognizes primarily carbohydrates and antigens with repeating epitopes and tends towards self-aggregation [reviewed in 50], activation of APCs, macrophages and some DCs, through antigen-bound IgG_3 interaction with their FcγRIs would contribute to innate responses and provide a link with the adaptive response by presenting for T cells, antigens from T-independent immune complexes [50,51]. Production of human IgG2 is considered to be relatively T-cell independent [reviewed in 52] so that low affinity interactions through FcγRIs may contribute similarly to innate and adaptive responses in humans. FcγRIs have been induced by INF-γ on human PMNs where they participated in ADCC and induction on human $CD34^+$ stem cell-derived mast cells lead to degranulation and cytokine release upon receptor aggregation [reviewed in 51].

FcγRII (CD32), a transmembrane molecule bears two IgSF domains and occurs in several isoforms, with some or all detected on human monocytes, macrophages, PMNs, platelets and B cells [reviewed in 48]. This is a low affinity IgG receptor, binding polymeric or aggregated IgG, with a low capacity for binding IgG2. Thus, this FcR should also contribute to innate and adaptive responses. Since binding of the T-independent IgG2 is lowest for FcγRI and FcγRII, as the adaptive response proceeds and T-dependent IgGs are produced they should compete more efficiently leading to an increasingly antigen-specific expansion and effector phase of the response.

FcγRIII (CD16) bears two IgSF domains and occurs in a transmembrane form in man and mouse and also a GPI-linked form in humans [reviewed in 48]. In humans, the transmembrane form is expressed on NK cells, macrophages and mast cells with the GPI-linked form on neutrophils. In mice the transmembrane form is expressed on NK cells, macrophages and neutrophils. FcγRI is a low-affinity receptor for aggregated IgG with the transmembrane form mediating phagocytosis and ADCC. The GPI-linked form on neutrophils appears to bind without any subsequent function or signal.

FcR-bearing APCs, bind and phagocytose antibody coated antigens. Additional effector cells: NK cells, mast cells, eosinophils and basophils, are stimulated through their Fc receptors to release their stored mediators leading to ADCC.

2.2.2. *NK transmembrane receptors*

IgSF activation receptors identified on NK cells include KIR2DS2, a short cytoplasmic tailed member of the Ig-like killing inhibitory receptors of the killer-cell Ig-like receptor (KIR) family which binds MHC-class-I [53], and NKp46, NKp44 and NKp30, receptors which do not bind classical or nonclassical MHC-I [11,25,54].

2.2.3. *Trem (triggering receptor expressed selectively in myeloid cells)*

Trem family receptors are transmembrane glycoproteins with a single extracellular immunoglobulin-like domain differentially expressed on myeloid cells [24,55,56]. TREMs signal through the ITAM-containing KARAP/DAP12 signalling adapter proteins upon exposure of TREM-bearing cells to bacteria or fungi. However, it is not clear whether the ligands are of microbial or host origin. Trem-1 activates neutrophils and monocytes/macrophages and amplifies TLR-initiated responses. Trems are distantly related to the novel Ig-like stimulatory receptor of NK cells NKp44 which signals through the same adapter proteins.

2.2.4. *DIgR1*

DIgR1 is a novel DC-derived Ig-like receptor I with a single extracellular Ig-like domain. It has been identified on murine dendritic cells and exhibits significant homology with the human CMRF-35 antigens of monocytes, neutrophils and some T and B lymphocytes, and the polymeric immunoglobulin receptors (pIgR) [57]. The extracellular V-Ig domains of CMRF-35A and CMRF-35H are highly homologous. However, the CMRF-35H contains three putative ITIM motifs suggesting an inhibitory role while the CMRF-35H has a very short cytoplasmic tail with no ITIM.

2.2.5. *Hemolin*

Hemolin, a four-Ig domain plasma protein Ig-superfamily member in insects is induced by microbial challenge and leads to binding and aggregation of bacteria and of yeast [58]. Hemolin has two distinct LPS binding sites, one being the phosphate groups of lipid A and the other the O-specific antigen and the outer-core carbohydrates of LPS [58].

2.2.6. *Transcription factors*

Iterative data-base searches revealed that the Ig-like DNA-binding domain of the transcription factors NFκB and NFAT is a member of a distinct superfamily of intracellular and extracellular domains with an immunoglobulin fold [59].

2.2.7. *Superantigens*

Superantigens rapidly activate a large proportion of lymphocytes independent of the antigen specificity of the variable domain of their receptor but dependent on conserved components of the receptor [60]. T cell superantigens are proteins of bacterial (pyrogenic toxin SAG family; staphylococcus aureus enterotoxins, SEs; staphylococcus aureus toxic shock syndrome toxin-1, TSST-1) or viral (Epstein-Barr virus, EBV; mouse mammary tumour virus, MMTV) origin which bind MHC outside of the peptide-binding groove and also interact with the T cell receptor immunoglobulin Vβ domain bringing an MHC-bearing APC together with a T cell through a trimolecular complex to activate up to 10 percent of T cells [61].

Unlike conventional antigen binding to B cell receptors which involves interactions of native antigen with the hypervariable regions of both heavy and light immunoglobulin chain V regions, superantigens recognise heavy chains, usually more conserved solvent exposed surfaces or framework regions. There are B cell superantigens of bacterial (staphylococcal protein A, SPA; staphylococcal enterotoxins, SEAs), viral (HIV gp 120) and endogenous (i/I carbohydrate red blood cell antigens) origin. SPA can bind 17% of B cells [62].

Thus, both T and B cells, the signatory cells of the adaptive immune response, can be persuaded to contribute to an innate immune response. Further, SEA has been shown to indirectly activate NK-type T cells and NK cells for INF-γ production and cytotoxicity through priming monocytes/macrophages for IL-12 production [63,64], demonstrating that lymphocytes of the innate immune system can also be activated by superantigens.

2.2.8. *Immunoglobulin*

The conventional role for polyclonal natural antibody (NAb) found in the circulation of normal, not-intentionally immunized individuals has been ascribed to early defence against infectious agents. However, a contribution to the early resistance against tumours has been suggested [65–67, rev in 68] and the autoreactivity of NAb has led several investigators to propose a regulatory function for NAb particularly regarding the immune system, and/or extending to organism homeostasis [69,70]. The multispecificity and low affinity for much of this NAb binding to cells have provided obstacles to the identification of cell surface targets and thus to the mechanisms of NAb-mediated cell regulation and a potentially unifying concept of NAb functions. However, analysis of pre-immune monoclonal antibodies has revealed a polyspecific autoreactive binding with apparently unrelated self-antigens including deoxyribonucleic acid and the highly conserved cellular proteins, actin and tubulin [71], and more recent reports suggest NAb binds to cell surface molecules including CD4 and the T cell receptor [rev. in 72].

2.3. Toll-like receptors (TLRs)

TLRs are a large family of pattern recognition receptors detected in several species, initially flies and subsequently rodents and humans, which exhibit some specificity in the recognition of particular invariant and ubiquitously expressed features of pathogens leading to the generation of inflammatory responses [73]. Several TLRs are employed simultaneously on immune cells to detect different types of epitopes on a pathogen. Analysis of murine cell lines revealed TLR mRNA transcripts predominantly in the cells of the innate immune system including, dendritic, macrophage, mast and neutrophil cell lines suggesting they play a dominant role in the first immune response to pathogens [74]. Ligands on pathogens can be protein, carbohydrate, lipid or nucleic acid in nature. However, reactivity with self ligands has also been discovered. The best characterized, TLR4 is a receptor for LPS. LPS is taken up by serum LPS-binding protein (LBP) allowing CD14 to interact with LPS. The LPS and CD14 form a complex with TLR4 and the extracellular accessory protein MD-2 which is required for TLR4 signalling in response to LPS. While high levels of TLR2, TLR4 and CD14 were expressed on human PBL monocytes, lower levels were detected on PMNs, only TLR2 and TLR4 on basophils and none of the three on eosinophils [75]. LPS was considered to play little role in regulating peripheral blood eosinophil or basophil function, and contaminating monocytes were thought likely to contribute to the observed PMN responses to LPS [75]. Fibroblast expression of TLR2, TLR4 and CD14 is consistent with their activation by LPS [76,77]. Leucine-rich repeats associated with protein-protein binding are found on the TLRs and on CD14. The TLRs exhibit a conserved cytoplasmic domain homologous with the IL-1 receptor (Toll/IL-1R homology; TIR) which accounts for similarities in TLR and IL-1R signalling. The intracellular propagation of the signal recruits the cytoplasmic adapter molecule MyD88 through TIR/TIR domain interaction activating the IRAK family of serine threonine kinases, which can then interact with TRAF6 which activates TAK1. Subsequently, the signal is split leading to activation of the JNK pathway and to translocation of NF-κB with activation of an inflammatory response. Differential recognition of cellular expression of TLRs is related to differential responses against the same pathogen [78]. Recognition of pathogens by combinations of different TLRs provides redundancy and specificity for the responses [79].

Endogenous ligands leading to an inflammatory response after interaction with TLR4 are heat-shock protein 60 (HSP60) and the extra domain A (EDA) region of fibronectin which appears due to alternative splicing in response to tissue injury [reviewed in 73]. HSPs are considered important as endogenous ligands for stimulation of TLRs when they are released upon cell necrosis. However, recognition of apoptotic cells by CD14 does not generate an inflammatory response [reviewed in 80].

2.4. Antimicrobial peptides

Numerous and diversely structured antimicrobial peptides are broadly expressed in nature [reviewed in 11]. The defensins, broadly reactive cationic antimicrobial peptides which must undergo enzymatic activation, exhibit a β-pleated structure with a hallmark six-cysteine motif which forms three intramolecular disulfide bonds [81]. The α-defensins are present in neutrophil granules and in Paneth cells beneath the epithelial stem cells at the base of the crypts in the small intestine. Human neutrophil protein (HNP) α-defensins were induced in IL-2 stimulated T- and NK-enriched human lymphocytes. β-defensins are made in epithelial cells of the skin, respiratory tract and heart skeletal muscle. They are induced in human epithelial cells by microorganisms and cytokines [82]. Circular Θ minidefensins have been found in rhesus monkeys. Defensins provide a direct antimicrobial action in a non-receptor-mediated manner by binding anionic microbial surface components via electrostatic interactions and damaging bacterial cell membranes. Additional functions suggest that they also contribute to immunostimulation of innate immune responses. This is evident in the ability of α-defensins to enhance phagocytosis by macrophages, to degranulate mast cells releasing histamine, to stimulate IL-8 production from epithelial cells, and to bind and activate complement, with support for receptor mediated interactions with eucaryotic cells for degranulation and IL-8 production [reviewed in 83]. Murine β-defensin-2 has been shown to activate immature DCs directly through TLR-4 [84]. α-defensins also contribute to adaptive immune responses through their selective chemotactic abilities observed at 1/10 to 1/100 their bactericidal concentration, HNP for $CD4^+$ $CD45RA^+$ T cells and $CD8^+$ T cells, β- defensins for $CD4^+$ $CD45RO^+$ T cells and α- and β- defensins for immature dendritic cells [reviewed in 83].

2.5. Complement and the complement receptor system

The complement system is important for activating the cells of the innate immune system. It consists of over 30 cell surface and plasma proteins, some with protease activity which can be activated by an earlier acting proteolytic component resulting in a cascading induction of potent biological activity including phagocytosis, lysis and generation of an inflammatory response [reviewed in 15]. C1q is a calcium-dependent carbohydrate-binding protein (C-type lectin), of the collectin family with collagen and C-type lectin domains. Complement components C3, C4 and C5 are considered to have originated from gene duplication of the ancestral α-2 macroglobulin gene [reviewed in 11]. Natural immune activation of complement likely involves the classical pathway employing in the main natural IgM and possibly natural IgG antibodies in addition to the evolutionarily ancient alternative pathway with the stabilization of the low concentration of C3b spontaneously activated by serum enzymes, or the lectin pathway initiated by mannose binding lectin (MBL) and ficolins. C3 a target component of all three activation pathways and essential for the development of the lytic pathway, contains a hidden thioester bond which is exposed on C3b after C3a is split off and is reactive, forming covalent bonds with hydroxyl and amine groups or is hydrolysed and inactivated by water. C3b, iC3b and C3d are ligands for the complement cell receptors CD35, CD21, CD11b and CD11c [85]. Complement receptor 1 (CR1), a large single transmembrane chain lectin-like molecule is a receptor for C3b, the homologous C4b, inactivated forms of C3b, plus C1q and MBL, but requires additional binding to mediate phagocytosis [86]. The lectin-like CR2 (CD21) and integrins CR3 (CD11b/CD18) and CR4 (CD11c/CD18) bind inactive forms of C3b, with CR3 and CR4 able to facilitate phagocytosis. Phagocytic activation of macrophages is associated with the release of proinflammatory mediators generating a local inflammatory response. Cellular receptors for the small, anaphylactic, split products C5a (C5aR) and C3a (C3aR) are seven-span receptors which interact with intracellular guanine-nucleotide-binding proteins to initiate activation signals.

2.6. Cytokines and their receptors

Cytokines of diverse structures including IL-1, IL-6, TNF-α, IL-12 and IL-8 are released from microbe-activated macrophages. These small molecular weight proteins can act locally in an autocrine or paracrine manner or at a distance after travelling through the circulation or tissue fluids. IL-6 of the large hemopoietin structural family, TNF-α (cachectin) of the TNF family and the unassigned IL-1, induce the liver to release acute phase reactants. IL-1α and IL-1β binding to the IL-1RI (CD121a) through the ligand binding domain consisting of three immunoglobulin-type (Ig-type) domains leads to intracellular signal transduction through the cytoplasmic TIR domain [87]. However, binding to IL-1RII (CD121b) which has a similar extracellular domain fails to activate due to its very short cytoplasmic domain. Sertoli cells are the main epithelial cells of the testes, surrounding the germinal cells and providing them with an immunologically protected environment [88]. Sertoli cells in adult rat testes constitutively express mRNA of IL-1α, dependent upon their contact with the germ cells and without producing inflammation [89] supporting the idea that IL-1α may play a physiological role for IL-1α as a germ cell growth factor in testes. TNF binds cellular TNFR-I and TNFR-II with homotrimer formation needed for signal induction for activating macrophages for NO production. IL-12 is also released and binds with IL-12Rβ1 and IL-12β2 stimulating NK cells.

2.7. Chemokines and their receptors

Over 50 small 8–10 kD, heparin-binding proteins with related amino acid sequences are divided into 4 chemokine subfamilies based on particular aminoacid sequence and the presence of cysteine [90,91]. With their chemokine receptors of the seven transmembrane receptor family, they direct the movement of cells and contribute to the activation of natural immune responses [91]. Depending on the combination of TLRs stimulated, tissue macrophages and dendritic cells release a subset of chemokines following NF-κB activation [92]. This can include IL-8 (CXCL8), MIP-1α (CCL3), MIP-1β (CCL4), RANTES (CCL5) and IP-10 (CXCL10). IL-8 binds and activates CXCR1/2 bearing PMNs. CCR5 bearing NK cells bind the CC chemokines and CXCR3 bearing activated T cells bind IP-10, so that all of these cells can be drawn from the circulation into the inflammatory site. Stimulation of immature dendritic cells through their constitutively expressed CCR1, CCR5 and CCR6 chemokine receptors leads to their maturation with downmodulation of CCR1, CCR5 and CCR6 and upregulation of CCR7 receptors directing the cells to migrate into the lymphatics. All bacteria produce proteins with amino terminal N-formylated methionine which act as chemoattractants for inflammatory cells particularly PMNs. The peptide f-Met-Leu-Phe (fMLP) acts similarly through the fMLPR [93] which is a seven-span receptor similar to the receptors for chemokines and for C3a and C5a, arguing that chemokines, complement components and bacterial products attract and activate PMNs through a common mechanism.

3. INHIBITION OF ACTIVATION BY SELF RECOGNITION

Ubiquitous activating activity combined with inhibiting activity against self is evident in the regulation of NK cell activation by target expression of MHC class I and in control of complement activation through target expression of sialic acid.

3.1. Inhibition based on MHC

NK cells [94] are cytotoxic toward "missing-self" targets [5]. NK cell activation depends on the balance of inhibitory signals initiated through MHC class I recognizing receptors and activating signals resulting from recognition of molecules other than MHC class I by several different receptors [36]. Inhibitory receptors bear cytoplasmic tails with immune tyrosine-based inhibitory motifs (ITIMs) and activating forms of the receptors appear to exhibit short cytoplasmic tails requiring for activation, interaction with adapter molecules bearing immune tyrosine-based activation motifs (ITAMs). The immunoglobulin superfamily and the c-type lectin family each contribute germline encoded activating and inhibitory receptor members [11,95].

3.2. Inhibition based on sialic acid

Sialic acid, the terminal carbohydrate residue on glycosylated molecules of higher vertebrates considered to be important for regulation of molecular and cellular interactions which can mask recognition sites shielding cells from their environment or act as recognition sites in multicellular organisms [92], has been proposed as a basis for self/nonself discrimination [44,97,98].

3.2.1. *Complement activation*

Cell surface sialic acids are important for regulation of complement, a potent biological effector mechanism considered "the major noncellular system of innate immunity in humans" [85]. The alternative pathway of complement is constitutively active in the form of the C3b component which is spontaneously generated through hydrolysis of C3 in the serum. Thus C3b is preformed, available systemically in the circulation and indiscriminately reactive with self or nonself particles through an active bond. The tagging of self structures for phagocytosis or for lysis through the alternative pathway is regulated by regulatory factor H which exhibits a decay-accelerating function and cofactor activity for factor I inactivation of C3b. Factor H has binding sites for C3b and polyanion binding sites for sialic acid which is thought to have arisen relatively late in evolution [99] and has been proposed as a basis of self/nonself discrimination [97,98]. Several studies have suggested that loss of cell surface sialic acid increased tumour and host lymphocyte sensitivity to NK cells [reviewed in 98].

3.2.2. *Siglecs*

Siglecs are sialic acid binding Ig-type transmembrane polypeptide lectins which are characterized by an N-terminal Ig V-set domain and have a cytoplasmic tail [98]. Members of the CD33 subgroup typically exhibit a consensus immunoreceptor tyrosine kinase inhibitory motif (ITIM). The family of siglecs is differentially expressed on haemopoietic cells including sialoadhesin found on macrophages, CD22 on B cells and CD33 on myeloid progenitors. Co-evolution of human CD33rSiglec specificity with the human sialylation pattern compared with that of chimpanzees and gorillas suggested that the natural functional ligands for siglecs were endogenous sialic acids [100]. Thus, similar to ITIM-bearing, MHC class-I-recognizing, receptors expressed on cells of the natural immune system, siglecs may be important for recognising broadly expressed 'self' in the form of sialic acid and inhibiting activation of the natural immune system [6,98].

3.2.3. *Tyro 3 family receptors*

Tyro 3 family receptors have been reported to limit the activation of macrophages. They are protein-tyrosine kinase (PTK) receptors, Tyro 3, Axl and Mer, which exhibit extracellular domains with two sequential Ig domains and two fibronectin III domains joined to a single-passe transmembrane domain and a cytoplasmic PTK domain [101]. Two ligands have been implicated, the products of the growth arrest specific gene (GAS)6 and the anti-coagulant Protein S which each have a 'Gla' domain rich in gamma carboxylated glutamic acid residues followed by four epidermal growth factor (EGF)-like domains and a large SHBG (androgen binding protein) domain.

3.2.4. *Natural antibodies*

3.2.4.1. *Multifaceted saccharide reactivity of the natural antibody/tumour interaction.* Evidence from several experimental approaches supports a role for polyclonal natural antibody (NAb) in the defence against small tumour inocula in mice. Knowledge of the NAb binding sites is essential for an understanding of their function. Pronase and neuraminidase treatment of the L5178Y-F9 T-cell lymphoma reduced and increased syngeneic DBA/2 NAb binding respectively and combined with monosaccharide inhibition, implicated asialo carbohydrates as targets of anti-tumour NAb. Tunicamycin pretreatment increased NAb acquisition but decreased the neuraminidase augmentation of NAb binding, arguing for N-linked oligosaccharide binding by NAb. Benzyl-α-GalNAc plus neuraminidase treatment suggested the binding of NAb to O-linked oligosaccharides. Inhibition of binding by preincubation of cells in GalNAc implicated cell surface lectins in the acquisition of NAb. In addition, the higher expression of asialo-GM1 and asialo-GM2 on an L5178Y-F9 variant selected through flow cytometry for high NAb binding, and higher expression of asialo-GM1 coupled with greater pronase resistance of NAb binding on neuraminidase treated cells were consistent with NAb also binding to cell surface glycolipids. Thus the saccharide reactivity of the anti-tumour/ NAb interaction is multifaceted, suggesting the essential nature and biological potency of NAb binding [Chow unpubl].

3.2.4.2. *NAb binding to activated cells,* NAb bound subconfluent syngeneic murine 10T½ fibroblasts better than confluent cells. In addition, ras transformation of 10T½ fibroblasts which increases their protein kinase C (PKC) activity, increased NAb binding [102,103] with an inverse correlation between NAb binding and tumourigenicity [104], providing evidence for an NAb-susceptible phase of oncogene-induced tumour development. Preneoplastic, rat PKC-β1 overexpressing 10T½ cells also exhibited higher NAb binding and a more rapid elimination in vivo of ^{131}I-dUrd-labelled cells [105]. Thus, constitutive increases in the basal activity of PKC seen in both the ras-transformation and PKC preneoplasia models argues for PKC upregulation of NAb binding structures and for NAb recognition of incipient neoplasia. In a direct assay, pre-incubation of tumour cells in serum NAb vs tumor-absorbed NAb reduced their tumourigenicity [106]. Furthermore, IV pretreatment of mice with syngeneic serum NAb, ammonium sulfate precipitated fractions of NAb, or human IVIG reduced the incidence and/or increased the latency of syngeneic tumours injected SC [102,107] and reduced the metastasis of tumours injected IV [108]. In our ras and PKC-β1 models, upregulation of NAb binding structures with the elevation of a dominant signalling activity, PKC, argued for NAb binding to activated cells in general.

In an in vitro model aimed at reversing progression and generating tumours with increased susceptibility uniquely to NAb, T-lymphomas were treated with the tumour promoter 12-O-tetradecanoylphorbol-13-acetate (TPA) to generate variants and were then selected for high NAb binding through fluorescence-activated cell-sorting (FACS). Three cycles of TPA treatment and sorting yielded the L5178Y-F9 TPA/NAb$^+$3 (LYNAb$^+$), which exhibited a reduced SC tumourigenicity [68]. The high NAb binding LYNAb$^+$ exhibited increases in CD44 [Chow unpubl], CD25, CD45RA and CD45RC but decreases in CD45RB and pan-CD45 expression [109]. The identification of a transitional, higher density CD45RA$^+$ naive adult T cell phenotype 1 to 2 days following mitogenic stimulation of T cells [110] which coincides with CD45RA expression on the most highly proliferating cells [111], suggests that highly proliferating cells which appear briefly, early after activation might be exquisitely sensitive to NAb regulation. This is consistent with the origin of the LYNAb$^+$ via selection for high NAb binding after TPA treatment which increased CD45RA in human T cells [112]. Natural monoclonal IgM bound to PHA stimulated normal CD3$^+$ T cells [113] and normal serum IgG rapidly bound to autologous PHA activated T lymphocytes [114], both in human systems. Increased neuraminidase activity 24–48 hours after T-cell activation [115] should ensure that the NAb-reactive asialo forms of CD45 are expressed. Similarly, IL-2R-α is expressed on activated T cells and IL-2Rβ [reviewed in 116], and CD44, particularly v6 variants [117,118] are increased on activated T cells [119]. These observations support the idea that NAb binds and regulates T cells undergoing activation.

The homeostatic action of polyclonal natural antibody (NAb) was further investigated using human Jurkat T leukemia cells selected in vitro for high binding of serum IgG plus IgM or IgG in intravenous immunoglobulin (IVIg). IVIg inhibited in vitro growth of the J4.1 and JIg3.1 variants obtained while enhancing Jurkat growth. The variants bound more monoclonal antibodies against activation-associated molecules including CD25, CD134, and CD45RA which rises transiently about 1 day after T cell activation. Binding of anti-CD45RB and anti-pan CD45 were increased with anti-CD45RO binding unchanged or slightly decreased. Immunoblotting revealed more of the higher molecular weight isoforms of CD45. Binding was decreased for antibodies against CD69, CD122, CD3 and FAS. Thus, similar to the findings from the murine model, markers which are increased about 1 day after activation, particularly the asialo forms, are likely targets of normal IgG and IgM. This further supports the idea that natural IgG and IgM directly regulate T cells during an early, possibly transient stage of normal activation likely critical for inflammation, autoimmunity and early neoplastic development [120].

4. NATURAL IMMUNE CELLULAR ACTIVATION

Macrophages are a heterogeneous group of cells including circulating monocytes and tissue resident macrophages. They are phagocytic, performing a major function contributing to the innate immune response by ingesting microbes and killing them intracellularly. Several different structural families contribute receptors which participate in phagocytosis [121,122]. Endocytosis has been demonstrated for FcRs (IgSF), CR3 (integrin) and the mannose-receptor (lectin), while CR1 (lectin) and CR4 (integrin), scavenger receptors MARCO and SR-A, leucine-rich repeat bearing CD14, and additional integrins recognizing fibronectin/vitronectin-opsonized particles, bind and increase the efficiency of particle internalization [86]. Phagocytosis of microbes is usually accompanied by the generation of an inflammatory response and the release of antimicrobial peptides. Some phagocytic receptors also stimulate inflammation such as FcRs. However, binding receptors such as TLRs which are not endocytic but localize to the phagosomes during phagocytosis, contribute to the regulation of the activation of inflammation. Trem-1 (IgSF) amplifies TLR-initiated responses to microbes and augments inflammatory chemokine and cytokine secretion [56]. A variety of cell surface receptors which participate in the phagocytosis of apoptotic cells have been identified on the professional phagocytes, macrophages and neutrophils, including FcRs, CR3, SR-A, CD14 and the vitronectin receptor as above, plus the class B scavenger receptor CD36, the glycoprotein macrosialin CD68, the ATP-binding cassette transporter 1, ABC1, the phosphatidylserine-receptor (PS-R), the Mer receptor tyrosine kinase and a protein complex of C1q and MBL with cell surface calreticulin and CD91 [reviewed in 123].

Dendritic cells are located in most tissues but particularly in the interface with the environment are considered to play a dual role in the generation of innate responses and in the initiation of adaptive immune responses [reviewed in 124]. Monocyte-derived, immature human DC express chemokine receptors CCR1, CCR2, CCR5 and CXCRI which would provide for DCs to follow concentration gradients of inflammatory chemokines such as MIP-1α, RANTES and MCP-1 to inflammatory sites. In peripheral tissue, immature DCs express cell surface molecules that mediate endocytosis including FcγRI, FcγRII, FcγRIII, CD14, mannose receptors (collectins), CR3 (Mac-1, integrin), MARCO (scavengerR), DEC205 and DC-SIGN [125] (multi-c-type lectins), which is linked with the induction of the inflammatory response to which TLR2/4 binding contributes. DC interaction with pathogens either directly through their PAMPs or the PAMP receptors leads to activation with production of inflammatory cytokines and chemokines attracting leukocytes, including granulocytes, macrophages, immature DCs and NK cells to the site of inflammation. DCs have been implicated in the activation of NK cells possibly through

DC production of IL-2 after microbial activation [126]. With the down regulation of CXCR1, CCR1 and CCR5 and upregulation of CCR7 expression, activated DCs migrate to the regional lymph nodes where they complete their maturation process, upregulate their costimulatory molecules and act as the APCs for priming T cells.

Neutrophils, polymorphonuclear cells (PMNs), the most abundant leukocyte in the circulation, originates from a myeloid progenitor. They are short-lived, 3–4 days, granulocytic and respond to many stimuli including those of bacterial, endogenous and immunologic origin, Several chemoattractants have been shown to arrest PMNs including IL-8, C5a, formyl peptides from bacteria, leukotriene LTB4 and platelet activating factor (PAF) [reviewed in 127]. Since high levels of chemoattractants can stop PMN rolling immediately [122], their extravasation into inflammatory tissues would be encouraged. Evidence of signalling in PMNs, through the G-protein-coupled chemokine receptors, Fc receptors, L-selectin and inflammatory adhesion molecules, β_2 integrins like Mac-1 and LFA-1 on PMNs which possibly bind ICAM-1 and P-selectin glycoprotein ligand for P-selectin and E-selectin on endothelial cells, suggests they are all important for activation. Consistent with the multiple activation pathways for conversion of rolling to adherent PMNs, the lack or only partial effect of blockade of each individual pathway supports the proposal that integration of multiple interactions at the cell surface provides a strategy for appropriate activation [127]. In further activation processes which would be important after extravasation, purified peripheral blood PMNs increase IL-8 mRNA within an hour after exposure to LPS in vitro consistent with their expression of TLR4, and they generate additional responses in the presence of contaminating monocytes [75]. PMNs can be activated through TLRs. They have Fcγ receptors for IgG and complement CR1 receptors for C3b and C4b which are important for their phagocytic function. Thus, PMNs exhibit several activation processes associated with their different functions.

Mast cells originate from a myeloid progenitor. They are found in a variety of tissues where they mature, including vascularized connective tissue and the submucosa. They are long-lived with a life span of months to years [reviewed in 45] and are capable of proliferation. They have been shown capable of phagocytosis in vitro through binding of CD48, a mannose-containing GPI-linked receptor binding to Fim-H, a mannose-binding lectin on fimbriae of bacteria [45,128,129]. Binding of complement components to their C3a/C4a receptors and C5a receptors leads to the release of active agents including preformed histamine, heparin and serine proteases, and newly synthesized cytokines and chemokines leading to the development of an inflammatory response. They have receptors for opsonins including CR3 for complement, $Fc_{\gamma}R$ and FcεRI. Mast cells can be activated directly through TLRs 2 and 4 [130]. Cross linking of the high affinity FcεRI by antigen binding to IgE of the adaptive response already bound to the FcR can also activate mast cells contributing to specific allergic responses.

Basophils are found in the circulation, have a short life span of hours to days and like other granulocytes and unlike mast cells they do not proliferate. Like mast cells they release proinflammatory mediators, although the cytokine repertoire is more limited [reviewed in 45,131]. Similar to mast cells, they express the cell surface CR3, FcγR and FcεRI. They recognize bacteria via IgE. Basophils express TLR2 and TLR4 but not CD14 and did not respond to LPS [75].

Eosinophils are located in the tissue of the lung, gastrointestinal and lower genitourinary tracts. They can release proinflammatory cytokines, chemokines, lipid mediators and toxic granule proteins including major basic protein [reviewed in 132]. Eosinophils did not express TLR2, TLR4 or CD14 and did not respond to LPS [75].

Epithelial cells provide a barrier that most microbial pathogens must breach. While the skin exhibits a more complex structure, the tubular mucosal surfaces of the gastrointestinal, respiratory and urogenital tract have only a single layer of epithelial cells to separate them from the external environment including commensal microbes [reviewed in 133], raising the question of how commensal and pathogenic microbes are distinguished. Although haematopoietic cells are the traditional mediators of innate immunity, a role for epithelial cells is clear from the evidence that activated epithelial cells rapidly secrete proinflammatory cytokines and chemokines after exposure to bacteria [reviewed in 130], in addition to their production of antimicrobial molecules. Microbes exhibit specific pathogen-epithelial interactions with a variety of receptors expressed on the apical (luminal) and/or the basolateral (BL) (facing basement membrane) surfaces of these polarized cells to facilitate their direct colonization or entry into epithelial cells, for transcytosing an epithelial cell, or for accessing directly the BL surface through cytolysis or by traversing tight junctions (TJs) for example, after inducing PMN transmigration [reviewed in 134]. Apical receptors which have been implicated include, the cystic fibrosis transmembrane receptor (CFTR), the phosphorylcholine-binding platelet activating factor receptor (PAFR), CD66 (for gonococcal opacity, Opa proteins) [135], CD46 (for gonococcal PilC1) and the polymeric immunolglobulin receptor (pIgR) (for ligand choline-binding protein A which binds bacterial phosphorylcholine) which is detected on apical and BL surfaces. Receptors on the BL surface include heparansulfate proteoglycans (HSPGs) (for Opa proteins), and the integrins which are engaged by vitronectin and fibronectin (as some Opa proteins bind these extracellular matrix proteins), β1-integrins on BL and TJ (for Inv and YadA of *Yersinia* and for intimin of *E. coli*, although the typical receptor is bacterially encoded and secreted into the host cell membrane by the bacterium), E-cadherins, (for leucine-rich repeat (LRR) family member internalin, In1A of *Listeria*) [136], and the fibronectin receptor and CD44 have been implicated in binding of Ipa-A complexes and IpaB complexes respectively of *Shigella*. InB1 (LRR family) of *Listeria* has three receptors, gC1qR, the receptor for complement C1q which is detected subcellularly, glycosaminoglycans and Met or the hepatocyte growth factor receptor (HGFR) [137] which is found predominantly on the BL but detected in low levels on the apical domain.

TLR2 and TLR4 are located on the apical surface of differentiated intestinal epithelial cells (IELs) optimally situated to survey the luminal contents [reviewed in 137]. However, TLR2 and TLR4 are also detected on the BL surface in immature IELs and TLR5 appears to be preferentially expressed on the BL surface [reviewed in 137]. Considering the efficiency of TLR in inducing inflammatory responses, it has been proposed that microbial stimulation of receptors on the BL side of epithelial cells would distinguish between commensal and pathogenic varieties. However, commensals may reduce the synthesis of inflammatory molecules by preventing IκB-α degradation and thus inhibiting the IκB/NK-κB signalling pathway, constant exposure to LPS may induce "cross-tolerance" against other signalling pathways for example those of TLR2 and TLR4, restricted apoptosis may contribute to this tolerance and the activation of cell survival mechanisms may all contribute to distinguish the response to commensals preventing a pathogenic induction of inflammation [reviewed in 137].

B1 cells, characterized by CD5 expression are localized to the peritoneal and pleural cavities. They can be activated by LPS, less so by anti-CD40 and not by anti-IgM [reviewed in 138] and the LPS activation was inhibited by anti-CD14 in a murine B1 cell line [139]. Activation of B cells by a variety of agents has increased CD5 expression suggesting that CD5 is a marker of B cell activation and not a marker for a distinct B cell subset. [reviewed in 140]. B1 cells have shown extensive reactivity against self including Ig, DNA, cytoskeletal molecules, phosphatidylcholine and cell surface proteins on red blood cells and thymocytes in addition to reactivity against microbial antigens including phosphorylcholine [141]. The B1 specificities are thought to be associated with their location, and with BCR-mediated signals from microenvironmental-antigen considered essential for survival of all B cells this suggests that the CD5 expressing B1 cells may provide an activated, self-renewing effector poised to respond to changes in the microenvironment or to pathogens. As such, B1 cells could be considered as part of a "natural memory" component of lymphocytes together with marginal zone B cells, NKT and γδ T cells, which can react within hours of exposure to antigen, after the earliest innate responses and well before the initiation of the adaptive response [138].

NK cells are important producers of cytokines, in particular INF-gamma, early during infections. Activation is initiated through members of the NKG2 C-type lectin-like family (NKG2D), the Ly49 C-type lectin family (Ly49D, LY49H) in mice, the killer-cell Ig-like receptor (KIR) family in humans (KIR2DS2) [53], and additional Ig superfamily receptors NKp46, NKp44 and NKp30 [reviewed in 11,25,54]. The last three are considered to be the main activation receptors for NK cells [25]. NKp46 interacts with sialic acid-binding haemagglutinin on virus-infected cells based on NKp46 bearing sialic acid [11]. Inhibitory receptors include the Ly49 C-type lectin family in mice, KIR Ig-like receptors in humans [53], the CD94/NKG2 heterodimer of C-type lectins in mice and primates [11] and the human leukocyte immunoglobulin-like receptor (LIR) (or ILT) family (LIR1 and LIR2), and the homologous, murine paired Ig-like receptors (PIR) (PIR-B) [11]. KIRs are a diverse, rapidly evolving receptor family which recognizes polymorphic determinants on MHC-class-I molecules [reviewed in 53]. CD94/NKG2A in humans recognizes a conserved class-I leader sequence peptide presented by HLA-E [reviewed in 53]. While different families of NK receptors bind different aspects of their MHC class I or MHC class I homologous ligands, their combinatorial expression provides an effective mechanism for surveying host cells for changes associated with infection or oncogenic transformation [25]. The balance of inhibitory signals from MHC Class-I specific receptors and signals from activating receptors with other specificities, determines the outcome of each NK-target cell interaction [reviewed in 25].

γδ T cells arise early in ontogeny with waves of cells expressing different Vγ and Vδ T cell receptor gene segments appearing in the murine foetal thymus and thought to home sequentially to the epidermis, reproductive epithelium and lymphoid organs, while intestinal epithelium γδ T cells arise distinctly [142]. In humans γδ T cells are also found in the epithelial-rich tissues of the intestinal and reproductive tracts, while comprising a small proportion of lymphocytes in the skin, blood and lymphoid organs [143]. While the Ig-superfamily Vγ and Vδ receptors of cells in the lymphoid tissue exhibit diversity, a lack of diversity is detected in the γδ T cell receptors of cells in the same epithelial site. In contrast with αβ T cell receptors, the γδ receptors do not recognize antigen as peptide/MHC complexes. γδ T cells are extensively self-reactive. Typical ligands are derived from local epithelium following infection, intact proteins including stress or heat-shock proteins, MHC class IB, and non-peptide phosphoantigens including nucleotide-conjugates and phospholipids which have been detected in association with microbes. NKG2D an NK C-type lectin receptor binds MHC-like molecules MIC A and MIC B expressed on intestinal epithelial cells in response to injury or stress. The constitutive expression of transcripts of genes associated with cytotoxic and regulatory activity and the rapid inducibility of cytotoxicity in intestinal intraepithelial γδ T cells, has raised the possibility that they may be primed effector cells capable of rapid responses [144]. Further, this state of activation may be controlled by inhibitory NK receptors [144].

NKT cells [145], provide an early antibacterial response and an early cytokine source leading to the differentiation to Th1 and Th2 and suppression of autoimmunity. Their αβ T cell receptors exhibit limited diversity recognizing CD1, not MHC. CD1 [90], a nonpolymorphic antigen presenting molecule is related structurally and functionally to MHC. However, it does not present peptide antigens but binds and presents lipids and glycolipids including structures from pathogenic mycobacteria. The CD1 binding groove is thought to bind the hydrophobic ligand components presenting the polar head groups for contact with the T cell receptors.

5. ACUTE PHASE RESPONSE

The acute phase response can be initiated rapidly through the release of soluble mediators into the circulation following stimulation of hepatocytes in the liver by the endogenous pyrogens IL-1, IL-6 and TNF-alpha released by activated macrophages. Thus the production of pro-inflammatory mediators from a local inflammatory response can lead to a systemic acute phase inflammatory response associated with fever and the increased production of acute phase proteins (APPs) in the liver. APPs include C-reactive protein (CRP) and serum amyloid P component (SAP), α-2-macroglobulin, mannose-binding lectin (MBL) and complement components.

α-2 macroglobulins, the universal protease inhibitors, have an intrachain thioester bond which becomes activated when the molecule is attacked by a protease. The protease is covalently bound and enfolded into the α-2 macroglobulin revealing a ligand for cell surface receptors which leads to internalization and degradation of the complex [reviewed in 11].

Thus, the acute phase response which is considered to be a systematic all-out last host defence against an invader provides a flood of diverse but in some cases homologous molecules which can react with invaders, facilitating their activation of natural immune cells directly or through activation of complement.

6. COMMON THEMES AND QUESTIONS

6.1. Repeating epitopes and polyvalent recognition

The affinity of many individual NAb interactions is considered weak. However, the binding of polyclonal natural antibodies to the multiple similar or different epitopes on the same cell surface molecule, or cross-linking of different molecules through binding of similar epitopes, plus subsequent crosslinking of bound NAb through anti-Ig reactivity of NAb can generate high functional binding activity. The oligomeric structures of ficolins and collectins, humoral lectins of the innate immune system, the latter typified by MBL, provides multiple binding receptors, which increase the potential for functional binding similar to IgM and C1q. Similarly, while the galectin binding to individual lactosamine moieties is a low affinity interaction, the avidity of galectin binding is increased for polylactosamines where the lactosamine units are repeated in chains [38].

6.2. Redundancy

Redundancy is a major aspect of the innate immune system, protecting against potentially harmful effects of individual molecular or cellular defects. Multiple solutions to self-nonself discrimination are evident in the different receptor/ligand systems. Many evolutionarily ancient structural families are employed in numerous roles in innate system recognition/activation and modulation of cell function suggesting the generation of diversity in the responses to the many challenges during evolution. Furthermore, the many structural families which provide receptors for activation also provide receptors for inhibition. The inhibition may be linked with ITIM motifs located on the cytoplasmic tail of the receptor, whereas the activating forms may bear ITAMs or have no tyrosine-based activation or inhibition motifs but interact with ITAM-bearing molecules.

6.3. Pre-activated state

Elements of the innate immune system can react very quickly employing constitutively expressed receptors and preformed molecules. Cells of the innate immune system also exhibit characteristics of activated cells. The asialo-GM1 marker which initially characterized the spontaneously cytotoxic NK cell was also detected on activated cells including activated macrophages and T cells, proliferating thymoblasts and functionally mature thymocytes [146]. Asialo-GM1 was proposed as a marker of early activation of resting cells. An N-linked carbohydrate marker was detected on resting neutrophils, PHA- or Con-A-activated CD45RO$^+$ lymphocytes and on neuraminidase treated T and NK cells [147]. These data raise questions regarding sialic acid in regulating binding and thus signalling. Is activation associated with desialylation ? Do the asialo residues act as targets for down regulation by the innate immune system for example by NAbs ? The relatively short lifespan of neutrophils and NK cells, approximately 4 days and two weeks respectively, would be consistent with a requirement to be present in an already activated stage.

6.4. Self-nonself discrimination

The basis of self/nonself discrimination is the major question regarding the activation and function of the natural immune system. Many strategies contribute. The theme of inhibition associated with self recognition is emerging. The expression of classical MHC Class I or sialic acid considered to distinguish mammalian cells from microbes, are the basis of two different strategies for inhibition of NK receptors and complement respectively. Recognition of self MHC by inhibitory NK cell receptors can be based on either conserved or polymorphic epitopes. The expression of multiple different epitopes on microbes and multiple receptors with different specificities on the cells of the host innate system provide for specificity. Quantitative expression of epitopes would contribute to achieving a threshold level of receptor stimulation for activation. Cooperation between TLRs for recognition of microbes provides for differential signalling which could tailor the inflammatory response to different pathogens [148]. Apoptotic cells generated through many essential physiological processes are clearly a major target of the innate immune system, taken up and disposed of by phagocytes without generating the inflammatory response which results from phagocytosis of pathogens. Are other categories of cells likely targets of innate immunity? The identification of receptors which bind exogenous and endogenous epitopes suggests the coevolutionarily conserved nature of these receptor/epitope systems. This raises a question regarding the relationship of the phenotypes of the epitope-expressing cells, microbial and mammalian cells. Is it an 'activated' phenotype? The expression of activation markers on susceptible host cells and the targeting of activation markers (CD45RA, MICA, MICB) suggests that activated cells would be regulated by the natural immune system. Cells undergoing activation with sufficient targets for susceptibility should be a minor population and the targeting of such markers for negative regulation should increase the specificity of a developing response. This could be important for regulating the development of a highly specific adaptive immune response. If the cells of the innate immune system are pre-activated and the innate response targets activated cells, then the innate immune system should also be self-regulating, contributing to the generalized homeostasis of the organism by the natural immune system. Thus, the natural immune system participates in the physiological homeostasis of the organism and provides a first and last line (APR) of defence against invading pathogens.

ACKNOWLEDGEMENTS

I wish to thank the Manitoba Medical Services Foundation and The Bayer, Canadian Blood Services, Héma Québec Partnership Fund for their support.

REFERENCES

1. Janeway CA, Jr. Approaching the asymptote? Evolution and revolution in immunology. Cold Spring Harb Symp Quant Biol 1989;54 Pt 1:1–13.
2. Janeway CA, Jr. The immune system evolved to discriminate infectious nonself from noninfectious self. Immunol Today 1992;13(1):11–6.
3. Medzhitov R, Janeway CA, Jr. On the semantics of immune recognition. Res Immunol 1996;147(4):208–14.
4. Medzhitov R, Janeway CA, Jr. Innate immunity: impact on the adaptive immune response. Curr Opin Immunol 1997;9(1):4–9.
5. Kärre K. How to recognize a foreign submarine. Immunol Rev 1997;155:5–9.
6. Medzhitov R, Janeway CA, Jr. Decoding the patterns of self and nonself by the innate immune system. Science 2002;296(5566):298–300.
7. Matzinger P. An innate sense of danger. Semin Immunol 1998;10(5):399–415.
8. Berczi I. Neurohormonal host defense in endotoxin shock. In: Annals New York Acad. Sci. 1998;840:787–801.
9. Berczi I, Bertok L, Chow DA. Natural immunity and neuroimmune host defense. Ann NY Acad Sci 2000;917:248–57.
10. Gordon S. Pattern recognition receptors: doubling up for the innate immune response. Cell 2002;111(7):927–30.
11. Magor BG, Magor KE. Evolution of effectors and receptors of innate immunity. Dev Comp Immunol 2001;25(8–9):651–82.
12. Christophides GK, Zdobnov E, Barillas-Mury C, Birney E, Blandin S, Blass C, et al. Immunity-related genes and gene families in Anopheles gambiae. Science 2002;298(5591): 159–65.
13. Kilpatrick DC. Animal lectins: a historical introduction and overview. Biochim Biophys Acta 2002;1572(2-3):187–97.
14. Holmskov U, Thiel S, Jensenius JC. Collections and ficolins: humoral lectins of the innate immune defense. Annu Rev Immunol 2003;21:547–78.
15. Fujita T. Evolution of the lectin-complement pathway and its role in innate immunity. Nat Rev Immunol 2002;2(5):346–53.
16. Turner MW. Mannose-binding lectin: the pluripotent molecule of the innate immune system. Immunol Today 1996;17(11):532–40.
17. Uemura K, Yokota Y, Kozutsumi Y, Kawasaki T. A unique CD45 glycoform recognized by the serum mannan-binding protein in immature thymocytes. J Biol Chem 1996;271(9): 4581–4.

18. Nagata T, Suzuki T, Ohta Y, Flajnik MF, Kasahara M. The leukocyte common antigen (CD45) of the Pacific hagfish, Eptatretus stoutii: implications for the primordial function of CD45. Immunogenetics 2002;54(4):286–91.
19. Irie-Sasaki J, Sasaki T, Matsumoto W, Opavsky A, Cheng M, Welstead G, et al. CD45 is a JAK phosphatase and negatively regulates cytokine receptor signalling. Nature 2001;409(6818):349–54.
20. Holmskov UL. Collectins and collectin receptors in innate immunity. APMIS Suppl 2000;100:1–59.
21. Tenner AJ. Membrane receptors for soluble defense collagens. Curr Opin Immunol 1999;11(1):34–41.
22. Taylor ME, Bezouska K, Drickamer K. Contributions to ligand binding by multiple carbohydrate-recognition domains in the macrophage mannose receptor. J Biol Chem 1992; 267(3):1719–26.
23. Martinez-Pomares L, Crocker PR, Da Silva R, Holmes N, Colominas C, Rudd P, et al. Cell-specific glycoforms of sialoadhesin and CD45 are counter-receptors for the cysteine-rich domain of the mannose receptor. J Biol Chem 1999 Dec 3; 274(49):35211–8.
24. Diefenbach A, Raulet DH. Innate immune recognition by stimulatory immunoreceptors. Curr Opin Immunol 2003;15(1):37–44.
25. Natarajan K, Dimasi N, Wang J, Mariuzza RA, Margulies DH. Structure and function of natural killer cell receptors: multiple molecular solutions to self, nonself discrimination. Annu Rev Immunol 2002;20:853–85.
26. Braud VM, Allan DS, McMichael AJ. Functions of nonclassical MHC and non-MHC-encoded class I molecules. Curr Opin Immunol 1999;11(1):100–8.
27. Zwirner NW, Dole K, Stastny P. Differential surface expression of MICA by endothelial cells, fibroblasts, keratinocytes, and monocytes. Hum Immunol 1999;60(4):323–30.
28. Molinero LL, Fuertes MB, Fainboim L, Rabinovich GA, Zwirner NW. Up-regulated expression of MICA on activated T lymphocytes involves Lck and Fyn kinases and signaling through MEK1/ERK, p38 MAP kinase, and calcineurin. J Leukoc Biol 2003;73(6):815–22.
29. Molinero LL, Fuertes MB, Rabinovich GA, Fainboim L, Zwirner NW. Activation-induced expression of MICA on T lymphocytes involves engagement of CD3 and CD28. J Leukoc Biol 2002;71(5):791–7.
30. Jinushi M, Takehara T, Kanto T, Tatsumi T, Groh V, Spies T, et al. Critical role of MHC class I-related chain A and B expression on IFN-alpha-stimulated dendritic cells in NK cell activation: impairment in chronic hepatitis C virus infection. J Immunol 2003;170(3): 1249–56.
31. Goke M, Kanai M, Podolsky DK. Intestinal fibroblasts regulate intestinal epithelial cell proliferation via hepatocyte growth factor. Am J Physiol 1998;274(5 Pt 1):G809–18.
32. Groh V, Bahram S, Bauer S, Herman A, Beauchamp M, Spies T. Cell stress-regulated human major histocompatibility complex class I gene expressed in gastrointestinal epithelium. Proc Natl Acad Sci U S A 1996;93(22):12445–50.
33. Shah M, Stanek J, Handwerger S. Differential localization of heat shock proteins 90, 70, 60 and 27 in human decidua and placenta during pregnancy. Histochem J 1998;30(7): 509–18.
34. Menon R, Gerber S, Fortunato SJ, Witkin SS. Lipopolysaccharide stimulation of 70 kilo Dalton heat shock protein messenger ribonucleic acid production in cultured human fetal membranes. J Perinat Med 2001;29(2):133–6.

35. Xiao X, Zuo X, Davis AA, McMillan DR, Curry BB, Richardson JA, et al. HSF1 is required for extra-embryonic development, postnatal growth and protection during inflammatory responses in mice. Embo J 1999;18(21):5943–52.
36. Long EO. Regulation of immune responses through inhibitory receptors. Annu Rev Immunol 1999;17:875–904.
37. Rabinovich GA, Rubinstein N, Toscano MA. Role of galectins in inflammatory and immunomodulatory processes. Biochim Biophys Acta 2002;1572(2-3):274–84.
38. Rabinovich GA, Baum LG, Tinari N, Paganelli R, Natoli C, Liu FT, et al. Galectins and their ligands: amplifiers, silencers or tuners of the inflammatory response? Trends Immunol 2002;23(6):313–20.
39. Cooper DN. Galectinomics: finding themes in complexity. Biochim Biophys Acta 2002;1572(2-3):209–31.
40. Sano H, Hsu DK, Apgar JR, Yu L, Sharma BB, Kuwabara I, et al. Critical role of galectin-3 in phagocytosis by macrophages. J Clin Invest 2003;112(3):389–97.
41. Mey A, Leffler H, Hmama Z, Normier G, Revillard JP. The animal lectin galectin-3 interacts with bacterial lipopolysaccharides via two independent sites. J Immunol 1996;156(4):1572–7.
42. Volanakis JE. Human C-reactive protein: expression, structure, and function. Mol Immunol 2001;38(2-3):189–97.
43. Chang MK, Binder CJ, Torzewski M, Witztum JL. C-reactive protein binds to both oxidized LDL and apoptotic cells through recognition of a common ligand: Phosphorylcholine of oxidized phospholipids. Proc Natl Acad Sci U S A. 2002 Oct 1;99(20):13043–8.
44. Uhlenbruck G, Sölter J, Janssen E, Haupt H. Two new, additional "combining sites" of C-reactive protein: lectin specificity of the anti-galactan type and anti-haemocyanin reactivity. Hoppe Seylers Z Physiol Chem 1981;362(8):1167–9.
45. Abraham SN, Arock M. Mast cells and basophils in innate immunity. Semin Immunol 1998;10(5):373–81.
46. Peiser L, Mukhopadhyay S, Gordon S. Scavenger receptors in innate immunity. Curr Opin Immunol 2002;14(1):123–8.
47. Davis RS, Dennis G, Jr., Odom MR, Gibson AW, Kimberly RP, Burrows PD, et al. Fc receptor homologs: newest members of a remarkably diverse Fc receptor gene family. Immunol Rev 2002;190:123–36.
48. Barclay AN, Brown MH, Law SK Alex, McKnight AJ, Tomlinson MG, van der Merwe P Anton. The leucocyte antigen factsbook. 2nd ed. London ; San Diego: Academic Press; 1997.
49. Ravetch JV. Fc receptors. Curr Opin Immunol 1997;9:121–5.
50. Gavin AL, Barnes N, Dijstelbloem HM, Hogarth PM. Identification of the mouse IgG3 receptor: implications for antibody effector function at the interface between innate and adaptive immunity. J Immunol 1998;160(1):20–3.
51. Tan PS, Gavin AL, Barnes N, Sears DW, Vremec D, Shortman K, et al. Unique monoclonal antibodies define expression of Fc gamma RI on macrophages and mast cell lines and demonstrate heterogeneity among subcutaneous and other dendritic cells. J Immunol 2003;170(5):2549–56.
52. Hutchins WA, Carlone GM, Westerink MA. Elderly immune response to a TI-2 antigen: heavy and light chain use and bactericidal activity to Neisseria meningitidis serogroup C polysaccharide. J Infect Dis 1999;179(6):1433–40.
53. Vilches C, Parham P. KIR: diverse, rapidly evolving receptors of innate and adaptive

immunity. Annu Rev Immunol 2002;20:217–51.
54. Pende D, Parolini S, Pessino A, Sivori S, Augugliaro R, Morelli L, et al. Identification and molecular characterization of NKp30, a novel triggering receptor involved in natural cytotoxicity mediated by human natural killer cells. J Exp Med 1999;190(10):1505–16.
55. Diefenbach A, Raulet DH. Innate immune recognition by stimulatory immunoreceptors. Curr Opin Immunol 2003;15(1):37–44.
56. Colonna M, Facchetti F. TREM-1 (triggering receptor expressed on myeloid cells): a new player in acute inflammatory responses. J Infect Dis 2003;187 Suppl 2:S397–401.
57. Luo K, Zhang W, Sui L, Li N, Zhang M, Ma X, et al. DIgR1, a novel membrane receptor of the immunoglobulin gene superfamily, is preferentially expressed by antigen-presenting cells. Biochem Biophys Res Commun 2001;287(1):35–41.
58. Yu XQ, Kanost MR. Binding of hemolin to bacterial lipopolysaccharide and lipoteichoic acid. An immunoglobulin superfamily member from insects as a pattern-recognition receptor. Eur J Biochem 2002 Apr;269(7):1827–34.
59. Aravind L, Koonin EV. Gleaning non-trivial structural, functional and evolutionary information about proteins by iterative database searches. J Mol Biol 1999 Apr 16;287(5): 1023–40.
60. Silverman GJ, Cary S, Graille M, Curtiss VE, Wagenknecht R, Luo L, et al. A B-cell superantigen that targets B-1 lymphocytes. Curr Top Microbiol Immunol 2000;252: 251–63.
61. Baker MD, Acharya KR. Superantigens structure, function and diversity. Methods in Mol Biol 2003;214:1–31.
62. Domiati-Saad R, Lipsky PE. B cell superantigens: Potential modifiers of the normal human B cell repertoire. Intern Rev Immunol 1997;14:309–24.
63. Ami K, Ohkawa T, Koike Y, Sato K, Habu Y, Iwai T, et al. Activation of human T cells with NK cell markers by staphylococcal enterotoxin A via IL-12 but not IL-18. Clin Exp Immunol 2002;128:453–9.
64. Dobashi H, Seki S, Habu Y, Ohkawa T, Takeshita S, Hiraide H, Sekine I. Activation of mouse liver natural killer cells and NK1.1(+) T cells by bacterial superantigen-primed Kupffer cells. Hepatology 1999;30:430–6.
65. Brunda M, Minden P. Antibodies to bacterial and tumor-derived antigens in sera from normal guinea pigs. J Immunol 1977;119:1374–7.
66. Gronberg A, Hansson M, Keissling R, Anderson B, Karre K, Roder J. Demonstration of natural antibodies in natural rabbit serum with similar specific pattern as mouse natural killers cells. J Natl Cancer Inst 1980;64:1113–9.
67. Castronovo V, Colin C, Parent B, Foidart JM, Lambotte R, Mahieu P. Possible role of human natural anti-alpha-galactosyl antibodies in the natural anti-tumor defense system. J Natl Cancer Inst 1989;81:212–6.
68. Tough DF, Chow DA. Tumorigenicity of murine lymphomas selected through fluorescence-detected natural antibody binding. Cancer Res 1988;48:270–5.
69. Stewart J. Immunoglobulins did not arise in evolution to fight infection. Immunol Today 1992;13(10):396–9.
70. Coutinho A, Kazatchkine MD, Avrameas S. Natural antibodies. Curr Opin Immunol 1995;7(6):812–8.
71. Avrameas S. Naturally occurring antibody against nine common antigens in human sera II. High incidence of murine immunoglobulin exhibit antibody activity against actin and tubulin and sharing antibody specificities with natural antibodies. J Immunol 1982;128:

2779–87.
72. Hurez V, Kaveri SV, Mouhoub A, Dietrich G, Mani JC, Klatzmann D, Kazatchkine MD. Anti-CD4 activity of normal human immunoglobulin G for therapeutic use (Intravenous immunoglobulin, IVIg). Ther Immunol 1994;1: 269–77.
73. Underhill DM, Ozinsky A. Toll-like receptors: key mediators of microbe detection. Curr Opin Immunol 2002;14(1):103–10.
74. Applequist SE, Wallin RP, Ljunggren HG. Variable expression of Toll-like receptor in murine innate and adaptive immune cell lines. Int Immunol 2002;14(9):1065–74.
75. Sabroe I, Jones EC, Usher LR, Whyte MK, Dower SK. Toll-like receptor (TLR)2 and TLR4 in human peripheral blood granulocytes: a critical role for monocytes in leukocyte lipopolysaccharide responses. J Immunol 2002;168(9):4701–10.
76. Putnins EE, Sanaie AR, Wu Q, Firth JD. Induction of keratinocyte growth factor 1 Expression by lipopolysaccharide is regulated by CD-14 and toll-like receptors 2 and 4. Infect Immun 2002 Dec;70(12):6541–8.
77. Vink A, Schoneveld AH, van der Meer JJ, van Middelaar BJ, Sluijter JP, Smeets MB, et al. In vivo evidence for a role of toll-like rece ptor 4 in the development of intimal lesions. Circulation 2002 Oct 8;106(15):1985–90.
78. Liu T, Matsuguchi T, Tsuboi N, Yajima T, Yoshikai Y. Differences in expression of toll-like receptors and their reactivities in dendritic cells in BALB/c and C57BL/6 mice. Infect Immun
2002 Dec; 70(12):6638–45.
79. Akira S. Mammalian Toll-like receptors. Curr Opin Immunol 2003;15(1):
80. Devitt A, Moffatt OD, Raykundalia C, Capra JD, Simmons DL, Gregory CD. Human CD14 mediates recognition and phagocytosis of apoptotic cells. Nature 1998;392(6675): 505–9.
81. Lehrer RI, Ganz T. Defensins of vertebrate animals. Curr Opin Immunol 2002;14(1): 96–102.
82. Harder J, Bartels J, Christophers E, Schroder JM. A peptide antibiotic from human skin. Nature 1997;387(6636):861.
83. Chertov O, Yang D, Howard OM, Oppenheim JJ. Leukocyte granule proteins mobilize innate host defenses and adaptive immune responses. Immunol Rev 2000;177:68–78.
84. Biragyn A, Ruffini PA, Leifer CA, Klyushnenkova E, Shakhov A, Chertov O, et al. Toll-like receptor 4-dependent activation of dendritic cells by beta-defensin 2. Science 2002;298(5595):1025–9.
85. Pangburn MK, Pangburn KL, Koistinen V, Meri S, Sharma AK. Molecular mechanisms of target recognition in an innate immune system: interactions among factor H, C3b, and target in the alternative pathway of human complement. J Immunol 2000;164(9):4742–51.
86. Underhill DM, Ozinsky A. Phagocytosis of microbes: complexity in action. Annu Rev Immunol 2002;20:825–52.
87. Sims JE. IL-1 and IL-18 receptors, and their extended family. Curr Opin Immunol 2002;14(1):117–22.
88. Silva FRMB, Leite LD, Wassermann GF. Rapid signal transduction in Sertoli cells. Eur J Endocrinology 2002;147:425–33.
89. Jonsson CK, Zetterström RH, Holst M, Parvinen M, Söder O. Constitutive expression of interleukin-1α messenger riboneucleic acid in rat Sertoli cells is dependent upon interaction with germ cells. Endocrinology 1999;140:3755–61.

90. Ulrichs T, Porcelli SA. CD1 proteins: targets of T cell recognition in innate and adaptive immunity. Rev Immunogenet 2000;2(3):416–32.
91. Matsukawa A, Hogaboam CM, Lukacs NW, Kunkel SL. Chemokines and innate immunity. Rev Immunogenet 2000;2(3):339–58.
92. Luster AD. The role of chemokines in linking innate and adaptive immunity. Curr Opin Immunol 2002;14(1):129–35.
93. Dalpiaz A, Spisani S, Biondi C, Fabbri E, Nalli M, Ferretti ME. Studies on human neutrophil biological functions by means of formyl-peptide receptor agonists and antagonists. Curr Drug Targets Immune Endocr Metabol Disord 2003;3(1):33–42.
94. Moretta L, Bottino C, Pende D, Mingari MC, Biassoni R, Moretta A. Human natural killer cells: their origin, receptors and function. Eur J Immunol 2002;32(5):1205–11.
95. Long EO. Regulation of immune responses through inhibitory receptors. Annu Rev Immunol 1999;17:875–904.
96. Kelm S, Schauer R. Sialic acids in molecular and cellular interactions. Int Rev Cytol 1997;175:137–240.
97. Pilatte Y, Bignon J, Lambre CR. Sialic acids as important molecules in the regulation of the immune system: pathophysiological implications of sialidases in immunity. Glycobiology 1993;3(3):201–18.
98. Crocker PR, Varki A. Siglecs in the immune system. Immunology 2001;103(2):137–45.
99. Angata T, Varki A. Cloning, characterization, and phylogenetic analysis of siglec-9, a new member of the CD33-related group of siglecs. Evidence for co-evolution with sialic acid synthesis pathways. J Biol Chem 2000;275(29):22127–35.
100. Sonnenburg JL, Altheide TK, Varki A. A uniquely human consequence of domain-specific functional adaptation in sialic acid-binding receptor. Glycobiology 2003;Dec 23 (Epub ahead of print)
101. Lemke G, Lu Q. Macrophage regulation by Tyro 3 family receptors. Curr Opin Immunol 2003;15(1):31–6.
102. Tough DF, Chow DA. Natural antibody recognition of v-H-ras induced 10T½ transformation. Natural Immun Cell Growth Regul 1991;10:83–93.
103. Tough DF, Haliotis T, Chow DA. Regulation of natural antibody binding and susceptibility to natural killer cells through Zn^{++}-inducible ras oncogene expression. Int J Cancer 1992;50:423–30.
104 Tough DF, Feng X, Chow DA. $p21^{ras}$ independent down-regulation of ras-induced increases in natural antibody binding during tumor progression. Nat Immun 1995;14:20–34.
105. Wang H, Chow DA. PKC expression in 10T½ cells associated increased acquisition of natural antibodies with surveillance of preneoplasia and homeostasis of the organism. Scand J Immunol 1999;49(4):381–90.
106. Chow DA, Wolosin LB, Greenberg AH. Murine natural antitumor antibodies II. The contribution of natural antibodies to tumor surveillance. Int J Cancer 1981;27:459–69.
107. Chow DA. Reduced tumorigenicity of threshold tumor inocula in xid-bearing mice treated with natural antibodies. Int J Cancer 1995;60:848–53.
108. Chow DA, Yuan X-y, Tough DF. Polyclonal natural antitumor antibody binding dynamics: Preferential release of surface membrane molecules and increased metastasis. Inv & Met 1992;12:218–32.
109. Zhang Z, Chow DA. Differential CD45 isoform expression accompanies reduced natural antibody binding in L5178Y-F9 tumor progression. J Immunol 1997;159(1):44–50.
110. Deans JP, Serra HM, Shaw J, Shen YJ, Torres RM, Pilarski LM. Transient accumulation

and subsequent rapid loss of messenger RNA encoding high molecular mass CD45 isoforms after T cell activation. J Immunol 1992;148:1898–1905.

111. Johannisson A, Festin R. Phenotype transition of CD4+ T cells from CD45RA to CD45RO is accompanied by cell activation and proliferation. Cytometry 1995;19:343–52.
112. Yamada A, Streuli M, Saito H, Rothstein DM, Schlossman SF, Morimoto C. Effect of activation of protein kinase C on CD45 isoform expression and CD45 protein tyrosine phosphatase activity in T cells. Eur J Immunol 1990;20:1655–60.
113. Bohn J, Roggenbuck D, Settmacher U, Docke W, Volk HD, Von-Baehr R, Jahn S. Binding of natural human IgM auto-antibodies to human tumor cell lines and stimulated normal T lymphocytes. Immunol Lett 1994;39:187–94.
114. Wolf-Levine R, Azuma T, Aoki K, Yagami Y, Okada H. Specific IgG autoantibodies are potent inhibitors of autoreactive T cells. J Immunol 1993;151:5864–77.
115. Landolfi NF, Leone J, Womack JE, Cook RG. Activation of T lymphocytes results in an increase in H-2-encoded neuraminidase. Immunogenetics 1985;22:159–67.
116. Karnitz LM, Abraham RT. Interleukin-2 receptor signaling mechanisms. Adv Immunol 1996;61:147–99.
117. Koopman , Heider K-H, Horst E, Adolf GR, van den Berg F, Ponta H, Herrlich P, Pals ST. Activated human lymphocytes and aggressive non-Hodgkin's lymphomas express a homologue of the rat metastasis-associated variant of CD44. J Exp Med 1993;177: 897–904.
118. Arch R, Wirth K, Hofmann M, Ponta H, Matzku S, Herrlich P, Zoller M. Participation in normal immune responses of a metastasis inducing splice variant of CD44. Science 1992;257:682–5.
119. Galluzzo E, Albi N, Fiorucci S, Merigiola C, Ruggeri L, Tosti A, Grossi CE, Velardi A. Involvement of CD44 variant isoforms in hyaluronate adhesion by human activated T cells. Eur J Immunol 1995;25:2932–9.
120. Chow DA, Li Y, Hebert S. Natural human antibody and intravenous immunolglobulin regulation of T cell activation. Cancer Detec Prev 2002;S176.
121. Xu Z, Weiss A. Negative regulation of CD45 by differential homodimerization of the alternatively spliced isoforms. Nat Immunol 2002;3(8):764–71.
122. Greenberg S, Grinstein S. Phagocytosis and innate immunity. Curr Opin Immunol 2002;14(1):136–45.
123. Franc NC. Phagocytosis of apoptotic cells in mammals, Caenorhabditis elegans and Drosophila melanogaster: molecular mechanisms and physiological consequences. Frontiers in Bioscience 2002;7:d1298–1313.
124. Rescigno M, Granucci F, Ricciardi-Castagnoli P. Dendritic cells at the end of the millennium. Immunol Cell Biol 1999;77(5):404–10.
125. Engering A, Geijtenbeek TB, van Vliet SJ, Wijers M, van Liempt E, Demaurex N, et al. The dendritic cell-specific adhesion receptor DC-SIGN internalizes antigen for presentation to T cells. J Immunol 2002;168(5):2118–26.
126. Granucci F, Zanoni I, Feau S, Ricciardi-Castagnoli P. Dendritic cell regulation of immune responses: a new role for interleukin 2 at the intersection of innate and adaptive immunity. Embo J 2003;22(11):2546–51.
127. Ley K. Integration of inflammatory signals by rolling neutrophils. Immunol Rev 2002;186: 8–18.
128. Malaviya R, Gao Z, Thankavel K, van der Merwe PA, Abraham SN. The mast cell tumor necrosis factor alpha response to FimH-expressing Escherichia coli is mediated by the

glycosylphosphatidylinositol-anchored molecule CD48. Proc Natl Acad Sci U S A 1999;96(14):8110–5.

129. Malaviya R, Ross EA, MacGregor JI, Ikeda T, Little JR, Jakschik BA, et al. Mast cell phagocytosis of FimH-expressing enterobacteria. J Immunol 1994;152(4):1907–14.

130. Supajatura V, Ushio H, Nakao A, Akira S, Okumura K, Ra C, et al. Differential responses of mast cell Toll-like receptors 2 and 4 in allergy and innate immunity. J Clin Invest 2002;109(10):1351–9.

131. Wedemeyer J, Tsai M, Galli SJ. Roles of mast cells and basophils in innate and acquired immunity. Curr Opin Immunol 2000;12(6):624–31.

132. Rothenberg ME, Mishra A, Brandt EB, Hogan SP. Gastrointestinal eosinophils. Immunol Rev 2001;179:139–55.

133. Kazmierczak BI, Mostov K, Engel JN. Interaction of bacterial pathogens with polarized epithelium. Annu Rev Microbiol 2001;55:407–35.

134. Kagnoff MF, Eckmann L. Epithelial cells as sensors for microbial infection. J Clin Invest 1997;100(1):6–10.

135. Hauck CR, Meyer TF. 'Small' talk: Opa proteins as mediators of Neisseria-host-cell communication. Curr Opin Microbiol 2003;6(1):43–9.

136. Cossart P, Pizarro-Cerda J, Lecuit M. Invasion of mammalian cells by Listeria monocytogenes: functional mimicry to subvert cellular functions. Trends Cell Biol 2003;13(1):23–31.

137. Cario E, Gerken G, Podolsky DK. "For whom the bell tolls!" -- innate defense mechanisms and survival strategies of the intestinal epithelium against lumenal pathogens. Z Gastroenterol 2002;40(12):983–90.

138. Martin F, Kearney JF. B1 cells: similarities and differences with other B cell subsets. Curr Opin Immunol 2001;13(2):195–201.

139. Koide N, Sugiyama T, Kato Y, Chakravortty D, Mu MM, Yoshida T, et al. Mouse B1 cell line responds to lipopolysaccharide via membrane-bound CD14. J Endotoxin Res 2001;7(1):39–43.

140. Kaplan D, Smith D, Meyerson H, Pecora N, Lewandowska K. CD5 expression by B lymphocytes and its regulation upon Epstein-Barr virus transformation. Proc Natl Acad Sci U S A 2001;98(24):13850–3.

141. Kantor AB, Herzenberg LA. Origin of murine B cell lineages. Annu Rev Immunol 1993;11:501–38.

142. Allison JP, Havran WL. The immunobiology of T cells with invariant γδ antigen receptors. Annu Rev Immunol 1991;9:679–705.

143. McVay LD, Carding SR. Generation of human gammadelta T-cell repertoires. Crit Rev Immunol 1999;19 (5-6):431–60.

144. Carding SR, Egan PJ. Gammadelta T cells: functional plasticity and heterogeneity. Nat Rev Immunol 2002;2(5):336–45.

145. Godfrey DI, Hammond KJ, Poulton LD, Smyth MJ, Baxter AG. NKT cells: facts, functions and fallacies. Immunol Today. 2000;21(11):573–83.

146. Stout RD, Schwarting GA, Suttles J. Evidence that expression of asialo-GM1 may be associated with cell activation. Correlation of asialo-GM1 expression with increased total cellular RNA and protein content in normal thymocyte and spleen cell populations. J Immunol 1977;139(7):2123–9.

147. Quinn MT, Swain SD, Parkos CA, Jutila KL, Siemsen DW, Kurk SL, et al. A carbohydrate neoepitope that is up-regulated on human mononuclear leucocytes by neuraminidase

treatment or by cellular activation. Immunology 2001;104(2):185–97.
148. Ozinsky A, Underhill DM, Fontenot JD, Hajjar AM, Smith KD, Wilson CB, et al. The repertoire for pattern recognition of pathogens by the innate immune system is defined by cooperation between Toll-like receptors. PNAS 2000;97:13766–71.

Natural Immunity
Edited by L. Bertók and D.A. Chow
© 2005 Elsevier B.V. All rights reserved

Signaling in Natural Immunity: Natural Killer Cells

LAURA N. ARNESON and PAUL J. LEIBSON

Department of Immunology, Mayo Clinic, Rochester, MN 55905, USA

ABSTRACT

Natural killer (NK) cells are large granular lymphocytes noted both for their cytotoxic role in innate immunity and for their linking of the innate immune system to the adaptive immune system through cytokine secretion. In both of these roles, NK cells make use of their ability to recognize tumour- and virus-associated ligands. These cells are identified by their phenotype: NK cells express CD16, the low-affinity Fc receptor (FcR) for IgG, but NK cells do not express T cell antigen receptors or the B cell-associated surface immunoglobulin (sIg).

Unlike T cells or B cells, NK cells do not have a single type of receptor through which they recognize antigens. Rather, clonal subpopulations of NK cells differ in their expression of receptors that recognize a variety of ligands on target cells throughout the body. NK cell binding of these ligands initiates signaling cascades within the NK cell that control its response to the target. Thus, understanding these receptors, their signals, and the interactions of the signaling pathways is key to understanding NK cell function.

1. NATURAL KILLER CELL FUNCTION

The role of an NK cell is two fold: to kill virally infected cells and tumour cells that are encountered within the body and to stimulate other arms of the immune system through cytokine release. NK cells can kill their targets by means of several different mechanisms (Fig. 1). Antibody-dependent cellular cytotoxicity (ADCC) is initiated by the binding of CD16 to the Fc portion of antibodies that are in turn bound to cell-associated antigens on potential targets. "Natural" or spontaneous cytotoxicity is the ability to kill without prior activation or proliferation and without antibody. This type of killing is controlled by a collection of receptors that bind ligands on target cells, determining whether these cells are stressed, tumorigenic, or virally infected rather than normal. NK cells can also kill via interactions between Fas ligand (FasL) and Fas. In this case, binding of FasL on NK cells to Fas on the target cells induces apoptosis of the target cells.

Another important feature of NK cells is their ability to produce cytokines that activate other elements of the immune response. When activated by their receptors, NK cells produce interferon-γ (IFN-γ) and tumour necrosis factor (TNF), cytokines with antiviral functions and the ability to stimulate inflammatory immune responses. NK cells are also regulated by cytokines; cytokines such as interleukin-2 (IL-2), IL-12 and IFN-α/β induce cytotoxic activity and stimulate cytokine production.

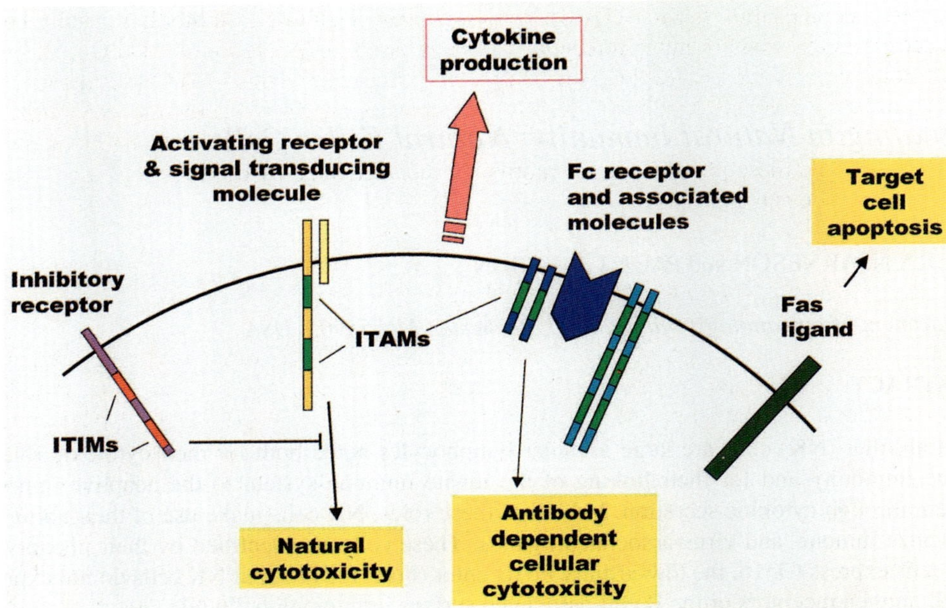

Figure 1. Types of receptors and their effects in NK cells. In addition to an Fc receptor and Fas ligand, NK cells express different types of activating and inhibitory receptors. When bound to ligand, the activating receptors send signals driving natural cytotoxicity, and inhibitory receptors may block these signals. The Fc receptor, when bound to the Fc portion of an antibody, signals for antibody dependent cellular cytotoxicity. The Fas ligand, upon binding to Fas on the target cells, results in signals within the target cell that drive its apoptosis. Activation of the NK cell also results in cytokine production that can activate other cells of the immune system.

2. MAJOR CLASSES OF NATURAL KILLER CELL RECEPTORS

NK cell receptors act as sensors for messages from outside the cell. The NK cell uses these receptors, which are categorized as either activating or inhibitory receptors, to monitor the ligands expressed by cells throughout the body. Activating receptors respond to the expression of exogenous ligands or ligands indicating that a target cell is pathologically "stressed" by initiating signals inside the NK cell that enhance its ability to kill the target. These signals are referred to as positive signals because they drive NK cell cytolytic function. Inhibitory receptors respond to the expression of normal, endogenous ligands on target cells by initiating signals inside the NK cell that inhibit killing of the targets. These signals are referred to as negative signals because they abrogate the signals initiated by activating receptors.

Once a message is detected by an NK cell receptor, it must be relayed inside the cell. This signal transduction takes place as a series of interactions between both catalytically-active signaling molecules and catalytically-inactive adapter proteins. Protein-protein interactions are mediated by domains within proteins that allow them to bind to specific motifs in other proteins. These motifs may be altered in the course of signaling, giving them more or less affinity for other members of the signaling pathway.

One of the most common interactions of this type is the binding of a Src homology 2 (SH2) domain-containing protein to a phosphorylated tyrosine [reviewed in 1]. For example, most of the pathways resulting in activation begin with receptor complexes that contain immunoreceptor tyrosine-based activation motifs (ITAM), while pathways resulting in inhibition usually begin with receptors that contain immunoreceptor tyrosine-based inhibitory motifs (ITIM) [reviewed in 2]. Both types of motifs become phosphorylated when the receptors bind their ligands, and this alteration increases their affinity for proteins containing SH2 domains that recognize the phosphorylated tyrosine in the context of the ITAM or the ITIM. The SH2 domain-containing proteins that bind these phosphorylated motifs are then activated by other modifications, and a signaling cascade is begun.

3. ACTIVATING RECEPTORS IN NK CELLS

The receptors that initiate activation of NK cells recognize a wide variety of ligands, many of which are still unidentified. Unlike T cell receptors, which can bind to antigens only when they are presented in the context of self (in major histocompatibility complexes, or MHCs), activating receptors in NK cells can directly recognize viral peptides as well as ligands on target cells that indicate target cell stress. As a result, NK cells can contribute to the initial defense against viruses and infections, greatly increasing the ability of the immune system to recognize problems in cells early and to respond to them quickly.

Despite this recognition of different ligands, many of the activating receptors contain highly conserved ITAMs within the receptor complex. Located on the cytoplasmic side of the receptors, an ITAM consists of the peptide sequence YxxL(I)x_{6-8}YxxL(I) [3,4]. One or more of these sequences may be found in the cytoplasmic tails of the adapter proteins that are noncovalently associated with the ligand binding immune recognition receptors. Once the receptor is bound by its ligand, the tyrosine in the ITAM is phosphorylated by a Src family protein tyrosine kinase (e.g., Lck, Fyn). Following phosphorylation, the ITAMs recruit and activate the Syk family tyrosine kinases (e.g., Syk, ZAP-70) through their SH2 domains [reviewed in 5]. Once activated, the Syk family tyrosine kinases are able to interact with adapter proteins and initiate the activation of a host of second messengers (Fig. 2).

The adapter proteins associated with activating receptors in NK cells are CD3ζ, FcεRIγ, and DAP12. To date, signaling pathways have not been completely traced from each receptor to the corresponding effector mechanism (e.g., granule exocytosis, cell-mediated cytotoxicity, and transcriptional regulation), but various pathways are known to be required for activation of particular effector mechanisms. By using pharmacologic inhibitors and genetic manipulation of effector cells, researchers have been able to determine many of the components of signaling pathways necessary for different types of activation. This work has provided insights into what is needed to activate and regulate different pathways, leading to an emerging understanding of the roles of different receptors in activating NK cells and the rest of the immune system. Next we briefly discuss the roles of several activating receptors.

3.1. FcγRIII

The human receptor involved in ADCC, FcγRIII, is a multimeric receptor complex consisting of the ligand-binding receptor CD16 (α subunit) which associates non-covalently with the ITAM-containing homodimers or heterodimers of ζ or γ [6–9]. The signaling of this receptor through ITAMs is very similar to that of the T cell receptor (TCR) on T lymphocytes. As in TCR signaling, after ligand binding, Src family kinases bind and phosphorylate tyrosine residues in the ITAMs. These phosphorylated tyrosines recruit Syk family protein tyrosine kinases

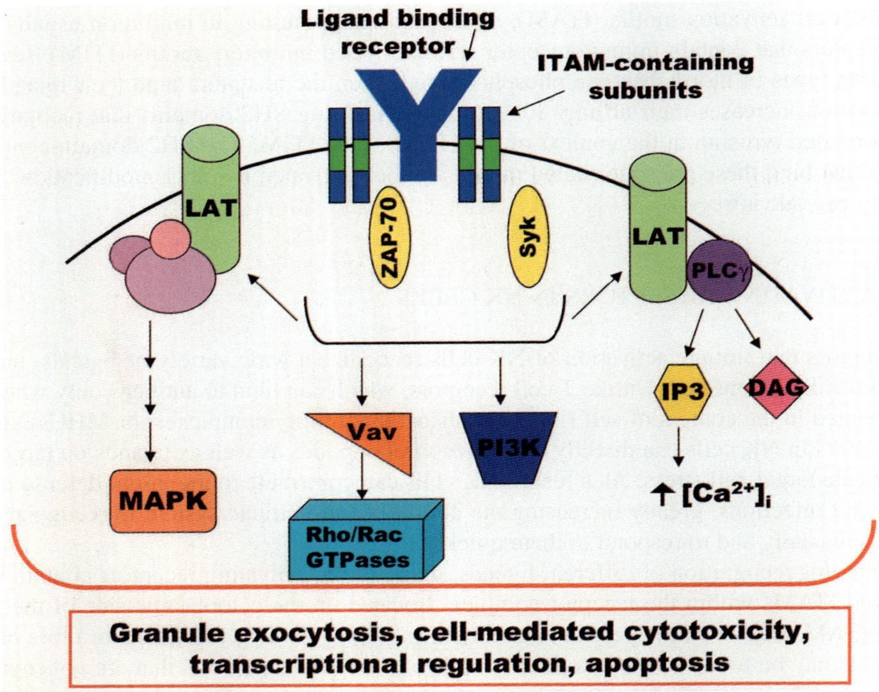

Figure 2. Signals from activating receptors containing ITAMs. Upon ligand binding to an ITAM-containing activating receptor, Src family kinases phosphorylate tyrosines in the ITAM. The phosphorylated ITAMs then recruit and activate the Syk family protein tyrosine kinases (Syk, ZAP-70) through their SH2 domains. Once activated, ZAP-70 and Syk recruit adaptors such as LAT and signalling molecules such as PI3K. The activation of major signalling pathways such as the MAPK, PI3K and PLCγ pathways along with activation of the Rho/Rac GTPases results in the activation of the NK cell and drives its effector functions.

through their SH2 domains, resulting in the phosphorylation and activation of the Syk family protein tyrosine kinases [10,11] to initiate downstream signaling through a variety of intracellular signaling molecules including activation of phospholipase (PLC)-γ [12,13]. This results in increased intracellular Ca^{2+} concentration, increased phosphatidylinositol-3-kinase (PI3K) activity [14,15], increased activity of the Rho/Rac GTPases [16,17], and stimulation of the MAP kinase pathway [18].

Although there are many similarities, signaling through FcγRIII is not identical to signaling from a TCR. For example, while the tyrosine phosphatase CD45 is crucial for T cell activation, CD45-deficient mice exhibit functional killing mediated by ADCC [19]. Moreover, mice with double knockouts of Src-family tyrosine kinases (Lck and Fyn), the first and crucial kinases activated after T cell engagement, have intact ADCC in NK cells [20]. These differences in signal transduction highlight the need to recognize the unique features of NK cell signaling in order to understand the differential regulation of separate subpopulations of lymphocytes and in order to develop drugs to specifically target distinct aspects of the immune system.

3.2. NKp30 and NKp46

The natural cytotoxicity receptors NKp30 and NKp46 are believed to initiate cytotoxicity upon binding to tumour cells [21,22]. NKp46 is also known to recognize hemagglutinins on virally infected cells [23], and it is involved in NK cell-mediated lysis of cells infected with an intracellular pathogen [24]. In humans, these receptors associate with ITAM-containing CD3ζ-homodimers. NKp46 can also associate with ITAM-containing FcεRIγ-CD3ζ heterodimers. Both of these types of ITAMs are phosphorylated by Src family tyrosine kinases, which recruit Syk and ZAP70 in a conventional manner. Cross-linking of NKp46 by antibodies drives an increase in intracellular calcium, cytokine production, and cytotoxic activity [25]. Identification of other ligands of NKp46 and NKp30 will serve to further elucidate how NK cells are activated and whether signals from different ligands to the same receptor vary.

3.3. NKp44 and KIR2DS2

The activating receptor NKp44 is expressed only on IL-2 activated NK cells [26]. Like NKp46, NKp44 can recognize hemagglutinins on virally infected cells [27]. NKp44 is known to be triggered during tumour cell lysis, and it is possible that it may recognize tumour-associated ligands [26]. This receptor associates with homodimers of the ITAM-containing adapter protein DAP12 (also known as KARAP), and this association is necessary for surface expression of NKp44 [28]. Once phosphorylated, DAP12 peptides bind ZAP70 and Syk protein tyrosine kinases [29].

3.4. 2B4 (CD244)

The proposed physiological ligand for the activating receptor 2B4 is CD48, a glycosyl-phosphatidyl-inositol (GPI)-anchored cell surface protein [30,31]. Upon binding to CD48 or when crosslinked with antibodies, 2B4 initiates increased cytotoxicity and cytokine secretion [32]. 2B4 itself does not, however, associate with any ITAM-containing polypeptides. Rather, it contains four TxYxxV(I) motifs that upon ligand binding are phosphorylated. Once phosphorylated, the motifs associate with the adaptor protein SAP and the p85 regulatory subunit of PI3K [33,34]. The phosphorylated TxYxxV(I) motifs may also bind via SH2 domains to the phosphatase SHP-2 or the adapter protein LAT [35]. Despite its lack of ability to activate protein tyrosine kinases through the ITAM pathway, 2B4 appears to play a role as a co-receptor by modulating other receptor-ligand interactions [36]. The possibility remains, however, that 2B4 may have the ability to independently activate NK cell functions.

3.5. NKG2D

The activating receptor NKG2D binds to the target cell ligands MICA [37] and MICB and the ULBP proteins [38,39] in humans and to H60, Rae-1, and MULT1 in mice [40–42]. The proteins MICA, MICB, H60, Rae-1, and MULT1 are stress-inducible molecules rarely expressed on normal cells. These proteins are highly expressed on certain types of tumours. ULBP proteins are, like MICA and MICB, distant members of the MHC class I family of proteins, but they are not believed to be able to present antigen. They are thought to play a role in fighting human cytomegalovirus (CMV), and one CMV protein can even block the ULBP-NKG2D association [39,43]. NKG2D-mediated binding to any of these ligands on target cells can then initiate activation of the NK cells and cytotoxicity.

NKG2D associates with the non-ITAM-containing adapter DAP10 [44]. DAP10 contains a YxxM motif that is phosphorylated by Src family protein tyrosine kinases but does not recruit Syk family tyrosine kinases. Once phosphorylated, the YxxM motif can recruit PI3K directly through the SH2 domain of its p85 regulatory subunit. This alternative method of activation provides a means for costimulation with ITAM-containing receptors [45]. Recent reports suggest that alternatively spliced forms of NKG2D may also associate in mice with the ITAM-containing adapter DAP12, allowing the receptor to act in an activating as well as a costimulatory fashion [46,47].

3.6. Activating receptors in the KIR and Ly49 families

The extracellular portions of some activating receptors are structurally similar to the extracellular portions of inhibitory receptors (killer cell Ig-like receptors, or KIRs, in humans and Ly49 in mice) and so are said to be in the same family despite their differences in function. These activating receptors have short cytoplasmic tails that do not contain an ITIM. Instead, these shortened receptors have a positively charged lysine residue in their transmembrane domain that allows them to interact with the ITAM-containing DAP12; thus, ligand binding results in cellular activation [29]. While the inhibitory receptors have high affinity for self MHC class I, the activating receptors have a decreased affinity for self and an increased affinity for specific class I-like molecules. For example, an activating isoform of Ly49 can recognize an MHC class I-like CMV protein [48]. This ability to recognize self-like proteins suggests that these activating isoforms may arise as a result of selective pressure imposed by pathogens.

4. SIGNALLING PATHWAYS FROM ACTIVATING RECEPTORS

As discussed above, many of the activating receptors in NK cells are associated with ITAM-containing adapter proteins through which they initiate signaling pathways. The receptors that do not associate with ITAM-containing proteins have novel ways of activating some of the same signaling pathways as the ITAM-containing receptors, via alternative mechanisms. Major pathways known to be activated by NK activating receptors include the PLCγ pathway, the MAP kinase pathway, the PI3 kinase pathway, and the Rho/Rac GTPase pathway.

4.1. PLCγ pathway

The activation of phospholipase C (PLC) γ begins with the recruitment of the transmembrane adapter LAT to the phosphorylated ITAM [49]. Once LAT itself is phosphorylated, it may recruit a variety of proteins through SH2 domains, including PLCγ. During certain forms of NK cell-mediated killing LAT is tyrosine phosphorylated [50]. However, in $LAT^{-/-}$ mice, NK cytotoxic function against certain tumours and via ADCC is normal [51]. These observations are consistent with the notion that redundant adapters may be able to replace or work in parallel with LAT in NK cells.

When PLCγ is recruited by LAT to the receptor complex, it is then phosphorylated by ZAP-70 or Syk, giving it the ability to cleave the membrane lipid phophatidylinositol-4,5-bisphosphate (PIP_2) to generate inositol-1,4,5-trisphosphate (IP_3) and diacylglycerol (DAG). IP_3 drives an increase in the intracellular concentration of Ca^{2+}. This increase in Ca^{2+} concentration is required for granule release, and it drives transcriptional changes by controlling the activation of Ca^{2+}-

sensitive transcription factors such as NFAT. DAG and the rise in Ca^{2+} recruit protein kinase C (PKC), which is involved both in the development of cytotoxicity and the phosphorylation of a variety of proteins involved in cell growth and differentiation, such as the MAP kinases.

4.2. MAP kinase pathway

MAP kinases play many roles in the immune response [reviewed in 52]. Generally speaking, MAP kinases in lymphocytes are involved in altering gene expression and thereby altering lymphocyte function. In NK cells, MAP kinases similarly amplify, transduce, and integrate signals from a variety of stimuli. However, in contrast to their role in other lymphocytes, MAP kinases in NK cells may also drive cytotoxic function without requiring transcriptional change [18,53–55]. This novel function may represent an alternative means of using the same signaling molecules to facilitate a more immediate response.

In another departure from other types of lymphocytes, NK cells activate a Ras-independent MAP kinase pathway [56]. While IL-2 activates a Ras-dependent pathway, ligation of targets activates a Ras-independent pathway that drives lytic function. The exact pathways by which MAP kinase is activated in NK cells are still under investigation, and further work will serve to clarify these differences in function and activation.

4.3. PI3K pathway

Phosphatidylinositol 3-kinase (PI3K) is an enzyme that, when recruited to the membrane, adds a phosphate to the inositol ring of phosphoinositides. The lipid products of PI3K phosphorylation affect a variety of targets, including guanine nucleotide exchange factors for the Rho/Rac GTPases, PKC, PLC, and a variety of protein kinases. In turn, a variety of cellular processes such as cell survival, proliferation, and migration may be controlled [reviewed in 57]. PI3K may be activated downstream of proximal protein tyrosine kinase activation, or, in the case of NKG2D/DAP10 activation, it may bind directly to the receptor [44]. The importance of PI3K in NK cell signaling is undisputed, but its exact role has not been determined. PI3K is involved in the regulation of several forms of NK cell cytotoxicity. ADCC and, in some instances, natural cytotoxicity are sensitive to PI3K inhibitors. PI3K may play a role upstream of the MAP kinase pathway [54,55].

4.4. Rac/Rho family of GTPases

Rac and Rho GTPases are GTP-binding proteins that act as molecular switches. When bound to GTP, the GTPases can interact with effector or target molecules and initiate signaling; however, when they are bound to GDP, this signal transduction is abrogated. The members of the Rac/Rho family have intrinsic GTPase activity, but cycling between the GTP- and GDP-bound states is also regulated by a large number of guanine nucleotide exchange factors (GEFs) [reviewed in 58].

The importance of the Rac/Rho family of GTPases in actin cytoskeleton organization is well known; furthermore, evidence of a significant role for these small GTPases and their exchange factors in a variety of signaling pathways is emerging [reviewed in 59]. The Rac/Rho GTPases have been found to play a role in signaling that activates transcription factors and cell cycle progression. In NK cells, the Rac/Rho GTPases and their exchange factors help regulate cytotoxicity [16,17,60]. For example, RhoA is involved in initiating the actin polarization necessary

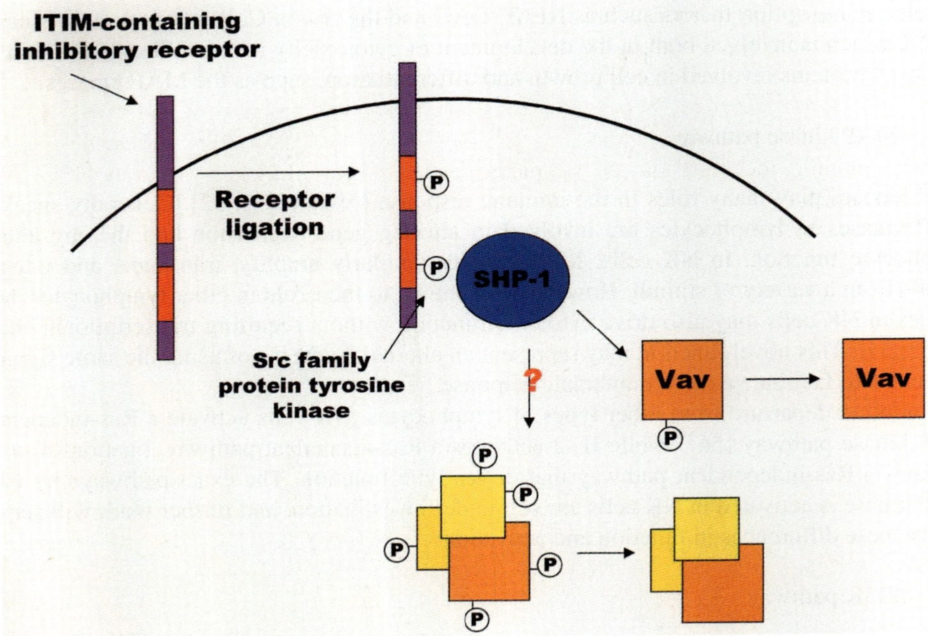

Figure 3. Signals from inhibitory receptors. Ligand binding to an inhibitory receptor results in the activation of Src family kinases, which phosphorylate the ITIM within the intracellular tail of the receptor. Once phosphorylated, the ITIM is able to recruit the phosphatase SHP-1 through its SH2 domain. SHP-1 is thought to act either by dephosphorylating and thereby deactivating a single major substrate such as Vav1 or by the dephosphorylation of a variety of substrates early in the activation cascade.

for granule release. Moreover, the Rac/Rho family GEFs Vav1 and Vav2 have been shown to control cell-mediated killing by NK cells [16,17]. This family of molecules control both actin accumulation and lipid polarization to the site of target cell contact, and other roles in signaling and granule delivery are likely.

5. SIGNALLING PATHWAYS FOR INHIBITION

Despite differences in their protein sequences and structural conformations, the different families of receptors that set in motion inhibition pathways recognize "self" by binding to MHC class I ligands. This recognition of MHC class I molecules provides a means of preventing the killing of normal cells. The known inhibitory receptors contain at least one ITIM through which they are able to suppress the activating signals initiated by ITAM-containing receptors.

ITIMs are found in the intracellular domains of the inhibitory receptors and have a consensus sequence of I(V/L/S)xYxxL(V) [reviewed in 61,62]. Similar to ITAMs, when the receptor binds its ligand, an ITIM is phosphorylated by Src family tyrosine kinases [63,64]. Once phosphorylated, however, ITIMs recruit SH2 domain-containing phosphatases rather than kinases. Instead of phosphorylating motifs and thereby facilitating their interaction with other proteins in the signaling cascade, the phosphatases inhibit progression of the signaling cascade (Fig. 3). SHP-1, a tyrosine phosphatase, directly removes phosphates from proteins phosphorylated by protein kinases. Two alternative views exist on the mechanism of SHP-1-mediated inhibition. SHP-1 may remove the activating phosphate from a central regulator of signaling (e.g., Vav1), or it may remove phosphates from multiple substrates (e.g., LAT, SLP-76, etc.) to affect inhibition. The tyrosine phosphatase SHP-2 can also bind to some ITIMs [65], and its functional role is still under investigation. If signaling through the ITIMs is strong enough, the activation initiated by ITAM-containing receptors may be completely blocked, preventing killing and cytokine release [reviewed in 2].

The ITIM-containing inhibitory receptors in NK cells are the KIR family in humans, the Ly49 family in mice, and the CD94/NKG2A receptor, found in both humans and mice. The expression of these inhibitory receptors on NK cells regulates the NK cell killing of self and provides an important regulatory component to NK cell function.

5.1. Killer cell Ig-like receptor family

Found in humans, members of the family of inhibitory killer cell Ig-like receptors (KIRs) recognize subgroups of the MHC class I molecules HLA-A, HLA-B, or HLA-C. The KIR family comprises at least a dozen genes that have evolved rapidly compared to other immune receptors. Not only do clonal subpopulations of NK cells within an individual present different combinations of inhibitory KIR receptors, but KIR expression among individuals differs significantly [66; reviewed in 67]. Because of these differences in expression, NK cells are able to recognize different combinations of "self," as presented by cells in the form of MHC class I molecules. Despite the variability of ligands that these receptors recognize, each contains ITIMs on the cytoplasmic side of the receptor. Binding of inhibitory KIRs to class I molecules results in inhibition of cytotoxicity through ITIM signaling cascades.

5.2. Ly49 family

Found in mice but not in humans, the Ly49 family of receptors, like the KIRs, recognizes subsets of MHC class I molecules [68]. The Ly49 family is composed of at least nine members, and inhibitory Ly49 family members are expressed on the surface of NK cells as homodimers. Like the KIRs, overlapping subsets of these genes are expressed on different clonal subpopulations of NK cells [reviewed in 69].

5.3. CD94/NKG2A

The CD94/NKG2A heterodimer [70] recognizes HLA-E in humans [71–73] or Qa1^b in mice [74,75]. Both HLA-E and Qa1^b present peptides derived from the leader sequences of other class I molecules (e.g., HLA-A, HLA-B, and HLA-C) that are usually used to present antigens to CD8+ T cells. The cell surface expression of HLA-E and Qa1^b is dependent upon binding to these leader sequences that are generated by proteolytic degradation in the endoplasmic reticulum. Since intact antigen processing is necessary for surface expression of HLA-E and Qa1^b, the expression of this peptide provides a means of gauging the integrity of the MHC class I antigen-presentation pathway. When expression of HLA-E is lost, the CD94/NKG2A receptor no longer sends inhibitory signals. Thus, the CD94/NKG2A receptor provides a means for NK cells to monitor the overall expression of MHC class I on a tissue and prevent the escape of a tumour or virally infected cell through down-regulation of MHC class I molecules.

HLA-E can also present a peptide derived from the leader sequence of human heat shock protein 60 (hsp60) [76]. CD94/NKG2A is unable to recognize HLA-E molecules bound to hsp60, thus the display of this peptide on the surface interferes with inhibitory effects of CD94/NKG2A-HLA-E binding. Human hsp60 is expressed by cells under stress, so the presentation of this peptide provides another means for NK cells to monitor the health of cells that it encounters.

6. STAGES OF NATURAL KILLER CELL ACTIVATION

Changes in the microscopic appearance of an NK cell can be used to mark different stages of activation. These changes in the spatial relationships of the cellular components result from intracellular signals that in turn result from signals from the NK cell receptors. During the stages of activation, changes in appearance and function are used to determine whether inhibition, overexpression, or knockout of a molecule is playing a role in NK cell processes.

The first step toward NK cell cytotoxicity is the physical association of the NK cell and its target. During conjugate formation, the NK cell attaches to ligands on the target via a variety of receptors and integrins. Determining if the number of NK:target cell conjugates is affected by a given molecule provides a way to determine if the molecule is involved in controlling the association of the two cells.

Shortly after the association of the NK cell and its target an immunological synapse is formed [77]. This assembly indicates a reorganization of the bound receptors into specific regions within the membranes between the target and the effector cell. Intracellular signaling is both a cause and an effect of this synapse formation; signaling is necessary for the membrane reorganization and is propagated by the synapse formation [78,79].

As part of this synapse formation and the resulting NK cell activation, microdomains enriched in sphingolipids and cholesterol, called lipid rafts, polarize to the site of NK:target cell contact [78]. The lipid rafts contain a different subset of proteins than the rest of the plasma membrane, and the composition of proteins in the lipid raft changes with lymphocyte activation. Thus, lipid rafts recruited as a result of signaling may then enhance signaling by aggregating activating receptors and other signaling and adapter molecules. Once aggregated, lipid rafts may also serve as a possible down-regulator of future signaling by recruiting phosphatases [80].

As proteins move into and out of the lipid rafts, other proteins must move about the NK cell to support its function. The cytoskeleton of the NK cell reorganizes as part of activation. This reorganization of the backbone of the cell facilitates the movement of other proteins about the cell, including proteins packaged in granules. After cytoskeleton reorganization, granules polarize to the site of target cell contact and are then exocytosed into the space between the NK cell and target cell. Both the microtubule organizing centre and the actin cytoskeleton participate in this reorganization. The dramatic changes in cell polarity that result from these cytoskeletal changes indicate the activation of the NK cell.

7. SIGNALS FOR DEACTIVATION AND APOPTOSIS

As one of the immune system's most powerful front-line defences, NK cells must be tightly regulated to prevent attacks on healthy cells or initiation of excessive immune responses. Several mechanisms serve to provide the needed regulation.

Once an NK cell kills its target it may go on to kill other targets, become inactivated, or undergo activation-induced cell death (AICD). Although the NK cell's ability to initiate signals in response to activating and inhibitory ligands on a target cell does not depend on its interactions with activating and inhibitory ligands on previously encountered cells, the NK cell's survival may nevertheless be influenced by its previous activation. For example, as part of their activation, NK cells upregulate Fas (in addition to FasL) [81,82]. Thus, like their targets that express Fas, NK cells are susceptible to killing through this death receptor pathway. The Fas receptor is upregulated by signaling through FcR and possibly other receptors [81,83], resulting in a suicide mechanism.

Many of the signals that initiate the NK cell's cytotoxic functions may also result in the cell's eventual death. For example, signaling through MAP kinases has been implicated in regulating cell survival and apoptosis in lymphocytes. Similarly, IL-2 not only activates NK cells; it also increases the likelihood that they will die by AICD [84]. These self-destructive mechanisms act as controls on NK cells.

8. CONCLUSIONS

NK cells use a variety of signaling pathways to make changes in their composition that support the killing of target cells and the release of cytokines. The variety of receptors and signaling pathways available to the NK cell provides a finely controlled response to a wide variety of target cells. The ability of an NK cell to survey the body on a cell-by-cell basis and carry out or induce killing on the basis of a balance of positive and negative signals provides a very powerful and sensitive monitoring tool for the immune system. Although the pathways involved in NK cell activation and apoptosis are still being explored, their importance in immune activation and regulation is already clear.

ACKNOWLEDGEMENTS

Many thanks to Bonnie Nestor for her editing of the manuscript.

REFERENCES

1. Tomlinson MG, Lin J, Weiss A. Lymphocytes with a complex: adapter proteins in antigen receptor signaling. Immunol Today 2000;21:584–91.
2. Billadeau DD, Leibson PJ. ITAMs versus ITIMs: striking a balance during cell regulation. J Clin Invest 2002;109:161–8.
3. Reth M. Antigen receptor tail clue. Nature 1989;338:383–4.
4. Cambier JC. New nomenclature for the Reth motif (or ARH1/TAM/ARAM/YXXL). Immunol Today 1995;16:110.
5. Weiss A. T cell antigen receptor signal transduction: a tale of tails and cytoplasmic protein-tyrosine kinases. Cell 1993;73:209–12.
6. Anderson P, Caligiuri M, Ritz J, Schlossman SF. CD3-negative natural killer cells express ζ TCR as part of a novel molecular complex. Nature 1989;341:159–62.
7. Lanier LL, Yu G, Phillips JH. Co-association of CD3ζ with a receptor (CD16) for IgG Fc on human natural killer cells. Nature 1989;342:803–5.

8. Orloff DG, Ra C, Frank SJ, Klausner RD, Kinet J-P. Family of disulphide-linked dimers containing the ζ and η chains of the T cells receptor and the γ chain of Fc receptors. Nature 1990;347:189–91.
9. Kurosaki T, Gander I, Ravetch JV. A subunit common to an IgG Fc receptor and the T-cell receptor mediates assembly through different interactions. Proc Natl Acad Sci USA 1991;88:3837–41.
10. Vivier E, da Silva AJ, Ackerly M, Levine H, Rudd CE, Andersson P. Association of a 70-kDa tyrosine phosphoprotein with the CD16:ζ: γ complex expressed in human natural killer cells. Eur J Immunol 1993;23:1872–76.
11. Ståhls A, Liwszyc GE, Couture C, Mustelin T, Anderson LC. Triggering of human natural killer cells through CD16 induces tyrosine phosphorylation of the $p72^{syk}$ kinase. Eur J Immunol 1994;24:2491–6.
12. Azzoni L, Kamoun M, Salcedo TW, Kanakaraj P, Perussia B. Stimulation of FcγRIIIA results in phospholipase C-γ1 tyrosine phosphorylation and $p56^{lck}$ activation. J Exp Med 1992;176:1745–50.
13. Ting AT, Karnitz LM, Schoon RA, Abraham RT, Leibson PJ. Fcγ receptor activation induces the tyrosine phosphorylation of both phospholipase C (PLC)-γ1 and PLC-γ2 in natural killer cells. J Exp Med 1992;176:1751–5.
14. Kanakaraj P, Duckworth B, Azzoni L, Kamoun M, Cantley LC, Perussia B. Phosphatidylinositol-3 kinase activation induced upon FcγRIIIA-ligand interaction. J Exp Med 1994;179:551–8.
15. Bonnema JD, Karnitz LM, Schoon RA, Abraham RT, Leibson PJ. Fc receptor stimulation of phosphatidylinositol 3-kinase in natural killer cells is associated with protein kinase C-independent granule release and cell-mediated cytotoxicity. J Exp Med 1994;180: 1427–35.
16. Billadeau DD, Brumbraugh KM, Dick CJ, Schoon RA, Bustelo XR, Leibson PJ. The Vav-Rac1 pathway in cytotoxic lymphocytes regulates the generation of cell-mediated killing. J Exp Med 1998;188:549–59.
17. Billadeau DD, Mackie SM, Schoon RA, Leibson PJ. The Rho family guanine nucleotide exchange factor Vav-2 regulates the development of cell-mediated cytotoxicity. J Exp Med 2000;192:381–91.
18. Wei S, Gamero AM, Liu JH, Daulton AA, Valkov NI, Trapani JA, et al. Control of lytic function by mitogen-activated protein kinase/extracellular regulatory kinase 2 (ERK2) in a human natural killer cell line: identification of perforin and granzyme B mobilization by functional ERK2. J Exp Med 1998;187:1753–65.
19. Yamada H, Kishihara K, Kong Y-Y, Nomoto K. Enhanced generation of NK cells with intact cytotoxic function in CD45 exon 6-deficient mice. J Immunol 1996;157:1523–8.
20. van Oers NSC, Lowin-Kropf B, Finlay D, Connolly K, Weiss A. $\alpha\beta$ T cell development is abolished in mice lacking both Lck and Fyn protein tyrosine kinases. Immunity 1996;5: 429–36.
21. Pessino A, Sivori S, Bottino C, Malaspina A, Morelli L, Moretta L, et al. Molecular cloning of NKp46: a novel member of the immunoglobulin superfamily involved in triggering of natural cytotoxicity. J Exp Med 1998;188:953–60.
22. Pende D, Parolini S, Pessino A, Sivori S, Augugliaro R, Morelli L, et al. Identification and molecular characterization of NKp30, a novel triggering receptor in natural cytotoxicity mediated by human natural killer cells. J Exp Med 1999;190:1505–16.
23. Mandelboim O, Lieberman N, Lev M, Paul L, Arnon TI, Bushkin Y, et al. Recognition

of haemagglutinins on virus-infected cells by NKp46 activates lysis by human NK cells. Nature 2001;409:1055–60.
24. Vankayalapati R, Wizel B, Weis SE, Safi H, Lakey DL, Mandelboim O, et al. The NKp46 receptor contributes to NK cell lysis of mononuclear phagocytes infected with an intracelullar bacterium. J Immunol 2002;168:3451–7.
25. Sivori S, Vitale M, Morelli L, Sanseverino L, Augugliaro R, Bottino C, et al. p46, a novel natural killer cell-specific surface molecule that mediates cell activation. J Exp Med 1997;186:1129–36.
26. Vitale M, Bottino C, Sivori S, Sanseverino L, Castriconi R, Marcenaro E, et al. NKp44, a novel triggering surface molecule specifically expressed by activated natural killer cells, is involved in non-major histocompatibility complex-restricted tumor cell lysis. J Exp Med 1998;187:2065–72.
27. Arnon TI, Lev M, Katz G, Chernobrov Y, Porgador A, Mandelboim O. Recognition of viral hemagglutinins by NKp44 but not by NKp30. Eur J Immunol 2001;31:2680–9.
28. Cantoni C, Bottino C, Vitale M, Pessino A, Augugliaro R, Malaspina A, et al. NKp44, a triggering receptor involved in tumor cell lysis by activated human natural killer cells, is a novel member of the immunoglobulin superfamily. J Exp Med 1999;189:787–95.
29. Lanier LL, Corliss BC, Wu J, Leong C, Phillips JH. Immunoreceptor DAP12 bearing a tyrosine-based activation motif is involved in activating NK cells. Nature 1998;391: 703–7.
30. Brown MH, Boles K, van der Merwe PA, Kumar V, Mathew PA, Barclay AN. 2B4, the natural killer and T cell immunoglobulin superfamily surface protein, is a ligand for CD48. J Exp Med 1998;188:2083–90.
31. Latchman Y, McKay PF, Reiser H. Identification of the 2B4 molecule as a counter-receptor for CD48. J Immunol 1998;161:5809–12.
32. Garni-Wagner BA, Purohit A, Mathew PA, Bennett M, Kumar V. A novel function-associated molecule related to non-MHC-restricted cytotoxicity mediated by activated natural killer cells and T cells. J Immunol 1993;151:60–70.
33. Tangye SG, Lazetic S, Woollatt E, Sutherland GR, Lanier LL, Phillips JH. Human 2B4, an activating NK cell receptor, recruits the protein tyrosine phosphatase SHP-2 and the adaptor signaling protein SAP. J Immunol 1999;162:6981–5.
34. Aoukaty A, Tan R. Association of the X-linked lymphoproliferative disease gene product SAP/SH2D1A with 2B4, a natural killer cell-activating molecule, is dependent on phohphoinesitide 3-kinase. J Biol Chem 2002;277;13331–13337.
35. Bottino C, Augugliaro R, Castriconi R, Nanni M, Biassoni R, Moretta L, et al. Analysis of the molecular mechanism involved in 2B4-mediated NK cell activation: evidence that human 2B4 is physically and functionally associated with the linker for activation of T cells. Eur J Immunol 2000;30:3718–22.
36. Nakajima H, Cella M, Langen H, Friedlein A, Colonna M. Activating interactions in human NK cell recognition: the role of 2B4-CD48. Eur J Immunol 1999;29:1676–83.
37. Bauer S, Groh V, Wu J, Steinle A, Phillips JH, Lanier LL, et al. Activation of NK cells and T cells by NKG2D, a receptor for stress-inducible MICA. Science 1999;285:727–9.
38. Steinle A, Li P, Morris DL, Groh V, Lanier LL, Strong RK, et al. Interactions of human NKG2D with its ligands MICA, MICB and homologs of the mouse RAE-1 protein family. Immunogenetics 2001;53:279–87.
39. Cosman D, Müllberg J, Sutherland CL, Chin W, Armitage R, Fanslow W, et al. ULBPs, novel MHC class I-related molecules, bind to CMV glycoprotein UL16 and stimulate NK

cytotoxicity through the NKG2D receptor. Immunity 2001;14:123–33.
40. Cerwenka A, Bakker AB, McClanahan T, Wagner J, Wu J, Phillips JH, et al. Retinoic acid early inducible genes define a ligand family for the activating NKG2D receptor in mice. Immunity 2000;12:721–7.
41. Diefenbach A, Jamieson AM, Liu SD, Shastri N, Raulet DH. Ligands for the murine NKG2D receptor: expression by tumor cells and activation of NK cells and macrophages. Nat Immunol 2000;1:119–26.
42. Carayannopoulos LN, Naidenko OV, Fremont DH, Yokoyama WM. Murine UL16-binding protein-like transcript 1: a newly described transcript encoding a high-affinity ligand for murine NKG2D. J Immunol 2002;169:4079–83.
43. Kubin M, Cassiano L, Chalupny J, Chin W, Cosman D, Fanslow W, et al. ULBP1, 2, 3: novel MHC class I-related molecules that bind to human cytomegalovirus glycoprotein UL16, activate NK cells. Eur J Immunol 2001;31:1428–37.
44. Wu J, Song Y, Bakker ABH, Bauer S, Spies T, Lanier LL, et al. An activating immunoreceptor complex formed by NKG2D and DAP10. Science 1999;285:730–2.
45. Wu J, Cherwinski H, Spies T, Phillips JH, Lanier LL. DAP10 and DAP12 form distinct, but functionally cooperative, receptor complexes in natural killer cells. J Exp Med 2000;192: 1059–67.
46. Diefenbach A, Tomasello E, Lucas M, Jamieson AM, Hsia JK, Vivier E, et al. Selective associations with signaling proteins determine stimulatory *versus* costimulatory activity of NKG2D. Nat Immunol 2002;3:1142–9.
47. Gilfillan S, Ho EL, Cella M, Yokoyama WM, Colonna M. NKG2D recruits two distinct adapters to trigger NK cell activation and costimulation. Nat Immunol 2002;3:1150–5.
48. Arase H, Mocarski ES, Campbell AE, Hill AB, Lanier LL. Direct recognition of cytomeglovirus by activating and inhibitory NK cell receptors. Science 2002;296:1323–6.
49. Zhang W, Sloan-Lancaster J, Kitchen J, Trible RP, Samelson LE. LAT: the ZAP-70 tyrosine kinase substrate that links T cell receptor to cellular activation. Cell 1998;92:83–92.
50. Jevremovic D, Billadeau DD, Schoon RA, Dick CJ, Irvin BJ, Zhang W, et al. A role for the adaptor protein LAT in human NK cell-mediated cytotoxicity. J Immunol 1999;162: 2453–6.
51. Zhang W, Sommers CL, Burshtyn DN, Stebbins CC, DeJarnette JB, Trible RP, et al. Essential role of LAT in T cell development. Immunity 1999;10:323–32.
52. Dong C, Davis RJ, Flavell RA. MAP kinases in the immune response. Ann Rev Immunol 2002;20:55–72.
53. Chini CCS, Boos MD, Dick CJ, Schoon RA, Leibson PJ. Regulation of p38 mitogen-activated protein kinase during NK cell activation. Eur J Immunol 2000;30:2791–8.
54. Jiang K, Zhong B, Gilvary DL, Corliss BC, Hong-Geller E, Wei S, et al. Pivotal role of phosphoinositide-3 kinase in regulation of cytotoxicity in natural killer cells. Nat Immunol 2000;1:419–25.
55. Jiang K, Zhong B, Gilvary DL, Corliss BC, Vivier E, Hong-Geller E, et al. Syk regulation of phophoinositide 3-kinase-dependent NK cell function. J Immunol 2002;168:3155–64.
56. Wei S, Gilvary DL, Corliss BC, Sebti S, Sun J, Straus DB, et al. Direct tumor lysis by NK cells uses a Ras-independent mitogen-activated protein kinase signal pathway. J Immunol 2000;165:3811–9.
57. Rameh LE, Cantley LC. The role of phosphoinositide 3-kinase lipid products in cell function. J Biol Chem 1999;274:8347–50.

58. Bishop AL, Hall A. Rho GTPases and their effector proteins. Biochem J 2000;348:241–55.
59. Ridley AJ. Rho family proteins: coordinating cell responses. Trends Cell Biol 2001;11: 471–7.
60. Lou Z, Billadeau DD, Savoy DN, Schoon RA, Leibson PJ. A role for RhoA/ROCK/LIM-kinase pathway in the regulation of cytotoxic lymphocytes. J Immunol 2001;167:5749–57.
61. Ravetch JV, Lanier LL. Immune inhibitory receptors. Science 2000;280:84–9.
62. Vivier E, Daëron M. Immunoreceptor tyrosine-based inhibition motifs. Immunol Today 1997;18:286–91.
63. Burshtyn DN, Scharenberg AM, Wagtmann N, Rajagopalan S, Berrada K, Yi T, et al. Recruitment of tyrosine phosphatase HCP by the killer cell inhibitory receptor. Immunity 1996;4:77–85.
64. Binstadt BA, Brumbaugh KM, Dick CJ, Scharenberg AM, Williams BL, Colonna M, et al. Sequential involvement of Lck and SHP-1 with MHC recognizing receptors on NK cells inhibits FcR-initiated tyrosine kinase activation. Immunity 1996;5:629–38.
65. Yusa S, Catina TL, Campbell KS. SHP-1- and phosphotyrosine-independent inhibitory signaling by a killer cell Ig-like receptor cytoplasmic domain in human NK cells. J Immunol 2002;168:5047–57.
66. Uhrberg M, Valiante NM, Shum BP, Schilling HG, Lienert-Weidenbach K, Corliss B, et al. Human diversity in killer cell inhibitory receptor genes. Immunity 1997;7:753–63.
67. Vilches C, Parham P. KIR: diverse, rapidly evolving receptors of innate and adaptive immunity. Annu Rev Immunol 2002;20:217–51.
68. Karlhofer FM, Ribaudo RK, Yokoyama WM. MHC class I alloantigen specificity of Ly-49^+ IL-2 activated natural killer cells. Nature 1992;358: 66–70.
69. Lanier LL. NK cell receptors. Ann Rev Immunol 1998;16:359–93.
70. Phillips JH, Chang C, Mattson J, Gumperz JE, Parham P, Lanier LL. CD94 and a novel associated protein (94AP) form a NK cell receptor involved in the recognition of HLA-A, HLA-B, and HLA-C allotypes. Immunity 1996;5:163–72.
71. Braud VM, Allan DS, O'Callaghan CA, Söderström K, D'Andrea A, Ogg GS, et al. HLA-E binds to natural killer cell receptors CD94/NKG2A, B and C. Nature 1998;391:795–9.
72. Borrego F, Ulbrecht M, Weiss EH, Coligan JE, Brooks AG. Recognition of human histocompatibility antigen (HLA)-E complexed with HLA class I signal sequence-derived peptides by CD94/NKG2A confers protection from natural killer cell-mediated lysis. J Exp Med 1998;187:813–8.
73. Lee N, Llano M, Carretero M, Ishitani A, Navarro F, López-Botet M, et al. HLA-E is a major ligand for the natural killer cell inhibitory receptor CD94/NKG2A. Proc Natl Acad Sci USA 1998;95:5199–209.
74. Kurepa Z, Hasemann CA, Forman J. Qa-1^b binds conserved class I leader peptides derived from several mammalian species. J Exp Med 1998;188:973–8.
75. Vance RE, Kraft JR, Altman JD, Jensen PE, Raulet DH. Mouse CD94/NKG2A is a natural killer cell receptor for the nonclassical major histocompatibility complex (MHC) class I molecule Qa-1^b. J Exp Med 1998;188:1841–8.
76. Michaëlsson J, de Matos CT, Achour A, Lanier LL, Kärre K, Söderström K. A signal peptide derived from hsp60 binds HLA-E and interferes with CD94/NKG2A recognition. J Exp Med 2002;196:1403–14.
77. Davis DM, Chui I, Fassett M, Cohen GB, Mandelboim O, Strominger JL. The human

natural killer cell immune synapse. PNAS 1999;96:15062–7.
78. Lou Z, Jevremovic D, Billadeau DD, Leibson PJ. A balance between positive and negative signals in cytotoxic lymphocytes regulates the polarization of lipid rafts during the development of cell-mediated killing. J Exp Med 2000;191:347–54.
79. Fassett MS, Davis DM, Valter MM, Cohen GB, Strominger JL. Signaling at the inhibitory natural killer cell immune synapse regulates lipid raft polarization but not MHC class I clustering. PNAS 2001;98:14547–52.
80. Galandrini G, Tassi I, Mattia G, Lenti L, Piccoli M, Frati L, et al. SH2-containing inositol phosphatase (SHIP-1) transiently translocates to raft domains and modulates CD16-mediated cytotoxicity in human NK cells. Blood 2002;100:4581–9.
81. Eischen CM, Schilling JD, Lynch DH, Krammer PH, Leibson PJ. Fc receptor-induced expression of Fas ligand on activated NK cells facilitates cell-mediated cytotoxicity and subsequent autocrine NK cell apoptosis. J Immunol 1996;156:2693–9.
82. Eischen CM, Leibson PJ. The Fas pathway in apoptosis. Adv Pharmacol 1997;41:107–32.
83. Spaggiari GM, Contini P, Dondero A, Carosio R, Puppo F, Indiveri F, et al. Soluble HLA class I induces NK cell apoptosis upon the engagement of killer-activating HLA class I receptors through FasL-Fas interaction. Blood 2002;100:4098–107.
84. Ross ME, Caligiuri MA. Cytokine-induced apoptosis of human natural killer cells identifies a novel mechanism to regulate the innate immune response. Blood 1997;89: 910–8.

Natural Immunity
Edited by L. Bertók and D.A. Chow
© 2005 Elsevier B.V. All rights reserved

Pathogen Recognition by Toll-like Receptors

TRUDE HELEN FLO and ALAN ADEREM

The Institute for Systems Biology, 1441 North 34th Street, Seattle, WA 98103-8904, USA

ABSTRACT

Macrophages are central in orchestrating the innate immune response to infection, representing both the janitor and the security guard. While performing their normal scavenging functions in various tissues they will, at the same time, survey the tissues for pathogenic intruders. This is not a trivial task: They must be able to discriminate microbes from self, and then initiate a proper response. The discovery of the Toll-like receptor (TLR) family of pattern-recognition receptors has provided a better understanding of how this can be done. TLRs are expressed on macrophages and other innate immune cells, where they collaborate to read the molecular fingerprint of different microbes and initiate inflammatory signalling pathways. It is becoming clear that the TLR family is important in infectious diseases, and there is also evidence that they may play a role in autoimmunity and degenerative diseases in the central nervous system. In this review we will give an overview of the current knowledge of pathogen recognition by TLRs.

1. INTRODUCTION

Cells of the mononuclear phagocyte system are widely distributed throughout every tissue of the body and their properties vary depending on their functional state and location. Macrophages are generated in the bone marrow and circulate in the blood as monocytes before crossing the vascular wall and entering the tissues. Once they have entered the tissue and have developed under the influence of the local environment, they are known as macrophages, or by more specialised names that were used prior to their identification as macrophages [1]. Thus liver macrophages are known as Kupffer cells, brain macrophages are microglial cells, and bone macrophages are osteoclasts. Importantly, tissue macrophages have very different functions depending on their locale. Thus spleen macrophages have a variety of functions that reflect their heterogeneity; the red pulp macrophages clear senescent red blood cells while the macrophages of the marginal zone and the lymphoid areas participate in the host response to infection. Similarly, the liver macrophages, or Kupffer cells, have a role in clearance of a wide variety of detritus. The osteoclasts are somewhat more exotic; they attach themselves to bone and remodel it by a specialised form of frustrated phagocytosis.

The homeostatic functions of tissue macrophages only partially represent the role of cells of the mononuclear phagocyte lineage. Macrophages are best known for their role in host defence and inflammation. Circulating monocytes are attracted to areas of infection by chemotactic agents; once there they become activated and acquire properties that facilitate effective defence against the pathogen. The cells bind pathogens via a variety of receptors, phagocytose them, and kill them within the ensuing vacuole [2]. The dead pathogen is degraded within the mature phagosome, also known as a phagolysosome, and microbial peptides are exported to the cell surface where they are presented to T cells. In this sense, macrophages, and their close relatives, the dendritic cells, initiate and orchestrate the adaptive immune response. This is a bi-directional relationship; activated T-cells produce cytokines like interferon-γ that activate the macrophage to become a voracious killing machine. Macrophage activation is a two-edged sword. It is absolutely required for effective host defence, but the inflammatory sequellae is also harmful. Unbridled macrophage-mediated inflammation is the effector of a multitude of pathological states including many autoimmune diseases and heart disease. Despite these negative effects, inflammatory mediators produced by macrophages mainly have positive functions as they participate in processes such as wound healing, tissue remodelling and angiogenesis.

Monocytes, macrophages, dendritic cells and the related microglial cells are critical for immune surveillance in the brain [3]. Although this surveillance is a normal homeostatic process, it can cause inflammation and pathology if it goes awry. This balance is tightly controlled by a variety of cytokines and protein mediators. For example, tumour necrosis factor (TNFα) enhances immune surveillance whereas transforming growth factor β (TGFβ) diminishes it. Similarly, pathogen-derived components such as bacterial lipopolysaccharides are capable of stimulating proinflammatory responses in the brain. A major goal of this review is the description of the mechanisms by which bacterial products stimulate proinflammatory responses.

2. RECOGNITION OF PATHOGENS BY PATTERN RECOGNITION RECEPTORS

Macrophages represent the cornerstone of the innate immune response to infection. They must be able to specifically define the threat and then formulate an appropriate, and measured, response. This requirement is not trivial; antigen recognition in the adaptive immune response is exquisitely tailored by mechanisms involving gene rearrangement and affinity maturation. How then can a macrophage, with only germ line receptors, precisely gauge the nature of the threat? The answer lies largely in pattern recognition receptors. The term "pattern recognition receptor" (PRR) was suggested by Janeway to describe a generic class of molecules that recognise structural features found on pathogens, but not the host. As the pattern recognition receptors are invariant molecules, this implies that the pathogen-derived components are necessary for the survival of the microbe, and thus cannot be mutated [4]. These structural features have been referred to as pathogen-associated molecular patterns, or PAMPS. However, it should be noted that these structures are also found on a variety of microbes that are not pathogenic, like the commensals inhabiting our intestines. In bacteria, the vast majority of PAMPS are associated with the cell wall (Fig. 1). These include the lipopolysaccharides (LPS) of Gram-negative bacteria and the lipoteichoic acids (LTA) of Gram-positive bacteria. However, host cells also recognise microbial molecules other than cell wall components. For example, the unmethylated CpG dinucleotide motif of bacterial DNA has immunostimulatory properties [5], as does flagellin, a protein component of the motile machinery of bacteria [6]. Other pathogens including viruses, fungi, and protozoan parasites also have immunostimulatory structures. These include different proteins, double-stranded RNA of viruses [7], and glycosyl-phosphatidyl inositol (GPI) anchors of protozoa [8].

PRRs can be membrane bound or soluble proteins. In some invertebrate species like the fruit

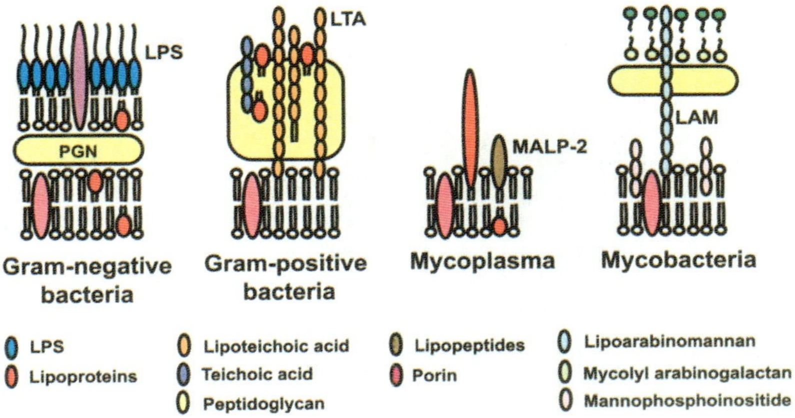

Figure 1. PAMPs in bacterial cell walls. The cell wall of Gram-positive bacteria consists of several layers of peptidoglycan (PGN) where proteins and carbohydrates like teichoic acids are covalently attached. Lipoteichoic acids (LTA) are inserted into the bacterial cell membrane together with other glycolipids and lipoproteins. An outer membrane covers the thin PGN layer of Gram-negative bacteria. Lipopolysaccharide (LPS) is anchored in the outer membrane together with various proteins and lipoproteins. The mycobacterial cell wall consists of several lipids, lipoproteins and glycolipids like lipoarabinomannan (LAM). Mycoplasma are special in that they do not have a cell wall, but they have lipoproteins and lipopeptides, such as MALP-2, inserted into their plasma membrane.

fly *Drosophila,* and the horseshoe crab *Limulus*, pathogens in the haemolymph are recognized by soluble PRRs that trigger proteolytic cascades that ultimately result in an immune response (reviewed in [9,10]). Similarly, the complement pathways in mammals are initiated by soluble PRRs that trigger proteolytic cascades that are central to host defence. Additional soluble PRRs used by the mammalian host to limit infection include the collectins and LPS-binding proteins. These molecules function as adaptors that facilitate the binding of pathogen components to innate immune receptors.

The mechanism by which the central nervous system (CNS) senses and responds to circulating microbial components is largely unknown. One explanation could be that activated endothelial cells produce proinflammatory mediators that further activate perivascular macrophages behind the blood-brain barrier. It is clear, however, that cells of the immune system are capable of crossing the barrier, and that they do so much more efficiently when PAMPs, or PAMP-induced cytokines are circulating in the blood or are generated in the CNS [3]. For infections originating in the CNS one can assume that microglia would recognise pathogen-derived molecules directly through PRRs. However, as the microglia are quiescent compared to other tissue macrophages, the threshold for activation and initiation of inflammation may also be higher. In addition to being involved in pathogen recognition, microglia are also involved in CNS disorders where they might recognise distorted self-structures formed during disease processes. It is tempting to speculate that neurodegenerative diseases result, in part, through the activation of proinflammatory responses that lead to neuronal destruction. For example, microglial cells are known to aggregate around the neurofibrilliary tangles that form in senile plaques during Alzheimer's disease [11].

The discovery of the role of the Toll-like receptor (TLR) family in regulating the activation of macrophages by microbes has opened a new field, demonstrating a remarkable specificity in microbial recognition by these pattern-recognition receptors. TLR transcripts are demonstrated

Table I Exogenous TLR ligands*.

TLR	Pathogen	Molecules
TLR2/TLR1	Bacteria *Neisseria*	Pam_3Cys lipopeptides/lipoproteins Soluble factor
TLR2/TLR6	Mycoplasma Yeast Gram-positive bacteria *Staphylococcus*	Pam_2Cys lipopeptides (MALP-2) Zymosan Peptidoglycan Modulin
TLR2/TLRX	Gram-positive bacteria Gram-negative bacteria *Leptospira*	Lipoteichoic acid Capsular polysaccharide Lipopolysaccharide
	Mycobacteria Measles virus Protozoan Spirochetes	Lipoarabinomannan, glycolipids Hemagglutinin protein Glycosyl-phosphatidyl inositol anchors Glycolipids
TLR3	Virus	dsRNA
TLR4	Gram-negative bacteria *Mycobacterium tuberculosis*	Lipopolysaccharide, capsular polysaccharide Heat-labile cell associated factor
	CMV virus, Murine retrovirus	F-protein, envelope protein
TLR5	Bacteria	Flagellin
TLR7, TLR8	?	Imidazoquinolines
TLR9	Bacteria	Unmethylated CpG DNA

* References are found in the text and in [19]. Some of the proposed TLR ligands have later been shown to contain contaminants (LPS, lipopeptides) [88–90]. This should be kept in mind when evaluating new TLR ligands that are isolated from a source that also contains an established ligand to the same TLR.

in cells of the CNS, including microglia, and this would certainly provide a mechanism for the initiation of proinflammatory responses in the brain [12–17]. Thus, the role of TLRs in CNS immunology and pathophysiology make up an exciting area of future research. Here we will review how macrophages utilise TLRs to recognise microbes and activate inflammation.

3. RECOGNITION BY TOLL-LIKE RECEPTORS (TLRS)

The TLRs are archetypal PRRs [18–20]. Toll was first discovered in *Drosophila* where it has a role in dorsoventral patterning. Subsequently it was demonstrated that dToll also functions as an immune receptor that participates in host defence to fungi and Gram-positive bacteria [9]. Since then, a large number of Toll-like receptors (TLRs) have been found in a wide array of species, and in most cases they act as PRRs in host defence. Like dToll, they are type I transmembrane proteins that have extracellular leucine rich repeats (LRR), and intracellular signalling domains that are homologous to the signalling domains of the interleukin-1 and interleukin-18 receptors (TIRs). As will be documented below, specific TLRs recognise specific PAMPs and stimulate specific inflammatory pathways (Table I and Fig. 2). In this review we will focus exclusively on mammalian TLRs. Both humans and mice have TLRs 1-9; TLR10 in humans is non-functional in mice. However, two additional mouse TLRs are found in databases (TLR11 and TLR12).

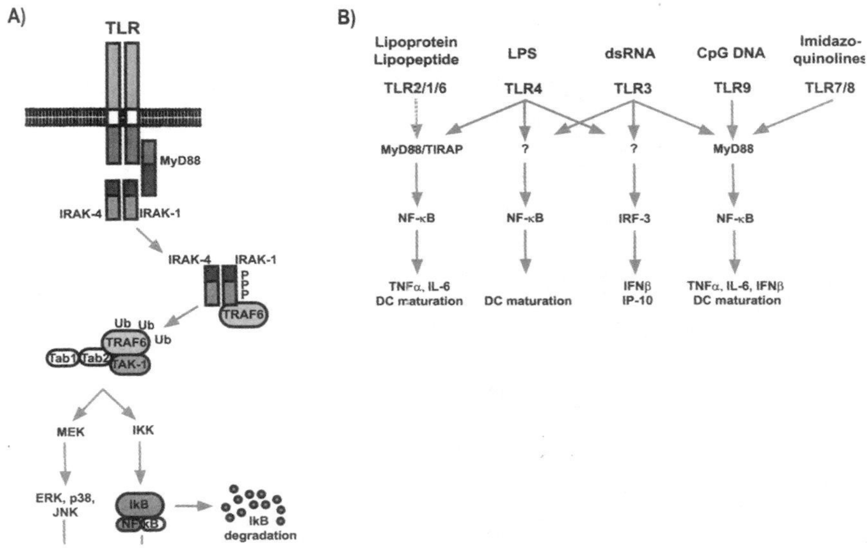

Figure 2. Signaling pathways from mammalian TLRs. A) A general signaling pathway emanating from MyD88. Engagement of the TLRs leads to recruitment of the adaptor MyD88 and activation of the IRAK family of kinases. Phosphorylated IRAK then dissociates from the receptor complex and activates TRAF6, which becomes ubiquitinated and activates TAB-1/TAB-2/TAK-1. TAK-1 subsequently triggers both the MAP kinase pathway, and degradation of IκB with subsequent translocation of NF-κB to the nucleus. Activation of this pathway leads to induction of genes for inflammatory cytokines like TNFα, and maturation of DCs. B) Diversity of TLR signaling. MyD88 is essential for signaling through most of the TLRs, but an additional adaptor, TIRAP, is involved in signaling by TLR2/1/6 and by TLR4. TLR4 and TLR3 also signal independently of MyD88 in pathways leading to delayed activation of NF-κB, and activation of another transcription factor, IRF-3. The MyD88 independent signaling results in upregulation of co-stimulatory molecules on DCs and induction of genes such as IFNβ and IP-10.

There are several controversial reports addressing the specificity of recognition by the mammalian TLRs, which is not surprising considering the relative purity of components that are isolated from microbial systems. Chemical synthesis is thus the safest way to go, and this has been done for some of the TLR ligands. However, this is also the joy of this field right now: We are becoming aware that TLRs can discriminate between subtle structural differences in complex molecules, thus imparting specificity to innate immunity.

3.1. TLR4

The first demonstration that TLRs act as PRRs in mammals was shown by genetic studies in mice [21,22]. The genetic lesions of two strains of LPS hyporesponsive mice were found to be due to mutations in TLR4, implicating this molecule in the recognition of LPS. These studies were supported by the demonstration that TLR4 null mice are non-responsive to LPS [23]. It is not clear whether LPS binds directly to TLR4, although recent evidence suggests that it might [24–27]. It is known that a number of additional proteins are required for LPS-dependent responses. TLR4 needs to bind MD2 in order to reach the surface of the cell, and these two proteins appear to form a functional unit since deletion of either gene in mice results in the loss of responsiveness to LPS [23,28,29]. In order for LPS to be detected by the TLR4 system it first binds an acute phase protein, LPS-binding protein (LBP). Subsequently LBP-LPS form a ternary complex with CD14, a GPI-linked protein found on macrophages and neutrophils. This ternary complex somehow interacts with the TLR4/MD2, which results in a functional signal. Signalling appears to emanate from the cell surface, although there is ample evidence for the internalisation and recycling of the TLR4 complex from the cell surface to intracellular membrane compartments [30].

Although TLR4 is primarily the "LPS receptor", there is also evidence that other ligands may signal through it. TLR4 has been implicated in the recognition of capsular polysaccharides (mannuronic acid polymers) from *Pseudomonas aeruginosa* [31]. TLR4 may also be important in anti viral defence; viral proteins from both respiratory syncytial virus and murine retroviruses are recognized by TLR4, and TLR4-mutant or TLR4-deficient mice show impaired inflammatory responses to the viruses [32–34]. Interestingly, an increasing number of endogenous molecules are reported to be recognized by TLR4 and other TLRs. These will be discussed in a later section.

3.2. TLR2

TLR2 is the most promiscuous TLR with respect to PAMP recognition. This is in part due to its capacity to combine with other TLRs; a property that results in an increased repertoire of recognition [35]. Intriguingly, TLR2 requires a partner in order to signal. Thus TLR2 can combine with TLR1 and TLR6, and probably with TLR10 based on homology. TLR2 combined with TLR1 recognises tri-acylated lipopeptides from various bacterial sources whereas TLR2 and TLR6 are specific for di-acylated lipopeptides [36–38]. TLR2/TLR6 also recognises other agonists including zymosan and bacterial modulin [35,39]. TLR2, in combination with as yet unknown TLRs recognises a wide array of PAMPs including additional lipoproteins, glycolipids, and protozoan components such as GPI-linked antigens [8,40,41] (Table I). TLR2 is the major receptor recognising mycobacteria and isolated mycobacterial cell wall components, such as lipoarabinomannan (LAM) [42,43]. However, although mycobacteria do not contain LPS, TLR4 also seem to have a role in recognition of live *M. tuberculosis* [43,44]. There are also a number of subtleties regarding TLR2. Whereas the data is incontrovertible that TLR4 is the primary receptor through which LPS is detected, there are some anomalies. For example, several reports indicate that TLR2 rather than TLR4 recognise LPS/lipid A from *Leptospira interrogans* [45]. This is explained by the structural differences between this LPS molecule and those of most Gram-negative bacteria such as the enteropathogens.

3.3. TLR3

Virus infections often result in the generation of RNA species that are recognized by the immune system, either as double-stranded RNA genomic fragments, or as replicative intermediates. dsRNA is known to activate the stress-kinase PKR, leading to activation of NF-κB and the MAPK pathways [7]. Recently, a study in TLR3-deficient mice demonstrates that dsRNA is also recognized by TLR3 [46]. The study further shows evidence that polyI:C, a synthetic dsRNA mimetic, induces the production of type I interferons in innate immune cells. Since type

I interferons are crucial in anti-viral immunity, it is likely that TLR3 plays an important role in anti-viral defence.

3.4. TLR5

Motility is required for the virulence of many bacteria, particularly those infecting mucosal surfaces. Bacterial motility is mediated by beating flagella that consist mainly of the protein flagellin. It has recently been shown that the immunostimulatory activity of flagellin is mediated by TLR5 [6,47]. Flagellin from different bacteria has conserved domains crucial for function, whereas the rest of the molecule is heterogeneous. Since the immunostimulatory activity of the molecule is found in the conserved domains, it is not surprising that TLR5 recognises this part of the molecule [48,49]. TLR5 is expressed on the basolateral surface of the polarised epithelial cells lining the mucosal surfaces, where it responds to translocated flagellin [50,51]. It is not known how flagellin is translocated across the epithelial barrier lining the intestine, but this translocation may be a possible answer to the conundrum as to how flagellin from pathogenic bacteria is immunostimulatory in an otherwise loaded commensal environment.

3.5. TLR7 and TLR8

TLR7 and TLR8 are tandem duplicated genes on the X-chromosome. TLR7 is known to respond to synthetic imidazoquinoline anti-viral compounds, although the natural ligand has not yet been discovered [52]. It is possible that these drugs act by mimicking a viral component, and that this component is the PAMP that stimulates TLR7. The imidazoquinoline compounds induce cytokines, including INFα, and dramatically increase the expression of co-stimulatory molecules on the dendritic cells of wild type mice, but not in TLR7 deficient mice. There is also preliminary evidence that one of the compounds, R-848, is recognized by human TLR8 [53], but this observation has not yet been reconciled with the finding that TLR7 null mice do not respond to the drug.

3.6. TLR9

Bacterial DNA has immunostimulatory properties and is recognized by TLR9 [5,54]. This recognition is due to the presence of unmethylated CpG dinucleotide motifs, a feature that discriminates bacterial DNA from primarily methylated sequences found in mammalian DNA [5]. Activation of immune cells by foreign DNA appears to require uptake into the cell by endocytosis, suggesting that its recognition by TLR9 occurs within this intracellular compartment [5,55].

3.7. Endogenous TLR ligands

It has previously been proposed that the innate immune system evolved in response to stress and danger [56]. The validity of this hypothesis can obviously not be discerned, but it is of great interest that a number of endogenous molecules have been identified as TLR agonists [57]. Like their bacterial counterparts, human heat shock proteins (Hsp) 60, Hsp70 and gp96 are reported to activate NF-κB and release TNF by engaging TLR2 and TLR4, events that also induce maturation of DCs [58,59]. There is also evidence that another stress protein, β-defensin 2, engages TLR4 in activation of DC maturation [60].

Tissue damage is known to be accompanied by an inflammatory response. It is of interest that damage of the extracellular matrix generates a variety of molecules that have been reported as TLR4 agonists. These include hyaluran, fibrinogen and degraded fibronectin [61–63]. The biological relevance of these studies awaits exploration.

4. TLR SIGNALLING

The intracellular signalling pathways of mammalian TLRs, IL-1R and IL-18R are mediated by their homologous TIR-domain. In general, these receptors stimulate the production of inflammatory cytokines and/or maturation of DCs, a feature required for successful initiation of adaptive immunity [64–66]. Induction of direct antimicrobial defence activity can also result from TLR activation [67]. A general TLR signalling pathway is depicted in Fig. 2A, although several divergent pathways and differences in usage of intracellular components have emerged from recent studies (for example, Fig. 2B).

In the common TIR signalling pathway, the adapter MyD88 is crucial in initiating a signalling cascade culminating in activation of mitogen-activated protein (MAP) kinases, translocation of NF-κB, and production of inflammatory cytokines. The TIR signalling pathways are reviewed in [64,65]. MyD88 associates with TLRs through TIR-domain interactions, and recruits a family of IL-1R associated kinases (IRAK) in complex with the adaptor protein, Tollip. The family of IRAK proteins consists of two active kinases, IRAK1 and 4, and two inactive kinases, IRAK2 and M [68]. Interaction of MyD88 and IRAK1/4 through their death domains leads to the phosphorylation of IRAK1, a process that may be controlled by IRAK4 [68]. IRAK4 is essential for TLR signalling, whereas, the related protein, IRAKM, negatively regulates TLR signalling [68–70]. Activated IRAK1/4 recruits a downstream adapter, TRAF6, that is subsequently ubiquitinated. Ubiquitinated TRAF6 then interacts with two adapter proteins TAB-1 and TAB-2, and a kinase called TAK-1. Activation of TAK-1 triggers two downstream pathways: It directly activates I-κB kinases that phosphorylate I-κB, a binding partner of the transcription factor NF-κB. This phosphorylation leads to the degradation of I-κB and the translocation of NF-κB to the nucleus. TAK-1 also activates the MAP kinase pathway, and the integration of NF-κB and MAP kinase activation eventually results in production of inflammatory cytokines like TNFα and IL-6 [64,65].

The general pathway described above has a great many subtleties. For example, TIRAP, an adaptor protein, is crucial in MyD88-dependent signalling by TLR2/1/6 and TLR4, but not by TLR3, TLR5, TLR7, TLR9, IL1R and IL18R [71,72]. Other signalling molecules such as the GTPase, rac1, and the phosphatidylinositol-3 kinase, PI3K, have also been implicated in the TLR pathway, but the role of these molecules needs to be clarified [73]. A new TIR-containing adaptor, TRIF, was recently reported [74]. MyD88, TIRAP and TRIF make up a fascinating area of research, as the interplay between these adaptors may be important in generating diversity of TLR signalling.

The adaptor, MyD88, has a critical role in host defence [64]. However, TLR4 and TLR3 also signal via one or more MyD88 (and TIRAP) independent pathways [46,75]. One such pathway leads to the expression of IFNβ that stimulates a variety of genes such as IP-10 and GARG-16, apparently via an autocrine loop [64,71,76]. TLR3 and TLR4 mediated increase of co-stimulatory molecules on dendritic cells can also occur independently of MyD88 and TIRAP [64,71,77].

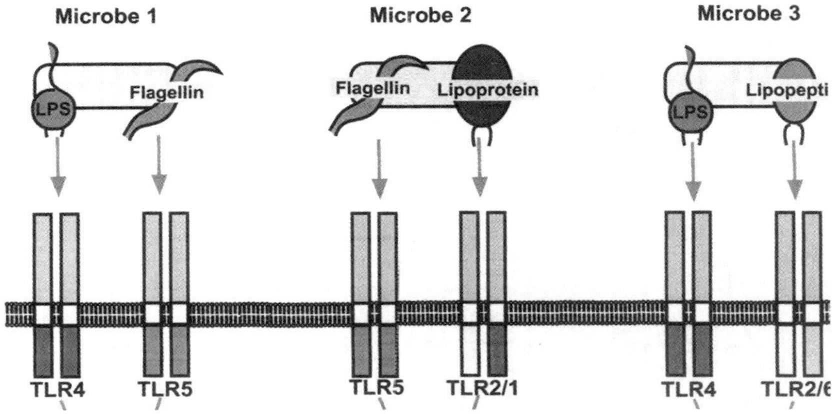

Figure 3. Integration of TLR signaling specifies the response to a particular microbe. Different immunostimulatory features on the same microbe will engage different host receptors that act in concert to read the microbial fingerprint. The ability of TLRs to form functional oligomers leaves the cell with a combinatorial repertoire for specific recognition of different pathogens. For instance, a motile Gram-negative bacterium (microbe 1) will be recognized by TLR4 (LPS) and TLR5 (flagellin), whereas a motile Gram-positive bacterium (microbe 2) engages TLR2+1 (lipoproteins) and TLR5 (flagellin). The final response will result from integration of the signaling pathways downstream of the different receptors. Diversity in specificity and outcome may also be fine-tuned by TLRs collaborating with other, non-TLR receptors, and by differential expression of TLRs in various cells.

5. TLRS FORMULATE APPROPRIATE RESPONSES TO SPECIFIC PATHOGENS

It has long been known that macrophages identify specific pathogens within their phagosomes and then formulate appropriate defensive responses. TLRs1, 2, and 6 are recruited to the phagosome, where they can sample the contents, and define the nature of the threat [35,78]. In principle, the macrophage can identify pathogens by integrating a variety of different TLR-mediated signals. It has been shown that TLR2 and TLR4 can discriminate between Gram-positive and Gram-negative bacteria. Also, as discussed above, TLR5 detects flagellin. Thus activation of TLR2 and TLR5 by a bacterium within the phagosome would imply the presence of a Gram-positive flagellated bacterium. Similarly, activation of TLR4 and TLR5 implies the presence of a Gram-negative flagellated bacterium. In principle, the host cell could use all of its TLRs to precisely read the molecular "bar code" displayed by the pathogen, integrate the information and formulate a specific response by, for example, the differential production of cytokines (Fig. 3). cDNA array experiments have revealed an extraordinarily complex set of responses initiated by each TLR. For example, activation of TLR4 results in the differential transcription of more than 2000 genes. TLR2 also activates a similar number of genes, but not all of these genes overlap (Sepsis GLUE consortium, unpublished observations). The common pathway specifies gene products such as TNFα that are required for a generalised defence against most pathogens. For example, TNFα and TNFα receptor gene deletions in mice lead to impaired resistance to a wide array of pathogens. One might speculate that the differential pathways induce the production of "modifying" signals that specify more specific host responses. This model would have the effect of limiting the non-specific inflammatory response, a prerequisite for normal function of the organism.

The specificity of the host response will also depend on the integration of many other signals in addition to those of TLRs. For example, different phagocytic receptors are required for the internalisation of different pathogens; one might well imagine a scenario where information from TLRs and phagocytic receptors are integrated. A recent report demonstrating cross-talk between the C3bi receptor and TLR4 supports this notion [79].

6. THE ROLE OF TLRS IN AUTOIMMUNITY

It is clear that the TLRs are required for an effective immune response to infections. What then happens when this response goes awry? It is likely that TLRs may play a role in a variety of inflammatory diseases including autoimmunity. A hallmark of autoimmune disease is the production of autoantibodies, including rheumatoid factor (RF), an autoantibody that binds to normal antibodies, as well as antinuclear antibodies, and antibodies to DNA. It has long been a mystery as to how B cells are induced to produce large amounts of autoantibodies like rheumatoid factor. Most efforts in understanding this process have focused on the adaptive immune system. However, a recent report suggests that, after tolerance is broken, the amplification of the autoreactive B cells and the secretion of autoantibodies occur in a T-cell independent manner, and that this is mediated via TLR9 [80]. These authors found that immune complexes containing self-DNA activate RF-specific B cells via two signals; first, the binding of the B cell antigen receptor through the Ig portion of the immune complex and second, the activation of TLR9 through the DNA portion of the immune complex. Not all human DNA is methylated, and it is possible that after the chromatin antibody complex is internalised into the endosomes, the CpG motifs are exposed and activate TLR9 that is known to be located in the endosome. If this hypothesis is true it would provide an explanation as to why so many autoantibodies are generated towards DNA or DNA-binding nuclear proteins. This data does not explain the breaking of tolerance, but it does provide a plausible explanation for amplification of autoreactive B cells.

7. THE ASSOCIATION OF TLRS WITH HUMAN DISEASE

The prominent role of TLRs in innate and adaptive immunity predicts that functional defects in any of these receptors will have a major impact on disease susceptibility. This has motivated several genetic studies of TLR polymorphisms in humans, especially on possible associations between single nucleotide polymorphisms (SNPs) and susceptibility to disease.

Several SNPs have been reported in both *Tlr2* and *Tlr4* that may influence the susceptibility to infectious diseases [81–83]. One TLR4 polymorphism, resulting in the amino acid substitution Asp299Gly, may be associated with increased susceptibility to Gram-negative bacterial infections, [81,84–86] and protection against atherosclerosis [87]. In a small study of leprosy patients in Korea, an Arg677Trp SNP in TLR2 was found to be associated with the lepromatous, but not the tuberculoid form of the disease [83]. The Arg677Trp mutation results in a form of TLR2 that is unable to signal, further supporting a functional link between this TLR and effective resistance to *M. leprae* (P-Y. Bochud, unpublished results). Recently a mutant, non-signalling, form of TLR5 that is expressed with high frequency in human populations was identified (T. Hawn, unpublished results). The presence of this allele is predicted to alter the susceptibility to infection with flagellated organisms. Systematic studies of the association of other TLR polymorphisms and specific diseases are currently being undertaken in a number of laboratories.

ACKNOWLEDGEMENTS

We would like to thank Drs. Adrian Ozinsky and Tom Hawn for critically reading and commenting on the manuscript, and Tatiana Gill for making the illustrations.

REFERENCES

1. Gordon S, Keshav S, Chung LP. Mononuclear phagocytes: tissue distribution and functional heterogeneity. Curr Opin Immunol 1988;1(1):26–35.
2. Underhill DM, Ozinsky A. Phagocytosis of microbes: complexity in action. Annu Rev Immunol 2002;20:825–52.
3. Hickey WF. Basic principles of immunological surveillance of the normal central nervous system. Glia 2001;36(2):118–24.
4. Janeway CA, Jr. Approaching the asymptote? Evolution and revolution in immunology. Cold Spring Harb Symp Quant Biol 1989;54 Pt 1:1–13.
5. Krieg AM, Wagner H. Causing a commotion in the blood: immunotherapy progresses from bacteria to bacterial DNA. Immunol Today 2000;21(10):521–6.
6. Smith KD, Ozinsky A. Toll-like receptor-5 and the innate immune response to bacterial flagellin. Curr Top Microbiol Immunol 2002;270:93–108.
7. Williams BR. Signal integration via PKR. Sci STKE 2001;2001(89):RE2.
8. Teixeira MM, Almeida IC, Gazzinelli RT. Introduction: innate recognition of bacteria and protozoan parasites. Microbes Infect 2002;4(9):883–6.
9. Imler JL, Hoffmann JA. Toll receptors in Drosophila: a family of molecules regulating development and immunity. Curr Top Microbiol Immunol 2002;270:63–79.
10. Muta T, Iwanaga S. The role of hemolymph coagulation in innate immunity. Curr Opin Immunol 1996;8(1):41–7.
11. Stoll G, Jander S. The role of microglia and macrophages in the pathophysiology of the CNS. Prog Neurobiol 1999;58(3):233–47.
12. Laflamme N, Rivest S. Toll-like receptor 4: the missing link of the cerebral innate immune response triggered by circulating gram-negative bacterial cell wall components. FASEB J 2001;15(1):155–163.
13. Bsibsi M, Ravid R, Gveric D, van Noort JM. Broad expression of Toll-like receptors in the human central nervous system. J Neuropathol Exp Neurol 2002;61(11):1013–21.
14. Dalpke AH, Schafer MK, Frey M, Zimmermann S, Tebbe J, Weihe E, et al. Immunostimulatory CpG-DNA activates murine microglia. J Immunol 2002;168(10): 4854–63.
15. Lehnardt S, Lachance C, Patrizi S, Lefebvre S, Follett PL, Jensen FE, et al. The toll-like receptor TLR4 is necessary for lipopolysaccharide-induced oligodendrocyte injury in the CNS. J Neurosci 2002;22(7):2478–86.
16. Kielian T, Mayes P, Kielian M. Characterization of microglial responses to Staphylococcus aureus: effects on cytokine, costimulatory molecule, and Toll-like receptor expression. J Neuroimmunol 2002;130(1-2):86–99.

17. Zekki H, Feinstein DL, Rivest S. The clinical course of experimental autoimmune encephalomyelitis is associated with a profound and sustained transcriptional activation of the genes encoding toll-like receptor 2 and CD14 in the mouse CNS. Brain Pathol 2002;12(3):308–19.
18. Underhill DM, Ozinsky A. Toll-like receptors: key mediators of microbe detection. Curr Opin Immunol 2002;14(1):103–10.
19. Lien E, Ingalls RR. Toll-like receptors. Crit Care Med 2002;30(1 Supp):S1–S11.
20. Kaisho T, Akira S. Toll-like receptors as adjuvant receptors. Biochim Biophys Acta 2002;1589(1):1–13.
21. Qureshi ST, Lariviere L, Leveque G, Clermont S, Moore KJ, Gros P, et al. Endotoxin-tolerant mice have mutations in Toll-like receptor 4 (Tlr4). J Exp Med 1999;189(4): 615–625.
22. Poltorak A, He X, Smirnova I, Liu MY, Van Huffel C, Du X, et al. Defective LPS signaling in C3H/HeJ and C57BL/10ScCr mice: mutations in Tlr4 gene. Science 1998;282(5396): 2085–8.
23. Hoshino K, Takeuchi O, Kawai T, Sanjo H, Ogawa T, Takeda Y, et al. Cutting edge: Toll-like receptor 4 (TLR4)-deficient mice are hyporesponsive to lipopolysaccharide: evidence for TLR4 as the Lps gene product. J Immunol 1999;162(7):3749–52.
24. Lien E, Means TK, Heine H, Yoshimura A, Kusumoto S, Fukase K, et al. Toll-like receptor 4 imparts ligand-specific recognition of bacterial lipopolysaccharide. J Clin Invest 2000;105(4):497–504.
25. Poltorak A, Ricciardi-Castagnoli P, Citterio S, Beutler B. Physical contact between lipopolysaccharide and toll-like receptor 4 revealed by genetic complementation. Proc Natl Acad Sci USA 2000;97(5):2163–7.
26. Hajjar AM, Ernst RK, Tsai JH, Wilson CB, Miller SI. Human Toll-like receptor 4 recognizes host-specific LPS modifications. Nat Immunol 2002;3(4):354–9.
27. da Silva Correia J, Soldau K, Christen U, Tobias PS, Ulevitch RJ. Lipopolysaccharide is in close proximity to each of the proteins in its membrane receptor complex. transfer from CD14 to TLR4 and MD-2. J Biol Chem 2001;276(24):21129–35.
28. Shimazu R, Akashi S, Ogata H, Nagai Y, Fukudome K, Miyake K, et al. MD-2, a molecule that confers lipopolysaccharide responsiveness on Toll- like receptor 4. J Exp Med 1999;189(11):1777–82.
29. Nagai Y, Akashi S, Nagafuku M, Ogata M, Iwakura Y, Akira S, et al. Essential role of MD-2 in LPS responsiveness and TLR4 distribution. Nat Immunol 2002;3(7):667–72.
30. Latz E, Visintin A, Lien E, Fitzgerald KA, Monks BG, Kurt-Jones EA, et al. Lipopolysaccharide rapidly traffics to and from the Golgi apparatus with the toll-like receptor 4-MD-2-CD14 complex in a process that is distinct from the initiation of signal transduction. J Biol Chem 2002;277(49):47834–43.
31. Flo TH, Ryan L, Latz E, Takeuchi O, Monks BG, Lien E, et al. Involvement of toll-like receptor (TLR) 2 and TLR4 in cell activation by mannuronic acid polymers. J Biol Chem 2002;277(38):35489–95.
32. Kurt-Jones EA, Popova L, Kwinn L., Haynes LM, Jones LP, Tripp RA, et al. Pattern recognition receptors TLR4 and CD14 mediate response to respiratory syncytial virus. Nat Immunol 2000;1(5):398–401.
33. Bieback K, Lien E, Klagge IM, Avota E, Schneider-Schaulies J, Duprex WP, et al. Hemagglutinin protein of wild-type measles virus activates toll-like receptor 2 signaling. J Virol 2002;76(17):8729–36.

34. Rassa JC, Meyers JL, Zhang Y, Kudaravalli R, Ross SR. Murine retroviruses activate B cells via interaction with toll-like receptor 4. Proc Natl Acad Sci U S A 2002;99(4): 2281–6.
35. Ozinsky A, Underhill DM, Fontenot JD, Hajjar AM, Smith KD, Wilson CB, et al. The repertoire for pattern recognition of pathogens by the innate immune system is defined by cooperation between toll-like receptors. Proc Natl Acad Sci USA 2000;97(25):13766–71.
36. Takeuchi O, Kawai T, Muhlradt PF, Morr M, Radolf JD, Zychlinsky A, et al. Discrimination of bacterial lipoproteins by Toll-like receptor 6. Int Immunol 2001;13(7):933–40.
37. Takeuchi O, Sato S, Horiuchi T, Hoshino K, Takeda K, Dong Z, et al. Cutting edge: role of Toll-like receptor 1 in mediating immune response to microbial lipoproteins. J Immunol 2002;169(1):10–4.
38. Alexopoulou L, Thomas V, Schnare M, Lobet Y, Anguita J, Schoen RT, et al. Hyporesponsiveness to vaccination with Borrelia burgdorferi OspA in humans and in TLR1- and TLR2-deficient mice. Nat Med 2002;8(8):878–84.
39. Hajjar AM, O'Mahony DS, Ozinsky A, Underhill DM, Aderem A, Klebanoff SJ, et al. Cutting edge: functional interactions between toll-like receptor (TLR) 2 and TLR1 or TLR6 in response to phenol-soluble modulin. J Immunol 2001;166(1):15–9.
40. Lien E, Sellati TJ, Yoshimura A, Flo TH, Rawadi G, Finberg RW, et al. Toll-like receptor 2 functions as a pattern recognition receptor for diverse bacterial products. J Biol Chem 1999;274(47):33419–25.
41. Campos MA, Almeida IC, Takeuchi O, Akira S, Valente EP, Procopio DO, et al. Activation of Toll-like receptor-2 by glycosylphosphatidylinositol anchors from a protozoan parasite. J Immunol 2001;167(1):416–23.
42. Underhill DM, Ozinsky A, Smith KD, Aderem A. Toll-like receptor-2 mediates mycobacteria-induced proinflammatory signaling in macrophages. Proc Natl.Acad Sci USA 1999;96(25):14459–63.
43. Means TK, Wang S, Lien E, Yoshimura A, Golenbock DT, Fenton MJ. Human toll-like receptors mediate cellular activation by Mycobacterium tuberculosis. JImmunol 1999;163(7):3920–7.
44. Abel B, Thieblemont N, Quesniaux VJ, Brown N, Mpagi J, Miyake K, et al. Toll-like receptor 4 expression is required to control chronic Mycobacterium tuberculosis infection in mice. J Immunol 2002;169(6):3155–62.
45. Werts C, Tapping RI, Mathison JC, Chuang TH, Kravchenko V, Saint Girons I, et al. Leptospiral lipopolysaccharide activates cells through a TLR2-dependent mechanism. Nat Immunol 2001;2(4):346–52.
46. Alexopoulou L, Holt AC, Medzhitov R, Flavell RA. Recognition of double-stranded RNA and activation of NF-kappaB by Toll- like receptor 3. Nature 2001;413(6857):732–8.
47. Hayashi F, Smith KD, Ozinsky A, Hawn TR, Yi EC, Goodlett DR, et al. The innate immune response to bacterial flagellin is mediated by Toll-like receptor 5. Nature 2001;410(6832): 1099–1103.
48. McSorley SJ, Cookson BT, Jenkins MK. Characterization of CD4+ T cell responses during natural infection with Salmonella typhimurium. J Immunol 2000;164(2):986–93.
49. Donnelly MA, Steiner TS. Two nonadjacent regions in enteroaggregative Escherichia coli flagellin are required for activation of toll-like receptor 5. J Biol Chem 2002;277(43): 40456–61.
50. Gewirtz AT, Simon PO Jr, Schmitt CK, Taylor LJ, Hagedorn CH, O'Brien AD, et al. Salmonella typhimurium translocates flagellin across intestinal epithelia, inducing a

proinflammatory response. J Clin Invest 2001;107(1):99–109.
51. Gewirtz AT, Navas TA, Lyons S, Godowski PJ, Madara JL. Cutting edge: bacterial flagellin activates basolaterally expressed TLR5 to induce epithelial proinflammatory gene expression. J Immunol 2001;167(4):1882–5.
52. Hemmi H, Kaisho T, Takeuchi O, Sato S, Sanjo H, Hoshino K, et al. Small anti-viral compounds activate immune cells via the TLR7 MyD88- dependent signaling pathway. Nat Immunol 2002;3(2):196–200.
53. Jurk M, Heil F, Vollmer J, Schetter C, Krieg AM, Wagner H, et al. Human TLR7 or TLR8 independently confer responsiveness to the antiviral compound R-848. Nat Immunol 2002;3(6):499.
54. Hemmi H, Takeuchi O, Kawai T, Kaisho T, Sato S, Sanjo H, et al. A Toll-like receptor recognizes bacterial DNA. Nature 2000;408(6813):740–5.
55. Ahmad-Nejad P, Hacker H, Rutz M, Bauer S, Vabulas RM, Wagner H. Bacterial CpG-DNA and lipopolysaccharides activate Toll-like receptors at distinct cellular compartments. Eur J Immunol 2002;32(7):1958–68.
56. Matzinger P. The danger model: a renewed sense of self. Science 2002;296(5566):301–5.
57. Beg AA. Endogenous ligands of Toll-like receptors: implications for regulating inflammatory and immune responses. Trends Immunol 2002;23(11):509–12.
58. Ohashi K, Burkart V, Flohe S, Kolb H. Cutting Edge: heat shock protein 60 is a putative endogenous ligand of the toll-like receptor-4 complex. J Immunol 2000;164(2):558–61.
59. Vabulas RM, Wagner H, Schild H. Heat shock proteins as ligands of toll-like receptors. Curr Top Microbiol Immunol 2002;270:169–84.
60. Biragyn A, Ruffini PA, Leifer CA, Klyushnenkova E, Shakhov A, Chertov O, et al. Toll-like receptor 4-dependent activation of dendritic cells by beta- defensin 2. Science 2002;298(5595):1025–9.
61. Okamura Y, Watari M, Jerud ES, Young DW, Ishizaka ST, Rose J, et al. The extra domain A of fibronectin activates Toll-like receptor 4. J Biol Chem 2001;276(13):10229–33.
62. Termeer C, Benedix F, Sleeman J, Fieber C, Voith U, Ahrens T, et al. Oligosaccharides of Hyaluronan activate dendritic cells via toll-like receptor 4. J Exp Med 2002;195(1): 99–111.
63. Smiley ST, King JA, Hancock WW. Fibrinogen stimulates macrophage chemokine secretion through toll-like receptor 4. J Immunol 2001;167(5):2887–94.
64. Takeuchi O, Akira S. MyD88 as a bottle neck in Toll/IL-1 signaling. Curr Top Microbiol Immunol 2002;270:155–67.
65. O'Neill LA. Signal transduction pathways activated by the IL-1 receptor/toll-like receptor superfamily. Curr Top Microbiol Immunol 2002;270:47–61.
66. Barton GM, Medzhitov R. Control of adaptive immune responses by Toll-like receptors. Curr Opin Immunol 2002;14(3):380–3.
67. Thoma-Uszynski S, Stenger S, Takeuchi O, Ochoa MT, Engele M, Sieling PA, et al. Induction of direct antimicrobial activity through mammalian toll-like receptors. Science 2001;291(5508):1544–7.
68. Suzuki N, Suzuki S, Yeh WC. IRAK-4 as the central TIR signaling mediator in innate immunity. Trends Immunol 2002;23(10):503–6.
69. Suzuki N, Suzuki S, Duncan GS, Millar DG, Wada T, Mirtsos C, et al. Severe impairment of interleukin-1 and Toll-like receptor signalling in mice lacking IRAK-4. Nature 2002;416(6882):750–6.
70. Kobayashi K, Hernandez LD, Galan JE, Janeway CA Jr, Medzhitov R, Flavell RA. IRAK-

M is a negative regulator of Toll-like receptor signaling. Cell 2002;110(2):191–202.
71. Yamamoto M, Sato S, Hemmi H, Sanjo H, Uematsu S, Kaisho T, et al. Essential role for TIRAP in activation of the signalling cascade shared by TLR2 and TLR4. Nature 2002;420(6913):324–9.
72. Horng T, Barton GM, Flavell RA, Medzhitov R. The adaptor molecule TIRAP provides signalling specificity for Toll- like receptors. Nature 2002;420(6913):329–33.
73. Arbibe L, Mira JP, Teusch N, Kline L, Guha M, Mackman N, et al. Toll-like receptor 2-mediated NF-kappaB activation requires a Rac1-dependent pathway. Nat Immunol 2000;1(6):533–40.
74. Yamamoto M, Sato S, Mori K, Hoshino K, Takeuchi O, Takeda K, et al. Cutting Edge: A novel Toll/IL-1 receptor domain-containing adapter that preferentially activates the IFN-beta promoter in the Toll-like receptor signaling. J Immunol 2002;169(12):6668–72.
75. Kawai T, Adachi O, Ogawa T, Takeda K, Akira S. Unresponsiveness of MyD88-deficient mice to endotoxin. Immunity 1999;11(1):115–22.
76. Toshchakov V, Jones BW, Perera PY, Thomas K, Cody MJ, Zhang S, et al. TLR4, but not TLR2, mediates IFN-beta-induced STAT1alpha/beta-dependent gene expression in macrophages. Nat Immunol 2002;3(4):392–8.
77. Hoshino K, Kaisho T, Iwabe T, Takeuchi O, Akira S. Differential involvement of IFN-beta in Toll-like receptor-stimulated dendritic cell activation. Int Immunol 2002;14(10): 1225–31.
78. Underhill DM, Ozinsky A, Hajjar AM, Stevens A, Wilson CB, Bassetti M, et al. The Toll-like receptor 2 is recruited to macrophage phagosomes and discriminates between pathogens. Nature 1999;401(6755):811–5.
79. Perera PY, Mayadas TN, Takeuchi O, Akira S, Zaks-Zilberman M, Goyert SM, et al. CD11b/CD18 acts in concert with CD14 and Toll-like receptor (TLR) 4 to elicit full lipopolysaccharide and taxol-inducible gene expression. J Immunol 2001;166(1):574–81.
80. Leadbetter EA, Rifkin IR, Hohlbaum AM, Beaudette BC, Shlomchik MJ, Marshak-Rothstein A. Chromatin-IgG complexes activate B cells by dual engagement of IgM and Toll-like receptors. Nature 2002;416(6881):603–7.
81. Arbour NC, Lorenz E, Schutte BC, Zabner J, Kline JN, Jones M, et al. TLR4 mutations are associated with endotoxin hyporesponsiveness in humans. Nat Genet 2000;25(2):187–91.
82. Lorenz E, Mira JP, Cornish KL, Arbour NC, Schwartz DA. A novel polymorphism in the toll-like receptor 2 gene and its potential association with staphylococcal infection. Infect Immun 2000;68(11):6398–401.
83. Kang TJ, Chae GT. Detection of Toll-like receptor 2 (TLR2) mutation in the lepromatous leprosy patients. FEMS Immunol Med Microbiol 2001;31(1):53–8.
84. Lorenz E, Mira JP, Frees KL, Schwartz DA. Relevance of mutations in the TLR4 receptor in patients with gram- negative septic shock. Arch Intern Med 2002;162(9):1028–32.
85. Agnese DM, Calvano JE, Hahm SJ, Coyle SM, Corbett SA, Calvano SE, et al. Human toll-like receptor 4 mutations but not CD14 polymorphisms are associated with an increased risk of gram-negative infections. J Infect Dis 2002;186(10):1522–5.
86. Smirnova I, Poltorak A, Chan EK, McBride C, Beutler B. Phylogenetic variation and polymorphism at the toll-like receptor 4 locus (TLR4). Genome Biol 2000;1(1): RESEARCH002.
87. Kiechl S, Lorenz E, Reindl M, Wiedermann CJ, Oberhollenzer F, Bonora E, et al. Toll-like receptor 4 polymorphisms and atherogenesis. N Engl J Med 2002;347(3):185–92.
88. Hirschfeld M, Ma Y, Weis JH, Vogel SN, Weis JJ. Cutting edge: repurification of

lipopolysaccharide eliminates signaling through both human and murine toll-like receptor 2. J Immunol 2000;165(2):618–22.

89. Ogawa T, Asai Y, Hashimoto M, Takeuchi O, Kurita T, Yoshikai Y, et al. Cell activation by Porphyromonas gingivalis lipid A molecule through Toll-like receptor 4- and myeloid differentiation factor 88-dependent signaling pathway. Int Immunol 2002;14(11):1325–32.

90. Gao B, Tsan MF. Endotoxin contamination in recombinant human heat shock protein 70 (Hsp70) preparation is responsible for the induction of tumor necrosis factor alpha release by murine macrophages. J Biol Chem 2003 Jan 3; 278(1):174–9.

IV. REGULATION OF NATURAL IMMUNITY

Natural Immunity
Edited by L. Bertók and D.A. Chow
© 2005 Elsevier B.V. All rights reserved

Molecular Control of Leukocyte Trafficking Internal Regulatory Circuits of the Immune System: Leukocyte Circulation and Homing

STEVEN E. BOSINGER[1,2,*], KAROLINE A. HOISAWA[1,2,*], CHERYL M. CAMERON[2], MARK E. DEVRIES[1,2], JEFF C. COOMBS[1], MARK J. CAMERON[1] and DAVID J. KELVIN[1,2,3]

[1]*Division of Experimental Therapeutics, University Health Network, Toronto General Research Institute, Toronto General Hospital, 200 Elizabeth Street, Toronto, Ontario, Canada, M5G 2C4;* [2]*Department of Microbiology & Immunology, University of Western Ontario, London, Ontario, Canada, N6A 5C1;* [3]*Department of Immunology, University of Toronto, Toronto, Ontario, Canada, M5S 1A8*

ABSTRACT

Leukocyte migration is essential for their ability to react to inflammatory stimuli at various locations within the body. However, leukocyte movement is also crucial during non-inflammatory processes such as haematopoietic development and routine passage through secondary lymphoid organs, which is the key to effective antigen presentation. The importance of cell migration in the establishment and maintenance of an intact immune system has been demonstrated by numerous observations of immune defects in chemokine receptor deficient mice. This review describes the role of chemokines, their receptors and adhesion molecules in the regulation of the immune response during inflammatory and homeostatic conditions. In particular, we describe the molecular events regulating the recruitment of innate cells in response to infection and inflammation, leukocyte trafficking during developmental processes such as haematopoiesis and thymic maturation of T cells, and regulatory circuits that ensure immune surveillance and communication between innate and adaptive components of immunity.

1. INTRODUCTION

The ability of leukocytes to phagocytose, produce superoxide, and selectively lyse cells is the backbone of the mammalian innate immune system. Knockout studies have demonstrated that the movement of neutrophils, monocytes and natural killer cells to sites of insult is central to the maintenance of intact innate immunity, and can mean the difference between routine clearance of an offending organism or a fatal infection. Beyond inflammation, strategic leukocyte homing to immunologically distal sites such as the gut and central nervous system is necessary to main-

---

*SEB and KAH contributed equally to this work.

tain adequate innate immunity in these sites. Homing mechanisms also regulate homeostasis of innate cells; how these cells maintain adequate numbers in the periphery and are cleared during senescence. An important function of cellular innate immunity is to provide stimulating signals for the activation of adaptive immunity, and migratory mechanisms regulate the movement of innate cells to the appropriate location in secondary lymphoid cells.

During haematopoiesis in the bone marrow and T cell differentiation in the thymus, leukocyte homing is critical for the manoeuvring of leukocytes into specific compartments for maturation. Furthermore, effective immune surveillance by T and B lymphocytes requires a constant cycle of migration between the primary and secondary lymphoid tissues, which allows for effective antigen presentation and initiation of adaptive immune responses.

Primarily, two families of molecules, chemokines plus their cognate receptors, and adhesion molecules regulate leukocyte migration. Chemokine gradients dictate the direction in which a cell will migrate and signal actin rearrangements within the cell, while adhesion molecules establish the cell-to-cell and cell-to-matrix interactions necessary for this movement.

The importance of these molecules is underscored by the observation that homozygous deletion of the chemokine CXCL12/SDF-1 in mice results in a lethal phenotype with defects in haematopoietic and cerebellar development [1,2]. This review will detail the current understanding of the role of chemokines and adhesion molecules in leukocyte homing and trafficking.

1.1. Chemokines and chemokine receptors

Chemokines are a subfamily of cytokines with chemotactic properties. While capable of acting on a variety of cell types including fibroblasts, endothelial cells, and smooth muscle cells, chemokines are best known for their ability to induce leukocyte chemotaxis. Chemokines are classified based on the positioning of conserved cysteine residues [3–5]. The CC, CXC and CX_3C families contain a set of four conserved cysteines in their amino-terminal regions and are distinguished by the absence (CC) or the presence of one (CXC) or three (CX_3C) intervening amino acids between the first two cysteines. The C family of chemokines (XC) contains only two conserved cysteines that correspond to the second and fourth cysteines of the other families [3]. Chemokines induce migration upon binding to their specific receptors. Chemokine receptors belong to the rhodopsin-like superfamily of seven transmembrane-spanning G protein-coupled receptors. The receptors themselves are classified based upon ligand specificity rather than amino acid similarity. Certain receptors are promiscuous, binding multiple chemokines and likewise certain chemokines can bind multiple receptors.

Chemokines and their receptors can be roughly divided based on their functionality. The receptors CXCR1, CXCR2, CXCR3, CCR1, CCR2, CCR3, CCR5, and CCR6 are typically associated with the inflammatory response, whereas the receptors CXCR4, CXCR5, CCR4, CCR7, CCR9, and CCR10 are regarded as homeostatic receptors [6]. In general, chemokines involved in leukocyte homing and trafficking bind only a single chemokine receptor.

1.2 Adhesion molecules

Adhesion molecules are proteins that regulate cell-to-cell and cell-to-matrix interactions. The binding of adhesion molecules allows cells to move along a substratum or to maintain contact with a target cell. Adhesion molecules can be divided into four families: selectins, integrins, vascular addressins, and immunoglobulins. The selectin and integrin subfamilies play the largest role in homeostatic immunity, particularly in T cell homing. Selectins are expressed both on leukocytes (CD62L/L-selectin) and on the endothelium (P- and E-selectin). Selectins share a core protein structure, but possess different extracellular lectin domains that determine specificity. L-selectin, for example, binds the sulphated sialyl Lewis^x sugar of the mucin-like vascular addressins common to the endothelium. Selectins provide the initial contact between leukocytes and vascular endothelium needed for leukocyte homing into tissues. This weak interaction participates in leukocyte rolling and acts in concert with integrins, which provide stronger adhesions capable of facilitating cell arrest and extravasation.

Integrins are heterodimeric proteins composed of α and β chains. The heterodimers are not specific, so that a particular β chain may associate with several different α chains and vice versa. Classification of the composite integrin is based on the β chain. Nearly all leukocytes express β2 integrins on their surface, however, T cells also express β1 integrins. These β1 integrins are termed very late activation antigens (VLAs) because they are only expressed late in the maturation process. Integrin binding partners also vary substantially. The integrin lymphocyte function-associated antigen (LFA)-1 is expressed on T-cells and binds to three members of the immunoglobulin superfamily: intercellular adhesion molecules (ICAM)-1,-2 and -3. The integrin vascular cell adhesion molecule (VCAM)-1, on the other hand, is expressed on activated endothelium and binds the T-cell VLA-4 integrin. The interaction between VCAM-1 and VLA-4 on lymphocytes provides a much stronger adhesion than selectins and allows for firm adhesion and arrest on the endothelium. Integrins and chemokines act in concert to regulate leukocyte homing: surface expression of integrins can be induced by signal transduction events initiated by chemokine receptor activation; conversely, cross-linking of integrins can stimulate chemokine production capable of acting in an autocrine fashion. For a comprehensive review of adhesion molecules in lymphocyte homing see Fabbri et al. [7].

2. MECHANISMS OF NEUTROPHIL HOMING

2.1. Introduction

Human polymorphonuclear neutrophils (PMNs) are the most numerous of the circulating phagocytes, composing 40–65% of the white blood cells [8]. Its phylogeny vastly predates lymphocytes, and as such PMNs represent an important arm of innate immunity. PMNs are the earliest leukocytes to arrive at a site of infection and function primarily to provide a rapid defence against invading pathogens and clearance of inflammatory debris [8]. In response to a diverse array of pro-inflammatory stimuli including cytokines, chemoattractants, opsonins and highly conserved bacterial structures, PMNs activate two central antimicrobial effector mechanisms: oxidative respiratory burst and mobilization of cytotoxic granules [9]. The respiratory burst mechanism consists of the formation of a multi-subunit NADPH oxidase complex in phagosomal membranes and the plasmalemma of the neutrophil, which exerts its antibiotic activity by the production of highly reactive superoxides [10]. Granules are intracellular vesicles containing primarily bactericidal and degradative enzymes [11,12]. Upon neutrophil activation, granules are mobilized and migrate from deep within the cytoplasm to fuse with phagosomes and the plasma membrane, releasing their components to the extracellular space and phagosomal lumen [11–13].

2.2. Regulation of neutrophil chemotaxis during inflammation

2.2.1. *Adhesion molecules in neutrophil transendothelial migration*

PMNs are segregated into two compartments: a mature subset circulating throughout the peripheral blood and an immature pool within the bone marrow. Because of their central role in acute inflammation, the mechanisms regulating neutrophil migration and effector function have been intensely studied. Migration of PMNs is regulated by three groups of surface molecules: adhesion molecules, receptors for pro-inflammatory cytokines/stimuli, and chemoattractant receptors [14].

Current models of the process by which leukocytes cross the endothelial cell wall and exit the circulation into inflamed tissue are separated into discrete steps, each governed by distinct molecular mechanisms. Monocytes, lymphocytes and granulocytes all utilize a similar process to emigrate from the peripheral blood, frequently utilizing related molecules at each stage. Upon encounter with a chemotactic stimulus, the initial stage in leukocyte migration is margination, whereby flowing cells "capture" the endothelial wall and commence "rolling" along the vessel wall [4]. PMNs utilize selectins for both capture and rolling. L-selectin is constitutively expressed on the surface of PMNs [15]. L-selectin on the surface of lymphocytes binds to endothelial CD34 [16]; the endothelial binding partner for L-selectin on PMNs is poorly characterized, but known to be a member of a family of sialomucin oligosaccharides [17]. Capture and rolling of PMNs has been demonstrated under non-inflammatory conditions, suggesting constitutive expression of an L-selectin endothelial ligand [18]. However, endothelial ligands for PMN L-selectin can also be induced by treatment with LPS and pro-inflammatory cytokines [19]. P-selectin and E-selectin regulate PMN capture by endothelial cells (ECs). P-selectin protein is stored within Weibel-Palade bodies of endothelial cells: stimulation by cytokines, complement components or superoxide products can induce their surface expression [20]. P-selectin glycoprotein ligand-1 (PSGL-1) is constitutively expressed on PMNs and likely contributes to the rolling process to re-enforce the more transient L-selectin mediated interactions [14,21]. E-selectin appears much later (4–6 h) on the endothelial surface, as it is transcribed *de novo* after stimulation with pro-inflammatory cytokines [22,23]. No definite PMN ligand for P-selectin has been described, but it is believed to belong to the same family of proteins as the PMN ligand for L-selectin [24]. Because of its late onset of surface presentation, E-selectin is believed to maintain rolling after P-selectin has been downregulated.

The second stage of leukocyte emigration across the endothelial barrier, "firm adhesion", is mediated by establishing associations with the endothelial wall that are longer lived than those mediated by selectins. This second step is mediated by integrins expressed on leukocytes and their cognate binding to endothelial-expressed ICAMs. PMN-endothelium are binding is predominately regulated by the β_2 integrin Mac-1 ($\alpha_M\beta_2$, CD11b/CD18), but is also mediated to a lesser degree by LFA-1 ($\alpha_L\beta_2$, CD11a/CD18) and p150, 95 ($\alpha_X\beta_2$, CD11c/CD18) [20,25]. Mac-1 is stored as a presynthesized protein within the membranes of secondary/specific and tertiary/gelatinase granules and secretory vesicles, and can be rapidly transported to the surface when cells are exposed to various secretagogues [12]. Inflammatory stimuli such as lipopolysaccharide (LPS) and pro-inflammatory cytokines are not classical stimuli of degranulation in that they are incapable of mobilizing the large, deeply embedded azurophil or specific granules; however they have been demonstrated to induce surface presentation of Mac-1 by inducing the release of the smaller secretory vesicles [12]. Upregulation of surface Mac-1, however, is not sufficient for activation of adhesion. Intracellular Mac-1 is unphosphorylated, but upon surface presentation, the CD18 subunit is phosphorylated [26]. Mac-1 activation can be stimulated by IL-8 treatment, selectin engagement and pro-inflammatory cytokine treatment [27,28]. The intracellular molecules regulating integrin activation are equally diverse: the small G protein Rho, cyohesin-1 and the actin-bundling protein L-plastin have all been implicated in integrin activation [27,29]. The ligand for Mac-1 is ICAM-1, expressed constitutively on endothelium, but with upregulation inducible by proinflammatory cytokines [7].

After establishing a strong association with the endothelial wall, leukocytes must pass between endothelial cells in a process termed "extravasation". This stage involves a receptor switch, as selectins are downregulated and a protein of the immunoglobulin family, platelet-endothelial cell adhesion molecule (PECAM-1) has been demonstrated to be vital to cell passage through endothelium [14]. PECAM-1 can form intercellular homodimers; thus, can act as its own ligand [30]. The role of PECAM-1 was most definitively demonstrated in studies involving neutralising anti-PECAM-1 antibodies; PMN extravasation within *in vitro* [31] and animal models [32] was inhibited, while cell adhesion was unaffected.

Extravascular passage of leukocytes, or transmigration, within the underlying tissues involves adhesion to both extracellular matrix and cell surfaces. Gelatinase granules within PMNs are released readily in response to secretagogues; the release of gelatinase B, a potent collagenase, has been postulated to facilitate neutrophil movement through the extracellular matrix [12]. The ability of protease inhibitors to reduce PMN chemotaxis *in vitro* has strengthened this hypothesis [33]. Counter to this model are observations that mice genetically deficient in gelatinase B do not show any abnormalities in PMN migration to lungs, skin or peritoneum [34].

The mechanisms by which PMNs adhere to resident cells as they navigate the subendothelial space has some redundancy with those used in the vascular lumen: ICAM-1 surface expression can be detected on parenchymal tissues [35], as well, antibodies against PECAM-1 are able to inhibit PMN movement across the basement membrane [36]. Activated PMNs express the β_1 integrins very late antigen 4 (VLA-4, $\alpha_4\beta_1$), VLA-5 ($\alpha_5\beta_1$), VLA-6 ($\alpha_6\beta_1$) and VLA-9 ($\alpha_9\beta_1$), all of which have been demonstrated to be required for PMN migration through lung and synovial barriers [37,38]. VLA-4 binds vascular VCAM-1 on endothelial cells *in vitro*; however, VLA-5 and 6 bind fibronectin and laminin, respectively [14]. VLA-9 is the most abundant β_1 integrin on PMNs, and is not expressed on monocytes or lymphocytes [38]. VLA-9 is capable of binding fibronectin, VCAM-1 and tenascin, making it an attractive candidate for regulation of PMN transmigration.

As described above, transendothelial migration of PMNs utilizes many different surface molecules. However, the timing of expression and activation of these receptors at the appropriate stages is equally important. The intracellular signalling pathways regulating neutrophil adhesion to endothelium have been intensely studied (for a full review see Wang and Doerschuk [39]). At each stage, the activation and expression of adhesion molecules can be modulated by chemoattractants and cytokines, however, this activation/upregulation is also regulated, at least partially, by adhesion molecules themselves in a domino like fashion, whereby receptors active at one stage serve to activate those regulating the next. Activation of L-selectin stimulates β_2 integrin-dependent adhesion, and this adhesion can be blocked by tyrosine kinase, and protein kinase C inhibitors, suggesting a putative pathway between L-selectin and Mac-1. In turn, activation of β_2 integrins can stimulate the phosphorylation of PECAM-1. It is unlikely that the complete process of transendothelial migration could be regulated autonomously by endogenous adhesion molecules; however it is clear that this internal cross-talk is necessary.

2.2.2. *Chemokine regulation of neutrophil inflammation*

Several soluble cytokines are capable of influencing PMN migration and can be divided into two categories [14]. The first are pro-inflammatory cytokines, which can stimulate expression/activation of adhesion receptors but are incapable of inducing chemotaxis alone. TNF-α, IL-1 and IFN-γ are representative members of this group. The second group, chemoattractants, induce trafficking independent of other stimuli. PMNs migrate in response to several stimuli: platelet activating factor (PAF), complement protein C5a, leukotriene B_4 (LTB_4), formylated bacterial peptides (fMLP) and chemokines. Of these, the regulatory mechanisms for chemokine and chemokine regulation have the most developed models.

Human PMNs express the chemokine receptors CXCR1, CXCR2, CCR1, CCR2 and CXCR4 [4,40]. CXCL8/IL-8 was the first chemokine to be discovered, based on its ability to induce PMN migration after LPS treatment of neutrophils; as such it has been the most intensely studied chemokine regulating PMN function [41]. CXCL8/IL-8 binds to both CXCR1 and CXCR2. Despite their prevalence in regulating human PMN biology, no murine counterpart to either molecule has been characterized [4]. IL-8 expression has been detected by endothelium, epithelium, monocytes, platelets, and a variety of parenchymal cells. In addition to IL-8, human PMNs also respond to the CXCL7/chemokines neutrophil-activating peptide-2 (NAP-2), 3 forms of melanoma growth stimulating activity (GRO-α,β,γ)/CXCL1, CXCL2, CXCL3, and CXCL5/ epithelial cell-derived neutrophil-activating peptide-78 (ENA-78) [4].

PMNs in mice and rats respond to the chemokines CXCL1/KC (a homologue of human GRO-β and γ), CXCL2/macrophage inflammatory protein-2 (MIP-2), CXCL15/LIX (an ENA-78 homologue) [4] and two novel chemokines in rat termed cytokine induced neutrophil chemoattractants, CINC-2α and CINC-2β, have been described [42]. CXCL1/KC and CXCL2/MIP-2 have been demonstrated to regulate PMN migration in rat models of lung and intestinal inflammation [43,44].

Granulocytes differ from lymphocytes in that the molecular signals for migration are closely linked to activation of their effector function; in PMNs, the same ligand can initiate migration, but can also stimulate degranulation and superoxide production. At low concentrations, (1 nM) IL-8 is capable of inducing PMN migration through classical heterotrimer signalling pathways [45]. At higher concentrations of IL-8, CXCR1 is desensitized to ligand, and rendered incapable of signalling along this pathway. Receptors are subsequently phosphorylated on serine residues within their cytoplasmic tails by G-protein coupled receptor kinases (GRKs), providing a signal for the association of the adapter molecule β-arrestin, which serves to internalize the CXCR1 from the membrane [45]. This model of receptor desensitization has been demonstrated for CCR5, CXCR1, CXCR4 and CCR2B [45–48]. After internalization, β-arrestin associated with CXCR1 has been demonstrated to bind to the activated form of the Src tyrosine-kinase Hck [49] and this complex could be detected on azurophil granules. Further, RBL-2H3 cells, a cell line model of PMNs, cotransfected with CXCR1 and dominant negative molecules of β-arrestin, demonstrated inhibited granule release in response to IL-8 stimulation. Thus, β-arrestin mediated signalling may represent a mechanism by which PMNs can migrate in response to lower ligand concentrations that might be present at sites distal from inflammation, and upon encounter with higher ligand concentrations that would be present at proximal locations, stop migration and switch to effector function.

3.3. Chemokine regulation of neutrophil homeostasis

Relative to lymphocytes, which have complex migratory pathways through the periphery, primary and secondary lymphoid organs, PMNs follow a simple route: development in the bone marrow, release to the periphery where they circulate until they are recruited into inflammatory sites. Bone marrow contains a large reserve of mature PMNs. Pro-inflammatory cytokines and chemoattractants in the blood can initiate rapid mobilization of this reserve compartment and increase the number of circulating PMNs [50]. Approximately 10^{11} PMNs are released into the blood per day [8]. Blood PMNs are short-lived ($t_{1/2}$ = 6 hr), thus a highly active homeostatic mechanism is required to maintain adequate PMN levels and clearance. At inflammatory sites, neutrophils have been demonstrated to undergo apoptosis and be phagocytosed by macrophages [51]. Circulating PMNs entering senescence have been postulated to undergo clearance by the liver, spleen and bone marrow. The expression of CXCR4 on PMNs has been debated, however conclusive evidence has demonstrated that PMNs maintain baseline levels of the receptor upon entry into the periphery, but that marked upregulation occurs as they age [40]. Using an *in vivo* bone marrow perfusion system, Martin et al demonstrated that the CXCR4 inhibitor, AMD-3100, could stimulate the migration of bone marrow resident PMNs into the circulation [40]. Further, *ex vivo* cultured PMNs drastically upregulated CXCR4. When re-introduced to mice either by IV or bone marrow perfusion, the cultured, $CXCR4^{high}$ PMNs were sequestered within the marrow at significantly higher numbers than freshly isolated $CXCR4^{low}$ PMNs.

3. MONOCYTE MIGRATION TO SITES OF INFLAMMATION

Monocytes play an important role in the immune network as one of the first lines of defence against inflammatory challenge. Monocytes develop in the bone marrow, enter the circulation, and subsequently enter tissues of the body where they differentiate into tissue macrophages and dendritic cells. Under inflammatory conditions, the number of monocytes leaving the circulation doubles that under homeostatic conditions [52]. CCL2/monocyte chemoattractant protein (MCP) -1 has been long known to mediate recruitment of monocytes into sites of inflammation. Lack of CCR2 expression in an experimental peritoneal inflammation model using a non-specific inflammatory stimulus, thioglycollate, results in an impaired recruitment of macrophages into the peritoneum [53]. In addition, CCR2 deficient mice are unable to clear infection by intracellular bacteria, *Listeria monocytogenes* [53]. Furthermore, macrophages play an important role in the development of protective cutaneous granulomas initiated by *Leishmania major* or *Mycobacterium leprae* [54]. Such early macrophage recruitment to sites of cutaneous granuloma formation has been shown to be mediated by MIP-1α/β chemokines released from neutrophils recruited by mast cell derived TNF-α [54].

Interestingly, CCL2/MCP-1 produced in inflamed skin is transported via lymph to the HEV of the draining lymph nodes, therefore mediating recruitment of monocytes into lymph nodes [55]. This suggests that chemokines have the potential to remotely control the immune network. CCL2/MCP-1 has also been implicated in macrophage trafficking to the central nervous system (CNS) under inflammatory conditions and in the pathogenesis of experimental autoimmune encephalomyelitis (EAE), where macrophages are thought to be the primary effector cells in mediating cellular pathology and tissue damage [56]. In particular, mice deficient in CCL2/MCP-1 or its cognate receptor CCR2, show resistance to EAE [57–59].

Other non-lymphoid tissues such as breast, kidney, skin and gut have been shown to express

CXCL14/BRAK, which selectively recruits circulating monocytes in homeostasis, as well as monocytes activated by prostaglandin E_2 (PGE_2). CXCL14/breast and kidney-expressed chemokine (BRAK), which is thought to be made constitutively by normal skin keratinocytes, dermal fibroblasts, as well as lamina propria cells [60]. Monocytes cultured with PGE_2 have been shown to gain chemotactic responsiveness to CXCL14/BRAK, while losing responsiveness to CCL2/MCP-1, CCL5/regulated upon activation, normal T cell expressed and secreted (RANTES), and CXCL12/stromal cell-derived factor (SDF) -1 [60]. The receptor for CXCL14/BRAK is yet unknown. The authors propose that once monocytes enter sites of inflammation, local secretion of PGE_2 polarizes monocytes to be responsive to high levels of CXCL14/BRAK.

Most recently, two functional subsets of monocytes with distinct migratory properties have been identified. Geissmann et al. [61] have identified a $CX_3CR1^{hi}CCR2^{-}GR1^{-}$ subset of monocytes characterized by CX_3CR1-dependent recruitment to non-inflamed tissues such as spleen, lung, liver, and brain; as well as a short-lived $CX_3CR1^{low}CCR2^{+}GR1^{+}$ subset that is actively recruited to sites of inflammation in a model of intraperitoneal thioglycollate injection. However, Ancuta et al. [62] have shown that Fractalkine, but not MCP-1, plays an important role in transendothelial migration of a $CD16^{+}$ subtype of monocytes, proposed to be dendritic cell precursors, via CX_3CR1 under inflammatory challenge. Further evidence supports the role of Fractalkine in monocyte recruitment under inflammatory challenge. Fractalkine protein has been detected in atherosclerotic lesions and CXCR3 deficient mice have impaired macrophage recruitment to the vessel wall and decreased atherosclerotic lesion formation [63]. In addition to Fractalkine, earlier evidence showed that KC (Gro-α), the ligand for CXCR2, but not MCP-1, significantly induced monocyte arrest on early atherosclerotic endothelium [64].

In addition to the above mentioned chemokines/chemokine receptors, other chemokines/receptors have been implicated in the trafficking of monocyte dendritic cell precursors such as CXCR1, CXCR4 and CCR6 [65]. Expression of inflammatory chemokines receptors CCR2, CCR5, CCR6, CXCR1, and CXCR2 allows immature dendritic cells to respond to inflammatory chemokines made by non-haematopoietic cells such as keratinocytes in the skin [65]. These signals direct dendritic cells to enter lymph and travel to T –cell areas of draining lymph nodes. Furthermore, Pashenkov et al. [66] have implicated CXCR4, the receptor for SDF-1, in mediating trafficking of dendritic cells to cerebrospinal fluid by showing partial inhibition of dendritic cells trafficking by CXCR4 neutralizing antibodies.

Overall, monocytes and macrophages are recruited to sites of foreign or self-antigen by CCL2/MCP-1 through their expression of CCR2. However, other chemokines such as CXCL14/BRAK and Fractalkine also have been shown to recruit monocytic macrophage precursors during both homeostasis and inflammation. Furthermore, monocyte dendritic cell precursors have been shown to be recruited by a number of chemokines such as IL-8, SDF-1 and MIP-3α in addition to MCP-1 and MIP-1α/β.

4. CHEMOKINE REGULATION OF HOMING WITHIN NATURAL KILLER CELL MEDIATED IMMUNITY

Natural killer (NK) cells are lymphoid-lineage cells that regulate innate immunity, primarily against tumour cells or virus infected host cells. Phenotypically, NK cells are defined by their surface expression of CD56 and lack of CD3 [67]. Approximately 90% of human NK cells in the periphery exhibit a $CD56^{dim}CD16\ (Fc\gamma RIII)^{hi}$ phenotype, while the remainder are $CD56^{bright}CD16^{-/low}$ [68]. Functional studies based on this phenotypic dichotomy have indicated that $CD56^{dim}CD16^{hi}$ are more efficient at cytotoxic killing, while the $CD56^{bright}CD16^{-/low}$ subset is more apt to produce immunoregulatory cytokines [68,69]. It is important to note that although mice have NK cells that function in a capacity analogous to those in humans, a murine counterpart to CD56 has not been reported, therefore, studies defining the two subsets have been limited to *in vitro* human studies [69].

NK cells act in a crucial capacity in the defence against select cytopathic viruses and intracellular pathogens [70]. NK cells are potent producers of interferon (IFN)-γ in mice, and represent the earliest and largest source of IFN-γ in response to murine cytomegalovirus (MCMV) infection and inoculation with LPS [71]. Via CD16, NK cells are capable of recognizing IgG immune complexes. NK cells are also capable of modulating the effector activity of monocytes, neutrophils and T and B cells via their production of cytokines and chemokines [67].

The molecular basis by which the cytotoxic activity of NK cells is activated has recently begun to be elucidated. Unlike its lymphoid counterparts, T and B cells, NK cells do not have a dominant, antigen specific receptor complex, nor do they require prior immunization or expression of autologous MHC molecules on target cells [71]. Activation of NK cytotoxicity is subject to the balance of signals of several different inhibitory and activating receptors. Insufficient expression of self-MHC, as frequently occurs in tumour or virus-infected cells, can provide an activating signal for NK cytolysis [69]. NK cell activation via HLA recognition has been the best characterized mechanism; however, there are alternate routes: NKG2D, a recently characterized activating NKR, is specific for MICA, MICB or ULBP proteins, typically induced in response to cell stress [72]. For reviews of NKRs and their activation pathways see Moretta et al. [71] or Cooper et al. [69]. In adult humans, NK cell development occurs within the bone marrow (for a comprehensive review on NK cell development see Colucci et al. [73]). Within the periphery, NK cells have been observed in the blood, in all lymphoid tissues and to a lesser extent within the liver and spleen [73]. Evidence has demonstrated that NK cells can migrate between compartments during disease or in response to inflammatory conditions [74]. However, the mechanisms by which NK cells recirculate during homeostatic conditions have not been determined. Several classes of molecules have been demonstrated to regulate NK cell migration: the neurotransmitters substance P and norepinephrine are able to increase or decrease NK chemokinesis *in vitro*, respectively [75]. Recent work has also demonstrated that a family of heptahelical receptors specific for various phospholipids can also regulate NK trafficking [76]. The role of chemokines and their receptors, however, has been the most closely studied.

The cell surface repertoire of chemokine receptors on NK cells has been comprehensively studied. Because NK cells are a heterogeneous population and change their receptor profile after activation, in some cases data within the literature is conflicting. Resting NK cells appear to have expression of CCR7, CXCR3, CXCR4 and XCR1 [77–79]. The expression of CCR7, however, has been reported to be only on $CD56^{bright}CD16^{-/low}$ cells [77,78]. The expression of CCR1, CCR4, CXCR1, CXCR2 and CX_3CR1 has also been reported, however contradictory data exists [74,80]. The reported expression of CXCR3, CXCR4 and XCR1 is supported by the observations that resting NK cells can migrate in response to CXCL10/IP-10, CXCL11/I-TAC or CXCL12/SDF-1 (CXCR3 and CXCR4 ligands respectively) [77–81]. Although CXCR1 and CXCR2 expression has been reported by several groups, data is also contradictory on the ability of resting cells to traffic in response to CXCL1 or CXCL8. Treatment of resting NK cells with the chemokines CCL2/MCP-1 (CCR2 and CCR4), CCL3/MIP-1α (CCR1, CCR4, CCR5), CCL4/MIP-1β (CCR5), CCL5/RANTES (CCR1, CCR2, CCR4, CCR5), CCL7/MCP-3 (CCR1) and CCL8/MCP-2 (CCR1, CCR2, CCR3) has been able to elicit chemotaxis, providing support for the expression of CCR1, and, paradoxically, for the presence of CCR5 on resting cells

[77,82–84]. In response to IL-2 or IL-15, activated NK cells have been demonstrated to upregulate expression of CCR2, CCR4, CCR5 and CXCR1. Some of the disagreement in the literature surrounding the expression of these receptors on resting cells has been proposed to be due to aberrant *in vitro* activation.

The role of chemokine controlled migration within innate NK cell immunity has been elegantly demonstrated using *in vivo* models. Mice infected with MCMV exhibit early activation of NK cells with a concurrent induction of IFN-γ production [85]. When challenged with MCMV, mice deficient in CCL3/MIP-1α demonstrate marked decreases in the NK cell trafficking to the liver and localized liver production of IFN-γ. CCL3/MIP-1$\alpha^{-/-}$ mice typically succumb to MCMV infection, in contrast to wild-type mice that can clear the virus. Treatment of wild-type mice with anti-CCL3/MIP-1α antibodies typically diminishes the accumulation of NK cells in the liver. IFN-γ levels in the serum are equivalent between knock-out and wild type mice, implying that it is the localized expression provided by the NK cells that is the controlling factor.

A second model takes advantage of the differential ability of strains with polarized Th1/Th2 responses to combat infection by the obligate intracellular pathogen *Leishmania major*. C57BL/6 mice develop a Th1 response and efficiently combat *L. major* infection, whereas the Balb/c strain is polarized to a Th2 response and typically succumb [86–88]. NK cells within draining lymph nodes in Balb/c mice demonstrate lower cytotoxic responses and level of activation compared to C57BL/6 mice [86]. Expression of XCL1/lymphotactin α, CCL2/MCP-1 and CXCL10/interferon-gamma-inducible protein-10 (IP-10) within draining lymph nodes could be detected within resistant mice during acute infection, but was absent in susceptible mice [86]. Injection of CXCL10/IP-10 at the site of infection improved NK cell cytotoxicity within the lymph nodes of Balb/c mice, however, no difference in the numbers of NK cells were detected between strains [86]. Therefore, it is unclear whether CXCL10/IP-10 is acting to augment NK migration within the lymph node architecture, or provide a stimulatory signal directly.

Several models of tumourigenesis have also demonstrated the role of chemokines in regulating NK mediated immunity. Transgene expression of CCL19/MIP-3β or CCL7/MCP-3 in murine breast or lung tumour-inducing cell lines, respectively, was able to reduce tumour survival *in vivo* and was correlated with recruitment of NK cells [89,90]. Mice deficient in CCR1 have defective recruitment of NK cells to granulomatous lesions and demonstrated decreased IFN-γ production [91].

The data from *in vivo* models of infectious disease and cancer provide convincing evidence that the migration of NK cells is crucial to their function. Based on the literature to date, it remains a reasonable hypothesis that the primary function of the inflammatory chemokine receptors on NK cells is to enable recruitment to primary sites of infection/tumourigenesis. Mature NK cells also express the homeostatic receptors CXCR4 and CCR7. These receptors may allow NK cells to localize to specific regions within secondary lymphoid organs to act as regulatory cells. Alternatively, CXCR4 expression has also been proposed to regulate the ability of NK cells to traffic to the bone marrow. Compared to the other major leukocyte subsets, the models describing chemokine regulation of NK cell migration are rather undeveloped. Further work in this burgeoning field will undoubtedly uncover novel aspects of NK cell biology and expand our understanding of their role in immunity as a whole.

5. HEMATOPOIETIC PROGENITOR TRAFFICKING WITHIN THE BONE MARROW

During embryonic development, blood forming stem cells travel from the yolk sac and the aorta gonad mesonephros region into the fetal liver and finally into the fetal bone marrow. As haematopoietic stem cells divide, some of the daughter cells remain as stem cells and continue dividing, while others become committed to specific cell lineages and lose their ability to self renew. Haematopoietic stem cells are constantly leaving and re-entering the bone marrow to replace cells lost through death or differentiation and ensuring that all of their corresponding bone marrow compartments are occupied [92]. Haematopoiesis itself is restricted to the extravascular compartments of the bone marrow, which are separated by a single layer of endothelial cells. Committed cells migrate from the haematopoietic stem cell compartments across this bone marrow endothelium into the extravascular compartments in response to homing signals. These new compartments provide a microenvironment designed to facilitate growth and differentiation of lymphoid and myeloid lineages. Stromal cells within these compartments secrete soluble mediators that trigger maturation of these committed cells [93].

Chemokines play a critical role in the haematopoietic process, both in homing of committed cells into the extravascular compartments, as well as serving as soluble mediators inducing differentiation. CXCL12/SDF-1 is one of the mediators produced by stromal cells and is essential for both myelopoiesis and B cell lymphopoiesis. In fact, deletion of this gene, or its corresponding receptor CXCR4, leads to a lethal phenotype with arrested B cell lymphopoiesis in the bone marrow, although myeloid development in the fetal liver is normal [1,94]. Ma et al. [93] reported that CXCR4 was required for the retention and subsequent maturation of both B lymphocytes and granulocytic precursors within the supportive fetal liver and bone marrow microenvironments. They suggested that in the absence of CXCR4, B cell and myeloid precursors fail to localize properly in association with stromal cells and exit the bone marrow before fully differentiating. This is supported by the fact that $CD34^+$ progenitor cells leaving the bone marrow exhibit reduced levels of CXCR4 expression in comparison to marrow-resident $CD34^+$ cells [95]. Additionally, Hattori et al. [96] reported that plasma elevation of CXCL12/SDF-1 induced mobilization of progenitor cells, precursor cells, and haematopoietic stem cells with repopulating capacity, further underscoring the role CXCL12/CXCR4 interactions play in haematopoiesis and homing within the bone marrow.

Adhesion molecules also play an important role in progenitor trafficking to the bone marrow. The integrins VCAM-1 and ICAM-1 are expressed by bone marrow stromal cells and endothelial cells [97]. Their corresponding receptors VLA-4 and LFA-1 are expressed in high levels on progenitor cells in the bone marrow but are downregulated on circulating progenitor cells in patients who receive granulocyte colony-stimulating factor after cytotoxic chemotherapy [98]. It is likely that these adhesion molecules are the ultimate effectors of CXCR4-induced homing and positioning within the bone marrow [3,99]. Similarly, stem cell factor is expressed as a membrane bound molecule on bone marrow stromal and endothelial cells, while its ligand, c-kit, is expressed at high levels in bone marrow haematopoietic progenitor cells but is subsequently downregulated in circulating progenitor cells, suggesting a similar role in cell mobilization and differentiation [100].

In summary, these signals act collectively to ensure localization of haematopoietic progenitor cells and stromal cells within extravascular bone marrow compartments. Only after sufficient maturation are these molecules downregulated and progenitor cells allowed to escape into the circulation.

6. THYMOCYTE TRAFFICKING

6.1. Entry into the thymus and trafficking to the subcapsule

The process by which undifferentiated lymphocyte precursors progress into fully mature self-tolerant T lymphocytes requires several changes in receptor expression and involves detailed movements through regions of the thymus [101–104]. A layer of connective tissue called the thymic capsule surrounds the thymus and extends into septa that divide the thymus into separate lobules. Lining the connective tissue is a layer of subcapsular epithelium that acts as a barrier to control cell movement to and from the thymus. A subset of haematopoietic progenitor cells having escaped from bone marrow, enter the thymus cortex from vessels within the septa and migrate to the subcapsular region. The exact entry point into the thymus has yet to be characterized. The earliest cells immigrating into the thymus have been localized to areas within the vasculature of the cortex, cortical-medullary junction (CMJ), and medulla [105]. Since an impermeable endothelial layer surrounds blood vessels in the cortex, some propose that progenitor cells enter the thymus into the medullary region and traverse "upstream" to the outer cortex/subcapsule [103]. Cells entering the subcapsular region are $CD4^-CD8^-$ double-negative (DN) progenitor cells. During their maturation, progenitor cells commit fully to the T lymphocyte lineage, where rearrangement of their TCR genes is supported by thymic stromal cell expression of IL-7 and c-kit [106,107]. The abundant expression of thymic CXCL12 /SDF-1 suggested CXCR4 as a candidate for thymocyte entry; however, several lines of evidence indicate the contrary: treatment of $CD34^+$ T cell precursors with anti-CXCR4 antibodies had no effect on the colonization of fetal thymic organ cultures [108], and CXCR4 is not expressed on $CD34^+$ progenitor cells within peripheral blood [95]. Although CXCR4 is not expressed on DN early immigrant cells, it is later upregulated during their maturation to $CD4^+CD8^+$ double-positive (DP) cells [101,109].

6.2. Transition from double-negative to double-positive cells

There are four distinct stages of maturation between DN cells and $CD4^+CD8^+$ DP cells. These stages are marked by the expression of the CD44 and CD25 cell surface molecules. Through these stages, cells progress from an early $CD44^+CD25^-$ phenotype to $CD44^+CD25^+$, $CD44^-CD25^+$, and finally back to a $CD44^-CD25^-$ profile. Upregulation of CD4 and CD8 expression coincides with the final acquisition of the $CD44^-CD25^-$ profile [103]. CXCR4 has been implicated in regulating the progression of cells to the DP state. Murine $CD44^+CD25^-$ early DN cells have been reported to migrate weakly in response to CXCL12/SDF-1, with the response increasing as the cells progress to $CD44^-CD25^-$ [110]. Similarly, Suzuki et al. [25] reported that $CD44^+CD25^-$ cells have low expression of CXCR4 that is upregulated upon progression to the more mature $CD44^+CD25^+$ phenotype but downregulated in CD4 or CD8 single-positive (SP) cells.

The chemokine receptor CCR9 and its ligand CCL25/thymus-expressed chemokine (TECK) have also been implicated in T lymphocyte development. CCL25/TECK induces migration in day 14 fetal thymocytes [111] and bone marrow cells from $CCR9^{-/-}$ mice were less efficient than wild-type animals at repopulating the thymi of irradiated $Rag\text{-}1^{-/-}$ mice [112]. While DN cells are $CCR9^-$, CCR9 expression is induced in the transition to DP cells and is maintained during the maturation to SP cells [103,113]. Similarly, expression of CCL25/TECK is strongest in the cortical epithelial cells that drive positive selection by selecting for thymocytes with TCRs capable of binding self-MHC [114].

6.3. Positive and Negative selection

During their maturation into DP cells, thymocytes undergo positive selection whereby cells with TCRs incapable of recognizing self-MHC are deleted [115]. Positively selected thymocytes migrate from the cortex to the CMJ where they interact with thymic antigen presenting cells (APCs) and undergo negative selection to eliminate thymocytes reactive with self MHC/peptide complexes on APCs [101]. Cell surface expression of CD69 is indicative of DP cells receiving a TCR signal [103]. Several observations support a role for the chemokine receptor CCR4 in regulating the migration of positively selected $CD4^+CD8^+$ DP thymocytes through the negative selection process. The transition from $CD69^-$ to $CD69^+$ cells coincides with responsiveness to the CCR4 ligand CCL22/MDC, as well as loss of responsiveness to CXCR4 [116,117]. This responsiveness is maintained as thymocytes progress through negative selection and first become $CD4^+$ SP or $CD8^+$ SP cells, but is lost as they progress to a more mature phenotype [116]. Expression of CCL22/macrophage-derived chemokine (MDC) by thymic epithelial cells and Hassal's corpuscles within the medulla suggests it recruits DP cells from the cortex into the medulla and it may play a role in negative selection [118]. CCL17/thymus and activation-regulated chemokine (TARC), another CCR4 and CCR8 ligand, is expressed by the thymic dendritic cells—which play a critical role in negative selection [119]. The role of other chemokine receptors and their ligands is less clear. CCL11/eotaxin and its receptor CCR3 may have a role in thymocyte negative selection since CCL11/eotaxin induces chemotaxis of DP and SP cells and CCR3 is expressed on thymic $CD8^+$ SP cells [120,121]. Similarly, the chemokines CCL18/PARC, CCL20/LARC, CXCL10/IP-10, CXCL11/I-TAC, CXCL9/MIG and their receptors CCR6 and CXCR3 are all expressed in the thymus but have not had their roles defined [103].

6.4. Exit from the thymus

Thymocytes which survive negative selection migrate deeper into the medulla where they reside for approximately 14 days and differentiate into mature $CD4^+$ or $CD8^+$ T cells before emigrating into the periphery [103]. During this maturation, SP cells progress from a $CD69^+$CD62L/L-selectin^{lo} phenotype to a $CD69^-$CD62L/L-selectin^{hi} phenotype [103]. Differentiation into $CD69^-$CD62L/L-selectin^{hi} cells is accompanied by a loss of responsiveness to the chemokine CCL25/TECK in $CD4^+$ cells, but not $CD8^+$ cells [122]. The acquisition of a SP phenotype is also accompanied by expression of the chemokine receptor CCR7 [101,103,116]. Both CCR7 ligands CCL19/ELC and CCL21/SLC are expressed in the thymus with CCL19/ELC being localized to medullary stromal cells [101,123]. Mature T lymphocytes are then thought to exit the thymus via draining lymphatics and/or medullary vessels [103].

The role of chemokines in T lymphocytes exiting the thymus has been difficult to establish conclusively. Treatment with pertussis toxin – which inhibits chemokine receptor signalling – abrogates thymic emigration [124]. When coupled with the expression of CCL21/SLC in the draining vessels, this led to the proposition that CCR7 mediates thymic emigration [123]. However, $CCR7^{-/-}$ mice exhibit no apparent defect in thymocyte development and export, as the amount of peripheral $CD4^+$ T cells increases by 6-fold [125]. In addition to a CCR7-mediated migration along a CCL21/SLC gradient, David Scadden's group proposed that T lymphocytes might in fact be moving along a decreased gradient of other chemotactic molecules [126]. This novel process, termed chemofugetaxis, has been demonstrated in an *in vitro* model of thymic emigration using mature SP cells and was blocked using antibodies to CXCL12/SDF-1. While this has yet to be confirmed *in vivo*, it suggests a possible model for not only thymic emigration, but lymphocyte movement out of secondary lymphoid tissues as well.

In summary, chemokines and chemokine receptors have definable roles in all stages of T cell development. One must be curious, however, about the lack of an obvious defect in T cell development within mice lacking CXCR4, CCR4, CCR7, or CCR9 receptors. This may be due to overlapping function and studies with multiple receptor knockouts must be pursued to confirm this hypothesis.

7. LEUKOCYTE HOMING WITHIN SECONDARY LYMPHOID ORGANS

Acquired immunity is perhaps the most significant evolutionary advancement of the vertebrate immune system. This system is dependent on the ability of circulating lymphocytes to migrate from the periphery to secondary lymphoid organs such as the lymph nodes, Peyer's patches, and spleen [127,128]. Constant circulation of lymphocytes through the lymphoid and circulatory systems provides an effective means to present captured foreign antigen to the lymphocyte repertoire. Homeostatic chemokines are largely responsible for regulating this aspect of acquired immunity.

During inflammation, chemokine release at the area of insult rapidly recruits tissue resident dendritic cells expressing CCR1, CCR5, CCR6, and CXCR1 chemokine receptors [127]. After antigen capture and dendritic cell stimulation, the profile of expressed chemokine receptors changes dramatically. The inflammatory receptors are downregulated and the homeostatic receptors CCR7, CXCR4, and CCR4 are upregulated [129]. This serves both to remove the chemotactic pressure to remain in the area of inflammation as well as to target the antigen-loaded dendritic cells to the draining lymph nodes.

Homing of both dendritic cells and T cells to secondary lymph nodes appears to be largely dependent on the CCR7 chemokine receptor. Mice possessing the paucity of lymph node T cells (*plt*) mutation—where T cell and dendritic cell migration to lymph nodes and splenic white pulps is impaired—show a defect in the expression of CCL21/SLC, the ligand of CCR7 [130]. In addition, CCR7 deficient mice exhibit severe defects in dendritic cell and T cell trafficking to lymph nodes and node microarchitecture. These mice also fail to mount primary T cell responses [125]. CCR7 has been identified as regulating the migration of $CD4^+$ Th1 cells to the T cell zone of secondary lymphoid organs [131]. Conversely, gene transfer of CCR7 to $CD4^+$ Th2 cells changed their localization from the splenic B cell zone to the periarteriolar lymphoid sheath (PALS) and severely impaired the B cell response to antigen [131]. Forster et al. [125] also demonstrated that non-primed $CCR7^{-/-}$ show inappropriate B cell stimulation, due to altered migration of T and B cells to PALS and B cell follicles, and that immunized $CCR7^{-/-}$ mice display delayed primary IgG isotype switching.

B cell trafficking is also highly dependent on chemokine expression. The means by which CXCL13/BLC and CXCR5 influence B cell function have been extensively studied. Mice deficient in CXCR5 or its ligand CXCL13/BLC both exhibit a severe developmental phenotype lacking most lymph nodes and Peyer's patches [132,133]. Furthermore, $CXCL13^{-/-}$ mice lack conventional B cell follicles in the lymph nodes and spleen and have defects in immigration of follicular dendritic cells [132]. $CXCR4^{-/-}$ B cells are capable of trafficking to lymphoid compartments, but ligand-induced desensitization of CXCR4 and CCR7 strongly inhibits B cell homing [134].

In summary, chemokines and their receptors are critical for trafficking of leukocytes for the process of antigen gathering. Furthermore, they contribute substantially to the organization of secondary lymphoid tissues, helping to dictate the various compartments within them.

8. LEUKOCYTE HOMING TO THE GASTROINTESTINAL SYSTEM

Associated with the gut are several unique lymphoid tissues including inductive sites (Peyer's patches and mesenteric lymph nodes) where lymphocytes undergo activation and effector sites (lamina propria of the intestinal villi) where lymphocytes carry out effector functions [135]. Peyer's patches are formed by aggregates of lymphoid follicles covered with M cells and are scattered throughout the small intestine. M cells trap, concentrate, and present antigens to lymphocytes in the adjoining B and T cell follicles. Naïve lymphocytes enter the Peyer's patches through high endothelial venules (HEV) where they undergo activation and differentiation to enteric antigens. These activated lymphocytes then traffic to mesenteric lymph nodes to undergo final maturation. Finally, activated lymphocytes enter the effector sites in the intestinal epithelial tissue and reside either between the epithelial cells or below epithelial cells in the core of the intestinal villi (lamina propria). These effector or memory cells either settle within the epithelium or lamina propria or emigrate via local collecting mesenteric lymph nodes before returning to the circulation. The lymphocytes found within the epithelium, called intraepithelial lymphocytes, are almost exclusively $CD8^+$ T cells, whereas lymphocytes in the lamina propria are predominantly IgA-antibody secreting B cells and $CD4^+CD45RO^+$ memory T cells [136]. These latter memory T cells display a much lower proliferative response to antigens than do circulating cells [136,137]. This is an evolutionary adaptation to the higher concentration of antigen within the mucosal environment. By requiring a higher activation threshold for T cells, potentially unnecessary and detrimental responses are avoided.

The intraepithelial cells on the other hand are mostly $CD8\alpha\alpha^+$ and have a $TCR\gamma\delta$ phenotype in comparison to the $TCR\alpha\beta$ phenotype of the memory T cells [138]. These $CD8\alpha\alpha^+TCR\gamma\delta$ T cells are thought to develop locally from cryptopatch precursor cells [138]. The intraepithelial lymphocyte compartment of the gut is highly enriched in $\gamma\delta$ T cells, yet their role in gastrointestinal immunity is not fully understood [139]. $\gamma\delta$ T cells are unique in that they are capable of different effector functions, including inflammatory cytokine production, cytolytic potential, as well as repair of epithelial tissue [139].

Chemokine mediated lymphocyte trafficking to Peyer's patches is similar to that of ordinary lymph nodes. CCR7, in conjunction with CXCR4, guides T cells and naïve B lymphocytes to Peyer's patches [134]. T cells lacking CCR7 show a defect in entering Peyer's patches [125]. Furthermore, T cells preferentially arrest in areas of the HEV where CCL21/SLC expression is high [140]. Expression of CCL19/ ELC/MIP-3β has also been reported in Peyer's patches [141]. As expected, T and B cells show selectivity as to which areas of the Peyer's patches vasculature they adhere. T cells have been shown to accumulate in the interfollicular HEV, while B cells accumulate in or near HEV follicles. This ensures appropriate segregation of B and T lymphocytes into the correct lymphoid compartments [140]. This difference is likely due to CXCR5 expression on B lymphocytes, since its ligand, CXCL13/BLC/BCA-1, is found selectively in Peyer's patches follicular HEV [134]. Together, this demonstrates that CCR7, CXCR4, and CXCR5 play an important role in trafficking of T and B cells into Peyer's patches.

Chemokine receptors are also important in directing migration of cells into the lamina propria. CCR9 is expressed on $CD4^+$ and $CD8^+$ memory T cells bearing the integrin $\alpha_4\beta_7$ in the lamina propria and within the intestinal epithelium of normal individuals [142]. Lymphocytes from all other normal and inflamed tissues have been shown to be $CCR9^-$ [143]. Indeed, CCL25/TECK, the ligand for CCR9, induces chemotactic function within lymphocytes from the small intestine, but not the colon. Coupled with the observation that mesenteric lymph nodes that drain the small intestine contain a higher percentage of $CCR9^+$ lymphocytes than do mesenteric lymph nodes draining the colon [144]. This suggests that CCR9 expression is uniquely induced in naïve T lymphocytes within the mucosal environment of the small intestine. Consistent with this hypothesis, CCL25/TECK is expressed in the small intestine by endothelial cells, epithelial cells, and a small subset of intestinal crypt cells within the lamina propria, but is not expressed in the colon, skin, lung or salivary glands [143,144]. Most recently, it was shown that $CD8^+$ cells activated in mesenteric lymph nodes maintained functional expression of CCR9, whereas CCR9 was rapidly downregulated on $CD8^+$ cells activated in the peripheral lymph nodes [145]. Furthermore, Svensson et al. [145] demonstrated that these $CCR9^+CD8^+$ cells preferentially migrate to the small intestinal mucosa and that *in vivo* neutralization of CCL25/TECK impaired the migration of these cells to small intestinal epithelium. Unfortunately, the mechanism of $\gamma\delta$ T cell recruitment to the intraepithelial lymphocyte compartment is still poorly understood. CCR9 deficient animals have been shown to have a significant decrease of intraepithelial $TCR\gamma\delta^+CD8^+$ T cells in the in the gut, although the number of $TCR\alpha\beta^+CD8^+$ or $TCR\alpha\beta^+CD4^+$ T cells remained unaltered [146]. This suggests that CCR9 mediates recruitment of $\gamma\delta$ T cells into the gut.

While CCR9 expression in the gut primarily consists of $CD3^+$ T cells, B cells and natural killer cells also express the receptor [144]. This expression on B cells is clearly relevant since Bowman et al. [147] recently reported that CCL25/TECK is a potent chemoattractant for IgA-antibody secreting cells, recruiting them from the spleen, Peyer's patches and mesenteric lymph nodes. Therefore, it is evident that CCL25/TECK and CCR9 play a critical role in homing of effector T and B lymphocytes to the small intestine.

In addition to the involvement of CCR9 in small intestinal homing a number of other chemokine receptors, which are widely known to play an important role in other tissues, are also expressed on T cells in the gastrointestinal system. For example, CXCR3, CCR5, and CCR2 chemokine receptors are expressed on lamina propria T lymphocytes, intraepithelial T lymphocytes, and $CD45RO^+\beta7^{hi}$ gut homing memory T cells [148]. CXCR3 has been shown to be a functional receptor on intraepithelial and lamina propria lymphocytes [148] and the expression of its ligand CXCL10/IP-10 has been reported in normal colon lamina propria [149]. Similarly, CCR5 has also been shown to be functional on intraepithelial and lamina propria lymphocytes and the expression of its ligand CCL5/RANTES has been reported in normal small intestine and colon epithelium and lamina propria [150]. Lastly, the CCR6 ligand CCL20/LARC is expressed in the small intestine and colon by epithelial cells, especially those lining the Peyer's patches and may attract lymphocytes and dendritic cells to the intestinal epithelium [151]. These data suggest that CXCR3, CCR5 and CCR2 also play a role in preferential homing of T lymphocytes to normal mucosa.

Moreover, dendritic cells also play a crucial role in the immune network by processing antigen and activating lymphocytes. Particularly, CCR6 mediates recruitment of immature dendritic cells to the sub-epithelial dome of Peyer's patches [152]. Furthermore, CCR6 has been found to be expressed in myeloid $CD11b^+$ dendritic cells found exclusively in the sub-epithelial dome region of Payer's patches, where its ligand MIP-3α is expressed [153]. Therefore, CCR6 and MIP-3α mediate recruitment of dendritic cells precursors to the gastrointestinal tract under non-inflammatory conditions.

While specific regulation of chemokines and their receptors is critical to directed cellular movement to and from Peyer's patches and lamina propria, differential expression of adhesion molecules is also of substantial importance. Peyer's patches uniquely expressed a modified mucosal addressin cell adhesion molecule, MadCAM-1, that adheres to CD62L/L-selectin preferentially expressed on naïve T and B lymphocytes. Unmodified MadCAM-1 is expressed on endothelial cells within the lamina propria and adheres to the $\alpha_4\beta_7$ integrins that are upregulated in activated gut-homing lymphocytes [154]. Kunkel et al. [155] show that although the leukocyte rolling flux was suppressed in CD62L/L-selectin knockouts, Payer's patches were of normal size and cellularity. In β_7 knockouts the rolling flux was normal, however the number of adherent leukocytes in HEV were greatly reduced [155].

It is clear that a variety of chemokines and chemokine receptors in conjunction with adhesion molecules are critical to immune homeostasis in the gastrointestinal system. CCR7, CXCR4 and CXCR5 mediate the homing of naïve T and B lymphocytes to the inductive Peyer's patches. Subsequently, CCR5, CXCR3, CCR9 and CCR6 play a major role in trafficking of effector $CD4^+$ and $CD8^+$ T cells, dendritic cells as well as IgA-antibody secreting cells to the lamina propria and epithelial cell effector sites in the intestines. These effector cells play a crucial role in immune surveillance at antigen-rich mucosal sites that are routinely exposed to potential pathogens.

9. LEUKOCYTE HOMING TO THE SKIN

While it is clear that immune responses in the skin have many unique characteristics, homing of lymphocytes to the skin is poorly understood. Naïve T cells that encounter antigen in skin-associated lymph nodes develop into skin-homing effector T cells. $\gamma\delta$ T cells have been shown to play an important role in innate immunity. Particularly, $\gamma\delta$ T cells have been shown to localize in large numbers to the epidermis of mice and cattle but not humans [156]. In the skin, these $\gamma\delta$ intraepithelial T cells show distinct dendritic cell morphology and are known as dendritic epidermal T cells [156]. However, little is known about trafficking of $\gamma\delta$ T cells to the skin. Most work on the role of chemokine mediated T cell trafficking to the skin focuses on $\alpha\beta$ T cells.

Skin-homing T cells are characterized by their expression of cutaneous lymphocyte antigen (CLA), an epitope which functions as a homing receptor for T cells in inflamed skin. Picker et al. [157] originally showed that the majority of T lymphocytes in inflammatory skin lesions expressed CLA, whereas very few T cells expressed CLA in extracutaneous sites of inflammation. The vascular CLA receptor, E-selectin, is highly expressed on endothelial cells in inflamed skin and mediates initial cell contact (tethering) and rolling. However, migration directed by CLA/E-selectin alone is insufficient to explain homing of memory T lymphocytes to skin. Neutrophils also express CLA but do not migrate to the skin and E-selectin is commonly expressed on extracutaneous epithelium [16]

The chemokine receptor CCR4 is involved in homing of cutaneous T memory lymphocytes to the vascular endothelium at cutaneous sites of inflammation. Systemic $\alpha_4\beta_7^-$ memory T cells in the blood, including all skin homing CLA^+ T cells, express CCR4 and respond to its ligands CCL17/TARC and CCL22/MDC. In addition, Campbell et al. [122] found $CCR4^+$ lymphocytes in chronically inflamed skin, but not in the gastrointestinal lamina propria and further demonstrated CCL17/TARC expression in cutaneous venules and skin epithelium but not mucosal epithelium. CCL17/TARC and CCL27/CTACK (cutaneous T cell-attracting chemokine) are expressed in the skin and can recruit CLA^+ memory T cells, but not naïve T cells, B cells, neutrophils or monocytes [158]. CCL27/CTACK mRNA is constitutively expressed in mouse epidermis and human keratinocytes, but is absent in all other tissues. This suggests that CCL27/CTACK plays a role in specific trafficking during normal immune surveillance, although its induction by proinflammatory cytokines suggests a role in inflammatory processes as well. Most recently, circulating skin-homing CLA$^+$ T cells, dermal microvascular endothelial cells, and fibroblasts were shown to express the CCL27/CTACK receptor CCR10. Neutralization of CCL27/CCR10 binding disrupts lymphocyte homing to the skin and can suppress allergen-induced skin inflammation [159]. However, Reiss et al. [160] recently demonstrated that blocking of either CCR4 or the CCR10 ligand CCL27/CTACK has no effect on T cell homing to inflamed skin, but blocking of CCL27/CTACK abrogated skin recruitment of CCR4 deficient T cells, showing that these receptors may have overlapping and redundant roles in T cell recruitment to the skin. In addition to T cells, Langerhans cells in the epidermis play a critical role in the immune network. Langerhans cells are immature dendritic cells which uptake and process foreign antigen in the skin, however they also traffic to the skin under homeostatic conditions. CCR6 has been shown to mediate trafficking of Langerhans cells to the epidermis in response to Mip-3α produced locally by keratinocytes [161].

It is becoming clear that a number of chemokine/receptors such as CCR4, CCR6 and CCR10, in conjunction with CLA contribute to the tissue-specific lymphocyte and dendritic cell homing in normal and inflamed cutaneous sites. Such chemokines and adhesion molecules are critical players in the immune network.

10. LEUKOCYTE TRAFFICKING WITHIN THE CENTRAL NERVOUS SYSTEM

Traditional immunological surveillance of the brain is restricted by the blood brain barrier, a customized vessel endothelium compacted by functional complexes that effectively eliminate any space between adjacent endothelial cells [162]. This barrier blocks the diffusion of blood-borne substances as well as immigration of circulating cells into the brain parenchyma. Typically, T, B and natural killer cells do not enter into neural tissue under homeostatic conditions [163]. However, violation of this barrier is a primary factor in several serious diseases of the central nervous system (CNS), such as multiple sclerosis and infection-induced encephalitis [163]. Ironically, in several CNS infections, the offending organism utilizes leukocytes as the vehicle for brain entry [164].

Several studies into the mechanisms of EAE have observed that only activated T cells adoptively transferred into rats could traffic to the neural parenchyma [165,166]. B cells are similarly implicated with several neuroinflammatory diseases exhibiting high levels of IgG antibody within the cerebrospinal fluid (CSF), which normally has IgG levels 1000 fold less than those observed in serum. The observation of "oligoclonal bands" of IgG – discrete bands detected by electrophoresis – within the CSF led to the hypothesis that activated B cells enter the CNS under activated conditions and even establish plasma cells inside the blood brain barrier [2]. Upon administration of antigen beyond an intact blood brain barrier via cannulization, in combination with peripheral immunization, Harling-Berg et al. [167] observed that antigen specific B cells could be detected within the rat brain. The general consensus is that B cells need a prerequisite activation signal similar to T cells before traversing the endothelial lining to the interior of the CNS. However, some resistance to this hypothesis exists based on the observation of some T and B lymphocytes within the CNS under steady-state conditions [164].

T cells found within the CSF have higher expression of CXCR3 than those in the periphery, and a neutralizing antibody against its ligand CXCL10/IP10 is capable of protection against EAE, however mice with a targeted deletion in CXCL10/IP10 are equally susceptible compared to wild-type mice [168–170]. Similarly, CCL3/MIP-1α or CCR5 knockout mice are not protected from EAE, despite data showing the protective effect of anti-CCL3/MIP-1α antibody [169,171].

$\gamma\delta$ T cells exhibiting an activated phenotype can be demonstrated in the CNS during EAE, however the mechanism of trafficking has not been characterized [172]. In a murine model of neurocysticercosis, $\gamma\delta$ T cells were the predominant subset recruited to the CNS, and animals depleted of $\gamma\delta$ lymphocytes had decreased severity of disease [173,174]. Increased expression of CCL2/MCP-1, CCL3/MIP-1α, CCL5/RANTES, CXCL2/MIP-2 and CCL11/eotaxin is correlated with disease onset [175]. TCR$\delta^{-/-}$ mice induced with neurocysticercosis demonstrated reduced expression of these chemokines and decreases in recruitment of NK, B, $\alpha\beta$ T and dendritic cells to the brain [175].

Unlike lymphocytes, macrophage/monocyte lineage cells are present within the CNS during resting conditions [163]. The types of macrophages that can be found within the CNS are expansive with several phenotypically distinct subsets occupying different regions of the brain. Some of these cell types, such as parenchymal microglial cells, appear early during fetal life with little or no replenishment from the bone marrow required. Other cell types, such as the meningeal and choroid plexus macrophages are replaced by new immigrating bone marrow derived cells [163].

While there is a large body of knowledge detailing the role of chemokines in the brain under inflammatory conditions, their role in regulating homeostatic leukocyte immigration into the CNS are ill defined. Nevertheless, the chemokines CCL2/MCP-1 and CX_3CL1/Fractalkine are implicated based on their constitutive expression within the CNS [176]. The chemokine receptor CXCR4 and its ligand CXCL12/SDF-1 have also been proposed to regulate homeostasis due to their cerebellar expression [1].

11. CONCLUDING REMARKS

The role of chemokines within the context of immunity extends beyond their function as inflammatory chemoattractants. Chemokines, their receptors, and adhesion molecules are fundamental components of the haematopoietic system, lymphoid organogenesis, and the maintenance of acquired immunity. Essential to leukocyte maturation in the bone marrow and thymus as well as activation and trafficking to lymphoid organs, chemokines provide both a common system of leukocyte movement and specific signals for specialized tissues.

As concepts of the role of chemokines have expanded, so have models of chemokine activity. For example, working on the assumption that leukocytes utilized an active process to halt chemotaxis and switch to effector activity, work from our group uncovered a role for the arrestin protein in blocking chemotactic signalling from chemokine receptors and converting it to a signal for degranulation [45,49]. Within the homeostatic model, the discovery of chemorepulsive activity mediated by CXCR4 provides a mechanism by which mature T cells may exit the thymus [1,126].

Our understanding of chemokine biology has evolved in circular fashion. The majority of early studies were directed at inflammatory neutrophil chemotaxis in the context of innate immunity; this model set the basis for investigating the migration of T and B cells as they scan antigen-presenting cells in the lymph node. As attention has shifted to the innate system in recent years, new questions have arisen: How do NK cells migrate between the circulation and secondary lymphoid organs? What signals do NK cells utilize to localize to tumours or infections, and is the mechanism different? Hopefully, the models of leukocyte migration established in adaptive immunity will provide a useful starting point for finding these answers.

ACKNOWLEDGEMENTS

This work was supported by grants from the Heart and Stroke Foundation of Canada, the Canadian Institutes of Health Research, and Genome Canada. SEB is funded by the National Sciences and Engineering Research Council of Canada and the Canadian Institutes of Health Research. KAH is funded by Ontario Graduate Scholarship Program.

REFERENCES

1. Zou YR, Kottmann AH, Kuroda M, Taniuchi I, Littman DR. Function of the chemokine receptor CXCR4 in haematopoiesis and in cerebellar development. Nature 1998;393(6685): 595–9.
2. Knopf PM, Harling-Berg CJ, Cserr HF, Basu D, Sirulnick EJ, Nolan SC et al. Antigen-dependent intrathecal antibody synthesis in the normal rat brain: tissue entry and local retention of antigen-specific B cells. J Immunol 1998;161(2):692–701.
3. Peled A, Grabovsky V, Habler L, Sandbank J, Arenzana-Seisdedos F, Petit I et al. The chemokine SDF-1 stimulates integrin-mediated arrest of CD34(+) cells on vascular endothelium under shear flow. J Clin Invest 1999;104(9):1199–1211.
4. Murphy PM, Baggiolini M, Charo IF, Hebert CA, Horuk R, Matsushima K et al. International union of pharmacology. XXII. Nomenclature for chemokine receptors. Pharmacol Rev 2000;52(1):145–176.
5. Zlotnik A, Yoshie O. Chemokines: a new classification system and their role in immunity. Immunity 2000;12(2):121–7.
6. Murphy PM. International Union of Pharmacology. XXX. Update on chemokine receptor nomenclature. Pharmacol Rev 2002;54(2):227–9.
7. Fabbri M, Bianchi E, Fumagalli L, Pardi R. Regulation of lymphocyte traffic by adhesion molecules. Inflamm Res 1999;48(5):239–46.
8. Gordon M. Origin and Development of Neutrophils. In: Hellewell PG, Williams TJ, editors. Immunopharmacology of neutrophils . San Diego: Academic Press, 1994:27–54.
9. Rosales C, Brown EJ. Neutrophil receptors and modulation of the immune response. In: Jon S.Abramson JGW, editor. The Neutrophil . New York: IRL Press at Oxford University Press, 2001:27–52.
10. Casimir C, Teahan C. The Respiratory Burst of Neutrophils and Its Deficiency. In: Hellewell PG, Williams TJ, editors. Immunopharmacology of neutrophils. San Diego: Academic Press, 2001:55–94.
11. Borregaard N, Lollike K, Kjeldsen L, Sengelov H, Bastholm L, Nielsen MH et al. Human neutrophil granules and secretory vesicles. Eur J Haematol 1993;51(4):187–98.
12. Borregaard N, Cowland JB. Granules of the human neutrophilic polymorphonuclear leukocyte. Blood 1997;89(10):3503–21.
13. Tapper H. The secretion of preformed granules by macrophages and neutrophils. J Leukoc Biol 1996;59(5):613–22.
14. Wagner JG, Roth RA. Neutrophil migration mechanisms, with an emphasis on the pulmonary vasculature. Pharmacol Rev 2000;52(3):349–74.

15. Matsuba KT, Van Eeden SF, Bicknell SG, Walker BA, Hayashi S, Hogg JC. Apoptosis in circulating PMN: increased susceptibility in L-selectin-deficient PMN. Am J Physiol 1997;272(6 Pt 2):H2852–8.
16. Tedder TF, Steeber DA, Chen A, Engel P. The selectins: vascular adhesion molecules. FASEB J 1995;9(10):866–73.
17. Varki A. Selectin ligands: will the real ones please stand up? J Clin Invest 1997;99(2): 158–62.
18. von Andrian UH, Chambers JD, McEvoy LM, Bargatze RF, Arfors KE, Butcher EC. Two-step model of leukocyte-endothelial cell interaction in inflammation: distinct roles for LECAM-1 and the leukocyte beta 2 integrins in vivo. Proc Natl Acad Sci U S A 1991;88(17):7538–42.
19. Spertini O, Luscinskas FW, Kansas GS, Munro JM, Griffin JD, Gimbrone MA, Jr. et al. Leukocyte adhesion molecule-1 (LAM-1, L-selectin) interacts with an inducible endothelial cell ligand to support leukocyte adhesion. J Immunol 1991;147(8):2565–73.
20. Malik AB, Lo SK. Vascular endothelial adhesion molecules and tissue inflammation. Pharmacol Rev 1996;48(2):213–29.
21. Ley K, Bullard DC, Arbones ML, Bosse R, Vestweber D, Tedder TF et al. Sequential contribution of L- and P-selectin to leukocyte rolling in vivo. J Exp Med 1995;181(2): 669–75.
22. Klein CL, Bittinger F, Kohler H, Wagner M, Otto M, Hermanns I et al. Comparative studies on vascular endothelium in vitro. 3. Effects of cytokines on the expression of E-selectin, ICAM-1 and VCAM-1 by cultured human endothelial cells obtained from different passages. Pathobiology 1995;63(2):83–92.
23. Scholz D, Devaux B, Hirche A, Potzsch B, Kropp B, Schaper W et al. Expression of adhesion molecules is specific and time-dependent in cytokine-stimulated endothelial cells in culture. Cell Tissue Res 1996;284(3):415–23.
24. Levinovitz A, Muhlhoff J, Isenmann S, Vestweber D. Identification of a glycoprotein ligand for E-selectin on mouse myeloid cells. J Cell Biol 1993;121(2):449–59.
25. Luscinskas FW, Lawler J. Integrins as dynamic regulators of vascular function. FASEB J 1994;8(12):929–38.
26. Buyon JP, Philips MR, Merrill JT, Slade SG, Leszczynska-Piziak J, Abramson SB. Differential phosphorylation of the beta2 integrin CD11b/CD18 in the plasma and specific granule membranes of neutrophils. J Leukoc Biol 1997;61(3):313–21.
27. Laudanna C, Campbell JJ, Butcher EC. Role of Rho in chemoattractant-activated leukocyte adhesion through integrins. Science 1996;271(5251):981–3.
28. Laudanna C, Campbell JJ, Butcher EC. Elevation of intracellular cAMP inhibits RhoA activation and integrin-dependent leukocyte adhesion induced by chemoattractants. J Biol Chem 1997;272(39):24141–4.
29. Jones SL, Wang J, Turck CW, Brown EJ. A role for the actin-bundling protein L-plastin in the regulation of leukocyte integrin function. Proc Natl Acad Sci U S A 1998;95(16): 9331–6.
30. Newman PJ. The biology of PECAM-1. J Clin Invest 1997;100(11 Suppl):S25–9.
31. Muller WA, Weigl SA, Deng X, Phillips DM. PECAM-1 is required for transendothelial migration of leukocytes. J Exp Med 1993;178(2):449–60.
32. Vaporciyan AA, DeLisser HM, Yan HC, Mendiguren II, Thom SR, Jones ML et al. Involvement of platelet-endothelial cell adhesion molecule-1 in neutrophil recruitment in vivo. Science 1993;262(5139):1580–2.

33. Lomas DA, Stone SR, Llewellyn-Jones C, Keogan MT, Wang ZM, Rubin H et al. The control of neutrophil chemotaxis by inhibitors of cathepsin G and chymotrypsin. J Biol Chem 1995;270(40):23437–43.
34. Betsuyaku T, Shipley JM, Liu Z, Senior RM. Neutrophil emigration in the lungs, peritoneum, and skin does not require gelatinase B. Am J Respir Cell Mol Biol 1999;20(6): 1303–9.
35. Feuerhake F, Fuchsl G, Bals R, Welsch U. Expression of inducible cell adhesion molecules in the normal human lung: immunohistochemical study of their distribution in pulmonary blood vessels. Histochem Cell Biol 1998;110(4):387–94.
36. Muller WA, Randolph GJ. Migration of leukocytes across endothelium and beyond: molecules involved in the transmigration and fate of monocytes. J Leukoc Biol 1999;66(5): 698–704.
37. Shang XZ, Issekutz AC. Beta 2 (CD18) and beta 1 (CD29) integrin mechanisms in migration of human polymorphonuclear leucocytes and monocytes through lung fibroblast barriers: shared and distinct mechanisms. Immunology 1997;92(4):527–35.
38. Shang T, Yednock T, Issekutz AC. alpha9beta1 integrin is expressed on human neutrophils and contributes to neutrophil migration through human lung and synovial fibroblast barriers. J Leukoc Biol 1999;66(5):809–16.
39. Wang Q, Doerschuk CM. The signaling pathways induced by neutrophil-endothelial cell adhesion. Antioxid Redox Signal 2002;4(1):39–47.
40. Martin C, Burdon PC, Bridger G, Gutierrez-Ramos JC, Williams TJ, Rankin SM. Chemokines acting via CXCR2 and CXCR4 control the release of neutrophils from the bone marrow and their return following senescence. Immunity 2003;19(4):583–93.
41. Yoshimura T, Matsushima K, Oppenheim JJ, Leonard EJ. Neutrophil chemotactic factor produced by lipopolysaccharide (LPS)-stimulated human blood mononuclear leukocytes: partial characterization and separation from interleukin 1 (IL 1). J Immunol 1987;139(3): 788–93.
42. Nakagawa H, Komorita N, Shibata F, Ikesue A, Konishi K, Fujioka M et al. Identification of cytokine-induced neutrophil chemoattractants (CINC), rat GRO/CINC-2 alpha and CINC-2 beta, produced by granulation tissue in culture: purification, complete amino acid sequences and characterization. Biochem J 1994;301(Pt 2):545–50.
43. Huang S, Paulauskis JD, Godleski JJ, Kobzik L. Expression of macrophage inflammatory protein-2 and KC mRNA in pulmonary inflammation. Am J Pathol 1992;141(4):981–8.
44. Ohno Y, Lee J, Fusunyan RD, MacDermott RP, Sanderson IR. Macrophage inflammatory protein-2: chromosomal regulation in rat small intestinal epithelial cells. Proc Natl Acad Sci U S A 1997;94(19):10279–84.
45. Barlic J, Khandaker MH, Mahon E, Andrews J, DeVries ME, Mitchell GB et al. beta-arrestins regulate interleukin-8-induced CXCR1 internalization. J Biol Chem 1999;274(23):16287–94.
46. Aramori I, Ferguson SS, Bieniasz PD, Zhang J, Cullen B, Cullen MG. Molecular mechanism of desensitization of the chemokine receptor CCR-5: receptor signaling and internalization are dissociable from its role as an HIV-1 co-receptor. EMBO J 1997;16(15): 4606–16.
47. Orsini MJ, Parent JL, Mundell SJ, Benovic JL, Marchese A. Trafficking of the HIV coreceptor CXCR4. Role of arrestins and identification of residues in the c-terminal tail that mediate receptor internalization. J Biol Chem 1999;274(43):31076–86.
48. Aragay AM, Mellado M, Frade JM, Martin AM, Jimenez-Sainz MC, Martinez A et al.

Monocyte chemoattractant protein-1-induced CCR2B receptor desensitization mediated by the G protein-coupled receptor kinase 2. Proc Natl Acad Sci U S A 1998;95(6):2985–90.
49. Barlic J, Andrews JD, Kelvin AA, Bosinger SE, DeVries ME, Xu L et al. Regulation of tyrosine kinase activation and granule release through beta-arrestin by CXCRI. Nat Immunol 2000;1(3):227–33.
50. Jagels MA, Hugli TE. Neutrophil chemotactic factors promote leukocytosis. A common mechanism for cellular recruitment from bone marrow. J Immunol 1992;148(4):1119–28.
51. Haslett C. Granulocyte apoptosis and its role in the resolution and control of lung inflammation. Am J Respir Crit Care Med 1999;160(5 Pt 2):S5–11.
52. Van Furth R, Diesselhoff-den Dulk MC, Mattie H. Quantitative study on the production and kinetics of mononuclear phagocytes during an acute inflammatory reaction. J Exp Med 1973;138(6):1314–30.
53. Kurihara T, Warr G, Loy J, Bravo R. Defects in macrophage recruitment and host defense in mice lacking the CCR2 chemokine receptor. J Exp Med 1997;186(10):1757–62.
54. von Stebut E, Metz M, Milon G, Knop J, Maurer M. Early macrophage influx to sites of cutaneous granuloma formation is dependent on MIP-1alpha /beta released from neutrophils recruited by mast cell-derived TNFalpha. Blood 2003;101(1):210–5.
55. Palframan RT, Jung S, Cheng G, Weninger W, Luo Y, Dorf M et al. Inflammatory chemokine transport and presentation in HEV: a remote control mechanism for monocyte recruitment to lymph nodes in inflamed tissues. J Exp Med 2001;194(9):1361–73.
56. Izikson L, Klein RS, Luster AD, Weiner HL. Targeting monocyte recruitment in CNS autoimmune disease. Clin Immunol 2002;103(2):125–31.
57. Izikson L, Klein RS, Charo IF, Weiner HL, Luster AD. Resistance to experimental autoimmune encephalomyelitis in mice lacking the CC chemokine receptor (CCR)2. J Exp Med 2000; 192(7):1075–80.
58. Fife BT, Huffnagle GB, Kuziel WA, Karpus WJ. CC chemokine receptor 2 is critical for induction of experimental autoimmune encephalomyelitis. J Exp Med 2000;192(6): 899–905.
59. Huang DR, Wang J, Kivisakk P, Rollins BJ, Ransohoff RM. Absence of monocyte chemoattractant protein 1 in mice leads to decreased local macrophage recruitment and antigen-specific T helper cell type 1 immune response in experimental autoimmune encephalomyelitis. J Exp Med 2001;193(6):713–26.
60. Kurth I, Willimann K, Schaerli P, Hunziker T, Clark-Lewis I, Moser B. Monocyte selectivity and tissue localization suggests a role for breast and kidney-expressed chemokine (BRAK) in macrophage development. J Exp Med 2001;194(6):855–61.
61. Geissmann F, Jung S, Littman DR. Blood monocytes consist of two principal subsets with distinct migratory properties. Immunity 2003;19(1):71–82.
62. Ancuta P, Rao R, Moses A, Mehle A, Shaw SK, Luscinskas FW et al. Fractalkine preferentially mediates arrest and migration of CD16+ monocytes. J Exp Med 2003;197(12):1701–7.
63. Lesnik P, Haskell CA, Charo IF. Decreased atherosclerosis in CX3CR1-/- mice reveals a role for fractalkine in atherogenesis. J Clin Invest 2003;111(3):333–40.
64. Huo Y, Weber C, Forlow SB, Sperandio M, Thatte J, Mack M et al. The chemokine KC, but not monocyte chemoattractant protein-1, triggers monocyte arrest on early atherosclerotic endothelium. J Clin Invest 2001;108(9):1307–14.
65. Cravens PD, Lipsky PE. Dendritic cells, chemokine receptors and autoimmune

inflammatory diseases. Immunol Cell Biol 2002;80(5):497–505.
66. Pashenkov M, Teleshova N, Kouwenhoven M, Smirnova T, Jin YP, Kostulas V et al. Recruitment of dendritic cells to the cerebrospinal fluid in bacterial neuroinfections. J Neuroimmunol 2002;122(1–2):106–16.
67. Robertson MJ, Ritz J. Biology and clinical relevance of human natural killer cells. Blood 1990;76(12):2421–38.
68. Lanier LL, Le AM, Civin CI, Loken MR, Phillips JH. The relationship of CD16 (Leu-11) and Leu-19 (NKH-1) antigen expression on human peripheral blood NK cells and cytotoxic T lymphocytes. J Immunol 1986;136(12):4480–6.
69. Cooper MA, Fehniger TA, Caligiuri MA. The biology of human natural killer-cell subsets. Trends Immunol 2001;22(11):633–40.
70. Biron CA, Nguyen KB, Pien GC, Cousens LP, Salazar-Mather TP. Natural killer cells in antiviral defense: function and regulation by innate cytokines. Annu Rev Immunol 1999;17:189–220.
71. Moretta L, Biassoni R, Bottino C, Cantoni C, Pende D, Mingari MC et al. Human NK cells and their receptors. Microbes Infect 2002;4(15):1539–44.
72. Sutherland CL, Chalupny NJ, Cosman D. The UL16-binding proteins, a novel family of MHC class I-related ligands for NKG2D, activate natural killer cell functions. Immunol Rev 2001;181:185–92.
73. Colucci F, Caligiuri MA, Di Santo JP. What does it take to make a natural killer? Nat Rev Immunol 2003;3(5):413–25.
74. Robertson MJ. Role of chemokines in the biology of natural killer cells. J Leukoc Biol 2002;71(2):173–83.
75. Lang K, Drell TL, Niggemann B, Zanker KS, Entschladen F. Neurotransmitters regulate the migration and cytotoxicity in natural killer cells. Immunol Lett 2003;90(2-3):165–72.
76. Kveberg L, Bryceson Y, Inngjerdingen M, Rolstad B, Maghazachi AA. Sphingosine 1 phosphate induces the chemotaxis of human natural killer cells. Role for heterotrimeric G proteins and phosphoinositide 3 kinases. Eur J Immunol 2002;32(7):1856–64.
77. Campbell JJ, Qin S, Unutmaz D, Soler D, Murphy KE, Hodge MR et al. Unique subpopulations of CD56+ NK and NK-T peripheral blood lymphocytes identified by chemokine receptor expression repertoire. J Immunol 2001;166(11):6477–82.
78. Inngjerdingen M, Damaj B, Maghazachi AA. Expression and regulation of chemokine receptors in human natural killer cells. Blood 2001;97(2):367–75.
79. Qin S, Rottman JB, Myers P, Kassam N, Weinblatt M, Loetscher M et al. The chemokine receptors CXCR3 and CCR5 mark subsets of T cells associated with certain inflammatory reactions. J Clin Invest 1998;101(4):746–54.
80. Maghazachi AA. G protein-coupled receptors in natural killer cells. J Leukoc Biol 2003;74(1):16–24.
81. Kim CH, Pelus LM, Appelbaum E, Johanson K, Anzai N, Broxmeyer HE. CCR7 ligands, SLC/6Ckine/Exodus2/TCA4 and CKbeta-11/MIP-3beta/ELC, are chemoattractants for CD56(+)CD16(-) NK cells and late stage lymphoid progenitors. Cell Immunol 1999;193(2):226–35.
82. Taub DD, Sayers TJ, Carter CR, Ortaldo JR. Alpha and beta chemokines induce NK cell migration and enhance NK-mediated cytolysis. J Immunol 1995;155(8):3877–88.
83. Allavena P, Bianchi G, Zhou D, Van Damme J, Jilek P, Sozzani S et al. Induction of natural killer cell migration by monocyte chemotactic protein-1, -2 and -3. Eur J Immunol 1994;24(12):3233–36.

84. Giancarlo B, Silvano S, Albert Z, Mantovani A, Allavena P. Migratory response of human natural killer cells to lymphotactin. Eur J Immunol 1996;26(12):3238–41.
85. Orange JS, Wang B, Terhorst C, Biron CA. Requirement for natural killer cell-produced interferon gamma in defense against murine cytomegalovirus infection and enhancement of this defense pathway by interleukin 12 administration. J Exp Med 1995;182(4):1045–56.
86. Vester B, Muller K, Solbach W, Laskay T. Early gene expression of NK cell-activating chemokines in mice resistant to Leishmania major. Infect Immun 1999;67(6):3155–9.
87. Scharton TM, Scott P. Natural killer cells are a source of interferon gamma that drives differentiation of CD4+ T cell subsets and induces early resistance to Leishmania major in mice. J Exp Med 1993;178(2):567–77.
88. Reiner SL, Zheng S, Wang ZE, Stowring L, Locksley RM. Leishmania promastigotes evade interleukin 12 (IL-12) induction by macrophages and stimulate a broad range of cytokines from CD4+ T cells during initiation of infection. J Exp Med 1994;179(2):447–56.
89. Braun SE, Chen K, Foster RG, Kim CH, Hromas R, Kaplan MH et al. The CC chemokine CK beta-11/MIP-3 beta/ELC/Exodus 3 mediates tumor rejection of murine breast cancer cells through NK cells. J Immunol 2000;164(8):4025–31.
90. Nokihara H, Yanagawa H, Nishioka Y, Yano S, Mukaida N, Matsushima K et al. Natural killer cell-dependent suppression of systemic spread of human lung adenocarcinoma cells by monocyte chemoattractant protein-1 gene transfection in severe combined immunodeficient mice. Cancer Res 2000;60(24):7002–7.
91. Shang X, Qiu B, Frait KA, Hu JS, Sonstein J, Curtis JL et al. Chemokine receptor 1 knockout abrogates natural killer cell recruitment and impairs type-1 cytokines in lymphoid tissue during pulmonary granuloma formation. Am J Pathol 2000;157(6):2055–63.
92. Wright DE, Wagers AJ, Gulati AP, Johnson FL, Weissman IL. Physiological migration of hematopoietic stem and progenitor cells. Science 2001;294(5548):1933–6.
93. Ma Q, Jones D, Springer TA. The chemokine receptor CXCR4 is required for the retention of B lineage and granulocytic precursors within the bone marrow microenvironment. Immunity 1999;10(4):463–71.
94. Nagasawa T, Hirota S, Tachibana K, Takakura N, Nishikawa S, Kitamura Y et al. Defects of B-cell lymphopoiesis and bone-marrow myelopoiesis in mice lacking the CXC chemokine PBSF/SDF-1. Nature 1996;382(6592):635–8.
95. Mohle R, Bautz F, Rafii S, Moore MA, Brugger W, Kanz L. Regulation of transendothelial migration of hematopoietic progenitor cells. Ann N Y Acad Sci 1999;872:176–85.
96. Hattori K, Heissig B, Tashiro K, Honjo T, Tateno M, Shieh JH et al. Plasma elevation of stromal cell-derived factor-1 induces mobilization of mature and immature hematopoietic progenitor and stem cells. Blood 2001;97(11):3354–60.
97. Jacobsen K, Kravitz J, Kincade PW, Osmond DG. Adhesion receptors on bone marrow stromal cells: in vivo expression of vascular cell adhesion molecule-1 by reticular cells and sinusoidal endothelium in normal and gamma-irradiated mice. Blood 1996;87(1):73–82.
98. Mohle R, Murea S, Kirsch M, Haas R. Differential expression of L-selectin, VLA-4, and LFA-1 on CD34+ progenitor cells from bone marrow and peripheral blood during G-CSF-enhanced recovery. Exp Hematol 1995;23(14):1535–42.
99. Peled A, Kollet O, Ponomaryov T, Petit I, Franitza S, Grabovsky V et al. The chemokine SDF-1 activates the integrins LFA-1, VLA-4, and VLA-5 on immature human CD34(+) cells: role in transendothelial/stromal migration and engraftment of NOD/SCID mice.

Blood 2000;95(11):3289–96.

100. Mohle R, Haas R, Hunstein W. Expression of adhesion molecules and c-kit on CD34+ hematopoietic progenitor cells: comparison of cytokine-mobilized blood stem cells with normal bone marrow and peripheral blood. J Hematother 1993;2(4):483–9.
101. Annunziato F, Romagnani P, Cosmi L, Lazzeri E, Romagnani S. Chemokines and lymphopoiesis in human thymus. Trends Immunol 2001;22(5):277–81.
102. Prockop S, Petrie HT. Cell migration and the anatomic control of thymocyte precursor differentiation. Semin Immunol 2000;12(5):435–44.
103. Norment AM, Bevan MJ. Role of chemokines in thymocyte development. Semin Immunol 2000;12(5):445–55.
104 Savino W, Mendes-da-Cruz DA, Silva JS, Dardenne M, Cotta-de-Almeida V. Intrathymic T-cell migration: a combinatorial interplay of extracellular matrix and chemokines? Trends Immunol 2002;23(6):305–13.
105. Cantor H, Weissman I. Development and function of subpopulations of thymocytes and T lymphocytes. Prog Allergy 1976;20:1–64.
106. Oosterwegel MA, Haks MC, Jeffry U, Murray R, Kruisbeek AM. Induction of TCR gene rearrangements in uncommitted stem cells by a subset of IL-7 producing, MHC class-II-expressing thymic stromal cells. Immunity 1997;6(3):351–60.
107. Godfrey DI, Zlotnik A, Suda T. Phenotypic and functional characterization of c-kit expression during intrathymic T cell development. J Immunol 1992;149(7):2281–5.
108. Hernandez-Lopez C, Varas A, Sacedon R, Jimenez E, Munoz JJ, Zapata AG et al. Stromal cell-derived factor 1/CXCR4 signaling is critical for early human T-cell development. Blood 2002;99(2):546–54.
109. Suzuki G, Sawa H, Kobayashi Y, Nakata Y, Nakagawa K, Uzawa A et al. Pertussis toxin-sensitive signal controls the trafficking of thymocytes across the corticomedullary junction in the thymus. J Immunol 1999;162(10):5981–5.
110. Kim CH, Pelus LM, White JR, Broxmeyer HE. Differential chemotactic behavior of developing T cells in response to thymic chemokines. Blood 1998;91(12):4434–43.
111. Wilkinson B, Owen JJ, Jenkinson EJ. Factors regulating stem cell recruitment to the fetal thymus. J Immunol 1999;162(7):3873–81.
112. Uehara S, Grinberg A, Farber JM, Love PE. A role for CCR9 in T lymphocyte development and migration. J Immunol 2002;168(6):2811–19.
113. Norment AM, Bogatzki LY, Gantner BN, Bevan MJ. Murine CCR9, a chemokine receptor for thymus-expressed chemokine that is up-regulated following pre-TCR signaling. J Immunol 2000;164(2):639–48.
114. Wurbel MA, Philippe JM, Nguyen C, Victorero G, Freeman T, Wooding P et al. The chemokine TECK is expressed by thymic and intestinal epithelial cells and attracts double- and single-positive thymocytes expressing the TECK receptor CCR9. Eur J Immunol 2000;30(1):262–71.
115. Chidgey AP, Boyd RL. Thymic stromal cells and positive selection. APMIS 2001;109(7-8):481–92.
116. Campbell JJ, Pan J, Butcher EC. Cutting edge: developmental switches in chemokine responses during T cell maturation. J Immunol 1999;163(5):2353–7.
117. Suzuki G, Nakata Y, Dan Y, Uzawa A, Nakagawa K, Saito T et al. Loss of SDF-1 receptor expression during positive selection in the thymus. Int Immunol 1998;10(8):1049–56.
118. Chantry D, Romagnani P, Raport CJ, Wood CL, Epp A, Romagnani S et al. Macrophage-derived chemokine is localized to thymic medullary epithelial cells and is a chemoattractant

for CD3(+), CD4(+), CD8(low) thymocytes. Blood 1999;94(6):1890–8.
119. Lieberam I, Forster I. The murine beta-chemokine TARC is expressed by subsets of dendritic cells and attracts primed CD4+ T cells. Eur J Immunol 1999;29(9):2684–94.
120. Franz-Bacon K, Dairaghi DJ, Boehme SA, Sullivan SK, Schall TJ, Conlon PJ et al. Human thymocytes express CCR-3 and are activated by eotaxin. Blood 1999;93(10):3233–40.
121. Zhang L, He T, Talal A, Wang G, Frankel SS, Ho DD. In vivo distribution of the human immunodeficiency virus/simian immunodeficiency virus coreceptors: CXCR4, CCR3, and CCR5. J Virol 1998;72(6):5035–45.
122. Campbell JJ, Haraldsen G, Pan J, Rottman J, Qin S, Ponath P et al. The chemokine receptor CCR4 in vascular recognition by cutaneous but not intestinal memory T cells. Nature 1999;400(6746):776–80.
123. Tanabe S, Lu Z, Luo Y, Quackenbush EJ, Berman MA, Collins-Racie LA et al. Identification of a new mouse beta-chemokine, thymus-derived chemotactic agent 4, with activity on T lymphocytes and mesangial cells. J Immunol 1997;159(11):5671–9.
124. Thelen M. Dancing to the tune of chemokines. Nat Immunol 2001;2(2):129–34.
125. Forster R, Schubel A, Breitfeld D, Kremmer E, Renner-Muller I, Wolf E et al. CCR7 coordinates the primary immune response by establishing functional microenvironments in secondary lymphoid organs. Cell 1999;99(1):23–33.
126. Poznansky MC, Olszak IT, Evans RH, Wang Z, Foxall RB, Olson DP et al. Thymocyte emigration is mediated by active movement away from stroma-derived factors. J Clin Invest 2002;109(8):1101–10.
127. Cyster JG. Chemokines and the homing of dendritic cells to the T cell areas of lymphoid organs. J Exp Med 1999;189(3):447–50.
128. Muller G, Hopken UE, Stein H, Lipp M. Systemic immunoregulatory and pathogenic functions of homeostatic chemokine receptors. J Leukoc Biol 2002;72(1):1–8.
129. Olson TS, Ley K. Chemokines and chemokine receptors in leukocyte trafficking. Am J Physiol Regul Integr Comp Physiol 2002;283(1):R7–28.
130. Gunn MD, Kyuwa S, Tam C, Kakiuchi T, Matsuzawa A, Williams LT et al. Mice lacking expression of secondary lymphoid organ chemokine have defects in lymphocyte homing and dendritic cell localization. J Exp Med 1999;189(3):451–60.
131. Randolph DA, Huang G, Carruthers CJ, Bromley LE, Chaplin DD. The role of CCR7 in TH1 and TH2 cell localization and delivery of B cell help in vivo. Science 1999;286(5447): 2159–62.
132. Ansel KM, Ngo VN, Hyman PL, Luther SA, Forster R, Sedgwick JD et al. A chemokine-driven positive feedback loop organizes lymphoid follicles. Nature 2000;406(6793): 309–14.
133. Forster R, Mattis AE, Kremmer E, Wolf E, Brem G, Lipp M. A putative chemokine receptor, BLR1, directs B cell migration to defined lymphoid organs and specific anatomic compartments of the spleen. Cell 1996;87(6):1037–47.
134. Okada T, Ngo VN, Ekland EH, Forster R, Lipp M, Littman DR et al. Chemokine requirements for B cell entry to lymph nodes and Peyer's patches. J Exp Med 2002;196(1): 65–75.
135. Nagler-Anderson C. Man the barrier! Strategic defences in the intestinal mucosa. Nat Rev Immunol 2001;1(1):59–67.
136. Agace WW, Higgins JM, Sadasivan B, Brenner MB, Parker CM. T-lymphocyte-epithelial-cell interactions: integrin alpha(E)(CD103)beta(7), LEEP-CAM and chemokines. Curr Opin Cell Biol 2000;12(5):563–8.

137. Eigenmann PA. T lymphocytes in food allergy: overview of an intricate network of circulating and organ-resident cells. Pediatr Allergy Immunol 2002;13(3):162–71.
138. Lambolez F, Azogui O, Joret AM, Garcia C, von Boehmer H, Di Santo J et al. Characterization of T cell differentiation in the murine gut. J exp Med 2002;195(4): 437–49.
139. Miller C, Roberts SJ, Ramsburg E, Hayday AC. gamma delta cells in gut infection, immunopathology, and organogenesis. Springer Semin Immunopathol 2000;22(3):297–310.
140. Warnock RA, Campbell JJ, Dorf ME, Matsuzawa A, McEvoy LM, Butcher EC. The role of chemokines in the microenvironmental control of T versus B cell arrest in Peyer's patch high endothelial venules. J Exp Med 2000;191(1):77–88.
141. Williams MB, Butcher EC. Homing of naive and memory T lymphocyte subsets to Peyer's patches, lymph nodes, and spleen. J Immunol 1997;159(4):1746–52.
142. Zabel BA, Agace WW, Campbell JJ, Heath HM, Parent D, Roberts AI et al. Human G protein-coupled receptor GPR-9-6/CC chemokine receptor 9 is selectively expressed on intestinal homing T lymphocytes, mucosal lymphocytes, and thymocytes and is required for thymus-expressed chemokine-mediated chemotaxis. J Exp Med 1999;190(9):1241–56.
143. Kunkel EJ, Campbell JJ, Haraldsen G, Pan J, Boisvert J, Roberts AI et al. Lymphocyte CC chemokine receptor 9 and epithelial thymus-expressed chemokine (TECK) expression distinguish the small intestinal immune compartment: Epithelial expression of tissue-specific chemokines as an organizing principle in regional immunity. J Exp Med 2000;192(5):761–8.
144. Papadakis KA, Prehn J, Nelson V, Cheng L, Binder SW, Ponath PD et al. The role of thymus-expressed chemokine and its receptor CCR9 on lymphocytes in the regional specialization of the mucosal immune system. J Immunol 2000;165(9):5069–76.
145. Svensson M, Marsal J, Ericsson A, Carramolino L, Broden T, Marquez G et al. CCL25 mediates the localization of recently activated CD8alphabeta(+) lymphocytes to the small-intestinal mucosa. J Clin Invest 2002;110(8):1113–21.
146. Wurbel MA, Malissen M, Guy-Grand D, Meffre E, Nussenzweig MC, Richelme M et al. Mice lacking the CCR9 CC-chemokine receptor show a mild impairment of early T- and B-cell development and a reduction in T-cell receptor gammadelta(+) gut epithelial lymphocytes. Blood 2001:98(9):2626–32.
147. Bowman EP, Kuklin NA, Youngman KR, Lazarus NH, Kunkel EJ, Pan J et al. The intestinal chemokine thymus-expressed chemokine (CCL25) attracts IgA antibody-secreting cells. J Exp Med 2002;195(2):69–275.
148. Agace WW, Roberts AI, Wu L, Greineder C, Ebert EC, Parker CM. Human intestinal lamina propria and intraepithelial lymphocytes express receptors specific for chemokines induced by inflammation. Eur J Immunol 2000;30(3):819–26.
149. Uguccioni M, Gionchetti P, Robbiani DF, Rizzello F, Peruzzo S, Campieri M et al. Increased expression of IP-10, IL-8, MCP-1, and MCP-3 in ulcerative colitis. Am J Pathol 1999;155(2):331–36.
150. Mazzucchelli L, Hauser C, Zgraggen K, Wagner HE, Hess MW, Laissue JA et al. Differential in situ expression of the genes encoding the chemokines MCP-1 and RANTES in human inflammatory bowel disease. J Pathol 1996;178(2):201–6.
151. Tanaka Y, Imai T, Baba M, Ishikawa I, Uehira M, Nomiyama H et al. Selective expression of liver and activation-regulated chemokine (LARC) in intestinal epithelium in mice and

humans. Eur J Immunol 1999;29(2):633–42.
152. Cook DN, Prosser DM, Forster R, Zhang J, Kuklin NA, Abbondanzo SJ et al. CCR6 mediates dendritic cell localization, lymphocyte homeostasis, and immune responses in mucosal tissue. Immunity 2000;12(5):495–503.
153. Iwasaki A, Kelsall BL. Localization of distinct Peyer's patch dendritic cell subsets and their recruitment by chemokines macrophage inflammatory protein (MIP)-3alpha, MIP-3beta, and secondary lymphoid organ chemokine. J Exp Med 2000;191(8):1381–94.
154. Brandtzaeg P, Farstad IN, Haraldsen G. Regional specialization in the mucosal immune system: primed cells do not always home along the same track. Immunology Today 1999;20(6):267–77.
155. Kunkel EJ, Ramos CL, Steeber DA, Muller W, Wagner N, Tedder TF et al. The roles of L-selectin, beta 7 integrins and P-selectin in leukocyte rolling and adhesion in high endothelial venules of Peyer's patches. J Immunol 1998;161(5):2449–56.
156. Hayday A, Tigelaar R. Immunoregulation in the tissues by gammadelta T cells. Nat Rev Immunol 2003;3(3):233–42.
157. Picker LJ, Michie SA, Rott LS, Butcher EC. A unique phenotype of skin-associated lymphocytes in humans. Preferential expression of the HECA-452 epitope by benign and malignant T cells at cutaneous sites. Am J Pathol 1990;136(5):1053–68.
158 Morales J, Homey B, Vicari AP, Hudak S, Oldham E, Hedrick J et al. CTACK, a skin-associated chemokine that preferentially attracts skin-homing memory T cells. Proc Natl Acad Sci U S A 1999;96(25):14470–5.
159. Homey B, Alenius H, Muller A, Soto H, Bowman EP, Yuan W et al. CCL27-CCR10 interactions regulate T cell-mediated skin inflammation. Nat Med 2002;8(2):157–65.
160. Reiss Y, Proudfoot AE, Power CA, Campbell JJ, Butcher EC. CC chemokine receptor (CCR)4 and the CCR10 ligand cutaneous T cell-attracting chemokine (CTACK) in lymphocyte trafficking to inflamed skin. J Exp Med 2001;194(10):1541–47.
161. Charbonnier AS, Kohrgruber N, Kriehuber E, Stingl G, Rot A, Maurer D. Macrophage inflammatory protein 3alpha is involved in the constitutive trafficking of epidermal Langerhans cells. J Exp Med 1999;190(12):1755–68.
162. Drewes LR. What is the blood-brain barrier? A molecular perspective. Cerebral vascular biology. Adv Exp Med Biol 1999;474:111–22.
163. Hickey WF. Leukocyte traffic in the central nervous system: the participants and their roles. Semin Immunol 1999;11(2):125–37.
164. Drevets DA, Leenen PJ. Leukocyte-facilitated entry of intracellular pathogens into the central nervous system. Microbes Infect 2000;2(13):1609–18.
165. Hickey WF, Hsu BL, Kimura H. T-lymphocyte entry into the central nervous system. J Neurosci Res 1991;28(2):254–60.
166. Takenaka A, Minagawa H, Kaneko K, Mori R, Itoyama Y. Adoptive transfer of experimental allergic encephalomyelitis with lectin-activated spleen cells. Part 2. Studies on T cell subsets and interleukin 2 production. J Neurol Sci 1986;72(2-3):337–45.
167. Harling-Berg C, Knopf PM, Merriam J, Cserr HF. Role of cervical lymph nodes in the systemic humoral immune response to human serum albumin microinfused into rat cerebrospinal fluid. J Neuroimmunol 1989;25(2-3):185–93.
168. Kivisakk P, Trebst C, Liu Z, Tucky BH, Sorensen TL, Rudick RA et al. T-cells in the cerebrospinal fluid express a similar repertoire of inflammatory chemokine receptors in the absence or presence of CNS inflammation: implications for CNS trafficking. Clin Exp Immunol 2002;129(3):510–8.

169. Fife BT, Kennedy KJ, Paniagua MC, Lukacs NW, Kunkel SL, Luster AD et al. CXCL10 (IFN-gamma-inducible protein-10) control of encephalitogenic CD4+ T cell accumulation in the central nervous system during experimental autoimmune encephalomyelitis. J Immunol 2001;166(12):7617–24.
170. Klein RS, Izikson L, Means T, Gibson HD, Lin E, Sobel RA et al. IFN-inducible protein 10/CXC chemokine ligand 10-independent induction of experimental autoimmune encephalomyelitis. J Immunol 2004;172(1):550–9.
171. Tran EH, Kuziel WA, Owens T. Induction of experimental autoimmune encephalomyelitis in C57BL/6 mice deficient in either the chemokine macrophage inflammatory protein-1alpha or its CCR5 receptor. Eur J Immunol 2000;30(5):1410–5.
172. Gao YL, Rajan AJ, Raine CS, Brosnan CF. gammadelta T cells express activation markers in the central nervous system of mice with chronic-relapsing experimental autoimmune encephalomyelitis. J Autoimmun 2001;17(4):261–71.
173. Cardona AE, Restrepo BI, Jaramillo JM, Teale JM. Development of an animal model for neurocysticercosis: immune response in the central nervous system is characterized by a predominance of gamma delta T cells. J Immunol 1999;162(2):995–1002.
174. Cardona AE, Teale JM. Gamma/delta T cell-deficient mice exhibit reduced disease severity and decreased inflammatory response in the brain in murine neurocysticercosis. J Immunol 2002;169(6):3163–71.
175. Cardona AE, Gonzalez PA, Teale JM. CC chemokines mediate leukocyte trafficking into the central nervous system during murine neurocysticercosis: role of gamma delta T cells in amplification of the host immune response. Infect Immun 2003;71(5):2634–42.
176. Ransohoff RM. The chemokine system in neuroinflammation: an update. J Infect Dis 2002;186 Suppl 2:S152–6.

Natural Immunity
Edited by L. Bertók and D.A. Chow
© 2005 Elsevier B.V. All rights reserved

Neuroendocrine Regulation of Natural Immunity

ISTVAN BERCZI

Department of Immunology, Faculty of Medicine, University of Manitoba, Winnipeg, Manitoba, R3E 0W3, Canada

ABSTRACT

Natural killer (NK) cells, γδ T lymphocytes and CD5+ B lymphocytes are key effector cells in the natural immune system. These cells utilize germ-line coded receptors that recognize highly conserved, homologous epitopes (homotopes). Cytokines, hormones and neurotransmitters regulate natural immunity. Under physiological conditions the natural immune system is regulated similarly to the adaptive immune system: growth and lactogenic hormones (GLH), insulin-like growth factor-I (IGF-I), insulin, leptin, some steroid (glucocorticoid at physiological concentrations, dehydroepiandrosterone and some of its derivatives) and thyroid hormones are stimulatory. The peptides of the hypothalamus-pituitary-adrenal axis (CRF, AVP, ACTH, αMSH, βEND) exert an immunosuppressive, anti-inflammatory and anti-pyretic effect. Opioid peptides and estradiol are immunomodulators that promote some immune activities while inhibiting others. High (pathophysiological) levels of glucocorticoids, progesterone and testosterone act as immunosuppressive hormones. Beta-adrenergic agents are immunosuppressive and anti-inflammatory, whereas cholinergic agents promote immunity and inflammation. Substance P and calcitonin-gene related peptide are pro-inflammatory and promote immunity, whereas somatostatin is an antagonoist of these neuropeptides.

Mild infection or a sublethal dose of endotoxin elicits a brief elevation of GH and PRL in the serum. Severe trauma, sepsis and shock results in the elevation of TNFα, IL-1 and IL-6 in the blood stream, the GLH-IGF-I axis is suppressed, whereas the hypothalamus-pituitary-adrenal axis is activated. LH, FSH, estrogens, androgens, progesterone, and thyroid hormones all decline during infection and endotoxin shock, as a rule. Leptin, insulin, glucagon, α-MSH, endorphin, and arginine vasopressin are increased during endotoxemia. A "sympathetic outflow" leads to elevated blood levels of catecholamines. Fever and catabolism prevails, whereas acute phase proteins in the liver, cell proliferation in the bone marrow, and protein synthesis by leukocytes are increased. This is an acute emergency reaction to save the organism after the adaptive immune system has failed to contain and eliminate the pathogenic agent. During sepsis and endotoxin shock, glucocorticoids potentiate the production of acute phase proteins and regulate pro-inflammatory cytokine production. Catecholamines also inhibit inflammatory responses and promote, even initiate, the acute phase response. Leptin regulates energy metabolism and it is a major stimulator of the immune system. If the acute phase reaction fails to protect the host, shock will develop and death will follow.

The acute phase response leads to *immunoconversion*, which involves the suppression of the T-cell regulated adaptive immune system and the amplification of natural immunity. Natural antibodies, C-reactive -, endotoxin binding- and mannose binding proteins are boosted and serve as polyspecific recognition molecules for leukocytes. The natural immune system provides the first and the last line of host defence and its functional integrity and massive activation is largely dependent on the neuroendocrine system.

1. INTRODUCTION

Natural immunity provides the first and last line of host defence against infectious disease, tissue injury and against a variety of noxious agents. Innate resistance may be divided into non-immune mechanisms and natural immune defence [1–6]. The natural immune defence system is comprised of highly specialized cells, such as natural killer (NK) cells, $\gamma\delta$ T lymphocytes, and CD5+ B cells that secrete natural antibodies (NAb). However, the adaptive $\alpha\beta$ T cells and B lymphocytes may also be activated by "superantigens" and other microbial mitogens, by the alternate complement pathway and cytokines during natural immune reactions. Neutrophilic, eosinophilic and basophilic leukocytes and mast cells also are integral to the natural immune system. Indeed, the entire immune system may be activated by natural immune mechanisms. The effector mechanisms of natural immune reactions are identical with those of adaptive immune reactions and include phagocytosis, cytotoxicity by the membrane attack pathway and by the induction of apoptosis, and most frequently, inflammation [5,7–10]. Non-immune mechanisms are diverse and it is beyond the scope of this chapter to discuss them in detail. Here we present the neuroendocrine regulation of the primary lymphoid organs (e.g., the bone marrow and thymus), of the cells involved in the natural immune system, and of the effector mechanisms, including inflammation, phagocytosis and cytotoxicity.

2. GROWTH AND LACTOGENIC HORMONES, INSULIN-LIKE GROWTH FACTOR AND INSULIN

2.1. Embryonic development of the immune system

In foetuses that lack the pituitary gland the immune system develops normally [11]. It is likely that placental GLH support the development of the foetal haemolymphopoietic system. Bone marrow function, thymus cellularity and various immune reactions can be restored in hypophysectomized (Hypox) rats by human placental lactogen (PL) [12,13]. Human PL is mitogenic for Nb2 rat thymic lymphoma cells [14]. Prolactin (PRL) and pituitary grafts placed onto the chorioallantoic membrane of decapitated chicken embryos stimulated the early maturation of thymocytes [15]. In neonatal rats anti-growth hormone (GH) serum significantly decreased thymus and spleen weights, cellularities and the antibody response, all of which were corrected by treatment with bovine GH [16].

2.2. Bone marrow

Hormones have long been known to regulate bone marrow function [17]. Jepson and Lowenstein [18] discovered the erythropoietic effect of PRL. The anaemia, impaired bone marrow DNA and RNA synthesis, leukocytopenia and thrombocytopenia of Hypox rats were restored by syngeneic pituitary grafts (SPG) or by PRL, GH or human PL [12,19–22]. PRL stimulated the phosphorylation of PRL-receptor-associated Janus tyrosine kinase (JAK)-2 in rat bone marrow and spleen cells, which led to the activation of signal transducer and activator of transcription (STAT) 5b protein, the interferon regulatory factor-1 (IRF-1) gamma activation sequence (GAS) and the IGF-I gene [23,24]. Recombinant human PRL enhanced bone marrow function, accelerated lymphoid and myeloid reconstitution and promoted immune function in animals [25].

Human haemopoietic progenitor cells formed granulocyte and erythroid colonies if stimulated with PRL in the presence of interleukin (IL)-3, granulocyte-macrophage colony stimulating factor (GM-CSF) and erythropoietin (EPO) [26]. Human GH increased the total number of macrophage precursors in bone marrow cultures [27]. IGF-I mediated the action of GH on the bone marrow, including B lymphocyte growth [28]. PRL regulated immunity and the function of the bursa of Fabricius in birds [29–30].

2.3. The thymus

The stimulatory effect of GH on thymus has long been established [31–33]. GH induced thymus growth and increased immunocompetence in hormone deprived and old animals. GH was mitogenic for thymocytes and stimulated the production of thymic hormones [21,34–36]. Many effects of GH on the thymus are mediated by IGF-I [37–39]. In mice with severe combined immunodeficiency (SCID), human GH promoted the engraftment of human thymocytes [40]. In Hypox rats SPG, or treatment with GH or PRL restored DNA synthesis, cell proliferation and weight of the thymus and reversed immunodeficiency [21]. Pituitary grafts increased thymus weight and the number of thymocytes in Ames dwarf mice [41]. In thymocytes, PRL stimulated the expression of the Thy-1, LT-34 (CD4), and TL antigens [36,42,43]. PL selectively increased thymus growth in Snell-Bagg pituitary dwarf mice and PRL stimulated thymic hormones [38,44,46].

2.4. The antibody response

The immunization of rats with sheep red blood cells (SRBC, a T cell-dependent antigen) increased hypothalamic thyrotropin releasing hormone (TRH) mRNA, pituitary TRH receptor mRNA and plasma PRL levels with no change in TSH or GH. The hypothalamus-pituitary-adrenal (HPA) suppressive response appeared 5–7 days after SRBC treatment. In contrast, after treatment with lipopolysaccharide (LPS, a T-independent antigen), TRH mRNA decreased and an early corticosterone peak was induced [45].

2.5. Cell mediated immunity

The T cell dependent induction of macrophage tumouricidal activity was prevented by bromocriptine (BRC) and reversed by PRL [46]. Physiological concentrations of PRL stimulated B, T and NK cell responses to mitogens, and 5 to 10-fold higher levels inhibited the T cell response to IL-2 [47,48]. PRL significantly increased interferon (IFN)γ secretion by human NK cells, which stimulated NK and lymphokine activated killer cell (LAK) cytotoxic activity [49]. PRL stimulated the growth and cytotoxic activity of purified NK cells, but there was no effect on NK activity in mixed populations of peripheral blood lymphocytes (PRL). This was due to the activation of suppressor cells in PBL. PRL did not induce novel cytotoxic NK cells, but stimulated novel LAK cytotoxicity. Both the NK and T cells participated in LAK induction. PRL had a diphasic (i.e. stimulatory and inhibitory) effect on NK cells with peaks either at 25 or 200 ng/ml, whereas LAK activation occurred only at 200 ng/ml. Physiological concentrations of PRL stimulated the generation of NK and LAK activities when combined with low doses of IL-2. Pathologically high concentrations of PRL reversibly inhibited the generation of LAK cells, whereas IL-2 activated NK cells were stimulated [50,51]. PRL enhanced the cytotoxicity of mouse tumour-associated macrophage, which correlated with elevated NO2(-) and O2(-) release and was enhanced by IFN-γ [52]. GH increased NK cells and cytotoxicity in normal and GH-deficient humans [53–56].

2.6. The effect of GLH on phagocytic cells

GH, PRL and GH releasing hormone (GHRH), at very high concentrations, enhanced H_2O_2 production in human monocytes stimulated with phorbol myristate acetate (PMA). IGF-I had no effect [57]. In neutrophils, GH stimulated lysosomal enzyme production, oxidative metabolism, adhesiveness, modulated chemotaxis, and priming for superoxide production [58,59]. GH treatment (100 ng/ml) of human polymorphonuclear cells (PMC) inhibited apoptosis and up-regulated the production of reactive oxygen intermediates and had no effect on apoptosis of monocytes and lymphocytes [60].

Neutrophilic leukocytes of aged rats show reduced superoxide anion secretion and bactericidal activity. This deficiency was corrected by treatment with IFN-γ or GH. Neutrophils from aged rats grafted with a syngeneic GH secreting pituitary tumour, GH3, responded normally to priming by IFN-γ for superoxide secretion [61]. The phagocytic activity of monocytes and PMC was increased significantly in children treated with GH for 6 months and in those on long term GH replacement therapy [62]. Neutrophils from patients with acromegaly and hyperprolactinemia showed a decrease in chemotactic activity [63].

2.7. The effect of GLH on cytokine production

In bovine foetal thymocytes at mid-gestation, GH down-regulated c-jun and c-fos mRNA and increased the transcript levels for IL-1α, -β, IL-6, and GM-CSF [64]. PRL enhanced IFN-γ production by murine spleen cells and by human peripheral blood mononuclear cells (PBMC) [46,65,and 66]. GH increased the release of IFN-γ and inhibited the enterotoxin A induced release of IL-1α from murine splenocytes. PRL also decreased IL-1α, but had no effect on IFN-γ release under these conditions [67]. Placental and pituitary GH reduced IL-5 production slightly and stimulated IFN-γ production in cultures of human peripheral blood lymphocytes (PBL). PRL also enhanced IFN-γ [68]. IRF-I gene expression and IFN-γ production were induced by PRL in Nb2 rat lymphoma cells and in T lymphocytes. GH stimulated the production of IL-2 by human lymphocytes and IL-1, TNF-α and superoxide anion production by monocytes [69–71]. GH activated monocytes for superoxide but not for TNF production, and for cell adherence or killing of *M. tuberculosis* [57].

Murine splenocytes were stimulated with protein A (PA), toxic shock syndrome toxin-1 (TSST-1) and streptolysin S (SLS). In splenocytes stimulated with PA, GH induced a 40% and 50% drop in IL-1α and IFN-γ release respectively, compared to controls, while no change was seen in IL-4 release. The release of IFN-γ by TSST-1-stimulated splenocytes fell by 30%, but no changes were shown in IL-1α and IL-4 release after GH treatment. The release of IL-1α by SLS-stimulated splenocytes increased by 50% in the presence of GH, and no changes were shown in IFN-γ and IL-4 release [72]. High dose GH (13 IU/m^2/day) did not affect TNF-α and IL-6 in patients undergoing laparoscopic surgery, nor did it in healthy individuals. The incubation of

PBL with the GH antagonist, B2036, had no effect on the production of these cytokines [73].

Enzymatically cleaved (16K)-PRL, but not full-length PRL, stimulated inducible nitric oxide synthase (iNOS) and nitric oxide (NO) by pulmonary fibroblasts and alveolar type II cells. The potency of 16K-PRL was comparable to that of IL-1β, IFN-γ, and TNF-α and occurred through a distinct receptor. Pulmonary fibroblasts endogenously produce 16K-PRL [74].

2.8. Experiments in genetically altered mice

PRL gene and PRL receptor deficient mice are immunocompetent [75,172]. In such animals GH must maintain immunocompetence. The over expression of IGF-II in FVB/N mice stimulated only T cell development. IGF-II transgenic Snell-dwarf mice are deficient in PRL, GH, TSH, and have low serum IGF-I. In these mice T cell development was stimulated to the same extent as in FVB/N mice. IGF-II also increased the number of nucleated bone marrow cells, including immature B lymphocytes. Mature B cells were not affected in the spleen [76,77].

2.9. Insulin (INS)

Insulin induced an anaphylactic inflammatory promoting factor, potentiated anaphylaxis and enhanced fibrinolysis and phagocytosis. Fc receptors of guinea pig macrophages were downregulated and antibody-dependent cytotoxicity (ADCC) was inhibited by INS. Insulin suppressed the production of IL-1 and IFN-γ induced in murine spleen cells by Staphylococcal entertoxin-A. Glucagon and somatostatin antagonized INS action in lymphoid tissue [36,68,78].

3. THE HYPOTHALAMUS-PITUITARY-ADRENAL AXIS AND OPIOID PEPTIDES

3.1. Corticotropin releasing factor (CRF)

CRF produced in the hypothalamus releases ACTH from the pituitary gland and also mediates, in part, the cytokine induced ACTH release. CRF integrates the stress response in the central nervous system (CNS) and also acts centrally as an immunosuppressive agent. This is mediated by the stimulation of *sympathetic outflow*. Immunocytes have CRF receptors and produce CRF [79,80]. Immune derived-CRF production increases during inflammatory responses and it is an important anti-inflammatory hormone, although some forms of inflammation may be enhanced by CRF [81]. T lymphocyte proliferation, IL-1, -2, and -6 secretion and NK cell activity are all influenced by CRF [82].

CRF type 1 receptor-deficient (CRFR1-0) mice show marked impairment of the HPA axis. Plasma ACTH concentrations of unstressed mutant mice are normal. Arginine vasopressin (AVP) is a major ACTH secretagogue in resting CRFR1-0 mice. Such mice are still able to mount an HPA response via mechanisms that do not depend critically on either CRF or AVP action [82,83]. In mice CRF overexpression leads to a profound impairment of lymphocyte development and function mediated by corticosteroids [84].

During immune/inflammatory reactions, cytokines, such as IL-1, -2, -6, -10, IFN-α, GM-CSF, leukaemia inhibitory factor (LIF) and oncostatin M [85–90] provide feedback signals for the activation/regulation of the HPA axis. IL-6 receptors are present on pituitary corticotrophs and on adrenocortical cells, which explains the ability of IL-6 to bypass CRF in the augmentation of adrenal function [91]. Radio-detoxification blunts the capacity of LPS to stimulate the HPA axis [92].

A single intracerebroventricular (icv) injection of IL-1β increased CRF, AVP, ACTH and β-endorphin in the spleens of both sham-operated and adrenalectomised (ADX) rats. IL-1β increased the thymic contents of CRF and ACTH in sham-operated but not in ADX rats [93]. Locally expressed CRF seems to release opioid peptides from immune cells in inflamed tissue, which inhibits pain sensation by peripheral nerves [94].

Urocortin (UCN) is a new mammalian member of the CRF family and is a candidate endogenous ligand for type 2 CRF receptors. UCN mRNA expression increases within the thymus after immune activation in a corticosterone-dependent manner, which is the consequence of HPA axis activation [95]. UCN given icv (1 ng) to rats produced a marked decrease in the proliferative response of splenocytes, which was mediated by the sympathetic nervous system [96].

3.2. Adrenotorticotropic hormone (ACTH)

ACTH has an anti-inflammatory effect and influences leukocyte recirculation in various species of mammals and birds, both are due largely to the stimulation of glucocorticoids in the adrenal gland. ACTH inhibited antibody formation, antibody mediated reactions (anaphylaxis, Arthus type hypersensitivity) and cell mediated immunity (graft rejection, tuberculin response) [36]. ACTH suppressed both the Ca^{++}-dependent and -independent phagocytosis of murine peritoneal macrophages [97]. ACTH exerts an anti-pyretic effect by acting on the CNS [98]. Acute stress and ACTH stimulated IL-18 mRNA in glucocorticoid-producing cells of the adrenal cortex of adult male Sprague-Dawley rats, which was not inhibited by cortisone [99].

3.3. Beta-endorphin (bEND) and other opioid peptides (OP)

Opioid receptors of κ-, δ- and μ-types are present on lymphocytes, monocyte/macrophages and on polymorphonuclear leukocytes [100–104]. Beta-END is derived in the pituitary gland and in other tissues from the proopiomelanocortin (POMC) peptide by enzymatic cleavage. CRF and cytokines, such as IL-1β and TNFα, regulate the production and secretion of βEND in the pituitary [105,106]. Lymphoid cells also produce βEND, especially in inflamed tissues. Opioids in general and βEND in particular exert an anti-inflammatory effect and downregulate the immune response [107,108].

Opioid peptides have a diverse effect on immune function. Antibody production, NK and LAK cell activity, cytotoxic T lymphocytes, the production of IL-1, -2, -4, -6, IFNγ and prostaglandins, mast cell degranulation and the activity of neutrophilic leukocytes were all affected by OP. Opioids modulate the immune system by acting through the CNS [109–118]. Opioid peptide-containing immune cells migrate to inflamed sites, where they release βEND which inhibits pain [119]. iNOS was expressed and cAMP levels were raised in human peripheral blood monocytes after incubation with βEND [120]. Met-enkephalin (MENK) and βEND enhanced chemiluminescence, induced a chemotactic response and up-regulated the expression of CD11b and CD18 by human neutrophils [121].

Endomorphine-1 (EMO-1) and EMO-2 are present in the nervous system, in spleen and thymus, and have a very high specificity for the μ receptor. EMO-1 and EMO-2 inhibited the production of super oxide anions by stimulated neutrophils [122,123]. Leucine-enkephalin (LENK) potentiates the immune response through the OP-1 (δ) receptor and suppresses it through the OP-2 (κ) receptor. The OP-3 receptor has a permissive effect for central immunomodulation of endogenous opioid peptides and LENK. MENK enhances immune function by OP-1 receptors independent of OP-3 [124].

3.4. Alpha-melanocyte stimulating hormone (α-MSH)

The POMC derived α-MSH is a major regulator of fever and inflammation. α-MSH is a cytokine antagonist and inhibits the pyrogenic and proinflammatory effects of IL-1, -6, TNF and IFNγ and promotes the secretion of IL-10. It acts within the brain to inhibit fever and peripheral inflammation. However, on the periphery α-MSH clearly exerts an anti-inflammatory effect [125–127]. Alpha-MSH inhibits inflammation by three general mechanisms: (i) inhibition of the production of inflammatory mediators; (ii) inhibition of inflammatory action of mediators; and (iii) inhibition of peripheral hosts cells [128]. Exogenous α-MSH antagonizes the stimulatory effects of IL-1 on the HPA axis. The ACTH response of rats to IL-1β was enhanced by icv infused α-MSH antiserum. [126,129–131].

α-MSH is produced by immune cells, by keratinocytes and is also present in the aqueous humour of the eye [132–135]. α-MSH inhibits thymocyte proliferation, induces neutrophilia and suppresses the production of acute phase proteins by the liver, TNF and IFN-γ production, the induction of prostaglandin E in fibroblasts and contact sensitivity reactions. The immunosuppressive effect of IL-1β, given icv, could be blocked by the simultaneous infusion of α-MSH [136–143]. A tripeptide from α-MSH strongly induced IL-10 in purified monocytes. T lymphocytes did not produce IL-10 in response to α-MSH [144,146]. The α-MSH derived peptide and its carboxy-terminal tripeptide α-MSH (1-13) have exerted a potent antiinflammatory effect in all major models of inflammation [129].

4. THE HYPOTHALAMUS-PITUITARY-THYROID AXIS

4.1. Thyrotropin releasing hormone (TRH)

B and T lymphocytes have receptors for TRH [145]. TRH treatment of rats significantly increased the proliferative response of spleen cells to Con-A [147]. TRH stimulated T cell development in the gut but not in the spleen [148]. In man TRH elevated serum IFN-γ levels [150]. Repeated TRH administration in critical illness resulted in a repetitive increase of TSH, PRL, GH, thyroxin (T4), and triiodothyronin (T3), without increasing reverse T3 [151].

4.2. Thyroid stimulating hormone (TSH)

TSH receptors (TSHR) are present in B and T cells, NK cells, monocytes and at high levels in dendritic cells (DC). TSHR are not detectable on foetal and neonatal immune cells. TSH significantly stimulated IL-2 and IL-12, IL-1β responses and enhanced the phagocytic activity of DCs from adult animals, enhanced the proliferative response of murine spleen cells to IL-2, significantly increased IL-2 induced NK cell cytotoxicity and enhanced the expression of MHC-II by human thyroid epithelial cells [149,152–156]. In bone marrow cells IL-6, IFNβ, TNFα, TNFβ, TGFβ2, and lymphotoxin-β responses were reproducibly induced by TSH [158]. Lymphocytes and monocytes synthesize TSH [149,158].

4.3. Thyroxin (T4) and Triiodothyronin (T3)

Lymphocytes and monocytes express nuclear receptors for both T3 and T4. Human lymphocytes convert T4 to biologically active T3. T3 regulates sodium exchange and glucose uptake in lymphocytes, stimulates thymus growth and hormone production, and promotes erythroid burst forming clones and B cell maturation in the bone marrow. In animals thyroid hormones have diverse effects on lymphocyte proliferation, antibody formation to various antigens, and on various cell mediated reactions, including NK cell activity. Thyroid deficiency was usually, but not always, associated with immune deficiency, which could be restored by treatment with T3. Hypothyroidism in man was associated with immunodeficiency. The supplemental treatment of normal animals with T3 yielded mostly negative results [36,158–166].

T4 inhibited the development of TCRαβ, CD8 in intestinal intraepithelial lymphocytes (IEL) in 6–8 week old euthymic mice [167]. The NK cell number and/or cytolytic activity of healthy subjects > 90 years old correlated positively with serum levels of vitamin D, while T3, FT4, i-PTH hormones and lean body mass were correlated only with NK cell number [168].

Dendritic cells inhibited the proliferation of rat thyroid follicles, which was mediated by IL-1β [169]. IL-1 in moderate to high concentrations inhibited thyroid cell (TEC) function, which was supported by TNF and IFNγ. IL-1 induced the release of NO and cGMP, inhibited the adenylate cyclase mediated pathways and stimulated the guanylate cyclase mediated pathways in TEC. IL-1 receptor antagonist counteracted these IL-1 effects [170]. The binding of thyroid hormone receptors to the DR4 thyroid hormone responsive element was markedly decreased in the spleens of rats with adjuvant arthritis (AA) or with AA + adrenalectomy [171]. Thyroid hormone deficient mouse strains showed a defective primary B cell development. Other haematopoietic cell lineages and mature B lymphocytes were normal [172].

5. NERVE GROWTH FACTOR, LEPTIN AND NEUROPEPTIDES

Nerve growth factor (NGF) shares tyrosine kinase receptors with other neurotropic factors that belong to the TNF receptor superfamily and are present in lymphoid cells and cells of the nervous system. NGF stimulates mast cells, haemopoietic colonies and neutrophilic leukocytes and locally exerts a proinflammatory effect. However, systematically applied NGF suppresses inflammation. Lymphocyte-derived NGF protects the nervous system and other tissues from inflammatory damage [173,174].

Leptin (LEP) is adipocyte-derived. It belongs to the GLH cytokine family and signals by a class I cytokine receptor. LEP regulates energy metabolism, reproductive function, lymphocyte development and function, and it up-regulates phagocytosis and proinflammatory cytokines. LEP stimulates the production of IL-1ra, which protected mice against LPS toxicity. In murine glial cells LEP stimulated IL-1β, it promoted wound healing and angiogenesis. During the acute phase response (APR), LEP increased rapidly in response to elevated TNF levels. LEP contributes significantly to survival in sepsis by moderating glucocorticoid and IL-6 production, stimulating IL-1ra and potentiating the immune response [175–184].

Arginine vasopressin (AVP) V_1 type receptors are present on human PBMC. AVP stimulated the production of prostaglandin E2 (PGE2) by human mononuclear phagocytes, and the production of βEND by human PBMC. AVP is antipyretic and it attenuates fever after central administration [6,185,186].

Substance P (SP) is produced in both the nervous- and in the immune systems. SP is a major mediator of neurogenic inflammation. SP induces mast cell discharge, increases capillary permeability and smooth muscle contraction, stimulates immune phenomena, bone marrow cytokines and the formation of granuloma tissue, increases Fcγ and ε receptors and decreases C3b receptors on eosinophils, releases TNFα from macrophages and modifies macrophage function during stress. In polymorphonuclear leukocytes SP stimulated the respiratory burst and chemotactic and phagocytic activities [187–194]. SP increased the release of PGE2 and collagenase from rheumatoid synoviocytes [195] and PGA and thromboxane B2 from astrocytes [196]. SP induced IL-3 and GM-CSF secretion by bone marrow cells, which was mediated by the stimulation of IL-1 and IL-6 [197]. SP activated platelet cytotoxicity against Shistosoma mansoni larvae and its receptor was necessary for the normal granulomatous response [198].

Calcitonin gene related peptide (CGRP) stimulates mast cell discharge and inflammation, inhibits antigen presentation, lymphocyte proliferation, IL-2 production, mRNA synthesis for TNFα, -β and IFN-γ and suppresses IFN-γ induced H_2O_2 production by human monocytes. T lymphocytes synthesize CGRP [199–201].

Somatostatin (SOM) is an antagonist of SP and inhibits inflammatory and immune reactions. SOM is beneficial in models of autoimmune disease and chronic inflammation. Lymphocyte proliferation, endotoxin induced leukocytosis, IgA secretion, and IFNγ production are inhibited by SOM. Its effect on antibody dependent cytotoxicity is variable. SOM exerts a regulatory influence on macrophages [190,191,202–204].

Vasoactive intestinal peptide (VIP) receptors are present on monocytes and lymphocytes. VIP stimulated macrophage chemotaxis and inhibited lymphocyte chemotaxis through the activation of adenylate cyclase [205], it enhanced phagocytosis by mouse peritoneal macrophages [206]. Immunoreactive VIP was detected in rat thymus, spleen and lymph nodes in both lymphoid and non-lymphoid cells [207].

Pituitary adenylate cyclase activating peptide (PACAP) and VIP inhibited the nuclear translocation of NFκB in stimulated macrophages. This antagonised the effect of IFN-γ and downregulated the inflammatory response. The production of TGF-β1, IL-4, -6, -12, TNF-α and NO were inhibited by both peptides [208–213]. IL-6 production was enhanced by VIP/PACAP in unstimulated macrophages [214].

Various immune cells express β-type adrenergic receptors. Beta-adrenergic agents inhibit allergic and asthmatic reactions and various immune phenomena. Acetylcholine and cholinergic agents, by acting on muscarinic receptors, enhance immune phenomena, including the release of histamine and other mediators from mast cells. Allergic patients show an increased sensitivity to cholinergic stimulation (214).

6. STEROID HORMONES

6.1. Glucocorticoids (GC)

Leukocytes express GC receptors (GR) [215,216]. GR are bound to heat shock protein 90 (HSP90) in the cytoplasm and function as nuclear transcription factors. GR modulate the transcription factors AP1, IκBα, and the cAMP-responsive element binding protein (CREB) [217–220]. Membrane GR initiate apoptosis [221]. Macrophage migration inhibitory factor (MIF) counter-acts GC action [222]. Lipocortin 1 is a GC-induced protein, which inhibits neurogenic inflammation. [223,224]. Cytokines that activate AP-1 may induce steroid resistance [225,226]. The thymic epithelium synthesizes GC, which inhibits T cell antigen receptor (TCR)-mediated apoptosis [227–229]. GC induce thymus involution [36,230,231]. Cytokines prevent their own toxicity by stimulating GC production, and by modifying target cell sensitivity for GC counter-regulatory action [232].

In the monocyte-macrophage lineage, metabolism, chemotaxis, phagocytosis, cytotoxic reactions, antigen presentation, IL-1, IL-1ra, IL-6 secretion and the ability to respond to lymphokines are inhibited by GC. In macrophages GC suppressed the production of collagenase, elastase, plasminogen activated TNFα, superoxide and NO [36,233–235].

GC increased HLA antigen and IFNγ receptor expression [236,237], and potentiated the induction of Fc-γ receptors in human monocytes by IFNγ [238]. Low concentrations of GC induced MIF production by macrophages. MIF could override the GC-mediated inhibition of cytokine secretion by LPS activated monocytes and antagonized the protective effect of GC in lethal endotoxemia [239].

Dexamethasone (DEX) inhibited the IL-12-induced IFNγ secretion and IFN regulatory factor-1 expression in NK and T cells [240]. GC inhibited NK cell-mediated cytotoxicity and ADCC, and this effect was potentiated by PGE2 and abrogated by IFN-γ or IL-2 [36,241].

GC have a powerful anti-inflammatory effect, including action against neurogenic inflammation. This is the result of GC action on cytokine and other mediator secretion, inhibition of leukocyte priming, reduction of vascular permeability, and synergism with other anti-inflammatory mediators, such as catecholamines, βEND and α-MSH [223,242–244]. The general hypersensitivity to GC is eliminated at the site of inflammation by locally produced cytokines [245].

GC induced mast cell destruction in rats and depleted cutaneous mast cells in man [246]. GC inhibited mediator release from mast cells and basophilic leukocytes [247]. Neonatal GC treatment reduced the corticosterone response to LPS in adult rats; LPS-stimulated macrophages of such rats produced less TNF-α and IL-1β and splenocytes showed increased mRNA levels for IFNγ and TNF-β [248].

The GC response peaked 36 hours after murine cytomegalovirus (MCMV) infection, coincident with elevated blood levels of IL-12, IFN-γ, TNF, and IL-6, and was dependent on IL-6 for maximal release. Adrenalectomised (ADX) mice were more susceptible than controls to MCMV-induced lethality, which was mediated by TNF and could be reversed by GC replacement. Lack of endogenous GC resulted in increased IL-12, IFN-γ, TNF, and IL-6 production as well as in mRNA expression for IL-1α and IL-1β. [249].

6.2. Aldosterone

Aldosterone, which is a GR-I agonist, significantly reduced the number of lymphocytes and monocytes and, unlike RU48362, also decreased the number of neutrophils. T helper cells and NK cells were decreased by aldosterone. Corticosterone at physiological doses behaved like a GR-II agonist in these experiments. The GR-II agonist RU48362 decreased T and B and NK cells to a very low absolute level in young adult rats. [250].

6.3. Sex hormones

6.3.1. Gonadotropins

Pyrogenic cytokines, especially IL-1β, are significantly influenced by exogenous gonadal steroids and gonadotropins. [251]. IL-1β, generated in the central nervous system (CNS) during inflammation, upregulates opioids and tachykinins in the hypothalamus which cause the suppression of hypothalamic luteinizing hormone releasing hormone (LHRH) and pituitary luteinizing hormone (LH) release [252].

6.3.2. *Sex hormone receptors and signalling*

Estrogen (ER) and androgen receptors (AR) are present in lymphoid tissues. The classical estrogen receptor (ERα) is detectable in lymphoid tissue, however, ERβ is more abundant in lymphoid cells. Progesterone (PS) also acts through GC receptors in addition to its own specific receptors (PR). At high concentrations estrogens and androgens also act on GR [253–256]. Membrane bound steroid receptors, which include the polyglycoprotein (PGP) pump also exist. [257]. ER binds to estrogen response elements (ERE) in target genes, recruits a coactivator complex called CBP-pl60 that mediates the stimulation of transcription, and also activates AP-1 sites that increases the activity of Jun/Fos [258,259]. ER interacts directly with the transcription factors NF-IL6 and NFκB, and inhibits their binding to DNA, which is likely to be the molecular basis for repression of IL-6 gene expression by estrogens. Unlike estrogens, the anti-estrogen, tamoxifen (TX) does not inhibit the induction of the IL-6 promoter [260].

Three dimeric species of PR, namely A/A, A/B, and B/B may be formed and bind to progesterone response elements (PRE) and subsequently regulate transcription. Receptor dimerization is obligatory for binding to PRE, but it is not sufficient to activate transcription without the hormone. In pure heterodimers, A receptors are dominant negative inhibitors of B receptors [261–263].

6.3.3. *Estrogens*

Estradiol (E2) causes thymic involution, suppresses bone marrow function, cell-mediated immune reactions, including the helper, suppressor and effector functions of T lymphocytes. Natural killer cells, neutrophils and mast cell degranulation are also inhibited by E2. Phagocytosis, antibody production and some autoimmune diseases of animals are enhanced by E2 [36,264,265].

In rat alveolar macrophages E2 and PS inhibited NO production [266]. In mice E2 inhibited the homing and activation of inflammatory cells and their production of TNFα and IFNγ [267], and reduced NK cell-mediated cytotoxicity [268]. In ovariectomized rhesus monkeys nine months after E2 replacement killer cell activity was reduced [269]. E2 modulated both pro- and anti-inflammatory cytokine activities [270]. In women, ovarian hyperstimulation led to neutrophil activation, which correlated with the degree of luteinization. Neutrophil L-selectin expression negatively correlated with serum progesterone levels [271].

6.3.3.1. *Immunomodulation by antiestrogens.* The non-steroidal antiestrogen, TX, has an antiproliferative effect on lymphocytes, interferes with the stimulatory effect of E2 on phagocytosis, inhibits giant cell formation by monocytes and blocks H_2O_2 production by human neutrophils. TX enhanced the LPS induced production of TNFα by human monocytes and by rat peritoneal cells [257,272–274].

TX and toremifene (TO) decrease serum PRL, GH and IGF-I levels, influence the expression of hormone receptors and their binding proteins, which also affect the immune system. TX-induced immunosuppression in rats could be reversed by treatment with either GH or PRL. TX also antagonized the stimulatory effect of PRL on lymphoid cells [257,275]. TX antagonized the inhibitory effect of E2 on NK cells. NK, LAK and CTL effector cells maintained their cytolytic activity after treatment with 1 μM TX or 5 μM TO, which are commonly achievable during cancer therapy. In murine tumour systems both TX and TO enhanced the immunotherapy (e.g., by NK, LAK or CTL effectors) of ERα negative tumours, which led to the cure and long-term survival of a significant proportion (50–75%) of animals with lethal cancer [276–282].

Antiestrogens enhanced the cytotoxic effect of anti-Fas monoclonal antibody in the majority of human ovarian carcinoma cells so examined. In Fas negative K562 target cells the NK mediated perforin/granzyme pathway of immune cytolysis was also enhanced [274,283,284].

6.4. Androgens

Human lymphocytes metabolize sex hormones and are capable of synthesizing androgens [285]. In general, testosterone (TS) suppresses immune reactions. The development of the bursa of Fabricius is prevented by TS in chicken embryos. TS has been proposed to selectively favour the differentiation of suppressor T lymphocytes in the thymus [36,286]. MHC-linked genes influence the effect of androgens on the immune system [287]. Androgens stimulate haemopoiesis [288]. In the thymus TS is converted to E2 by aromatase and E2 is a powerful inducer of thymic involution [289]. Dihydrotestosterone (DHT) and dehydroepiandrosterone (DHEA) restored the capacity of T cells to produce IL-2, IL-4 and IFN-γ in aged mice to the levels of young animals [290].

TS inhibited NO release and stimulated the release of reactive oxygen intermediates from rat peritoneal macrophages [233], inhibited inducible NO synthesis in the RAW 264.7 murine macrophage cell line [291]. In guinea pigs, androgens (TS, DHT and mesterolone) impaired the clearance of IgG-coated cells by decreasing splenic macrophage FcγR expression. Antiandrogens (flutamide, nilutamide, cyproterone acetate, spironolactone, and finasteride) counteracted the inhibitory effects of androgens [292].

In women, androgens slightly decreased free urinary cortisol levels and enhanced the mitogen-induced IFNγ/IL-4 ratio and TNFα production. [293]. Bioactive TGF-β_1 fell to approximately 50% after castration of male mice and was normalized 1 week after TS treatment. TS modulated the production of TGF-β by thymocytes [294]. In male mice DHT significantly decreased the releases of IL-1β and IL-6 by splenic and peritoneal macrophages after trauma-haemorrhage. DHT-treated animals exhibited increased IL-10 and Kupffer cell IL-6 release. Estrogen prevented this immunodepression in castrated male mice [295,296].

Both pregnenolone (PREG) and DHEA are metabolized by the spleen and the derivatives, which include testosterone, DHT, androstenediol (AED) and androstenetriol (AET), are much more potent immunoregulators than DHEA itself. [297]. Human monocytes express receptors for DHEA. In monocytes DHEA enhanced the induction of cytotoxicity, IL-1 secretion, reactive nitrogen intermediate release, and the expression of complement receptor-1 and TNFα protein [298].

Plasma levels of DHEA-S, AED and TS are suppressed in chronically ill patients and in those treated with DEX. This is corrected by ACTH [299]. DHEA-S is depressed in postmenopausal women with rheumatoid arthritis [300]. In postmenopausal women treated with physiologic doses of DHEA for 3 weeks, $CD4^+$ T cells were decreased and $CD8^+/CD56^+$ (natural killer) cells increased. T cell mitogenic and IL-6 responses were inhibited, whereas NK cell cytotoxicity was dramatically increased [301].

6.5. Progesterone (PS)

PS is immunosuppressive. It suppressed lymphocyte proliferation [302] and the anti-*Candida* activity of neutrophils from mice [303]. PS significantly inhibited nitrite release and stimulated the release of reactive oxygen intermediates [304] and stimulated TNF release from rat peritoneal macrophages [234]. Human PBMC, stimulated with LPS, produced less IL-1 upon exposure to PS, whereas IL-6 secretion was not altered. However, PS failed to inhibit IL-1 secretion by PBMC from male donors with rheumatoid arthritis [305].

PS protects the foetus against maternal immune reactions [306,307] and lymphocyte sensitivity to PS is increased during pregnancy, due to the expression of PR by $\gamma\delta$ T lymphocytes in response to foetal antigens, leading to the production of a progesterone-induced blocking factor (PIBF). PIBF acts on the phospholipase A2 enzyme, interferes with arachidonic acid metabolism, induces a Th2 biased immune response, and exerts an anti-abortive effect by controlling NK activity [308]. PS treatment of mice suppressed glucocorticoid-induced thymocyte apoptosis [309] and decreased host resistance against viral and fungal infections [310,311].

6.6. 1,25-Dihydroxivitamin-D3 (VD3)

The VD3 precursor, cholecalciferol, is present in the diet and induced in the skin by UV radiation. 25-Hydroxyvitamin D3 is generated in the liver, which is processed further by 1-hydroxylase in the kidney, in monocyte/macrophages, in keratinocytes, bone marrow, placenta, glia cells and pneumocytes [312–314].

The VD3 receptor (VDR) interacts with VD3 responsive elements (VDRE) on DNA and also with the retinoic X receptor (RXR). Stimulation and inhibition are both possible through VDRE. Protein kinase C is involved in VDR mediated signalling and VD3 regulates the DNA binding subunit of NFκB. Monocyte/macrophages, activated T lymphocytes, and bone marrow cells express VDR [312–315]. The GM-CSF enhancer is transcriptionally repressed [316] and the IFNγ promoter is down-regulated by VD3. [317].

VD3 is a potent anti-proliferative and pro-differentiation mediator for macrophages, lymphocytes and other cells [318]. In monocytes/macrophages, adherence, chemotaxis, phagocytosis, cytotoxicity, H_2O_2, oxygen radicals, and HSP production are stimulated by VD3. Antigen presentation, the production of IL-1, -2, -6, -12, TNFα, IFN-γ and the function of Th-1 cells are inhibited. Suppressor T cell function, B cell proliferation and Ig secretion are inhibited. Natural killer cell cytotoxicity is stimulated [312,313].

The NK cell number and/or cytolytic activity of healthy subjects greater than 90 years old was positively associated with serum levels of vitamin D, while T3, FT4, i-PTH hormones and lean body mass were associated only with NK cell number [168].

The regulation by neurohormonal regulatory factors of natural immunity is summarized in Table I.

7. IMMUNOCONVERSION IN THE ACUTE PHASE RESPONSE

7.1. Introduction

The healing power of fever has been recognised in ancient Egypt, Greece the Roman and Persian empires and fever therapy was practised during the first half of the 19th century [319] using whole

Table I Major hormonal and neural regulators of natural immunity.

Hormone Mediator	NK	γδT	$CD5^+$B/NAb	CTK	PHAG	CTX	APP	INFL
HPT axis								
TRH				↑ IFNγ			↑	
TSH	↑			↑ IL1,2,6,12,IFNβ,TNFα,TGFβ	↓			
T4/T3	↑		↑				↓	
GLH hormones								
GH	↑			↑ IL1,2,6, IFNγ,TNFα; ↓ IL5	↑	↑		
PRL	↑			↑ IFNγ; ↓ IL1α	↑	↑		
IGF-I	↑				↑			
INS				↓ IL1, IFNγ	↑	↓ ADCC		
GLU				↑ IFNγ			↑	
HPA axis								
CRF	↓			↑ IL18; ↓ IL1,2,5				↓
ACTH				↑ IL18	↓			↓
GC	↓		↑	↑ IL10; ↓ IL1,6,TNFα	**0** ↓	↓	↑	↓
αMSH			↑	↑ IL10; ↓ IL1,6,TNF,IFNγ			↓	↓
βEND	↑↓				↑			↓
CAT					↑		↑	↓
Steroid hormones								
E2	↓		↑	↑ IL6; ↓TNFα, IFNγ	↑	↓		
TS					↑			
DHEA	↑		↑	↑ IL2,4, IFNγ		↑		
PS		↑		↑ IL1; ↓TNF	↓			
VD3	↑			↓ Il1,2,6,12,TNFα, IFNγ		↑		
Neurotransmitters/peptides								
SP				↑ IL1,3,6,TNFα,GMCSF	↑			↑
CGRP								↑
SOM								↓
NGF					↑			↑↓
LEP				↑ IL1,6,IL1Ra,TNF				↑

Legend: ↑ = increase; ↓ = decrease; ↑↓ = variable effect; **0** = no effect
Abbreviations not used in the text: CTK = cytokine, PHAG = phagocytosis, CTX = Cytotoxicity, INFL = inflammation.

Gram-negative bacteria until Boivin et al. [320] purified *endotoxin* from such bacteria. Numerous beneficial effects can be induced by sublethal doses of endotoxin in animals [321–329].

Glucosuria, hyperglycaemia and insulin resistance have long been recognised in infectious disease. Subsequently the pyrogenic leukocyte derived endogenous mediator (LEM) was discovered, which induced acute phase reactants in the liver during severe infectious disease. Pyrogens also induced ACTH release. By 1975 infection was known to influence GC, mineralcorticoids, INS, glucagon, GH, and metabolism [330–332]. Subsequently, IL-1 was identified as an endogenous pyrogen. Because endogenous pyrogens released ACTH, the hypothesis was proposed that IL-1 is an immune derived mediator that acts on the pituitary gland [333]. Indeed, IL-1 was shown subsequently to activate the HPA axis [334–338]. Today it is clear that IL-1 and other cytokines induce the neuroendocrine and metabolic responses to infection and to other forms of injury, which is designated as the *acute phase response* (APR).

Hans Selye discovered that infection and injury activated the HPA axis. He concluded that various noxious agents elicit *stress*, which leads to a *general adaptation syndrome (GAS).*

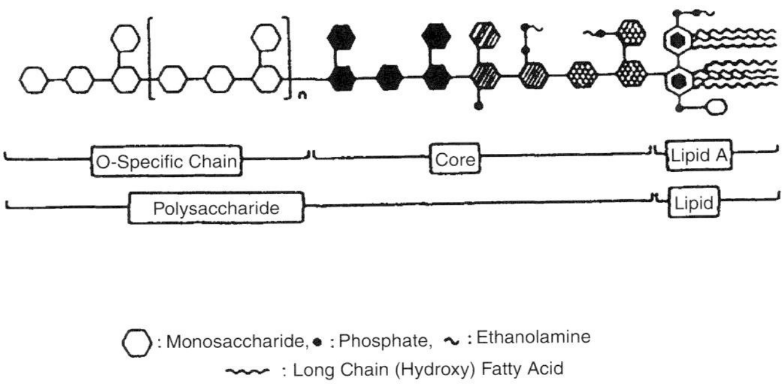

Figure 1. The molecular structure of bacterial lipolysaccharide [After Westphal et al., 351].

Stressed animals showed an initial alarm reaction, followed by adaptation when the organism was resistant towards various insults including the stressor, and the endocrine and other parameters returned to normal. With lasting stress, exhaustion would occur which could lead to death [339–342]. Selye also discovered the anti-inflammatory effects of GC [343] and the influence of sex hormones on lymphoid tissue [344]. It is now apparent that Selye's general adaptation syndrome is analogous to the *acute phase response* [345–348].

7.2. The response to endotoxin

In a broad sense physical, chemical and biological agents may cause injury. Injured cells release chemokines and cytokines, which in turn attract and activate leukocytes. This leads to immune activation and inflammation and is in most instances followed by regeneration and healing [349].

7.2.1. *Bacterial endotoxin*

Lipopolysaccharide, or *endotoxin,* is present in the outer cell membrane of all Gram-negative bacteria and divided into *polysaccharide* and core glycolipid, which consists of *lipid A* (LA) plus the core polysaccharide. The core glycolipid is the "toxic" moiety and it is an *obligatory component* of the bacterial cell wall (Fig. 1) [350]. The polysaccharide chain exhibits *heterologous epitopes* that stimulate specific antibodies, which are used for the serological classification of Gram-negative bacteria [246]. LA is highly conserved and shows extensive cross-reactivity amongst all Gram negative bacterial strains. Therefore LA functions as a *homologous epitope*, or *homotope*, which identifies all Gram-negative bacteria towards the immune system [351,352].

Lipopolysaccharide binding proteins (LBP) bind LA (10^{-9} M) in the serum of multiple species [353]. It is a 60 kDa glycoprotein with normal serum level of 0.5–10 μg/ml, but it may surpass 200 μg/ml during APR [354,355]. LBP mediates the interaction of LPS with CD14, which is present on monocytes, macrophages and neutrophilic granulocytes, and enables them to respond to extremely low levels of LPS. CD 14 lacks a transmembrane sequence [356,357]. CD14 mediates TNF, IL-6 and IL-8 responses in monocytes and macrophages. VD3 induced CD14 in a premonocytic cell line. IL-4 decreased CD14 expression, and IL-4 or IFN inhibited CD14 release by monocytes. TNF and LPS enhanced CD14 expression by monocytes. In human neutrophils, TNF, GM-CSF, G-CSF and formyl peptides increased CD14 expression [358].

The CD14 concentration increases in hospitalized patients, especially in those with autoimmune disease. Soluble CD14 inhibits the biological activities of LPS and is assumed to present LPS to endothelial cells [358]. The Toll-like receptor 4 is involved in signal transduction by LPS-CD14 complexes, leading to NFκB activation [359]. An integrin, CD18, also mediates LPS signalling. Three forms exist, CD11a/CD18, CD11b/CD18, and CD11c/CD18. All three bind LPS, participate in phagocytosis but are not essential for cellular responses. CD11b/CD18 expression by human neutrophils was up-regulated by LPS [359].

Frog and fish show extreme resistance to LPS, whereas mammals are very sensitive [360]. However, in Tilapia oreochnomis mossanbicus (Teleosti) LPS elicits integumental and cortisol responses [361]. In the horseshoe crab (Limulus polyphemus) LPS causes fatal intravascular coagulation by activating clottable proteins in the blood, which is produced by amoebocytes [362]. It seems apparent that lipid A is not inherently toxic to animal cells, but rather, the immune system has evolved in higher animals to recognize LA as a target (homotope) for the purpose of natural immune host defence . Numerous other homotopes are present on microbes, self-components and cancer cells [345,349].

7.2.2. The cytokine response to LPS

In normal mice, blood TNF is significantly increased at 1–2 hours after systemic LPS administration, which is followed by a decline and return to normal levels at around 4 hours. In ADX animals the TNF response was 60 times higher and sensitivity to LPS toxicity increased about 500 times compared to controls. Pre-treatment with DEX prevented these excessive responses. The inhibition of cortisone synthesis in the adrenals by metyrapone also increased susceptibility to LPS (~15 times higher than controls) [364–366]. Similar kinetics of TNF release were found in man after LPS infusion [366].

Blood IL-1 reaches the maximum at 4 hours in mice after LPS administration and remains elevated up to 24 hrs [365]. In man IL-6 peaked at 120 minutes after LPS administration, which was not inhibited by glucocorticoids or by repeated LPS administration [352,367,368]. Leukaemia inhibitory factor (LIF) rose moderately in mice after a sub-lethal injection of LPS and rose progressively during lethal septic shock induced by E-coli. LIF induced catabolism and had a protective effect if given prior to the administration of bacteria [369]. Additional cytokines/mediators that participate in endotoxin shock include IL-8 [370], IL-10 [371], IFNγ [372], TNF synthesis inhibitor [373], IL-1ra [374], platelet activating factor, colony stimulating factor, prostaglandins and thromboxanes [352,375,376].

7.2.3. Neuroendocrine response to endotoxin

Wexler et al. [377] discovered that in rats that LPS stimulated the release of ACTH. Endotoxin, infectious disease, and various forms of injury elicit a neuroendocrine response by the stimulation of cytokines and chemokines [353,376,377]. Profound changes occur in serum hormone levels (Table II), which are likely to be much more complicated than is indicated in the table. Dynamic and diurnal changes of hormones also play a role. Although much remains to be elucidated, it is very clear that the HPA axis exerts a powerful suppressive effect on the adaptive immune system and on inflammatory cytokines. Thus adaptive immune reactions are profoundly suppressed, whereas the induction of acute phase proteins in the liver and the production of natural antibodies by CD5+ B cells are stimulated by cytokines glucocorticoids and cathecolamines [349,352,378–380]. PRL and GH are immunostimulatory and usually rise within the first hour after endotoxin injection. This is followed by a decline to low normal to subnormal levels in

Table II Major neuroendocrine changes induced by endotoxins.

HPT and GLH hormones	Response	The HPA axis	Response	Gonadotropins & sex hormones	Response
TRH	↓	CRF	↑	LH	↑↓
TSH	**0**↓	AVP	↑	FSH	↓
T4	↓	ACTH	↑	E2	↑↓
T3	↓	GC	↑	TS	↑↓
PRL	↑↓	αMSH	↑	DHEA	↓?
GH	↑↓	βEND	↑	PS	↑↓
IGF-I	↓	CAT	↑		
INS	↑				
GLU	↑				
LEP	↑				

Please see legends to Table I. **0** = no effect. This table is modified from reference [350].

endotoxin shock. LH, FSH, estrogens, androgens, progesterone, and thyroid hormones also decline, whereas leptin, insulin, glucagon, α-MSH, β-endorphin, and arginine vasopressin are increased during endotoxemia [179,352,375,376].

7.2.4. The acute phase response induced by endotoxin

Geller et al. [381] discovered that cortisone treatment protected mice against a lethal dose of LPS. Since then, the protective effect of GC against endotoxin shock has been confirmed repeatedly in various species [381–383]. The systemic response to LPS is a typical APR. Moreover, during severe trauma and shock LPS absorbs from the intestines and may aggravate the condition [374]. In mice approximately 7% of genes were activated in the liver by LPS. The pathways for cholesterol, fatty acid, and phospholipid synthesis were suppressed and gene expression for innate defence were enhanced, which resulted in the coordinate induction of the MHC class I antigen presentation machinery, illustrating an interaction between innate and adaptive immunity [384].

Animals exposed to LPS will produce fewer cytokines in response to a second dose, which is known as *endotoxin tolerance.* Pathological changes are reduced and resistance to endotoxin, to infectious agents and to toxic and other noxious insults is significantly increased in LPS-tolerant animals [370,385,386]. LPS toxicity and tolerance is mediated by macrophages [387]. The hormones of the HPA axis play an important role in the development of LPS tolerance [358,378,389]. LPS injected into rats ip increased IL-1 levels in the hypothalamus, hippocampus, dorsal vagal complex, cerebellum, posterior cortex, and pituitary 2 hrs after injection [390]. CRP protected mice from a lethal LPS dose by binding to Fcγ-receptors (FcγR)-I and FcγRII, which results in the enhanced secretion of the anti-inflammatory cytokine, IL-10 and in the down-regulation of IL-12 [391].

In mice transgenic for human CRP and deficient in the C3 or C5 components of complement, there was a diminished induction of CRP and serum amyloid P-component (SAP) by LPS. LPS induced IL-6, but not IL-1 in complement-deficient mice. Human C5a induced IL-1β and caused significant elevation of both serum CRP and SAP in human CRP transgenic mice. However, in human CRP transgenic IL-6-deficient mice, recombinant human C5a was ineffective [392]. A transgenic human CRP protected C57BL/6 mice against experimental allergic encephalomyelitis (EAE). Human CRP inhibited the encephalitogenic peptide-induced proliferation of T cells, the production of TNF-α, IFN-γ and chemokines (macrophage-inflammatory protein-1α, RANTES, monocyte chemoattractant protein-1), and increased IL-10 production [393].

Newly synthesized acute phase proteins are essential for the development of endotoxin tolerance and these proteins exert anti-microbial and immunoregulatory functions [375]. The importance of the liver in the development of endotoxin tolerance is emphasized by the observation that D-galactosamine (GalN), which profoundly increases endotoxin sensitivity, intoxicates the liver [394]. Moreover, GalN- treated mice cannot develop endotoxin tolerance [389]. Metallothionein (MT), a low-molecular weight, cysteine-rich, metal-binding protein, is also induced in APR. MT-null mice were more sensitive to LPS/GalN-induced lethality than wild-type mice. Messenger RNA levels of APP in response to LPS/GalN were decreased in MT-null mice compared to wild-type mice [167].

Treatment of rats with the cyclooxygenase inhibitors either attenuated (meloxicam) or abolished (diclofenac) LPS-induced fever, but had no effect on plasma cortisol or IL-6. The TNF response was enhanced by both drugs. Thus the prostaglandin-dependent inflammatory pathway for fever induction is distinct from the pathway of HPA axis activation [396]. The expression of the G protein-coupled prostanoid receptors EP2-R, EP4-R, and DP-R, but not the IP-R, was up-regulated by treatment of rat hepatocytes with IL-6. In such hepatocytes PGE2 attenuated the IL-6-induced alpha-2-macroglobulin formation [397].

IL-6 induces DNA-binding of STAT transcription factors on regulatory elements in target genes. TNFα is involved in several models of liver failure as a mediator of both cytotoxicity and cell proliferation. It activates NFκB, thereby triggering inflammatory processes [398] IL-1 concomitantly induces NFκB activation and dephosphorylates IL-6-activated STAT1. The latter mechanism could account for the inhibition by IL-1 of the IL-6-dependent induction of type II acute-phase genes [399]. Soluble gp130 is the natural inhibitor of IL-6 responses [400].

The nuclear hormone receptors, *peroxisome proliferator-activated receptor alpha* (PPAR) and liver RXR play key roles in regulation of hepatic lipid metabolism. LPS markedly decreased both basal and Wy-14,643-induced expression of acyl-CoA synthetase, a well characterized PPAR target [401]. LPS elicits a dramatic increase in the synthesis and secretion of triglyceride (TG)-rich lipoproteins by the liver and the inhibition of lipoprotein lipase. This cytokine-induced "lipemia of sepsis" was considered to represent the mobilization of lipid stores to fuel the host response to infection. However, since lipoproteins can also bind and neutralize LPS, it is hypothesized that lipoproteins (VLDL and chylomicrons) are also components of an innate immune response to infection [402].

Elevation of IL-6, soluble TNFα and soluble IL-6 receptors was detected during liver regeneration [403]. In mice with acute liver failure induced by GalN, a single low dose of a hyper-IL-6-encoding adenoviral vector maintained liver function, prevented the progression of liver necrosis, induced liver regeneration, and dramatically enhanced survival [404]. In mice IL-1Ra was up-regulated in the liver after systemic LPS and local turpentine injections. After LPS stimulation, the hepatic production of sIL-1Ra correlated with the increase in plasma IL-1Ra levels. The total amount of LPS-induced soluble IL-1Ra present in the liver was six fold and tenfold higher than in the lung and spleen. In IL-6(-/-) mice exogenous IL-6 mediated the turpentine-induced production of IL-1Ra mRNA by the liver [405].

In bone marrow donors treated with G-CSF, IL-6 induced bone metabolism and an acute-phase reaction along with mobilization of CD34+ cells in the peripheral blood [406]. IL-6 treatment of rabbits caused an accelerated release of polymorphonuclear cells from the bone marrow [407].

Serum MIF levels were significantly elevated on day 1 in patients with septic shock, as opposed to trauma patients and controls. MIF paralleled cortisol, but contrasted with ACTH and was significantly higher in non-survivors than in survivors. Patients with septic adult respiratory distress syndrome (ARDS) showed higher MIF levels than those without ARDS. MIF and ARDS were independent predictors of adverse outcome. Significant correlations were established between MIF and cortisol and MIF and IL-6 and disease severity scores. No relation was found between MIF and acute phase proteins (APP, e.g., procalcitonin, CRP, and LBP). In multitrauma patients MIF levels were not elevated. During immune-mediated inflammation (such as septic shock) MIF is a contraregulator of the immunosuppressive effects of glucocorticoids [408].

Anti-inflammatory cytokines, including the IL-1ra [374], the TNF synthesis inhibitor [375], IL-10 [371] and LIF [369], participate in the down regulation of the noxious effects of endotoxin. Interferon-γ antagonizes the development of endotoxin tolerance [372].

Previte et al. [409] discovered that ionizing radiation detoxifies endotoxin. Bertok and coworkers [410] demonstrated that radiodetoxified endotoxin is capable of boosting host resistance against infectious agents, radiation, septic shock, tourniquet shock, intestinal ischemic shock, hemorrhagic shock, X-irradiation and even against immunosuppression by anti-lymphocytic serum [411]. Radiodetoxified endotoxin has been tested clinically for the treatment of infectious disease [412]. Monophosphoryl lipid A preparations of low toxicity were also studied in animals and in man for boosting host resistance to infections and traumatic events [413,414].

7.3. The acute phase response (APR)

The APR is a neuroimmune defence reaction to injury caused by physical, chemical and biological agents. It is characterized by fever, loss of appetite, inactivity and sleepiness. Cytokines, primarily IL-1, -6 and TNFα, which act on the CNS, the endocrine system and virtually on all other tissues and organs initiate the neuroendocrine and metabolic changes characteristic of APR. Later several other cytokines have been found to be involved in APP. ACTH and GC, LEP, IN, EP, NEP, GLN, AVP, and ALD are elevated during the APR, whereas GH, estrogens, androgens and thyroid hormones may be either elevated or suppressed, depending on the severity of the condition (Table II) [416–419].

C reactive protein (CRP) is an important acute phase protein. It binds to C-type pneumococcal cell walls in the presence of Ca^{2+}. This protein is present in mammals, birds, fish and crabs. In the serum, 5 identical subunits (23 kDa) of CRP form a ring-shaped molecule called *pentraxin* [421]. Pentameric CRP recognizes multiple homotopes, such as phosphocholine, polysaccharides containing galactose. Monomeric CRP binds some biologic polycations, such as protamine, poly-*L-lysin* and myelin basic protein. These determinants are frequently present on the surface of bacteria, fungi, parasites and damaged cells and tissues. After combination with the specific ligand, CRP activates complement by the classical pathway, induces chemotaxis and enhances phagocytosis by neutrophilic leukocytes and monocytes and elicits tumouricidal activity in macrophages, all of which are complement dependent. In addition, CRP stimulates the synthesis of IL-1, TNF, and potentiates the cytotoxic activity of T lymphocytes, natural killer (NK) cells and platelets. CRP localizes *in vivo* at sites of inflammation. It binds platelet activating factor (PAF) and blocks its activity. The clinical determination of CRP is diagnostic of infectious and inflammatory disease [422–424]. A third conformation is referred to as neoCRP, which functions as galactose-specific receptors on NK cells and macrophages. It also accumulates at sites of injury. Monocyte/macrophages express specific CRP receptors and proteolytic fragments of CRP activate macrophages and neutrophils [421]. Human CRP protected mice from an otherwise lethal *S. pneumoniae* infection [424]. In patients with APR, CRP concentrations correlated with an increased cortisol/cortisone ratio, which was the result of a shift towards the active cortisol [425].

LBP opsonizes LPS bearing particles, and thus may be required for the activation of complement by endotoxin through the alternate pathway. LBP-LPS complexes are potent stimulators of cytokines from monocytes and macrophages after combining with CD14 on the surface of these cells [353].

Other APP are *proteinase inhibitors*, such as α2-macroglobulin, α1-acid glycoprotein, antithrombin III, α1-acute phase globulin, and α1-proteinase inhibitor, which are present in the rat. Kupffer cells stimulated α2-macroglobulin synthesis by hepatocytes *in vitro* in the presence of 10^{-9} M DEX [426]. Fibrinogen is an important APP. Alpha-macrofetoprotein (αMFP) is a strong inhibitor of inflammatory mediators, such as histamine, bradykinin, serotonin, PGE2 and also polymorphonuclear cell chemotaxis. Catecholamines and GC induce αMFP in normal rats. Some other APP, such as haptoglobin and α1-major acute phase protein, were affected differently by these hormones [427]. Haptoglobin is an APP that binds haemoglobin, thus preventing iron loss and renal damage. Haptoglobin is an antioxidant, has antibacterial activity and plays a role in modulating many aspects of the acute phase response [428]. α1-acid glycoprotein and α1-antitrypsin exert antiapoptotic and anti-inflammatory effects and contribute to the delayed type protection associated with ischemic preconditioning in the kidney and in other insults [429].

In 10 laboratory mouse strains mannan-binding lectins (MBL)-A and MBL-C varied between 4 μg/ml to 12 μg/ml, and 16 μg/ml to 118 μg/ml, respectively. After ip injection of casein or LPS, MBL-A increased approximately 2-fold, with a maximum at 32 h, while MBL-C did not change. Serum amyloid A peaked at 15 h with an approximately 100-fold increase [430]. MBL is characterized by both collagenous and lectin domains. It binds to repeating sugar arrays on microbes. Following binding, MBL activates the complement system via an associated serum protease, MASP-2. There is an increased incidence of infections in individuals with mutations of MBL and an association with SLE and rheumatoid arthritis [431].

IL-6 is a major inducer of APP synthesis. Additional cytokines, namely IFNγ, LIF, TGFβ and OSM, were found to be inducers of APP from the liver. IL-6 activates the genes of APP through the DNA binding protein called NF-IL-6, which is a pleiotropic mediator of many inducible genes involved in the acute-phase-, immune- and inflammatory responses, similarly to NFκB. Both NF-IL-6 and NFκB binding sites are present in the inducible genes, such as IL-6, IL-8 and several acute phase genes [418].

Adrenalin evokes a high level of IL-6 in rats, which can be antagonized by propranolol. When IL-6 release is blocked, the fast reacting APP, α2-macroglobulin and cysteine protease inhibitor are strongly depressed. Isoprenalin, a β2-adrenergic receptor agonist, also causes very high levels of IL-6 [431].

APR causes a rapid thymus involution. Thymus-derived (T) lymphocytes govern adaptive immune reactions through their regulatory function. The thymus is an endocrine organ and is subject to complex neuroendocrine control mechanisms. During APR, HPA axis activation and the suppression of the GH/PRL-IGF-1 axis result in the suppression of the T-cell-dependent adaptive immune response. Catecholamines and glucocorticoids, which are released in large quantities during APR, induce apoptosis in the thymus with a striking efficiency. The elevated levels of TNF and zinc deficiency, which develop during APR, also contribute to thymic involution and to the suppression of the adaptive immune system [348].

In patients with APR the GH-IGF-I axis is suppressed and GH action is attenuated. TNF, IL-1 and IL-6 inhibit GH-signalling pathways, which results in the reduced expression of GH-responsive genes [126]. These observations prompted the treatment of acutely ill patients with GH with the aim of preventing the severe catabolic state and improving immunocompetence. However, so far the results are not encouraging. A controlled clinical trial revealed that deaths attributed to "septic shock or uncontrolled infection" occurred nearly four times more commonly in GH treated patients compared to placebo receiving patients [433]. These findings suggest strongly that the suppression of the GH/PRL – IGF-I axis in APR is required for the development of intense catabolism, which must be fundamental to the rapid release of large amounts of nutrients and of energy to support maximally the acute phase immune host defence system. During APR the CNS, the HPA axis, the sympathetic nervous system, the bone marrow, CD5+ B lymphocytes, leukocytes and the liver are metabolically activated and functionally altered [345,347,433]. The adaptive immune system is controlled by T lymphocytes and it needs 7–10 days to develop an effective host defence. During APR no time is available for an adaptive immune reaction, and therefore, this system is shut down, primarily by the cytokine and neuroendocrine alterations that take place. Thymus and T cell function is heavily dependent on the GH/PRL–IGF-I axis and it is suppressed profoundly by the elevated levels of glucocorticoids and catecholamines [345,347,348]. GH inhibited the production of acute phase proteins in rats with burn injury and in human hepatocytes [348,434,435]. On the basis of this information one may argue that the rapid breakdown of bodily tissues is the only way to fuel the acute systemic effort for host survival during APR. Clearly, GH is a powerful anabolic hormone and acts as an antagonist of the HPA axis that promotes APR [332,346,348,433,434,438]. This hypothesis is further supported by the results of GH treatment in burn injury. The catabolic effect and wasting has been reduced [439], serum IGF-I, IGFBP-3 and free fatty acids, constitutive hepatic proteins and P-selectin were increased, whereas TNFα, IL-1β, CRP and amyloid-A were decreased [438–442].

Chronic APR may lead to *cachexia* [443] or *anorexia of infection* [444]. The presence of APP predict future risk for coronary disease in healthy subjects [445]. A minimal APR is present during a*ging* [446,447], and may underlie the *metabolic syndrome* that leads to type 2 diabetes [448–453]. Polymorphism of the IL-6 gene influences the relationship among insulin sensitivity, post load glucose levels and peripheral white blood cell count [453]. APR plays a role in the pathogenesis of *rheumatoid arthritis* [454–458] in *IgA nephropathy* [457] and in numerous other inflammatory diseases. Various insults, including irritation, trauma or toxic agents, are also capable of immune activation by nonspecific pathways which can lead to APR [448].

Adaptive or natural immune activation will lead to shared host defence reactions that include inflammation, phagocytosis, cytotoxicity and neutralization of viruses, toxins etc. During systemic reactions the immune-effector function is supported by neuroendocrine and metabolic responses. Once the pathogen has been eliminated, the immune system participates in the healing process [9,347–349,448–459].

7.4. Concluding remarks

The current consensus is that endotoxin is harmful. However, LPS itself is devoid of toxicity in some lower animal species. The toxicity of LPS is due to the stimulation of immune-derived cytokines, which kills the host. Many other microbial pathogens induce such "polyclonal lymphocyte activation" [461]. Some are known as "*superantigens*" [362–364]. Many of these substances are pyrogenic [464] and induce APR.

In a natural setting immune mechanisms are activated locally at the site of pathogen penetration. This provides instantaneous defence at the site of invasion. The target is promptly identified by one of the innate mechanisms (e.g., natural antibodies, serum proteins, leukocytes) that recognize the homotopes of the pathogen. This is followed by the activation of effector mechanisms that may involve complement, blood clotting and various subsets of the white blood cell series. Blood coagulation at the focus of infection is a defence reaction, whereas disseminated intravascular coagulation may lead to disaster [345,348].

When the immune system fails to control the infection/insult locally, APR will develop. APR is an emergency reaction, which represents a switch of the immune system from the specific, adaptive mode of reactivity, which is under the control of thymus derived T lymphocytes to a less specific, but very rapid and intense natural immune reaction. Natural antibodies and APP play a major role in the identification of the target and the activation and regulation of immune effector mechanisms during APR. Febrile illness represents the mobilization of all resources of the host in the interest of defeating/eliminating the pathogen and achieving survival/recovery. By and large, APR is very successful, as in the overwhelming majority of cases febrile illness will lead to healing and recovery. On this basis, one may suggest that APR is truly beneficial and only in rare and extreme cases will it result in severe disease, shock and death [345,348]. LPS has affects on the immune system, CNS, endocrine organs and on many other tissues and organs in the body [363–366]. All tissues contain "resident macrophages" or related cells such as the glia cells in the CNS, the Kupffer cells in the liver, Langerhans cells in the skin, etc., which have the capacity to react to LPS with cytokine production [469,470]. Consequently, systemically applied LPS has the capacity to activate the immune and the neuro-endocrine systems, and also the liver via locally induced cytokines. This is supplemented by the effect of blood borne cytokines and also by neural communication. For instance, the *vagus nerve* plays a role in the activation of the ACTH-adrenal axis and the initiation of a behavioural response after the intraperitoneal injection of LPS [471,472].

Endotoxin is always present in the gastrointestinal tract, even in germ free animals [23]. However, bile acids normally destroy LPS and thus prevent its absorption from the gut of rats even when mucosal damage is inflicted [473,474]. The liver is an important clearance organ of LPS via bile secretion [475]. Therefore, bile provides a physico-chemical defence barrier against LPS toxicity in vertebrate animals [476].

LPS has an enormous potential to boost host resistance by its ability to stimulate immunity and APR. The absorption of LPS from the intestine during acute illness may represent an important pathophysiological mechanism that evolved in higher animals for the rapid conversion of the immune system from the adaptive mode of reactivity to the amplification of natural immune mechanisms. This *immunoconversion* may be achieved simply by the control of bile secretion. Indeed, there is good evidence to illustrate that intestinal endotoxin is readily absorbed after X-irradiation, trauma or even after stressful situations [348]. Liver regeneration was stimulated by intestinal endotoxin as was granulopoiesis and healing in the central nervous system [26]. However, intestinal endotoxin was blamed for death in trauma patients [345,348].

The adaptive immune system fails gradually in many people due to aging, during disease or as the result of various insults to the body. Stressful insults initially mobilize the adaptive immune system to enhance immune reactivity in peripheral tissues. If the pathogenic insult continues *immunoconversion* occurs from adaptive to natural immune host defence [342,345–349,352].

REFERENCES

1. Janeway CA, Travers P, Walport M, Shlomochik M.Innate immunity. In Immunobiology, 5th edition, Garlnad Publishing, New York, 2001. Pp.35–91.

2. Bertok L. Stimulation of nonspecific resistance by radio-detoxified endotoxin. In Beneficial effects of endotoxins. A. Nowotny, Editor, Plenum Press, New York, 1983;213–226.
3. Berczi I. Neuroendocrine defence in endotoxin shock. Acta Microbiol. Hung. 1993;40: 265–302.
4. Sabbadini ER, Berczi I. The submandibular gland: a key organ in the neuro-immunoregulatory network? Neuroimmunomodulation 1985;2:184–202.
5. Berczi I. Neurohormonal host defence in endotoxin shock Ann NY Acad Sci 1998;840: 787–802.
6. Berczi I, Nagy E. Neurohormonal control of cytokines during injury. In Brain control of the response to injury. Rothwell, N.J.& F. Berkenbosch, Editors, Cambridge University Press 1995;32–107.
7. Medzhitov R, Janeway CA, Innate immunity: impact on the adaptive immune response. Curr Opin Immunol 1997;9:4–9.
8. Boismenu R, Havran WL. An innate view of $\gamma\delta$T cells. Curr. Opin. Immunol. 1997;9: 57–63.
9. Berczi I, Chow DA, Sabbadini ER. Neuroimmunoregulation and natural immunity. Domestic Animal Endocrin 1998;15:273–281.
10. Berczi I, Bertok L, Chow DA. Natural immunity and neuroimmune host defence. Ann NY Acad Sci 2001;917:248–257.
11. Potter EL, Craig JM. Pathology of the fetus and the infant, 3rd Edition. Chicago:Year Book;1975.
12. Nagy E. Berczi I, Friesen HG. Regulation of immunity in rats by lactogenic and growth hormones. Acta Endocrinol 1983;102:351–357.
13. Berczi I, Nagy E. Human placental lactogen is a hemopoeitic hormone. Brit J Haematol 1991;79:355–358.
14. Nickel BE, Kardami E, Cattini, PA. The human placental growth hormone variant is mitogenic for rat lymphoma Nb2 cells. Endocrinology 1990; 126: 971–976.
15. Moreno J, Vicente A, Heijnen I, Zapata AG. Prolactin and early T-cell development in embryonic chicken. Immunol Today 1994;15:524–526.
16. Crilly PR, Johnson PC, Gardner MJ, Flint DJ. Immunoneutralisation of GH in neonatal rats results in defects in lymphatic tissues and the humoral immune response. Endocrine J 1994;2:105–109.
17. Crafts RC, Meinecke HA. The anemia of hypophysectomized animals. Ann NY Acad Sci 1959;77:501–517.
18. Jepson JH, Lowenstein L. The effect of testosterone, adrenal steroids and prolactin on erythropoiesis. Acta Haematol 1967:38:292–299.
19. Berczi I, Nagy E. The effect of prolactin and growth hormone on hemolyphopoietic tissue and immune function. In: Berczi I, Kovacs K, editors. Hormones and Immunity. Lancaster, England: MTP Press, 1987;145–171.
20. Nagy E, Berczi I. Pituitary dependence of bone marrow function. Brit J Haematol 1989;71: 457–462.
21. Berczi I, Nagy E, DeToledo SM, Matusik RJ, Friesen HG. Pituitary hormones regulate c-myc and DNA synthesis in lymphoid tissue. J Immunol 1991:146:2201–6.
22. Murphy WJ, Durum SK, Anver MR, Longo DL. Immunologic and hematologic effects of neuroendocrine hormones. J Immunol 1992;148:3799–3805.
23. Dogusan Z, Book ML, Verdood P, Yu-Lee LY, Hooghe-Peters EL. Prolactin activates interferon regulatory factor-1 expression in normal lympho-hemopoietic cells. Eur

Cytokine Netw 2000;11:435–42.
24. Morales P, Carretero MV, Geronimo H, Copin SG, Gaspar ML, Marcos MA,
25. Richards SM, Murphy WJ. Use of human prolactin as a therapeutic protein to potentiate immunohematopoietic function. J. Neuroimmunol. 2000;109:56–62.
26. Bellone G, Geuna M, Carbone A. Regulatory action of prolactin on the in vitro growth of CD34+ve human hemopoietic progenitor cells. J Cell Physiol 1995;163:221–231.
27. Guicheux J, Heymann D, Gouin F, Pilet P, Faivre A, Daculsi G. Growth hormone stimulates multinucleated cell formation in long-term bone marrow cultures. Eur J Cell Biol 1998;7559–65.
28. Merchav S, Tatarsky I, Hochberg Z. Enhancement of erythropoiesis in vitro by human growth hormone is mediated by insulin-like growth factor-I. Brit J Haematol 1988b;70: 267–271.
29. Bhat G, Gupta SK, Maiti BR. Influence of prolactin on mitogenic activity of the bursa of Fabricius of the chick. Gen Comp Endocrinol 1983;52:452–5.
30. Skwarlo-Sonta K, Sotowaska-Brochocka J. Rosolowska-Huszcz D. Effect of prolactin on the diurnal changes in immune parameters and plasma corticosterone in white leghorn chickens. Acta Endocrinol 1987;116:172–178.
31. Frænkel-Conrat H, Li CH. Hormonal effects on the nucleic acid and phospholipid turnover of rat liver and thymus. Endocrinology 1949;44:487–91.
32. Baroni CD, Fabris N, Bertoli G. Effects of hormones on development and function of lymphoid tissues: Synergistic action of thyroxin and somatotropic hormone in pituitary dwarf mice. Immunology 1969;17:303–14.
33. Baroni CD, Pesando PC, Bertoli G. Effects of hormones on development and function of lymphoid tissues II: Delayed development of immunological capacity in pituitary dwarf mice. Immunology 1971;21:455–61.
34. Pandian MR, Talwar GP. Effect of growth hormone on the metabolism of thymus and on the immune response against sheep erythrocytes. J Exp Med 1971;134:1095–113.
35. Kelley KW, Brief S. Westly HJ. GH_3 pituitary adenoma cells can reverse thymic aging in rats. Proc Natl Acad Sci USA 1986;83:5663–5667.
36. Berczi I. Pituitary Function and Immunity. Boca Raton, Florida:CRC Press; 1986.
37. Timsit J, Savino W, Safieh B. Growth hormone and insulin-like growth factor-I stimulate hormonal function and proliferation of thymic epithelial cells. J Clin Endocrinol Metab 1992;75:183–8.
38. Savino W. Mello-Coelho V, Dardenne M. Neuroendocrine control of the thymic microenvironment: role of pituitary hormones. In: Berczi I, Szelenyi J, editors. Advances in Psychoneuroimmunology. New York:Plenum Press, 1994;75–82.
39. Yamada M, Hato F, Kinoshita Y. The indirect participation of growth hormone in the thymocyte proliferation system. Cell Mol Biol Noisy le Grand 1994;40:111–121.
40. Taub DD, Tsarfaty G, Lloyd AR. Growth hormone promotes human T cell adhesion and migration to both human and murine matrix proteins in vitro and directly promotes xenogeneic engraftment. J Clin Invest 1994;94:293–300.
41. Esquifino AI, Vallanua MA, Szary A, Yau J, Bartke A. Ectopic pituitary transplants restore immunocompetence in Ames dwarf mice. Acta Endocrinol 1991;125:67–72.
42. Singh U, Owen JJT. Studies on the maturation of the thymus stem cells: The effects of catecholamines, histamines and peptide hormones on the expression of T cell alloantigens. Eur J Immunol 1976;6:59–62.
43. Russell DH, Mills KT, Talamantes RJ, Bern HA. Neonatal administration of prolactin

antiserum alters the developmental pattern of T- and B- lymphocytes in the thymus and spleen of BALB/c female mice. Proc Natl Acad Sci USA 1988; 85:7404–7.
44. Arezzini C, DeGori V, Tarli P, Neri P. Weight increase of body and lymphatic tissues in dwarf mice treated with human chorionic somatomammotropin (HCS). Proc Soc Exp Biol Med 1972;141:98–100.
45. Perez Castro C, Penalva R, Paez Pereda M, Renner U, Reul JM, Stalla GK, Holsboer F, Arzt E. Early activation of thyrotropin-releasing-hormone and prolactin plays a critical role during a T cell-dependent immune response. Endocrinology 1999;140:690–7.
46. Bernton EW, Meltzer MT, Holaday JW. Suppression of macrophage activation and T-lymphocyte function in hypoprolactinemic mice. Science 1988;239:401–4.
47. Matera L, Cesano A, Bellone G, Oberholtzer E. Modulatory effect of prolactin on the resting and mitogen-induced activity of T, B and NK lymphocytes. Brain Behav Immun 1992;6:409–17.
48. Athreya BH, Pletcher J, Zulian F. Subset-specific effects of sex hormones and pituitary gonadotropins on human lymphocyte proliferation in vitro. Clin Immunol Immunopathol 1993;66:201–211.
49. Matera L, Contarini M, Bellone G, Forno B, Biglino A. Up-modulation of interferon-γ mediates the enhancement of spontaneous cytotoxicity in prolactin-activated natural killer cells. Immunology 1999;98:386–92.
50. Matera L, Cesano A, Muccioli G, Veglia F. Modulatory effect of prolactin on the DNA synthesis rate and NK activity of large granular lymphocytes. Int J Neurosci 1990;51: 265–67.
51. Cesano A, Oberholtzer E, Contarini M. Independent and synergistic effect of interleukin-2 and prolactin on development of T- and NK-derived LAK effectors. Immunopharmacology 1994;28:67–75.
52. Majumder B, Biswas R, Chattopadhyay U. Prolactin regulates antitumor immune response through induction of tumoricidal macrophages and release of IL-12. Int J Cancer 2002;97: 493–500.
53. Rogen-Westerlaken C, Rijkers GT, Scholtens EJ. Immunologic studies in Turner syndrome before and during treatment with growth hormone. J Pediat 1991;119:268–272.
54. Crist DM, Peake GT, Mackinnon LT. Exogenous growth hormone treatment alters body composition and increases natural killer cell activity in women with impaired endogenous growth hormone secretion. Metabolism 1987;36:1115–7.
55. Crist DM, Kraner JC. Supplemental growth hormone increases the tumor cytotoxic activity of natural killer cells in healthy adults with normal growth hormone secretion. Metabolism 1990;39:1320–1324.
56. Bidlingmaier M, Auernhammer CJ, Feldmeier H, Strasburger CJ. Effects of growth hormone and insulin-like growth factor I binding to natural killer cells. Acta Paediatr Suppl 1997;423:80–1.
57. Warwick-Davies J, Lowrie DB, Cole PJ. Growth hormone is a human macrophage activating factor priming of human monocytes for enhanced release of H_2O_2. J Immunol 1995;154:1909–1918.
58. Rovensky J, Ferencikova J, Vigas M. Effect of growth hormone on the activity of some lysosomal enzymes in neutrophilic polymorphonuclear leukocytes of hypopituitary dwarfs. Int J Tissue React 1985;7:153–59.
59. Wiedermann CJ, Niedermuhlbicher M, Geissler D. Priming of normal human neutrophils by recombinant human growth hormone. Brit J. Hæmatol 1991;78:19–22.

60. Matsuda T, Saito H, Inoue T, Fukatsu K, Han I, Furukawa S, Ikeda S, Muto T. Growth hormone inhibits apoptosis and up-regulates reactive oxygen intermediates production by human polymorphonuclear neutrophils. J Parenter Enteral Nutr 1998; 22:368–74.
61. Fu YK, Arkins S, Li YM. Reduction in superoxide anion secretion and bactericidal activity of neutrophils from aged rats : reversal by the combination of gamma interferon and growth hormone. Infect Immun 1994;62:1–8.
62. Manfredi R, Turnietto F, Azzaroli L. Growth hormone (GH) and the immune system : imparied phagocytic function in children with idiopathic GH deficiency is corrected by treatment with biosynthetic GH. J Pediat Endocrinol 1994;7:245–251.
63. Cecilia-Fornari M, Fernanda-Palacios M, Diez RA, Intebi AD. Decreased chemotaxis of neutrophils in acromegaly and hyperprolactinemia. Eur J Endocrinol 1994;130:463–468
64. Chen HT, Schuler LA, Schultz RD. Growth hormone receptor and regulation of gene expression in fetal lymphoid cells. Mol Cell Endocrinol 1998;137:21–9.
65. Rapaport R, Oleske J, Ahdieh H. Suppression of immune function in growth hormone deficient children during treatment with human growth hormone. J Pediat 1986;109: 434–439.
66. Cesario TC, Yousefi S, Carandang G. Enhanced yields of gamma interferon in prolactin treated human peripheral blood mononuclear cells. Proc Soc Exp Biol Med 1994;205: 89–95.
67. Thellin O, Coumans B, Devos S, Hooghe-Peters EL, Zorzi W, Igout A, Heinen E, Hooghe R. Limited effects of placental and pituitary growth hormone on cytokine expression in vitro Eur Cytokine Netw 2000;11:452–5.
68. Galdiero M, Donnarumma G, Cipollareo de L'Ero G, Marcatili A, Scarfogliero P, Sommesse L. Effect of growth hormone, prolactin and insulin on the release of the IL-1 alpha, IFN-gamma and IL-4 by staphylococcal enterotoxin A-stimulated splenocytes. Euro Cytokine Netw 1995;6:187–94.
69. Edwards CK, Ghiasuddin SM, Yunger LM. In vivo administration of recombinant growth hormone or gamma-interferon activates macrophages: Enhanced resistance to experimental Salmonella-typhimurium infection is correlated with generation of reactive oxygen intermediates. Infec Immun 1992;60:2514–2521.
70. Kelley KW, Arkins S, Li YM. Growth hormone, prolactin and insulin-like growth factors: New jobs for old players. Brain Behav Immun 1992;6:317–26.
71. Horseman ND, Yu-Lee LY. Transcriptional regulation by the helix bundle peptide hormones: growth hormone, prolactin and hematopoietic cytokines. Endocrine Rev 1994;15:627–649.
72. Galdiero M, Vitiello M, Scarfogliero P, Sommese L. Growth hormone release of interleukin-1 alpha, interferon-gamma and, interleukin-4 from murine splenocytes stimulated with staphylococcal protein A, toxic shock syndrome toxin-1 and streptococcal lysin S. Eur Cytokine Netw 1997;8:83–90.
73. Zarkesh-Esfahani SH, Kolstad O, Metcalfe RA, Watson PF, von Laue S, Walters S, Revhaug A, Weetman AP, Ross RJ. High-dose growth hormone does not affect proinflammatory cytokine (tumor necrosis factor-alpha, interleukin-6, and interferon-gamma) release from activated peripheral blood mononuclear cells or after minimal to moderate surgical stress. J Clin Endocrinol Metab 2000;85:3383–90.
74. Corbacho AM, Nava G, Eiserich JP, Noris G, Macotela Y, Struman I, Martinez De La Dardenne M, Mello-Coelho V, Gagnerault MC, Postel-Vinay MC. Growth hormone receptors and immunocompetent cells. Ann N Y Acad Sci 1998;840:510–7.

75. Bouchard B, Ormandy CJ, Di Santo JP, Kelly PA. Immune system development and function in prolactin receptor-deficient mice. J Immunol 1999;163:576–82.
76. Kooijman R, Buul-Offers SC van, Scholtens EJ, Schuurman HJ, Brande JL Van den, Zegers ZJM. Cell development in insulin-like growth factor II transgenic mice. J Immunol 1995;154:5736–45.
77. Kooijman R, Buul-Offers SC van, Scholtens LE, Reijnen-Gresnight RG, Zegers BJM. and B cell development in pituitary deficient insulin-like growth factor-II transgenic dwarf mice. J Endocrinol 1997;155:165–170.
78. Berczi I. Hormonal interactions between the pituitary and immune system. In: Grossman CJ, editor. Bilateral Communication Between the Endocrine and Immune Systems. Berlin: Springer, 1994;96–144.
79. Besedovsky HO, del Rey A, Klusman I, Furukawa H, Monge Arditi G, Kabiersch A. Cytokines as modulators of the hypothalamus-pituitary-adrenal axis. J Steroid Biochem Mol Biol 1991;40:613–8.
80. Tsagarakis S, Grossman A. Corticotropin-releasing hormone: interactions with the immune system. Neuroimmunomodulation 1994;1:329–34.
81. Karalis K, Sano H, Redwine J. Autocrine or paracrine inflammatory actions of corticotropin-releasing hormone in vivo. Science 1991;254:421–23.
82. Turnbull AV, Smith GW, Lee S, Vale WW, Lee KF, Rivier C. CRF type I receptor-deficient mice exhibit a pronounced pituitary-adrenal response to local inflammation. Endocrinology 1999;140:1013–7.
83. Harbuz MS, Conde GL, Marti O, Lightman SL, Jessop DS. The hypothalamic-pituitary-adrenal axis in autoimmunity. Ann N Y Acad Sci 1997;823:214–24.
84. Boehme SA, Gaur A, Crowe PD, Liu XJ, Tamraz S, Wong T, Pahuja A, Ling N, Vale W, De Souza EB, Conlon PJ. Immunosuppressive phenotype of corticotropin-releasing factor transgenic mice is reversed by adrenalectomy. Cell Immunol 1997;176:103–12.
85. Menzies R, Phelps C, Wiranowska M, Oliver J, Chen L, Horvath E, Hall N. The effect of interferon-alpha on the pituitary-adrenal axis. J Interferon Cytokine Res. 1996;16: 619–29.
86. Raber J, Koob GF, Bloom FE. Interferon-alpha and transforming growth factor-beta 1 regulate corticotropin-releasing factor release from the amygdala: comparison with the hypothalamic response. Neurochem Int 1977;30:455–63.
87. Smith EM, Hughes TK, Cadet P, Stefano GB. Corticotropin-releasing factor-induced immunosuppression in human and invertebrate immunocytes. Cell Mol Neurobiol 1992;12:473–81.
88. Kim DS, Melmed S. Stimulatory effect of leukemia inhibitory factor on ACTH secretion of dispersed rat pituitary cells. Endocr Res 1999;25:11–9.
89. Kim DS, Choi HS, Park YS, Kim TW. Effects of oncostatin M on hormone release of rat pituitary cells in primary culture. J Korean Med Sci 2000;15:323–6.
90. Zylinska K, Mucha S, Komorowski J, Korycka A, Pisarek H, Robak T, Stepien H. Influence of granulocyte-macrophage colony stimulating factor on pituitary-adrenal axis (PAA) in rats in vivo Pituitary. 1999;2:211–692.
91. Bethin KE, Vogt SK, Muglia LJ. Interleukin-6 is an essential, corticotropin-releasing hormone-independent stimulator of the adrenal axis during immune system activation. Proc Natl Acad Sci U S A 2000;97:9317–22.
92. Barna I, Bertok L, Koenig JI, Makara GB. Radiodetoxified Lipopolysaccharide Fails to Activate the Hypophyseal-Pituitary-Adrenal Axis in the Rat. Neuroimmunomodulation

2000;8:128–131.
93. Jessop DS, Douthwaite JA, Conde GL, Lightman SL, Dayan CM, Harbuz MS. Effects of Acute Stress or Centrally Injected Interleukin-1beta on Neuropeptide Expression in the Immune System. Stress 1997;2:133–144.
94. Schafer M, Mousa SA, Stein. Corticotropin-releasing factor in antinociception and inflammation. Eur J Pharmacol 1997;323:1–10.
95. Kageyama K, Bradbury MJ, Zhao L, Blount AL, Vale WW. Urocortin messenger ribonucleic acid: tissue distribution in the rat and regulation in thymus by lipopolysaccharide and glucocorticoids. Endocrinology 1999;140:5651–8.
96. Okamoto S, Ishikawa I, Kimura K, Saito M. Potent suppressive effects of urocortin on splenic lymphocyte activity in rats. Neuroreport 1998;9:4035–9.
97. Ichinose M, Sawada M, Mæno T. Suppression of phagocytosis by adrenocorticotropic hormone in murine peritoneal macrophages. Immunol Lett 1994;42:161–5.
98. Zimmer JZ, Lipton JM. Central and peripheral injections of ACTH (1–24) reduce fever in adrenalectomized rabbits. Peptides 1981;2:413–417.
99. Conti B, Sugama S, Kim Y, Tinti C, Kim H, Baker H, Volpe B, Attardi B, Joh T. Modulation of IL-18 production in the adrenal cortex following acute ACTH or chronic corticosterone treatment. Neuroimmunomodulation 2000;8:1–7.
100. Gaveriaux C, Peluso J, Simonin F, Laforet J, Kieffer B. Identification of kappa and delta-opioid receptor transcripts in immune cells. FEBS Lett 1995;369–272–6.
101. Chuang TK, Killam KR, Chuange LF, Kumg HF, Sheng WS, Chao CC, Yu L, Chuange RY. Mu opioid receptor gene expression in immune cells. Biochem Biophys Res Comm 1995;216:922–30.
102. Sedqi M, Roy S, Ramakrishnan S, Elde R, Loh HH. Complementary DNA cloning of a mu-opioid receptor from rat peritoneal macrophages. Biochem Biophys Res Commun 1995;209:563–74.
103. Wick MJ, Minnerath SR, Roy S, Ramakrishnan S, Loh HH. Differential expression of opioid receptor genes in human lymphoid cell lines and peripheral blood lymphocytes. J Neuroimmunol 1996;64:29–36.
104. Sharp BM, Roy S, Bidlack JM. Evidence for opioid receptors on cells involved in host defense and the immune system. J Neuroimmunol 1998;83:45–56.
105. Ruzicka BB, Akil H. Differential cellular regulation of pro-opiomelanocortin by interleukin-1β and corticotropin-releasing hormone. Neuroendocrinology 1995;61:136–51.
106. Sacerdote P, Brini AT, Locatelli L, Radulovic J, Panerai AE. Tumor necrosis factor alpha differentially regulates beta-endorphin concentrations and proopiomelanocortin RNA in the anterior and neurointermediate pituitary in vivo. Neuroimmunomodulation 1994;1: 357–6.
107. Panerai AE, Radulovic J, Monastra G, Manfredi B, Locatelli L, Sacerdote P. Beta-endorphin concentrations in brain areas and peritoneal macrophages in rats susceptible and resistant to experiemental allergic encephalomyelitis; a possible relationship between tumor necrosis factor alpha and opioids in the disease. J Neuroimmunol 1994;51:169–75.
108. Stein C, Schafer M, Hassan AHS. Peripheral opioid receptors. Ann Med 1995;27:219–21.
109. Plotnikoff NP, Faith RE, Murgo AJ, Good RA. Enkephalins and Endorphins: Stress and the Immune System. New York:Plenum Press;1986.
110. Gilmore W, Weiner LP. Beta-Endorphin enhances interleukin-2 (IL-2) production in

murine lymphocytes. J Neuroimmunol 1988;18:125–38.
111. Stefano GB. Role of opioid neuropeptides in immunoregulation. Prog Neurobiol 1989;33: 149–59.
112. Weber RJ, Pert A. The periaqueductal gray matter mediates opiate-induced immunosuppression. Science 1989;245:188–190.
113. Apte RN, Durum SK, Oppenheim JJ. Opioids modulate interleukin-1 production and secretion by bone-marrow macrophages. Immunol Lett 1990;24:141–48.
114. Millar DB, Hough CJ, Mazorow DL, Gootenberg JE. Beta-endorphin's modulation of lymphocyte proliferation is dose, donor and time dependent. Brain Behav Immun 1990;4: 232–242.
115. Chiappelli F, Nguyen L, Bullington R, Fahey JL. Beta-Endorphin blunts phosphatidylinosoitol formation during in vitro activation of isolated human lymphocytes: Preliminary report. Brain Behav Immun 1992;6:1–10.
116. Bergh van den P, Dobber R, Ramlal S. Role of opioid peptides in the regulation of cytokine production by murine CD4$^+$ T cells. Cell Immunol 1994;154:109–122.
117. Hiddinga HJ. Isaak DD, Lewis RV. Enkephalin-containing peptides processed from proenkephalin significantly enhance the antibody-forming cell responses to antigens. J Immunol 1994;152:3748–59.
118. Mazorow DL, Simpkins CO, Millar DB. Beta-endorphin modulates calcium channel activity in human neutrophils. J Neuroimmunol 1994;50:77–83.
119. Machelska H, Cabot PJ, Mousa SA, Zhang Q, Stein C. Pain control in inflammation governed by selectins Nat Med 1998;4:1425–8.
120. Aymerich MS, Bengoechea-Alonso MT, Lopez-Zabalza MJ, Santiago E, Lopez-Moratalla. Inducible nitric oxide synthase (iNOS) expression in human monocytes triggered by beta-endorphin through an increase in cAMP. Biochem Biophys Res Commun 1988;245: 717–21.
121. Pasnik J, Tchorzewski H, Baj Z, Luciak M, Tchorzewski M. Priming effect of met-enkephalin and beta-endorphin on chemiluminescence, chemotaxis and CD11b molecule expression on human neutrophils in vitro. Immunol Lett 1999;67:77–83.
122. Jessop DS, Major GN, Coventry TL, Kaye SJ, Fulford AJ, Harbuz MS, De Bree FM. Novel opioid peptides endomorphin-1 and endomorphin-2 are present in mammalian immune tissues. J Neuroimmunol 2000;106:53–9.
123. Azuma Y, Want P, Shinohara M, Ohura K. Immunomodulation of the neutrophil respiratory burst by endomorphins 1 and 2. Immunol Lett 2000;75:55–9.
124. Dimitrijevic M, Stanojevic S, Kovacevic-Jovanovic V, Miletic T, Vujic-Redzic V, Radulovic J. Modulation of humoral immune responses in the rat by centrally applied Met-Enk and opioid receptor antagonists: functional interactions of brain OP1, OP2 and OP3 receptors. Immunopharmacology. 2000;49:255–62.
125. Catania A, Lipton JM. The neuropeptide alpha-melanocyte-stimulating hormone: a key component of neuroimmunomodulation. Neuroimmunomodulation 1994;1:93–99.
126. Papadopoulos AD, Wardlaw SL. Endogenous alpha-MSH modulates the hypothalamic-pituitary-adrenal response to the cytokine interleukin-1beta. J Neuroendocrinol 1999;11: 315–9.
127. Brzoska T, Kalden DH, Scholzen T, Luger TA. Molecular basis of the α-MSH/IL-1 antagonism. Ann NY Acad Sci 1999;885:230–8.
128. Lipton JM, Catania A. Mechanisms of antiinflammatory action of the neuroimmunomodulatory peptide α-MSH. Ann NY Acad Sci 1998;840:373–80.

129. Blalock JE. Proopiomelanocortin and the immune-neuroendocrine connection. Ann NY Acad Sci 1999;885:161–72.
130. Luger TA, Kalden D, Scholzen TE, Brzoska T. α-MSH as a mediator of tolerance induction. Pathobiology 1999a;67:318–21.
131. Luger TA, Schwarz T, Kalden H, Scholzen T, Schwarz A, Brzoska T. Role of epidermal cell-derived α-MSH in ultraviolet light mediated local immunosuppresion. Ann NY Acad Sci 1999; 885:209–16.
132. Jessop DS, Jukes KE, Lightman SL. Release of alpha-melanocyte-stimulating hormone from rat splenocytes in vitro is dependent on protein synthesis. Immunol Lett 1994;41: 191–94.
133. Schauer E, Trautinger F, Kock A. Proopiomelanocortin-derived peptides are synthesized and released by human keratinocytes. J Clin Invest 1994;93:2258–62.
134. Taylor AW, Streilein JW, Cousins SW. Immunoreactive vasoactive intestinal peptide contributes to the immunosuppressive activity of normal aqueous humor. J Immunol 1994a;153:1080–86.
135. Slominski A, Wortsman J, Luger T, Paus R, Solomon S. Corticotropin releasing hormone and proopiomelanocortin involvement in the cutaneous response to stress. Physiol Rev 2000;80:979–1020.
136. Glyn-Ballinger JR, Bernardini GL, Lipton JM. Alpha-MSH injected into the septal region reduces fever in rabbits. Peptides 1983;4:199.
137. Murphy MT, Richards DB, Lipton JM. Antipyretic potency of centrally administered alpha-melanocyte stimulating hormone. Science 1983;221:192–93.
138. Cannon JG, Tatro JB, Reichlin S, Dinarello CA. Alpha melanocyte stimulating hormone inhibits immunostimulatory and inflammatory actions of interleukin 1. J Immunol 1986;337:2232–36.
139. Dardenne M, Itoh T, Homo-Delarche F. Presence of glucocorticoid receptors in cultured thymic epithelial cells. Cell Immunol 1986;100:112–118.
140. Robertson B, Dostal K, Daynes RA. Neuropeptide regulation of inflammatory and immunologic responses: The capacity of α-melanocyte-stimulating hormone to inhibit tumor necrosis factor and IL-1-inducible biologic responses. J Immunol 1988;140:4300–4307.
141. Sundar SK, Becker KJ, Cierpial MA. Intracerebro-ventricular infusion of interleukin 1 rapidly decreases peripheral cellular immune responses. Proc Natl Acad Sci USA 1989;6398–402.
142. Goelst K, Mitchell D, Laburn H. Effects of α-melanocyte stimulating hormone on fever caused by endotoxin in rabbits. J Physiol 1991;441:469–476.
143. Taylor AW, Streilein JW, Cousins SW. Alpha-melanocyte-stimulating hormone suppresses antigen-stimulated T cell production of gamma-interferon. Neuroimmunomodulation 1994b;1:188–194.
144. Bhardwaj RS, Schwarz A, Becher E, Mahnke K, Aragane Y, Schwarz T, Luger TA. Pro-opiomelanocortin-derived peptides induce IL-10 production in human monocytes. J Immunol 1996;156:2517–21.
145. Luger TA, Scholzen T. Brzoska T, Becher E, Slominski A, Paus R. Cutaneous immunomodulation and coordination of skin stress responses by α-MSH. Ann NY Acad Sci 1998;840:381–94.
146. Mellado M, Fernandez-Agullo T, Rodriguez-Frade JM, San Frutos MG, de la Pena P, Martinez-A C, Montoya E, Expression analysis of the thyrotropin-releasing hormone

receptor (TRHR) in the immune system using agonist anti-TRHR monoclonal antibodies. FEBS Lett 1999;451:308–14.
147. Luger TA, Scholzen T. Brzoska T, Becher E, Slominski A, Paus R. Cutaneous immunomodulation and coordination of skin stress responses by α-MSH. Ann NY Acad Sci 1998;840:381–94.
148. Raiden S, Polack E, Nahmod V, Labeur M, Holsboer F, Larzt E. TRH receptor on immune cells: in vitro and in vivo stimulation of human lymphocyte and rat splenocyte DNA synthesis by TRH. J Clin Immunol 1995;15:242–49.
149. Wang J, Klein JR. Thymus-neuroendocrine interactions in extrathymic T cell development. Science 1994;265:1860–62.
150. Komorowski J, Zylinska K, Pawlikowski M, Stepien H. Stimulatory effect of thyrotropin (TSH) on interleukin-2 (IL-2) release from human peripheral blood lymphocytes. A dose-response study in vitro. Hormones Metab Res 1993;25:598–99.
151. Grasso G, Massai L, De Leo V, Muscettola M. The effect of LHRH and TRH on human interferon-gamma production in vivo and in vitro. Life Sci 1998;62:2005–14.
152. Van den Berghe G, de Zegher F, Vlasselaers D, Schetz M, Verwaest C, Ferdinande P, Lauwers P. Thyrotropin-releasing hormone in critical illness: from a dopamine-dependent test to a strategy for increasing low serum triiodothyronine, prolactin, and growth hormone concentrations. Crit Care Med 1996;24:590–5.
153. Bagriacik EU, Klein JR. The thyrotropin (thyroid-stimulating hormone) receptor is expressed on murine dendritic cells and on a subset of CD45RB high lymph node T cells: functional role for thyroid-stimulating hormone during immune activation. J Immunol 2000;164:6158–65.
154. Harbour DV, Leon S, Keating C, Hughes K. Thyrotropin modulates B-cell function through specific bioactive receptors. Prog Neuroendocrinimmunol 1990;3:266–76.
155. Coutelier JP, Kehrl JH, Bellur SS. Binding and functional effects of thyroid stimulating hormone on human immune cells. J Clin Immunol 1990;10:204–10.
156. Provinciali M, Di Stefano G, Fabris N. Improvement in the proliferative capacity and natural killer cell activity of murine spleen lymphocytes by thyrotropin. Int J Immunopharmacol 1992;14:865–70.
157. Todd I, Pujol-Borrell R, Hammond LJ, McNally JM, Feldman M, Bottazzo GF. Enhancement of thyrocyte HLA class II expression by thyroid stimulating hormone. Clin Exp Immunol 1987;69:524–31.
158. Whetsell M, Bagriacik EU, Seetharamaiah GS, Prabhakar BS, Klein JR. Neuroendocrine-induced synthesis of bone marrow-derived cytokines with inflammatory immunomodulating properties. Cell Immunol 1999;192:159–66.
159. Peele ME, Carr FE, Baker Jr JR, Wartofsky L, Burman KD. TSH beta subunit gene expression in human lymphocyte. Am J Med Sci 1993;305:1–7.
160. Fabris N, Mocchegiani E, Provinciali M. Pituitary-thyroid axis and immune system: a reciprocal neuroendocrine-immune interaction. Horm Res;1995:43:29–38.
161. Haddad EE, Mashaly MM. In vivo effects of TRH, T3 and cGH on antibody production and lymphocytes-T and lymphocytes-B proliferation in immature male chickens. Immunol Invest 1991;20:557–68.
162. Stein-Streilein J, Zakarija M, Papic M, McKenzie JM. Hyperthyroxinemic mice have reduced natural killer cell activity: Evidence for a defective trigger mechanism. J Immunol 1987;139:2502–07.
163. Turaihi K, Khan FA, Baron DN, Dandona P. Effect of short term triiodothyronine

administration on human leukocyte Fb (K) influx and Na efflux. J Clin Endocrinol Metab 1987;65:1031–34.
164. Schoenfeld PS, Myers JW, Myers L, LaRocque JC. Suppression of cell-mediated immunity in hypothyroidism. South Med J 1995;88:347–49.
165. Ohashi H, Itoh M. Effects of thyroid hormones on the lymphocyte phenotypes in rats: changes in lymphocyte subsets related to thyroid function. Endocr Regul 1994;18:117–23.
166. Cole NA, Allowvan RH, Rodrigues SL, Purdy CW. Influence of triiodothyronine injections on calf immune response to an infectious bovine rhinotracheitis virus challenge and nitrogen balance of lambs. J Amin Sci 1994;72:1263–73.
167. Ingram KG, Crouch DA, Douez DL, Croy BA, Woodward B. Effects of triiodothyronine supplements on splenic natural killer cells in malnourished weanling mice. Int J Immunopharmacol 1995;17:21–31.
168. Wang J, Klein JR. Hormone regulation of murine T cells: potent tissue-specific immunosuppressive effects of thyroxine targeted to gut T cells. Int Immunol 1996;8: 231–5.
169. Mariani E, Ravaglia G, Forti P, Meneghetti A, Tarozzi A, Maioli F, Boschi F, Pratelli L, Pizzoferrato A, Piras F, Facchini A. Vitamin D, thyroid hormones and muscle mass influence natural killer (NK) innate immunity in healthy nonagenarians and centenarians. Clin Exp Immunol 1999;117:206.
170. Simons PJ, Delemarre FG, Drexhage HA. Antigen-presenting dendritic cells as regulators of the growth of thyrocytes: a role of interleukin-1beta and interleukin-6. Endocrinology 1998;139:3148–56.
171. Rasmussen AK. Cytokine actions on the thyroid gland. Dan Med Bull 2000;47:94–114.
172. Brtko J, Jurcovicova J, Schmutzler C, Rokyta R, Svik K, Bobal'ova J. Adjuvant arthritis in the rat is associated with decreased binding of nuclear receptors to thyroid hormone responsive element in spleen extracts. Gen Physiol Biophys 1998;17:341–7.
173. Dorshkind K, Horseman N. The roles of prolactin, growth hormone, insulin-like growth factor-I and thyroid hormones in lymphocyte development and function: insights from genetic models of hormone and hormone receptor deficiency. Endocrine Rev 2000;21: 292–312.
174. Gee AP, Boyle MDP, Munger KL. Nerve growth factor: stimulation of polymorphonuclear leukocyte chemotaxis in vitro. Proc Natl Acad Sci USA 1983;80:7213–18.
175. Boyle MDP, Lawman MJP, Gee AP, Young M. Nerve growth factor: a chemotactic factor for polymorphonuclear leukocytes in vivo. J Immunol 1985;135:564–68.
176. Bornstein SR, Licinio J, Tauchnitz R, Engelmann L, Negrao AB, Gold P, Chrousos GP. Plasma leptin levels are increased in survivors of acute sepsis: associated loss of diurnal rhythm, in cortisol and leptin secretion. J Clin Endocrinol Metab 1998;83:280–3.
177. Giovambattista A, Chisari AN, Corro L, Gaillard RC, Spinedi E. Metabolic, neuroendocrine and immune functions in basal conditions and during the acute-phase response to endotoxic shock in undernourished rats. Neuroimmunomodulation 2000;7:92–8.
178. Okamoto S, Irie Y, Ishikawa I, Kimura K, Masayuki Saito. Central leptin suppresses splenic lymphocyte functions through activation of the corticotropin-releasing hormone-sympathetic nervous system. Brain Res 2000;855:192–97.
179. Chautard T, Spinedi E, Voirol M, Pralong FP, Gaillard RC. Role of glucocorticoids in the response of the hypothalamo-corticotrope, immune and adipose systems to repeated endotoxin administration. Neuroendocrinology 1999;69:360–69.

180. Torpy DJ, Bornstein SR, Chrousos GP. Leptin and interleukin-6 in sepsis. Horm Metab Res 1998;30:726–9.
181. Faggioni R, Fantuzzi G, Gabay C, Moser A, Dinarello CA, Feingold KR, Grunfeld C. Leptin deficiency enhances sensitivity to endotoxin-induced lethality. Am J Physiol 1999;276:R136–42.
182. Takahashi N, Waelput W, Guisez Y. Leptin is an endogenous protective protein against the toxicity exerted by tumor necrosis factor. J Exp Med 1999;189:207–12.
183. Finck BN, Kelley KW, Dantzer R, Johnson RW. In vivo and in vitro evidence for the involvement of tumor necrosis factor-alpha in the induction of leptin by lipopolysaccharide. Endocrinology 1998;139:2278–83.
184. Loffreda S, Yang SQ, Lin HZ, Karp CL, Brengman ML, Wang DJ, Klein AS, Bulkley GB, Bao C, Noble PW, Lane MD, Diehl AM. Leptin regulates proinflammatory immune responses. FASEB J 1998;12:57–65.
185. Fantuzzi G, Faggioni R. Leptin in the regulation of immunity, inflammation, and hematopoiesis. J Leukoc Biol 2000;68:437–46.
186. Malkinson, TJ, Bridges TE, Lederis K, Veale WL. Perfusion of the septum of the rabbit with vasopressin antiserum enhances endotoxin fever. Peptides 1987;8:385–89.
187. Torres BA, Johnson HW. Arginine vasopressin (AVP) replacement of helper cell requirement in IFN-γ production: evidence for a novel AVP receptor on mouse lymphocytes. J Immunol 1988;140:2179–83.
188. Lee HR, Ho WZ, Douglas SD. Substance P augments tumor necrosis factor release in human monocyte-derived macrophages. Clin Diagn Lab Immunol 1994;1:419–223.
189. Nair MPN, Schwartz SA. Immunomodulatory effects of corticosteroids on natural killer and antibody-dependent cellular cytotoxic activities of human lymphocytes. J Immunol 1984;132:2876–82.
190. Chancellor-Freeland C, Zhu GF, Kage R, Beller DI, Leeman SE, Black PH. Substance P and stress-induced changes in macrophages. Ann NY Acad Sci 1995;771:472–84.
191. Payan DG, McGillis JP, Renold FK, Mitsuhashi M, Goetzl EJ. The immunomodulating properties of neuropeptides. In: Berczi I, Kovacs K, editors. Hormones and Immunity. Lancaster, England: MTP Press;1987.
192. Foreman, JC. Neuropeptides and the pathogenesis of allergy. Allergy 1987;42:1–11.
193. Shanahan F, Lee TDG, Bienenstock J, Befus AD. Mast cell heterogeneity: Effect of anti-allergic compounds on neuropeptide-induced histamine release. Int Arch Allergy Appl Immunol 1986;80:424–26.
194. Jancso G, Obal Jr. F, Toth-Kasa I, Katona M, Husz S. The modulation of cutaneous inflammatory reactions by peptide-containing sensory nerves. Int J Tissue React 1985;7: 449–57.
195. Serra M, Bazzoni F, Della Bianca V, Greskowiak M, Rossi F. Activaiton of human neutrophils by substance P: Effect on oxidative metabolism, exocytosis, cytosolic Ca^{2+} concentration and inositol phosphate formation. J Immunol 1988;141:2118–24.
196. Lotz M, Carson DA, Vaughan JH. Substance P activation of rheumatoid synoviocytes: Neural pathway in pathogenesis of arthritis. Science 1987;235:893–95.
197. Hartung HP, Heininger K, Schafer B, Toyka KV. Substance P and astrocytes: stimulation of the cyclooxygenase pathway of arachidonic acid metabolism. Fed Am Soc Exp Bio J 1988;2:48–51.
198. Rameshar P, Ganea D, Gascon P. Induction of IL-3 and granulocyte-macrophage colony-stimulating factor by substance P in bone marrow cells is partially mediated through the

release of IL-1 and IL-6. J Immunol 1994;152:4044–54.
199. Damonneville M, Monte D, Auriault C, Capron A. The neuropeptide substance-P stimulates the effector functions of platelets. Clin Exp Immunol 1990;81:346–51.
200. Nong YH, Titus RG, Ribeiro JMC, Remold HG. Peptides encoded by the calcitonin gene inhibit macrophage function. J Immunol 1989;145:45–49.
201. Wang F, Millet I, Bottomly K, Vignery A. Calcitonin gene-related peptide inhibits interleukin 2 production by murine T lymphocytes. J Biol Chem 1992;267:21052–57.
202. Wang J, Klein JR. Thymus-neuroendocrine interactions in extrathymic T cell development. Science 1994;265:1860–62.
203. Foris G, Gyimesi E, Komaromi I. The mechanism of antibody-dependent cellular cytotoxicity stimulation by somatostatin in rat peritoneal macrophages. Cell Immunol 1985;90:217–25.
204. Muscettola M, Grasso G. Somatostatin and vasoactive intestinal peptide reduce interferon gamma production by human peripheral blood mononuclear cells. Immunobiology 1990;180:419–30.
205. Church MK, El-Lati S, Caulfied JP. Neuropeptide-induced secretion from human skin mast cells. Int Arch Allergy Appl Immunol 1991;94:310–18.
206. Fuente de la M, Delgado M, del Rio M, Garrido E, Leceta J, Hernanz A, Gomariz RP. Vasoactive intestinal peptide modulation of adherence and mobility in rat peritoneal lymphocytes and macrophages. Peptides 1994;15:1157–63.
207. Ichinose M, Asai M, Imai K, Sawada M. Enhancement of phagocytosis in mouse macrophages by pituitary adenylate cyclase activating polypeptide (PACAP) and related peptides. Immunopharmacology 1995;30:217–24.
208. Leceta J, Martinez MC, Delgado M, Garrido E, Gomariz RP. Lymphoid cell subpopulations containing vasoactive intestinal peptide in the rat. Peptides 1994;15:791–97.
209. Delgado M, Ganea D. Inhibition of IFN-gamma-induced janus kinase-1-STAT1 activation in macrophages by vasoactive intestinal peptide and pituitary adenylate cyclase-activating polypeptide. J Immunol 2000; 165:3051–7.
210. Sun W, Tadmori I, Yang L, Delgado M, Ganea D. Vasoactive intestinal peptide (VIP) inhibits TGF-beta1 production in murine macrophages. J Neuroimmunol 2000;107: 88–99.
211. Xin Z, Sriram S. Vasoactive intestinal peptide inhibits IL-12 and nitric oxide production in murine macrophages. J Neuroimmunol 1998; 89:206–12.
212. Kawamura N, Tamura H, Obana S, Wenner M, Ishikawa T, Nakata A, Yamamoto H. Differential effects of neuropeptides on cytokine production by mouse helper T cell subsets. Neuroimmunomodulation 1998;5:9–15.
213. Martinez C, Delgado M, Pozo D, Leceta J, Calvo JR, Ganea D, Gomariz RP. Vasoactive intestinal peptide and pituitary adenylate cyclase-activating polypeptide modulate endotoxin-induced IL-6 production by murine peritoneal macrophages. J Leukoc Biol 1998; 63:591–601.
214. Tang H, Sun L, Xin Z, Ganea D. Down-regulation of cytokine expression in murine lymphocytes by PACAP and VIP. Ann N Y Acad Sci 1996;805:768–78.
215. Berczi I. Neuroimmune Biology: An introduction. In "Neuroimmune Biology Volume 1: New foundation of Biology" I. Berczi I, Gorczynski R, Editors, Elsevier, 2001; pp. 3–45.
216. Homo-Delarche F. Duval D. Glucocorticoid receptors in lymphoid tissue. In Hormones and Immunity, Berczi I, Kovacs K, editors, Lancaster, England, MTP Press, 1987; 1–19.
217. Miller AH, Spencer RL, Husain A, Rhee R, McEwen BS. Stein M. Differential expression of

type I adrenal steroid receptors in immune tissues is associated with tissue-specific regulation of type II receptors by aldosterone, Endocrinology 1993; 133: 2133–40.
218. Karin M. Ynag-Yen H-F, Chambard J-C, Deng T, Saatcioglu F. Various modes of gene regulation by nuclear receptors for steroid and thyroid hormones. Eur J Clin Pharmacol 1993;45:S9–15.
219. Scheinman RI, Cogswell PC, Lofquist AK, Baldwin Jr. AS. Role of transcriptional activation of IκBα in mediation of immunosuppression by glucocorticoids, Science 1995;270: 283–6.
220. Auphan N, DiDonato JA, Rosette C, Helmberg A, Karin M. Immunosuppression by glucocorticoids: inhibition of NF-κB activity through induction of IκB synthesis, Science 1995;270: 286–90.
221. Adcock IM, Brown CR, Gelder GM, Shirasaki H, Peters MJ, Barnes PJ. Effects of glucocorticoids on transcription factor activation in human peripheral blood mononuclear cells. Am J Physiol 1995;268: C331–8.
222. Watson CS, Gametchu B. Membrane estrogen and glucocorticoid receptors—implications for hormonal control of immune function and autoimmunity. Int Immunopharmacol 2001;1: 1049–63.
223. Angeli A, Masera RG, Sartori ML, Fortunati N, Racca S, Dovio A, Staurenghi A, Frairia R. Modulation by cytokines of glucocorticoid action. Ann N Y Acad Sci 1999;876:210–20.
224. Ahluwalia A, Newbold P. Brain SD, Flower RJ. Topical glucocorticoids inhibit neurogenic inflammation: involvement of lipocortin 1. Eur J Pharmacol 1995;283: 193–8.
225. Taylor AD, Loxley HD, Flower RJ, Buckingham JC. Immunoneutralization of lipocortin 1 reverses the acute inhibitory effects of dexamethasone on the hypothalamo-pituitary-adrenocortical responses to cytokines in the rat in vitro and in vivo. Neuroendocrinology 1995;62: 19–31.
226. Barnes PJ. Adcock IM. Steroid resistance in asthma. QJ Med 1995;88:455–68.
227. Herrlich P. Cross-talk between glucocorticoid receptor and AP-1. Oncogene 2001;20: 2465–75.
228. Vacchio MS, Papadopoulos, Ashwell JD. Steroid production in the thymus: implications for thymocyte selection. J Exp Med 1994;179:1835–846.
229. King LB, Vacchio MS, Dixon K, Hunziker R, Margulies DH, Ashwell JD. A targeted glucocorticoid receptor antisense transgene increases thymocyte apoptosis and alters thymocyte development. Immunity 1995;3: 647–56.
230. Vacchio MS, Lee JY, Ashwell JD. Thymus-derived glucocorticoids set the thresholds for thymocyte selection by inhibiting TCR-mediated thymocyte activation. J Immunol 1999;163:1327–33.
231. Thompson EB. Apoptosis and steroids. Mol Endocrinol 1994;8:665–73.
232. Homo-Delarche F, Duval D, Papiernik M. Prostaglandin produciton by phagocytic cells of the mouse thymic reticulum in culture and its modulation by indomethacin and corticosteroids. J Immunol 1985;135:506–12.
233. Arzt E, Kovalovsky D, Igaz LM, Costas M, Plazas P, Refojo D, Paez-Pereda M, Reul JM, Stalla G, Holsboer F. Functional cross-talk among cytokines, T-cell receptor, and glucocorticoid receptor transcriptional activity and action. Ann N Y Acad Sci 2000;917: 672–77.
234. Chao TC, Van-Alten PJ, Walter RJ. Steroid and sex hormones and macrophage function: modulation of reactive oxygen intermediates and nitrite release. Amer J Reprod Immunol 1994;32:43–52.
235. Munck A, Naray-Fejes-Toth A, Guyre PM. Mechanisms of glucocorticoid actions on the

immune system. In: Berczi I, Kovacks K, editors. Hormones and Immunity. Lancaster, England:MTP Press;1987.
236. Sauer J, Castren M, Hopfner U, Holsboer F, Stalla GK, Arzt E. Inhibition of lipopolysaccharide-induced monocyte interleukin-1 receptor antagonist synthesis by cortisol: involvement of the mineralocorticoid receptor. J Clin Endocrinol Metab 1996;81: 73–79.
237. Gerrard TL, Cupps TR, Jurgensen CH, Fauci AS. Increased expression of HLA-DR antigens in hydrocortisone-treated monocytes. Cell Immunol 1984;84:311–16.
238. Strickland RW, Wahl LM, Finbloom DS. Corticosteroids enhance the binding of recombinant interferon-gamma to cultured human monocytes. J Immunol 1986;137:1577–80.
239. Girard MT, Jhaltadottir S, Fejes-Toth AN, Guyre PM. Glucocorticoids enhance the γ-interferon augmentation of human monocyte immunoglobulin G Fc receptor expression. J Immunol 1987;138:3235–3241.
240. Calandra T, Bernhagen J, Metz CN, Spiegel LA, Bacher M, Donnelly T, Cerami A, Bucala R. MIF as a glucocorticoid-induced modulator of cytokine production. Nature 1995;377: 68.
241. Franchimont D, Galon J, Gadina M, Visconti R, Zhou Y, Aringer M, Frucht DM, Chrousos GP, O'Shea JJ. Inhibition of Th1 immune response by glucocorticoids: dexamethasone selectively inhibits IL-12-induced Stat4 phosphorylation in T lymphocytes. J Immunol 2000;164:1768–74.
242. Gatti G, Cavallo R, Sartori ML, Marinone C, Angeli A. Cortisol at physiological concentrations and prostagladin E_2 are additive inhibitors of human natural killer cell activity. Immunopharmacology 1986;11:119–28.
243. Schleimer RP. An overview of glucocorticoid anti-inflammatory actions. Eur J Clin Pharmacol 1993;45:S3–7.
244. Sternberg EM. Neuroendocrine factors in susceptibility to inflammatory disease: focus on the hypothalamic-pituitary-adrenal axis. Horm Res 1995;43:159–61.
245. Karalis K, Sano H, Redwine J. Autocrine or paracrine inflammatory actions of corticotropin-releasing hormone in vivo. Science 1991;421–423.
246. Molijn GJ, Spek JJ, vanUffelen JCJ, de Jong FH, Brinkmann AO, Bruining HA, Lamberts SWJ, Koper JW. Differential adaption of glucocorticoid sensitivity of peripheral blood mononuclear leukocytes in patients with sepsis or septic shock. J Clin Endocrinol Metab 1995;80:1799–1803.
247. Lavker RM, Schechter NM. Cutaneous mast cell depletion results from topical corticosteroid usage. J Immunol 1985;135:2368–373.
248. Bergstrand H, Bjornsson A, Lundquist B, Nilsson A, Brattsand R. Inhibitory effect of glucocorticosteroids on anti-IgE-induced histamine release from human basophilic leukocytes: Evidence for a dual mechanism of action. Allergy 1983;39:217–30.
249. Bakker JM, Kavelaars A, Kamphuis PJ, Cobelens PM, van Vugt HH, van Bel F, Heijnen CJ. Neonatal dexamethasone treatment increases susceptibility to experimental autoimmune disease in adult rats. J Immunol 2000;165:5932–37.
250. Ruzek MC, Pearce BD, Miller AH, Biron CA. Endogenous glucocorticoids protect against cytokine-mediated lethality during viral infection. J Immunol 1999;162:3527–33.
251. Miller AH, Spencer RL, Hassett J, Kim C, Rhee R, Ciurea D, Dhabhar F, McEwen B, Stein M. Effects of selective type I and II adrenal steroid agonists on immune cell distribution. Endocrinology 1994;135:1934–44.
252. Cannon JG. Adaptive interactions between cytokines and the hypothalamic-pituitary-

gonadal axis. Ann N Y Acad Sci 1998;856:234–42.
253. Kalra PS, Edwards TG, Xu B, Jain M, Kalra SP.The anti-gonadotropic effects of cytokines: the role of neuropeptides. Domest Anim Endocrinol 1998;15:321–32.
254. Grossman CG, editor. Bilateral Communication between the Endocrine and Immune Systems. New York:Springer-Verlag, 1994.
255. Stimson WH. Sex steroids, steroid receptors and immunity. In: Berczi I, Kovacs K, editors. Hormones and Immunity. Lancaster, England:MTP Press, 1987;43–53.
256. Myers JM, Heim MC, Hirsch KS, Queener SF, Peterson BH. Translocatable estrogen receptors in rat splenocytes. Life Sci 1986;39:313–320.
257. Kovacs WJ, Olsen NJ. Androgen receptors in human thymocytes. J Immunol 1987;139–490–93.
258. Baral E, Nagy E, Berczi I. The effect of tamoxifen on the immune response. In: Kellen JA, editor. Tamoxifen beyond the antiestrogen. Boston:Birkhauser, 1996;137–78.
259. Kushner PJ, Agard DA, Greene GL, Scanlan TS, Shiau AK, Uht RM, Webb P. Estrogen receptor pathways to AP-1. J Steroid Biochem Mol Biol 2000;74:311–7.
260. Kato S S.Estrogen receptor-mediated cross-talk with growth factor signaling pathways. Breast Cancer 2001;8:3–9.
261. Ray P, Ghosh SK, Zhang DH, Ray A. Repression of interleukin-6 gene expression by 17 beta-estradiol: inhibition of the DNA-binding activity of the transcription factors NF-IL6 and NF-kappa B by the estrogen receptor. FEBS Lett 1997;409:79–85.
262. DeMarzo AM, Beck CA, Onate SA, Edwards DP. Dimerization of mammalian progesterone receptors occurs in the absence of DNA and is related to the release of the 90-k-Da heat shock protein. Proc Natl Acad Sci USA 1991;88:72–76.
263. Mohamed MK, Tung L, Takimoto GS, Horwitz KB. The leucine zippers of c-fos and c-jun for progesterone receptor dimerization: A-dominance in the A/B heterodimer. J Steroid Biochem Mol Biol 1994;51:241–50.
264. Conneely OM. Perspective: female steroid hormone action. Endocrinology 2001;142: 2194–99.
265. Nelson JL, Steinberg AD. Sex steroids, autoimmunity and autoimmune disease. In: Berczi I, Kovacs K, editors. Hormones and Immunity. MTP Press:Lancaster, England, 1987, pp93–119.
266. Berczi I, Chalmers IM, Nagy E, Warrington RJ. The immune effects of neuropeptides. Bailliere Clin Rheumatol 1996;10:227–57.
267. Robert R, Spitzer JA. Effects of female hormones (17beta-estradiol and progesterone) on nitric oxide production by alveolar macrophages in rats. Nitric Oxide 1997;1:453–62.
268. Salem ML, Hossain MS, Nomoto K. Mediation of the immunomodulatory effect of beta-estradiol on inflammatory responses by inhibition of recruitment and activation of inflammatory cells and their gene expression of TNF-alpha and IFN-gamma. Int Arch Allergy Immunol 2000;121:235–45.
269. Nilsson N, Carlsten H. Estrogen induces suppression of natural killer cell cytotoxicity and augmentation of polyclonal B cell activation. Cell Immunol 1994;158:131–39.
270. Keller ET, Zhang J, Yao Z, Qi Y. The impact of chronic estrogen deprivation on immunologic parameters in the ovariectomized rhesus monkey (Macaca mulatta) model of menopause. J Reprod Immunol 2001;50:41–55.
271. Gilmore W, Weiner LP, Correale J. Effect of estradiol on cytokine secretion by proteolipid protein-specific T cell clones isolated from multiple sclerosis patients and normal control subjects. J Immunol 1997;158:446–51.

272. Orvieto R, Ben-Rafael Z, Abir R, Bar-Hava I, Fisch B, Molad Y. Controlled ovarian hyperstimulation: a state of neutrophil activation. Am J Reprod Immunol 1999;42:288–91.
273. Berczi I, Chow DA, Baral E, Nagy E. Neuroimmunoregulation and cancer. Int J Oncol 1998;13:1049–1051.
274. Nagy E, Baral E, Berczi I. Immune System. In: Oettel M, editor. Handbook of Experimental Pharmacology: Estrogens and anti-estrogens. Section IV. Physiology and Pathophysiology of Estrogens. Jena,Germany:Springer-Verlag 1999;135/I:343–351.
275. Nagy E, Berczi I, Baral E. Combination immunotherapy of cancer. In: Berczi I, Gorczynski R, editors. Neuroimmune Biology: New Foundations of Biology. Amsterdam: Elsevier, 2001; pp. 417–432.
276. Nagy E, Berczi I. Immunomodulation by tamoxifen and pergolide. Immunopharmacology 1986;12:145–153.
277. Baral E, Nagy E, Berczi I. Modulation of natural killer cell mediated cytotoxicity by tamoxifen and estradiol. Cancer 1995;75:591–99.
278. Baral E, Nagy E, Berczi I. Modulation of lymphokine-activated killer cell-mediated cytotoxicity by estradiol and tamoxifen. Int J Cancer 1996;66:214–18.
279. Baral E, Nagy E, Kangas L, Berczi I. Anti-estrogens enhance the therapeutic effect of lymphokine activated killer cells on the P815 murine mastocytoma. Int J Cancer 1996; 67: 580–85.
280. Baral E, Nagy E, Kangas L, Berczi I. Immunotherapy of the SL2–5 murine lymphoma with natural killer cells and tamoxifen or toremifene. Anticancer Res. 1997;17:77–84.
281. Baral E, Nagy E, Kangas L, Berczi I. Combination therapy of the H2712 murine mammary carcinoma with cytotoxic T lymphocytes and anti-estrogens. Anticancer Res 1997;17: 3647–52.
282. Baral E, Nagy E, Kangas L, Berczi I. Combination immunotherapy of the P815 murine mastocytoma with killer cells, IL-2 and anti-estrogens. Anticancer Res. 1997;17:3653–58.
283. Haeryfar SMM, Nagy E, Baral E, Krepart GE, Lotocki R J, Berczi I. Antiestrogens affect both pathways of killer cell-mediated oncolysis. Anticancer Res 2000;20:1849–53.
284. Nagy E, Baral E, Kangas L, Berczi I. Anti-estrogens potentiate the immunotherapy of the P815 murine mastocytoma by cytotoxic T lymphocytes. Anticancer Res 1997;17:1083–1088.
285. Baral E, Nagy E, Krepart GE, Lotocki RJ, Unruh HW, Berczi I. Antiestrogens sensitize human ovarian and lung carcinomas for lysis by autologous killer cells. Anticancer Res 2000;20:2027–31.
286. Zhou Z, Shackleton CH, Pahwa S, White PC, Speiser PW. Prominent sex steroid metabolism in human lymphocytes. Mol Cell Endocrinol 1998;138:61–69.
287. Ravache ES, Steiberg AD. Sex hormones in autoimmunity. In Pituitary Function and Immunity, Berczi I. Editor, CRC Press, Boca Raton, CA 1986; pp.283–301.
288. Ahmed SA, Talal N, Christadoss P. Genetic regulation of testosterone-induced immune suppression. Cell Immunol 1987;104:91–98.
289. Fried W, Morley C. Effects of androgenic steroids on erythropoiesis. Steroids 1985;46: 799–826.
290. Greenstein BD, de Bridges EF, Fitzpatrick FT. Aromatase inhibitors regenerate the thymus in aging male rats. Int J Immunopharmacol. 1992;14:541–53.
291. Araneo BA, Dowell T, Diegel M, Daynes RA. Dihydrotestosterone exerts a depressive influence on the production of interleukin-4 (IL-4), IL-5 and γ-interferon, but not IL-2 by

activated murine T cells. Blood 1991;78:688–99.

292. Friedl R, Brunner M, Moeslinger T, Spieckermann PG. Testosterone inhibits expression of inducible nitric oxide synthase in murine macrophages. Life Sci 2000;68:417–29.
293. Gomez F, Ruiz P, Lopez R, Rivera C, Romero S, Bernal JA. Effects of androgen treatment on expression of macrophage Fcgamma receptors. Clin Diagn Lab Immunol 2000;7:682–6.
294. Giltay EJ, Fonk JC, von Blomberg BM, Drexhage HA, Schalkwijk C, Gooren LJ. In vivo effects of sex steroids on lymphocyte responsiveness and immunoglobulin levels in humans. J Clin Endocrinol Metab 2000;85:1648–57.
295. Olsen NJ, Zhou P, Ong H, Kovacs WJ. Testosterone induces expression of transforming growth factor-beta 1 in the murine thymus. J Steroid Biochem Mol Biol. 1993;45:327–32.
296. Angele MK, Knoferl MW, Schwacha MG, Ayala A, Cioffi WG, Bland KI, Chaudry IH. Sex steroids regulate pro- and anti-inflammatory cytokine release by macrophages after trauma-hemorrhage. Am J Physiol 1999;277(1 Pt 1):C35–42.
297. Angele MK, Schwacha MG, Ayala A, Chaudry IH. Effect of gender and sex hormones on immune responses following shock. Shock 2000;14:81–90.
298. Morfin R, Courchay G. Pregnenolone and dehydroepiandrosterone as precursors of native 7-hydroxylated metabolites which increase the immune response in mice. J Steroid Biochem Molec Biol 1994;50:91–100.
299. McLachlan JA, Serkin CD, Bakouche O. Dehydroepiandrosterone modulation of lipopolysaccharide-stimulated monocyte cytotoxicity. J Immunol 1996;156:328–35.
300. Regelson W, Loria R, Kalimi M. Dehydroepiandrosterone (DHEA) - the "mother steroid". I immunologic action. Ann NY Acad Sci 1994;719:553–63.
301. Hall GM, Perry LA, Spector TD. Depressed levels of dehydroepiandrosterone sulphate in postmenopausal women with rheumatoid arthritis but no relation with axial bone density. Ann Rheum Dis 1993;52:211–14.
302. Casson PR, Andersen RN, Herrod HG, Stentz FB, Straughn AB, Abraham GE, Buster JE. Oral dehydroepiandrosterone in physiologic doses modulates immune function in postmenopausal women. Am J Obstet Gynecol 1993;169:1563–69.
303. Kalo-Klein A, Witkin SS. Regulation of the immune response to Candida albicans by monocytes and progesterone. Am J Obstet Gynecol 1991;164:1351–54.
304. Nohmi T, Abe S, Dobashi K, Tansho S, Yamaguchi H. Suppression of anti-Candida activity of murine neutrophils by progesterone in vitro: a possible mechanism in pregnant women's vulerability to vaginal candidiasis. Microbiol Immunol 1995;39:405–09.
305. Chao TC, Van Alten PJ, Greager JA, Walter RJ. Steroid sex hormones regulate the release of tumor necrosis factor by macrophages. Cell Immunol 1995;160:43–49.
306. Li ZG, Danis VA, Brooks PM. Effect of gonadal steroids on the production of IL-1 and IL-6 by blood mononuclear cells in vitro. Clin Exp Rheumatol 1993;11:157–62.
307. Scarpellini F, Scarpellini L, Dino N, Benvenuto P. Progesterone immunosuppressive levels and luteal steroid profiles in the cycles induced with clomiphene citrate. Clin Exp Obstet. Gynecol 1993;20–182–88.
308. Check JH, Tarquini P, Gandy P, Lauer C. A randomized study comparing the efficacy of reducing the spontaneous abortion rate following lymphocyte immunotherapy and progesterone treatment versus progesterone alone in primary habitual aborters. Gyncecol Obstet Invest 1995;39:257–61.
309. Szekeres-Bartho J, Barakonyi A, Par G, Polgar B, Palkovics T, Szereday L. Progesterone as an immunomodulatory molecule. Int Immunopharmacol 2001;1:1037–48.

310. McMurray RW, Wilson JG, Bigler L, Xiang L, Lagoo A. Progesterone inhibits glucocorticoid-induced murine thymocyte apoptosis. Int J Immunopharmacol 2000;22: 955–65.
311. Fleming MW, Gamble HR. Consequences of dose-dependent immunosuppression by progesterone on parasitic worm burdens in lambs. Am J Vet Res 1993;54:1299–302.
312. Parr MB, Kepple L, McDermott MR, Drew MD, Bozzola JJ, Parr EL. A mouse model for studies of mucosal immunity to vaginal infection by herpes simplex virus type 2. Lab Invest 1994;70:369–80.
313. Manolagas SC, Yu X-P, Girasole G, Bellido T. Vitamin D and the hematolymphopoietic tissue: a 1994 update. Sem Nephrol 1994;14:129–43.
314. Bouillon R, Garmyn M, Verstuyf A, Segaert S, Casteels K, Mathieu C. Paracrine role for calcitriol in the immune system and skin creates new therapeutic possibilities for vitamin D analogs. Euro J Endocrinol 1995;133:7–16.
315. Jones G, Strugnell SA, DeLuca HF. Current understanding of the molecular actions of vitamin D. Physiol Rev 1998;78:1193–231.
316. Veldman CM, Cantorna MT, DeLuca HF. Expression of 1,25-dihydroxyvitamin D(3) receptor in the immune system. Arch Biochem Biophys 2000;374:334–8.
317. Twers TL, Staeva TP, Freedman LP. A two-hit mechanism for vitamin D3-mediated transcriptional repression of the granulocyte-macrophage colony-stimulating factor gene: vitamin D receptor competes for DNA binding with NFAT1 and stabilizes c-Jun. Mol Cell Biol 1999;19:4191–9.
318. Cippitelli M, Santoni A. Vitamin D3: a transcriptional modulator of the interferon-gamma gene. Eur J Immunol 1998;28:3017–30.
319. Holick MF. Noncalcemic actions of 1,25-dihydroxyvitamin D3 and clinical applications. Bone 1995;17:107S–111S .
320. Nowotny, A. In search of active sites in endotoxins. In: Nowotny A, editor Beneficial Effects of Endotoxins. New York: Plenum Press, 1983;1–55.
321. Boivin A, Mesrobeanu J, Mesrobeanu L. Technique pour la preparation des polysaccharides microbiens specifiques. CR Soc Biol 1933;113:490.
322. Greisman SE. Induction of endotoxin tolerance. In: Nowotny A, editor. Beneficial Effects of Endotoxins. New York: Plenum Press, 1983;149–178.
323. Behling UH. The radioprotective effect of bacterial endotoxin. In: Nowotny A, editor. Beneficial Effects of Endotoxins. New York: Plenum Press, 1983;127–148.
324. Parant M. Effect of LPS on nonspecific resistance to bacterial infections. In: Nowotny A, editor. Beneficial Effects of Endotoxins. New York: Plenum Press, 1983;179–196.
325. Johnson AG. Adjuvant action of bacterial endotoxins on antibody formation. A historical perspective. In: Nowotny A, editor. Beneficial Effects of Endotoxins. New York: Plenum Press,1983;249–253.
326. Butler RC. Enhancement of nonspecific resistance to tumor by endotoxin. In: Nowotny A, editor. Beneficial Effects of Endotoxins. New York: Plenum Press, 1983;497–512.
327. Walker RI. Possibilities for use of endotoxin in compromised subjects. In: A. Nowotny, editor. Beneficial Effects of Endotoxins. New York: Plenum Press, 1983;197–212.
328. Abdelnoor AM. Effect of LPS on the clotting system. In: Nowotny A, editor. Beneficial Effects of Endotoxins. New York: Plenum Press,1983;75–90.
329. Cornell RP. Restriction of gut-derived endotoxin impairs DNA synthesis for liver regeneration. Am J Physiol. 1985;249(5 Pt 2):R563–9.
330. Windle WF, Chambers WW. Regeneration in spinal cord of cat and dog. J Comp Neurol.

1950;93:241–258.
331. Williams JL, Dick GF. Decreased dextrose tolerance in acute infectious disease. Arch Intern Med 1932;50:801.
332. Fox MJ, Kuzma JF, Washam WT. Transitory diabetic syndromes associated with meningococcic meningitis Arch Intern Med 1947;79:614.
333. Beisel WR. Metabolic response to infection. Ann Rev Med. 1975;26:9–20.
334. Berczi I. The influence of pituitary-adrenal axis on the immune system. In: Berczi I, editor. Pituitary function and immunity. Boca Raton, FL: CRC Press, 1986;49–132.
335. Berkenbosch F, van Oers J, del Rey A, Tilders F, Besedovsky H. Corticotropin-releasing factor-producing neurons in the rat activated by interleukin-1. Science. 1987;238:524–6.
336. Sapolsky R, Rivier C, Yamamoto G, Plotsky P, Vale W. Interleukin-1 stimulates the secretion of hypothalamic corticotropin-releasing factor. Science. 1987;238:522–4.
337. Uehara A, Gottschall PE, Dahl RR, Arimura A. Interleukin-1 stimulates ACTH release by an indirect action which requires endogenous corticotropin releasing factor. Endocrinology. 1987 ;121:1580–2.
338. Bernton EW, Beach JE, Holaday JW, Smallridge RC, Fein HG. Release of multiple hormones by a direct action of interleukin-1 on pituitary cells. Science. 1987;238:519–21.
339. Nakamura H, Motoyoshi S, Kadokawa T. Anti-inflammatory action of interleukin 1 through the pituitary-adrenal axis in rats. Eur J Pharmacol. 1988;151:67–73.
340. Selye H. A syndrome produced by diverse nocuous agents. Nature 1936;138:32.
341. Selye H. Thymus and the adrenals in response of the organism to injuries and intoxications. Br J Exp Pathol 1936;17:234–248.
342. Selye H. The general adaptation syndrome and the diseases of adaptation. J Clin Endocrinol 1946;6:117–230.
343. Selye H. Stress and disease. Science 1955;122:625.
344. Selye H. Effect of ACTH and cortisone upon an "anaphylactoid reaction". Can Med Assoc J 1949;61:553–556.
345. Selye H. Morphological changes in the fowl following chronic overdosage with various steroids. J Morphol 1943;73:401–421.
346. Berczi I. Neurohormonal host defence in endotoxin shock. Ann NY Acad Sci 1998;840: 787–802.
347. Berczi I. The stress concept and neuroimmunoregulation in modern biology. Ann NY Acad Sci 1998;851:3–12.
348. Haeryfar SMM, Berczi I. The thymus and the acute phase response. Cell Mol Biol 2001;47:145–156.
349. Berczi I, Bertok L, Chow D. Natural immunity and neuroimmune host defence. Ann NY Acad Sci 2001;917:248–257.
350. Berczi I, Szentivanyi A. The acute phase response. In Neuroimmmune Biology, Volume 4: The Immune-Neuroendocrine Circuitry. History and Progress. Berczi I. Szentivanyi A. Editors, Elsevier, Amsterdam, 2003.
351. Westphal O, Jann K, Himmelspach K. Chemistry and immunochemistry of bacterial lipopolysaccharides as cell wall antigens and endotoxins. Prog Allergy. 1983;33:9–39.
352. Ramachandra RN, Berczi A, Sehon AH, Berczi I. Inhibition of lipid A and lipopolysaccharide (LPS) induced cytokine secretion, B cell mitogenesis and lethal shock by lipid A specific murine monoclonal antibodies. J Infect Dis 1993;167:1151–1159.
353. Berczi I. Neuroendocrine defence in endotoxin shock. (A review) Acta Microbiol Hung

1993;40:265–302.

354. Raetz CRH, Ulevitch RJ, Wright SD, Sibley CH, Ding A, Nathan CF. Gram-negative endotoxin: An extraordinary lipid with profound effects on eukaryotic signal transduction. FASEB J 1991;5:2652–2660.
355. Tobias PS, Mathison J, Mintz D, Lee JD, Kravchenko V, Kato K, Pugin J, Ulevitch RJ. Participation of lipopolysaccharide-binding protein in lipopolysaccharide-dependent macrophage activation. Am J Respir Cell Mol Biol. 1992;7:239–45.
356. Schumann RR. Function of lipopolysaccharide (LPS)-binding protein (LBP) and CD14, the receptor for LPS/LBP complexes: a short review. Res Immunol. 1992;143:11–5.
357. Mathison JC, Tobias PS, Wolfson E, Ulevitch RJ. Plasma lipopolysaccharide (LPS)-binding protein. A key component in macrophage recognition of gram-negative LPS. J Immunol. 1992;149:200–6.
358. Haziot A, Chen S, Ferrero E, Low MG, Silber R, Goyert SM. The monocyte differentiation antigen, CD14, is anchored to the cell membrane by a phosphatidylinositol linkage. J Immunol. 1988;141:547–52.
359. Kielian TL, Blecha F. CD14 and other recognition molecules for lipopolysaccharide: a review. Immunopharmacology. 1995;29(3):187–205.
360. Rivest S, Nadeau S, Lacroix S, Laflamme N. Proinflammatory signal transduction pathways in the CNS during systemic immune response. In New Foundation of Biology, Berczi I, Gorczynski RM Editors, Neuroimmune Biology, Volume I. Berczi I, Szentivanyi A. Series editors, Elsevier 1991, pp. 163–173.
361. Berczi I, Bertok L, Bereznay T. Comparative studies on the toxicity of Escherichia coli lipopolysaccharide endotoxin in various animal species. Can J Microbiol 1966;12:1070–71.
362. Balm PH, van Lieshout E, Lokate J, Wendelaar Bonga SE. Bacterial lipopolysaccharide (LPS) and interleukin 1 (IL-1) exert multiple physiological effects in the tilapia Oreochromis mossambicus (Teleostei). J Comp Physiol [B]. 1995;165:85–92.
363. Levin J, Bang FB. The role of endotoxin in the extracellular coagulation of limulus blood. Bull Johns Hopkins Hosp 1964;115:265–274.
364. Ramachandra RN, Sehon AH, Berczi I. Neuro-hormonal host defence in endotoxin shock. Brain Behav Immun 1992;6:157–169
365. Parant M, Le Contel C, Parant F, Chedid L. Influence of endogenous glucocorticoid on endotoxin-induced production of circulating TNF-alpha. Lymphokine Cytokine Res. 1991;10:265–71.
366. Zuckerman SH, Shellhaas J, Butler LD. Differential regulation of lipopolysaccharide-induced interleukin 1 and tumor necrosis factor synthesis: effects of endogenous and exogenous glucocorticoids and the role of the pituitary-adrenal axis. Eur J Immunol. 1989;19:301–5.
367. Richardson RP, Rhyne CD, Fong Y, Hesse DG, Tracey KJ, Marano MA, Lowry SF, Antonacci AC, Calvano SE. Peripheral blood leukocyte kinetics following in vivo lipopolysaccharide (LPS) administration to normal human subjects. Influence of elicited hormones and cytokines. Ann Surg. 1989;210:239–45.
368. Flohe S, Heinrich PC, Schneider J, Wendel A, Flohe L. Time course of IL-6 and TNF alpha release during endotoxin-induced endotoxin tolerance in rats. Biochem Pharmacol. 1991;41:1607–14.
369. Barber AE, Coyle SM, Marano MA, Fischer E, Calvano SE, Fong Y, Moldawer LL, Lowry SF. Glucocorticoid therapy alters hormonal and cytokine responses to endotoxin in man. J

Immunol. 1993;150:1999–2006.
370. Waring PM, Waring LJ, Billington T, Metcalf D. Leukemia inhibitory factor protects against experimental lethal Escherichia coli septic shock in mice. Proc Natl Acad Sci U S A. 1995;92:1337–41.
371. Granowitz EV, Porat R, Mier JW, Orencole SF, Kaplanski G, Lynch EA, Ye K, Vannier E, Wolff SM, Dinarello CA. Intravenous endotoxin suppresses the cytokine response of peripheral blood mononuclear cells of healthy humans. J Immunol. 1993;151:1637–45.
372. Berg DJ, Kuhn R, Rajewsky K, Muller W, Menon S, Davidson N, Grunig G, Rennick D. Interleukin-10 is a central regulator of the response to LPS in murine models of endotoxic shock and the Shwartzman reaction but not endotoxin tolerance. J Clin Invest. 1995;96: 2339–47.
373. Matic M, Simon SR. Effects of gamma interferon on release of tumor necrosis factor alpha from lipopolysaccharide-tolerant human monocyte-derived macrophages. Infect Immun. 1992;60:3756–62.
374. Schade FU, Franke C, Schlegel J, Rietschel ET. Formation of a TNF synthesis inhibitor in endotoxin tolerance. Prog Clin Biol Res. 1995;392:513–21.
375. Henricson BE, Neta R, Vogel SN. An interleukin-1 receptor antagonist blocks lipopolysaccharide-induced colony-stimulating factor production and early endotoxin tolerance. Infect Immun. 1991;59:1188–91.
376. Berczi I, Nagy E. Neurohormonal control of cytokines during injury. In: Rothwell NJ, Berkenbosch F, editors. Brain Control of Responses to Trauma. Cambridge University Press, 1994;32–107.
377. Berczi I, Szentivanyi A. The pituitary gland, psychoneuroimmunology and infectious disease. In: Friedman H, Klein T, Friedman AL, editors Psychoneuroimmunology, stress and infectious disease. Boca Raton, FL: CRC Press, 1996;79–109.
378. Wexler BC, Dolgin AE, Tryczynski EW. Effects of bacterial polysaccharide (Piromen) on the pituitary-adrenal axis: Adrenal ascorbic acid, cholesterol and histological alterations. Endocrinology 1957;61:300–308.
379. Wilder RL. Neuroendocrine-immune system interactions and autoimmunity. Annu Rev Immunol. 1995;13:307–38.
380. Torpy DJ, Chrousos GP. In: Chikanza IC, editor. Neuroendocrine Immune Mechanisms of Rheumatic Diseases. Bailliere's Clin Rheumatol London: Bailliere Tindall 1996;10: 181–198.
381. Berczi I, Chalmers IM, Nagy E, Warrington RJ. In: Chikanza IC Editor. Neuroendocrine Immune Mechanisms of Rheumatic Diseases. Bailliere's Clin Rheumatol, London: Bailliere Tindall,1996;10:227–157.
382. Geller P, Merrill ER, Jawetz E. Effects of cortisone and antibiotics on lethal action of endotoxins in mice. Proc Soc Exp Biol Med 1954;86:716–719.
383. Jansen NJG, Vanoeveren W, Hoiting BH, Wildevuur CRH. Methylprednisolone prophylaxis protects against endotoxin-induced death in rabbits. Inflammation 1991;15: 91–101.
384. Izumi T, Bakhle YS. Modification by steroids of pulmonary oedema and prostaglandin E2 pharmacokinetics induced by endotoxin in rats. Brit J Pharmacol 1988;93:955–963.
385. Yoo JY, Desiderio S. Innate and acquired immunity intersect in a global view of the acute-phase response. Proc Natl Acad Sci U S A 2003;100:457–62.
386. Cavaillon JM. The nonspecific nature of endotoxin tolerance.Trends Microbiol. 1995 ;3: 320–4.

387. Mengozzi M, Ghezzi P. Cytokine down-regulation in endotoxin tolerance. Eur Cytokine Netw. 1993;4:89–98.
388. Freudenberg MA, Galanos C. Induction of tolerance to lipopolysaccharide (LPS)-D-galactosamine lethality by pretreatment with LPS is mediated by macrophages. Infect Immun. 1988;56:1352–7.
389. Evans GF, Zuckerman SH. Glucocorticoid-dependent and -independent mechanisms involved in lipopolysaccharide tolerance. Eur J Immunol. 1991;21:973–9.
390. Szabo C, Thiemermann C, Wu CC, Perretti M, Vane JR. Attenuation of the induction of nitric oxide synthase by endogenous glucocorticoids accounts for endotoxin tolerance in vivo. Proc Natl Acad Sci U S A. 1994;91:271–5.
391. Hansen MK, Nguyen KT, Goehler LE, Gaykema RP, Fleshner M, Maier SF, Watkins LR. Effects of vagotomy on lipopolysaccharide-induced brain interleukin-1beta protein in rats. Auton Neurosci 2000;85:119–26
392. Mold C, Rodriguez W, Rodic-Polic B, Du Clos TW. C-reactive protein mediates protection from lipopolysaccharide through interactions with Fc gamma R. J Immunol 2002;169: 7019–25.
393. Szalai AJ, van Ginkel FW, Wang Y, McGhee JR, Volanakis JE. Complement-dependent acute-phase expression of C-reactive protein and serum amyloid P-component. J Immunol 2000;165:1030–5.
394. Szalai AJ, Nataf S, Hu XZ, Barnum SR. Experimental allergic encephalomyelitis is inhibited in transgenic mice expressing human C-reactive protein. J Immunol 2002;168: 5792–7.
395. Galanos C, Freudenberg MA, Reutter W. Galactosamine-induced sensitization to the lethal effects of endotoxin. Proc Natl Acad Sci U S A. 1979;76:5939–43.
396. Kimura T, Itoh N, Takehara M, Oguro I, Ishizaki JI, Nakanishi T, Tanaka K. Sensitivity of metallothionein-null mice to LPS/D-galactosamine-induced lethality. Biochem Biophys Res Commun 2001;280:358–62.
397. Roth J, Hubschle T, Pehl U, Ross G, Gerstberger R. Influence of systemic treatment with cyclooxygenase inhibitors on lipopolysaccharide-induced fever and circulating levels of cytokines and cortisol in guinea-pigs. Pflugers Arch 2002;443:411–417.
398. Fennekohl A, Lucas M, Puschel GP. Induction by interleukin 6 of G(s)-coupled prostaglandin E(2) receptors in rat hepatocytes mediating a prostaglandin E(2)-dependent inhibition of the hepatocyte's acute phase response. Hepatology 2000;31:1128–34.
399. Streetz KL, Wustefeld T, Klein C, Manns MP, Trautwein C. Mediators of inflammation and acute phase response in the liver. Cell Mol Biol (Noisy-le-grand) 2001;47:661–73.
400. Shen X, Tian Z, Holtzman MJ, Gao B. Cross-talk between interleukin 1beta (IL-1beta) and IL-6 signalling pathways: IL-1beta selectively inhibits IL-6-activated signal transducer and activator of transcription factor 1 (STAT1) by a proteasome-dependent mechanism. Biochem J 2000;352 Pt 3:913–9.
401. Jostock T, Mullberg J, Ozbek S, Atreya R, Blinn G, Voltz N, Fischer M, Neurath MF, Rose-John S. Soluble gp130 is the natural inhibitor of soluble interleukin-6 receptor transsignaling responses. Eur J Biochem 2001;268:160–7.
402. Beigneux AP, Moser AH, Shigenaga JK, Grunfeld C, Feingold KR. The acute phase response is associated with retinoid X receptor repression in rodent liver. J Biol Chem 2000;275:16390–9.
403. Harris HW, Gosnell JE, Kumwenda ZL. The lipemia of sepsis: triglyceride-rich lipoproteins as agents of innate immunity. J Endotoxin Res 2000;6:421–30.

404. Fulop AK, Pocsik E, Brozik M, Karabelyos C, Kiss A, Novak I, Szalai C, Dobozy O, Falus A. Hepatic regeneration induces transient acute phase reaction: systemic elevation of acute phase reactants and soluble cytokine receptors. Cell Biol Int 2001;25:585–92.
405. Hecht N, Pappo O, Shouval D, Rose-John S, Galun E, Axelrod JH. Hyper-IL-6 gene therapy reverses fulminant hepatic failure. Mol Ther 2001;3(5 Pt 1):683–7.
406. Gabay C, Gigley J, Sipe J, Arend WP, Fantuzzi G. Production of IL-1 receptor antagonist by hepatocytes is regulated as an acute-phase protein in vivo. Eur J Immunol 2001;31: 490–9.
407. Carstanjen D, Regenfus M, Muller C, Salama A. Interleukin-6 is a major effector molecule of short-term G-CSF treatment inducing bone metabolism and an acute-phase response. Exp Hematol 2001;29:812–21.
408. Suwa T, Hogg JC, Klut ME, Hards J, van Eeden SF. Interleukin-6 changes deformability of neutrophils and induces their sequestration in the lung. Am J Respir Crit Care Med 2001;163:970–6.
409. Beishuizen A, Thijs LG, Haanen C, Vermes I. Macrophage migration inhibitory factor and hypothalamo-pituitary-adrenal function during critical illness. J Clin Endocrinol Metab 2001;86:2811–6.
410. Previte JJ, Chang Y, El-Bisi HM. Detoxification of Salmonella typhimurium lipopolysaccharide by ionizing radiation. J Bacteriol 1967;93:1607.
411. Fust G, Bertok L, Juhasz-Nagy S. Interactions of radio-detoxified Escherichia coli endotoxin preparations with the complement system. Infect Immun. 1977;16:26–31.
412. Bertok L. Stimulation of nonspecific resistance by radiation-detoxified endotoxin. In:. Nowotny A, editor. Beneficial Effects of Endotoxin. New York: Plenum Press, 1983;213–226.
413. Banhegyi D, Varnai F, Horvath A, Bertok L. Treatment of severe immune deficiency with radio-detoxified endotoxin. J Med. 1992;23:154–6.
414. Gustafson GL, Rhodes MJ, Hegel T. Monophosphoryl lipid A as a prophylactic for sepsis and septic shock. Prog Clin Biol Res. 1995;392:567–79.
415. Astiz ME, Rackow EC, Still JG, Howell ST, Cato A, Von Eschen KB, Ulrich JT, Rudbach JA, McMahon G, Vargas R, et al. Pretreatment of normal humans with monophosphoryl lipid A induces tolerance to endotoxin: a prospective, double-blind, randomized, controlled trial. Crit Care Med. 1995;23:9–17.
416. Jamieson JC, Lammers G, Janzen R, Woloski BMRNJ. The acute phase response to inflammation: The role of monokines in changes in liver glycoproteins and enzymes of glycoprotein metabolism. Comp Biochem Physiol 1987;87B:11–15.
417. Berczi I. Neurohormonal immunoregulation. Endocr Pathol 1990;1:197–219.
418. Spangelo BL, Macleod RM. Immunopeptide regulation of anterior pituitary function. Int J Neurosci. 1990;51:369–70.
419. Akira S, Kishimoto T. IL-6 and NF-IL6 in acute-phase response and viral infection. Immunol Rev 1992;127:26–50.
420. Baue AF. Neuroendocrine response to severe trauma and sepsis. In: Faist E, Ninnemann J, Green D, editors. Immune consequences of trauma, shock and sepsis. Springer Verlag, 1989;17–32.
421. Bornstein SR, Licinio J, Tauchnitz R, Engelmann L, Negrao AB, Gold P, Chrousos GP. Plasma leptin levels are increased in survivors of acute sepsis: associated loss of diurnal rhythm, in cortisol and leptin secretion. J Clin Endocrinol Metab 1998;83:280–3
422. Kolb-Bachofen V. A review on the biological properties of C-reactive protein.

Immunobiology. 1991;183:133–45.
423. Ballou SP, Kushner I. C-reactive protein and the acute phase response. Adv Intern Med. 1992;37:313–36.
424. Young B, Gleeson M, Cripps AW. C-reactive protein: a critical review. Pathology. 1991;23: 118–24.
425. Mold C, Nakayama S, Holzer TJ, Gewurz H, Du Clos TW. C-reactive protein is protective against Streptococcus pneumoniae infection in mice. J Exp Med. 1981;154:1703–8.
426. Vogeser M, Zachoval R, Felbinger TW, Jacob K. Increased ratio of serum cortisol to cortisone in acute-phase response. Horm Res 2002;58:172–5.
427. Bauer J, Birmelin M, Northoff GH, Northemann W, Tran-Thi TA, Ueberberg H, Decker K, Heinrich P. Induction of rat β2-macroglobulin in vivo and in heaptocyte primary cultures: synergistic action of glucocorticoids and a Kupffer cell derived factor. FEBS Lett 1984;177:89–94.
428. van Gool J, Boers W, Sala M, Ladiges NC. Glucocorticoids and catecholamines as mediators of acute-phase proteins, especially rat alpha-macrofoetoprotein. Biochem J. 1984;220:125–32.
429. Wassell J. Haptoglobin: function and polymorphism. Clin Lab 2000;46(11–12):547–52.
430. Daemen MA, Heemskerk VH, van't Veer C, Denecker G, Wolfs TG, Vandenabeele P, Buurman WA. Functional protection by acute phase proteins alpha(1)-acid glycoprotein and alpha(1)-antitrypsin against ischemia/reperfusion injury by preventing apoptosis and inflammation. Circulation 2000;102:1420–6.
431. Liu H, Jensen L, Hansen S, Petersen SV, Takahashi K, Ezekowitz AB, Hansen FD, Jensenius JC, Thiel S. Characterization and quantification of mouse mannan-binding lectins (MBL-A and MBL-C) and study of acute phase responses. Scand J Immunol 2001;53:489–97.
432. Turner MW, Hamvas RM. Mannose-binding lectin: structure, function, genetics and disease associations. Rev Immunogenet 2000;2:305–22.
433. Van Gool J, Van Vugt H, Helle M, Aarden LA. The relation among stress, adrenalin, interleukin 6, and acute phase proteins in the rat. Clin Immunol Immunopathol 1990;57: 200–210.
434. Takala J, Ruokonen E, Webster NR, et al. Increased mortality associated with growth hormone treatment in critically ill adults. N Engl J Med 1999;341:785–92.
435. Jaschke MG, Herndon DN, Wolf SE, et al. Recombinant human growth hormone alters acute phase reactant proteins, cytokine expression, and liver morphology in burned rats. J Surg Res 1999;83:122–29.
436. Derfalvi B, Igaz P, Fulop KA, Szalai C, Falus A. Interleukin-6-induced production of type II acute phase proteins and expression of junB gene are downregulated by human recombinant growth hormone in vitro. Cell Biol Int 2000;24:109–14.
437. Berczi I, Nagy E, Asa SL, Kovacs K. Pituitary hormones and contact sensitivity in rats. Allergy 1983;38:325–330.
438. Berczi I, Nagy E, Asa SL, Kovacs K. The influence of pituitary hormones on adjuvant arthritis. Arthritis Rheum 1984;27:682–688.
439. Ramirez RJ, Wolf SE, Herndon DN. Is there a role for growth hormone in the clinical management of burn injuries? Growth Horm IGF Res 1998 ;8 Suppl B:99–105.
440. Jaschke MG, Barrow RE, Herndon DN. Recombinant human growth hormone treatment in pediatric burn patients and its role during the hepatic acute phase response. Crit Care Med 2000;28:1578–84.

441. Jaschke MG, Herndon DN, Barrow RE. Insulin-like growth factor I in combination with insulin-like growth factor binding protein 3 affects the hepatic acute phase response and hepatic morphology in thermally injured rats. Ann Surg 2000;231:408–16.
442. Jeschke MG, Barrow RE, Herndon DN. Insulinlike growth factor I plus insulinlike growth factor binding protein 3 attenuates the proinflammatory acute phase response in severely burned children. Ann Surg 2000;231:246–52.
443. Basoglu M, Kiziltunc A, Yildirgan MI, Gumustekin K, Gumus M, Yildirim A, Atamanalp SS. Recombinant human growth hormone modulates the hepatic acute-phase response and P-selectin in burned rats. Burns 2002;28:760–4.
444. Kotler DP. Cachexia. Ann Intern Med 2000;133:622–34.
445. Langhans W. Anorexia of infection: current prospects. Nutrition 2000;16:996–1005.
446. Yudkin JS, Kumari M, Humphries SE, Mohamed-Ali V. Inflammation, obesity, stress and coronary heart disease: is interleukin-6 the link? Atherosclerosis 2000;148(2):209–14.
447. Kushner I. C-reactive protein elevation can be caused by conditions other than inflammationand may reflect biologic aging. Cleve Clin J Med 2001;68:535–7.
448. Bruunsgaard H, Pedersen M, Pedersen BK. Aging and proinflammatory cytokines. Curr Opin Hematol 2001;8:131–6.
449. Duncan BB, Schmidt MI. Chronic activation of the innate immune system may underlie the metabolic syndrome. Sao Paulo Med J 2001;119:122–7.
450. Richardson AP, Tayek JA. Type 2 diabetic patients may have a mild form of an injury response: a clinical research center study. Am J Physiol Endocrinol Metab 2002;282: E1286–90.
451. Fernandez-Real JM, Vayreda M, Richart C, Gutierrez C, Broch M, Vendrell J, Ricart W. Circulating interleukin 6 levels, blood pressure, and insulin sensitivity in apparently healthy men and women. J Clin Endocrinol Metab 2001;86:1154–9.
452. Arnalich F, Hernanz A, Lopez-Maderuelo D, Pena JM, Camacho J, Madero R, Vazquez JJ, Montiel C. Enhanced acute-phase response and oxidative stress in older adults with type II diabetes. Horm Metab Res 2000;32:407–12.
453. Pickup JC, Chusney GD, Thomas SM, Burt D. Plasma interleukin-6, tumour necrosis factor alpha and blood cytokine production in type 2 diabetes. Life Sci 2000;67:291–300.
454. Fernandez-Real JM, Broch M, Vendrell J, Gutierrez C, Casamitjana R, Pugeat M, Richart C, Ricart W. Interleukin-6 gene polymorphism and insulin sensitivity. Diabetes 2000;49: 517–20.
455. Boss B, Neeck G. Correlation of IL-6 with the classical humoral disease activity parameters ESR and CRP and with serum cortisol, reflecting the activity of the HPA axis in active rheumatoid arthritis. Z Rheumatol 2000;59 Suppl 2:II/62–4.
456. Sakane T, Suzuki N. Neuro-endocrine-immune axis in human rheumatoid arthritis. Arch Immunol Ther Exp (Warsz) 2000;48:417–27.
457. O'Hara R, Murphy EP, Whitehead AS, FitzGerald O, Bresnihan B. Acute-phase serum amyloid A production by rheumatoid arthritis synovial tissue. Arthritis Res 2000;2(2): 142–4.
458. Janssen U, Bahlmann F, Kohl J, Zwirner J, Haubitz M, Floege J. Activation of the acute phase response and complement C3 in patients with IgA nephropathy. Am J Kidney Dis 2000;35:21–8.
459. Anisman H, Baines MG, Berczi I, et al. Neuroimmune mechanisms in health and disease: 1. Health. Can Med Assoc J 1996;155:867–874.
460. Anisman H, Baines MG, Berczi I, et al. Neuroimmune mechanisms in health and disease:

2. Disease. Can Med Assoc J 1996;155:1075–1082.
461. Banck G, Forsgren A. Many bacterial species are mitogenic for human blood B lymphocytes. Scand J Immunol. 1978;8:347–54.
462. Fleischer B, Gerlach D, Fuhrmann A, Schmidt KH. Superantigens and pseudosuperantigens of gram-positive cocci. Med Microbiol Immunol (Berl). 1995;184:1–8.
463. Levinson AI, Kozlowski L, Zheng Y, Wheatley L. B-cell superantigens: definition and potential impact on the immune response. J Clin Immunol. 1995;15(6 Suppl):26S-36S.
464. Zumla A. Superantigens, T cells and microbes. Clin Infect Dis 1992;15:313–320.
465. Kotb M. Bacterial pyrogenic exotoxins as superantigens. Clin Microbiol Rev. 1995;8: 411–26.
466. Spangelo BL, deHoll PD, Kalabay L, Bond BR, Arnaud P. Neurointermediate pituitary lobe cells synthesize and release interleukin-6 in vitro: effects of lipopolysaccharide and interleukin-1 beta. Endocrinology. 1994;135:556–63.
467. Chao HS, Poisner AM, Poisner R, Handwerger S.Lipopolysaccharides inhibit prolactin and renin release from human decidual cells. Biol Reprod. 1994;50:210–4.
468. Di Santo E, Sironi M, Pozzi P, Gnocchi P, Isetta AM, Delvaux A, Goldman M, Marchant A, Ghezzi P. Interleukin-10 inhibits lipopolysaccharide-induced tumor necrosis factor and interleukin-1 beta production in the brain without affecting the activation of the hypothalamus-pituitary-adrenal axis. Neuroimmunomodulation. 1995;2:149–54.
469. Faggioni R, Fantuzzi G, Villa P, Buurman W, van Tits LJ, Ghezzi P. Independent down-regulation of central and peripheral tumor necrosis factor production as a result of lipopolysaccharide tolerance in mice. Infect Immun. 1995;63:1473–7.
470. Das KP, McMillian MK, Bing G, Hong JS. Modulatory effects of [Met5]-enkephalin on interleukin-1 beta secretion from microglia in mixed brain cell cultures. J Neuroimmunol. 1995;62:9–17.
471. Scotte M, Hiron M, Masson S, Lyoumi S, Banine F, Teniere P, Lebreton JP, Daveau M. Differential expression of cytokine genes in monocytes, peritoneal macrophages and liver following endotoxin- or turpentine-induced inflammation in rat. Cytokine. 1996;8: 115–20.
472. Gaykema RP, Dijkstra I, Tilders FJ. Subdiaphragmatic vagotomy suppresses endotoxin-induced activation of hypothalamic corticotropin-releasing hormone neurons and ACTH secretion. Endocrinology. 1995;136:4717–20.
473. Laye S, Bluthe RM, Kent S, Combe C, Medina C, Parnet P, Kelley K, Dantzer R. Subdiaphragmatic vagotomy blocks induction of IL-1 beta mRNA in mice brain in response to peripheral LPS. Am J Physiol. 1995;268(5 Pt 2):R1327–31.
474. Berczi I, Bertok L, Baintner K, Jr, Veress B. Failure of oral Escherichia coli endotoxin to induce either specific tolerance or toxic syndromes in rats. J Path Bact 1968;96:481–486.
475. Kocsar LT, Bertok L, Varteresz V. Effect of bile acids on the intestinal absorption of endotoxin in rats. J Bacteriol. 1969;100:220–3.
476. Mimura Y, Sakisaka S, Harada M, Sata M, Tanikawa K. Role of hepatocytes in direct clearance of lipopolysaccharide in rats. Gastroenterology. 1995;109:1969–76.
477. Bertok L. Physico-chemical defence of vertebrate organisms: the role of bile acids in defence against endotoxins. Persp Biol Med 1977;21:70–76.

Natural Immunity
Edited by L. Bertók and D.A. Chow
© 2005 Elsevier B.V. All rights reserved

Natural Immunity – Effect of Exercise

BENTE KLARLUND PEDERSEN

The Copenhagen Muscle Research Centre and The Department of Infectious Diseases, Rigshospitalet, University of Copenhagen, Copenhagen, Denmark

ABSTRACT

Natural immunity is influenced by exercise. Physical activity induces increased circulating levels of a number of cytokines. IL-6 more than any other cytokine is produced in large amounts in response to exercise. Recently, it has been demonstrated that IL-6 is produced locally in contracting skeletal muscles and that the net release from the muscle can account for the exercise-induced increase in arterial IL-6 concentration. IL-6 stimulates the production of a number of anti-inflammatory cytokines such as IL-1ra and IL-10 and works in a hormone-like fashion. IL-6 also stimulates cortisol production. In the recovery phase of heavy exertion, a cortisol-induced shift in leukocyte subsets is seen. Thus, dominant features in the post-exercise period are lymphopenia, neutrophilia and a marked suppressed natural killer cell activity are seen. In addition secretory IgA is inhibited.

This chapter focuses on the effect of exercise on natural immunity. Over the past 20 years a variety of studies have demonstrated that exercise induces considerable changes in the immune system. The interactions between exercise, stress and the immune system provide a unique opportunity to link basic and clinical physiology, and to evaluate the role of underlying stress and immunophysiological mechanisms. It has been suggested that exercise represents a quantifiable model of physical stress [1,2] as many clinical physical stressors (e.g., surgery, trauma, burn, sepsis) and environmental factors such as hyperthermia and hypoxia induce a pattern of hormonal and immunological responses that have similarities to the cellular response to exercise [3].

1. THE ACUTE PHASE RESPONSE TO EXERCISE

Initially, it was thought that the cytokine response to exercise represented a reaction to exercise-induced muscle injury or transposition of lipopolysacharide (LPS) to the gut. However, recent data suggest that the massive response of IL-6 to exercise may primarily mediate important exercise-related metabolic changes [4,5]. Several cytokines can be detected in plasma during and after strenuous exercise [6–8]. Most studies report that exercise does not induce an increase in plasma levels of TNF-α except a few studies demonstrating that strenuous, prolonged exercise, such as marathon running results in a small increase in the plasma concentration of TNF-α [7–10]. Thereby, the cytokine cascade due to exercise differs from the cytokine response to infections. The first cytokine that is present in the circulation following exercise is IL-6, which may increase 100 fold. The increase in IL-6 is followed by a marked increase in the concentration of IL-1ra [4,6]. The cytokine inhibitors (IL-1ra and sTNF-R) as well as the anti-inflammatory cytokine IL-10 [6] increase, and also the concentrations of the chemokines, IL-8, MIP-1alpha and MIP-1beta, are elevated after a marathon race [11,12]. Interleukin 8 (IL-8) is produced by various cells upon stimulation and influences a variety of functions of leukocytes in particular neutrophils. Systemic administration of IL-8 induces a rapid neutropenia associated with sequestration of neutrophils in the lung which is followed by a neutrophilia characterised by the rapid release of neutrophils from the bone marrow. These cells are released predominantly from the bone marrow venous sinusoids [13]. Increased levels of plasma-chemokines in response to exercise have only been described if the exercise has been extremely exhaustive suggest as in a marathon [11,12], whereas even 2.5 hours of treadmill running did not cause an increase in plasma-chemokines [5]. Thus, it is not known if chemokines are involved in post-exercise neutrophilia.

When blood mononuclear cells are sampled during or following strenuous exercise and stimulated in vitro to produce cytokines, it has been reported that the in vitro cytokine production is either impaired [14,15], not changed or enhanced [16]. These findings are likely to be explained by exercise-induced altered blood mononuclear cell composition.

In addition to cytokines, serum levels of non-cytokine acute phase reactants, including serum amyloid A inducer (SAA), C-reactive protein (CRP), serum amyloid A, haptoglobulin, ceruloplasmin, transferrin and α_{2}-macroglobulin, also change with inflammation [17]. Many of these acute phase reactants have essential roles in host defence; for example, ceruloplasmin and transferrin may have antioxidant functions [18]. With respect to exercise models, the serum levels of these acute reactants have not been well characterised with the exception of transferrin.

The concentration of serum transferrin, a β_1-globulin carrier protein of iron which is synthesised in the liver, decreases with inflammation and trauma [19]. Transferrin may play a role in nonspecific host defence against bacterial pathogens through the 'iron binding' hypothesis [20]. However, when samples were corrected for plasma volume shifts, transferrin concentrations did not change immediately after, 30, 60 or 120 minutes after high intensity swimming or treadmill exercise in athletes [21]. In contrast, blood concentration of a related acute phase iron transport molecule, ferritin, was significantly decreased at 5 and 7 days post exercise compared with immediately and 1 day post exercise [22]. Iron-binding capacity and percentage of saturation of transferrin did not change after 12 weeks of moderate endurance walking/running or cycling exercise in 31 women [23]. In rangers participating in an eight week USA training course, and who had associated energy deficit of about 1000 kcal/d, there were no effects on serum transferrin concentrations [24]. In contrast, transferrin concentration decreased significantly in male recruits undergoing prolonged physical stress during survival training [25]. It is not possible, however, to disentangle the effects of the physical exercise from restricted water and food intake on the levels of serum transferrin that were observed in this study. C-reactive protein (CRP) concentration was unchanged after either uphill running or 24 hours after downhill running [26]. However, CRP levels increased in elderly subjects following an intensive training programme [27].

2. THE IL-6 RESPONSE TO EXERCISE

Interleukin-6 is produced in larger amounts than any other cytokine in relation to exercise. IL-6 is produced by many different cells, but the main sources in vivo are stimulated monocytes/macrophages, fibroblasts and vascular endothelial cells [28], indicative of its role in modulation of the immune system. Other cells known to express IL-6 include keratinocytes, osteoblasts, T cells, B cells, neutrophils, eosinophils, mast cells, smooth muscle cells [28] and skeletal muscle cells [29]. Until now, IL-6 has been considered a cytokine with immunomodulatory effects and immune cells have been regarded as the main cell source of production. However, during the past few years it has also been demonstrated that the level of circulating IL-6 increases dramatically (up to 100 fold) in response to exercise [2,30,31]. Northoff and Berg [32] were the first to suggest that IL-6 might be involved in the generation of the acute phase response post-exercise. They found an increase in IL-6 levels immediately after a marathon run. The finding of increased levels of IL-6 after exercise is a remarkably consistent finding [4–6,8–11,14,33–46]. The finding of markedly increased levels of IL-6 after strenuous exercise has consistently been found in many studies [4–6,9,14,32,34,35–37,47–48]. A two-fold increase in plasma-IL-6 was demonstrated after six minutes intense exercise [43]. In treadmill running, the IL-6 level in blood was significantly enhanced 30 min after the start of running with the IL-6 peaking at the end of 2.5 hours of running [5]. In other studies where IL-6 was not measured during the running but at several time points after, maximal IL-6 levels were found immediately after the exercise followed by a rapid decline. Thus, following a marathon run maximal IL-6 levels (100 fold increase) were measured immediately after the 3–3.5 hour race [4,6]. Data from the Copenhagen Marathon (1996, 1997 and 1998, n=56) suggest that there is a correlation between the intensity of exercise and the increase in plasma IL-6 [11]. A previous study suggested that the appearance of IL-6 in the circulation was related to muscle damage [49], however, more recent studies clearly demonstrate that muscle contractions without any muscle damage induce marked elevation of plasma IL-6 [5,6,50,51]. In a recent study, we demonstrated that despite marked increases in both creatine kinase and myoglobin five days after eccentric exercise, the plasma IL-6 peaked into recovery only a few folds in both groups [51]. Apart from exercise intensity, duration and mode, it has also been suggested that the exercise-induced increase in plasma IL-6 is related to the sympatho-adrenal response [34,45,52]. A study performed in animals suggested that the increase in epinephrine during stress was responsible for the increase in IL-6 [53]. However, recent data from our group showed that when adrenaline was infused into volunteers to closely mimic the increase in plasma-adrenaline during 2.5 h of running exercise, plasma IL-6 increased only 4-fold during the infusion, but 30-fold during the exercise [42]. Thus, it seems that epinephrine only plays a minor role in the exercise-induced increase in plasma IL-6. It was previously demonstrated that peak plasma IL-6 during exercise correlated with plasma lactate [5].

2.1. Exercise-induced IL-6 – where is it produced?

A number of studies [48,54] have demonstrated that IL-6 mRNA in monocytes, the blood mononuclear cells responsible for the increase in plasma IL-6 during sepsis [2], did not increase as a result of exercise. While determining intracellular cytokine production, it was demonstrated that the number, percentage and mean fluorescence intensity of monocytes staining positive for IL-6 either does not change during cycling exercise [55], or in fact, decreases during prolonged running [8]. To test the possibility that working muscle produces IL-6, muscle biopsies were collected before and after exercise [4]. Before exercise, IL-6 mRNA could not be detected in muscle but we did detect IL-6 in the post-exercise samples. The observation that intramuscular IL-6 gene expression increases in skeletal muscle in response to exercise, was confirmed in a rat exercise model using the quantitative competitive RT-PCR method [56]. In this model, rats were subjected to electrically-stimulated eccentric or concentric contractions of one hind leg, while the other leg remained at rest. Both the eccentric and concentric contractions resulted in elevated levels of IL-6 mRNA in the exercised muscle, whereas the level in the resting leg was not elevated. It appears, therefore, that the local IL-6 production is connected with contracting muscle, and is not due to a systemic effect, because IL-6 mRNA was elevated only in the muscle from the exercising leg and not in the resting leg. As discussed, in these previous studies, we were unable to detect IL-6 mRNA in resting skeletal muscle. Of note, the finding of similar levels of IL-6 mRNA in both concentric and eccentric exercised muscle [39,56] supports the idea that the cytokine production cannot be as closely related to muscle damage as first thought. More recent studies [39,41] utilising the real time RT-PCR technique have shown that IL-6 mRNA is present in resting skeletal muscle and is enhanced up to 30-fold in contracting muscle, thus indicating that exercise is responsible for the IL-6 gene-induction. Recently, it was shown that the IL-6 gene is not only activated in working muscle, but that the IL-6 protein is released in large amounts from a contracting limb and markedly contributed to the exercise-induced increase in arterial plasma concentrations [40]. By obtaining arterial-femoral venous differences over an exercising leg we found that exercising limbs released IL-6. In addition, during the last two hours of exercise the release per unit time was approximately 17-fold higher than the amount accumulating in the plasma. We have recently confirmed that IL-6 is released from a contracting limb during both knee extensor [41] and bicycle [57] exercise. Although IL-6 appears to be produced in the contracting skeletal muscle, it is still not fully clear which cell type within the muscle is responsible for the production. While myoblasts have been shown to be capable of producing IL-6 [58,59], endothelial cells [60], fibroblasts [59] and smooth muscle cells [61] have also been shown to produce IL-6 under certain circumstances. In order to determine which cells produce the IL-6, Keller and colleagues isolated nuclei from muscle biopsies obtained before, during and after exercise. Using RT-PCR it was demonstrated that the transcription rate for IL-6 increased rapidly and markedly after the onset of exercise [62]. This suggested that a factor associated with muscle contraction increases the IL-6 transcriptional rate. The finding that human muscle cell lines can be stimulated to produce IL-6 further supports the hypothesis that myocytes are the origin of IL-6. Other sources of IL-6 include the human brain, which releases a small amount of IL-6 during exercise [65], tendons [66], and adipose tissue [67]. However, it appears that most of the IL-6 produced during exercise originates from the contracting limbs. The recent finding that muscle fibres express high amounts of IL-6 protein after exercise, but not at rest, strongly suggests that muscle fibres per se are the source of origin [68].

2.2. Carbohydrate loading, muscle glycogen content and IL-6 production.

Several studies have reported that carbohydrate ingestion attenuates elevations in plasma IL-6 during both running and cycling [34,45]. Recently, it was reported that carbohydrate ingestion did attenuate the increase in plasma IL-6 in response to both cycling and running [39]. However, the IL-6 gene expression in the contracting muscles was not affected by carbohydrate ingestion. Thus, during exercise carbohydrate ingestion exerts its effect at the post-transcriptional level of IL-6, although it is not known yet whether this effect occurs through translation and/or the release of IL-6.

In a recent study, an elevated plasma IL-6 response was observed when subjects exercised in a glycogen-depleted state [65]. Subjects completed 1 h of single-legged bicycle exercise followed by 1 h of double-arm cranking 16 h prior to performing 4–5 h of exhaustive two-legged knee extensor exercise. In the intervening 16 h, subjects consumed a low carbohydrate diet. This protocol was designed to deplete glycogen content in one leg and it allowed us to test the hypothesis that pre-exercise glycogen availability affected IL-6 production. The model was advantageous because delivery of substrates and hormones to each limb was the same. Subjects commenced exercise with a 40% lower glycogen content in the low-glycogen compared with the high-glycogen leg [41]. It was found that in the post-exercise samples, those with the lowest glycogen content expressed the highest levels of IL-6 mRNA. In addition, the release of IL-6 from the low-glycogen exercising leg occurred after only 60 min of exercise whereas it occurred after 120 min in the other limb [41]. Thus, muscle glycogen content was a determining factor for the production of IL-6 across contracting limbs. However, one potential concern from this previous study was that the exercise performed the day before would influence the results the day after. To rule out this possibility, subjects performed exercise on two different occasions, once with a normal and once with a low pre-exercise muscle glycogen content [62]. The study demonstrated that prolonged exercise activates transcription of the IL-6 gene in skeletal muscle of humans, a response that was dramatically enhanced under conditions in which muscle glycogen concentrations were low. Therefore, pre-exercise intramuscular glycogen content appears to be an important stimulus for the IL-6 gene transcription.

2.3. *Biological roles of muscle-derived IL-6*

As discussed, the increase in the IL-6 mRNA [41,62], its nuclear transcriptional activity [62] and protein release from skeletal muscle [41] is augmented when muscle glycogen availability is reduced. Furthermore, the increased expression of IL-6 was associated with increased glucose uptake during exercise [41]. This suggests that IL-6 may be involved, at least in part, in mediating glucose uptake during exercise. Of note, work from Stouthard and co-workers have shown a more direct relationship between IL-6 and glucose transport. In the first of these studies Stouthard et al. [66] demonstrated that infusion of recombinant human IL-6 (rhIL-6) into human subject, increased whole body glucose disposal and subsequent oxidation compared with a control trial. Even though endogenous glucose production was increased with rhIL-6 infusion, the metabolic clearance rate of glucose was higher in this trial suggesting that relative hyperglycaemia was not responsible for the augmented glucose disposal. Moreover, in a follow up study, Stouthard et al. [67] demonstrated that IL-6 increased both basal and insulin stimulated glucose uptake in cultured 3T3-L1 adipocytes. These authors concluded that IL-6 acted by increasing glucose transporter intrinsic activity. Recent evidence from others also provides a mechanism as to how IL-6 may act to increase glucose uptake. Increased glucose transport was found in jejunal tissue incubated with IL-6 compared with controls [68]. Moreover, IL-6 also seems to be able to increase the absorption of glucose in the gut, thereby increasing the plasma glucose levels [68]. Although speculative, these studies suggest the possibility that muscle-derived IL-6 may act, at least in part, to contribute to contraction-mediated glucose uptake.

Beside the possible glucoregulatory effect of IL-6, emerging evidence suggests that this cytokine may also be involved in other metabolic pathways. Concomitantly with the increase in liver glucose output during IL-6 infusion, Stouthard et al. [67] found an increase in circulating free fatty acids (FFA) with rhIL-6 infusion. It must be noted, however, that in this previous study, epinephrine was elevated and, therefore, the authors could not determine whether IL-6 acted directly on adipocytes, since epinephrine is a powerful lipolytic hormone. Infusion of IL-6 into rats increased serum triglyceride and FFA levels in a dose-dependent manner [69]. The hypertriglyceridaema was due to increased secretion by the liver and not decreased clearance. In a recent study from our group (unpublished data), IL-6 was infused into normal healthy volunteers at a dose that did not influence catecholamine and glucagon levels. Physiological concentrations of rhIL-6 induced a pronounced lipolysis indicating that IL-6 should be classified as a novel lipolytic hormone. The suggestion that IL-6 is strongly involved in fat metabolism is supported by a very important study be Wallenius et al. [70], who recently demonstrated that IL-6-deficient mice developed mature-onset obesity compared with wild type control mice. In addition, when the mice were treated with IL-6 for 18 days, there was a significant decrease in body weight in the transgenic, but not wild-type mice. Thus it is evident that IL-6 is a powerful lipolytic fac_tor and suggests that during exercise, the increase in arterial FFA concentration is mediated at least in part by IL-6 released from the muscle. Hence, it is likely that muscle-derived IL-6 acts in a neuro-endocrine hormone-like manner.

Today, interleukin IL-6 is thought by many authors to be the link between inflammation, obesity, stress and coronary heart disease [71]. However, given the finding that working muscles produce and release IL-6 in large amounts and the many beneficial effects of physical exercise on health [30], it is hard to believe that muscle-derived IL-6 is detrimental to health. An alternative explanation is that TNF-α, rather than IL-6, is the actual driver behind the metabolic syndrome. Thus, since TNF induces the production of IL-6, a high concentration of TNF will induce a high production of IL-6. Increased levels of both TNF-α and IL-6 have been observed in ageing [72], in obese individuals [73] and in non-insulin-dependent diabetes mellitus [74–77]. Furthermore, in several population-based studies, plasma concentrations of IL-6 have been shown to predict total and cardiovascular mortality [78]. Nevertheless, although adipose tissue produces and releases both TNF-α and IL-6 [79,80], there is experimental evidence that adipose TNF-α-expression, but not expression of IL-6, plays a mechanistic role in insulin resistance [81]. Hotamisligil [80] was the first to report a close relationship between increased adipose tissue TNF-α-expression and features of insulin resistance in rodent models of obesity and type 2 diabetes mellitus. The mechanisms by which TNF-α induces insulin resistance may be several. Long-term exposure of differentiated human adipocytes to TNF-α in vitro resulted in marked reduction of GLUT-4 [82] although later studies suggested that TNF-α-mediation of GLUT-4mRNA expression may not be responsible for insulin resistance [83]. TNF-α impairs insulin receptor signalling [84]. TNF-α also inhibits lipoprotein lipase (LPL) and stimulates lipolysis in adipocytes [85]. The resulting increase in circulating nonesterified fatty acids would be expected to contribute to insulin resistance [86]. TNF-α was elevated in elderly patients with atherosclerosis compared with age-matched subjects without this diagnosis [72]. However, although TNF-α correlated with IL-6 [72], the latter cytokine was not associated with atherosclerosis. TNF-α and IL-6 are tightly linked, with TNF-α stimulating IL-6 production. On the other hand, in vitro studies [87] as well as animal studies [88,89] suggest that IL-6 may inhibit TNF-α production. Therefore, exercise-induced IL-6 production may inhibit TNF-α-induced insulin resistance.

Finally, exercise-induced IL-6 production may also have an indirect role in mediating leukocyte trafficking of natural killer (NK) cells and neutrophils [90]. As described below, it appears that the acute exercise effect on NK cells is mediated by catecholamines, in particular epinephrine [42]. However, the post-exercise decline of NK cell activity and post-exercise neutrophilis is mediated by cortisol. The latter hormone is of particular interest, if the exercise is of long duration. The increase in cortisol is mediated by IL-6 [91]. Linking exercise-induced changes in NK cells and neutrophils to an effect of IL-6 on cortisol production, is further supported by several studies demonstrating that carbohydrate loading during exercise attenuates the exercise effect on function [34,92,93].

3. ACUTE EXERCISE AND LEUKOCYTES

Responses of blood leukocyte subpopulations to an episode of acute exercise are highly stereotyped. Neutrophil concentrations increase during and post exercise whereas lymphocyte concentrations increase during exercise and fall below prevalues after long duration physical work [90]. Several reports describe exercise-induced changes in subsets of blood mononuclear cells (BMNC) [94–102]. Increased lymphocyte concentration is likely due to the recruitment of all lymphocyte subpopulations to the vascular compartment: CD4+ T cells, CD8+ T cells, CD19+ B cells, CD16+ NK cells, and CD56+ NK cells.

3.1. Neutrophil function

Neutrophils represent 50% to 60% of the total circulating leukocyte pool. These cells are part of the innate immune system, are essential for host defence, and are involved in the pathology of various inflammatory conditions. This latter inflammatory involvement reflects tissue peroxidation resulting from incomplete phagocytosis. One of the more pronounced features of physical activity on immune parameters is the prolonged neutrocytosis following acute long-term exercise [90]. There are a number of reports showing that exercise triggers a series of changes in the neutrophil population and may affect certain subpopulations differentially. A reduction in the expression of L-selectin (CD62L) immediately after exercise followed by an increase during recovery has been reported [103]. There were no concomitant changes in CD11a or CD11b expression. In contrast, however, increased expression of CD11b in response to exercise was found [104]. Increased expression of the cell-adhesion molecules following exercise may contribute to neutrophil extravasation into damaged tissue, including skeletal muscle.

Regarding the function of neutrophils, exercise has both short- and long-term effects. The neutrophil response to infection includes adherence, chemotaxis, phagocytosis, oxidative burst, degranulation and microbial killing. In general, moderate exercise boosts neutrophil functions, including chemotaxis, phagocytosis and oxidative burst activity. Extreme exercise on the other hand reduces these functions, with the exception of chemotaxis and degranulation which are not affected [101,105–107].

The movement of neutrophils from marginal pools located intravascularly and from extravascular storage pools contributes to exercise-related neutrocytosis. The role of the lung vasculature in neutrophilic granulocyte sequestration has been demonstrated [108]. With respect to the lymphocytosis of exercise, the role of margination is less clear. The spleen may contribute to lymphocytosis since it encloses a major storage pool of lymphocytes with approximately 2.5 x 10^{11} cells per day circulating between the blood and the splenic pulpa [109]. It has been demonstrated that splanchnic sympathectomy reduces the splenic NK cell activity [110]. Splenectomized subjects demonstrate a low lymphocyte count in response to injection of adrenaline [111] and subjects without a spleen show a smaller increase in lymphocyte numbers during exercise [112]. However, there are also studies suggesting that the spleen does not play a role in exercise-leukocytosis [113].

Based on the available data, we hypothesise the following model of lymphocyte recirculation with exercise. Lymphocytes are recruited to the circulation from other tissue pools during exercise. The organs involved include the spleen, the lymph nodes and the gastrointestinal tract.

Since the cells mobilised to the blood have short telomere lengths, it is not likely that these cells are mobilised from the bone marrow or from the thymus. The number of cells that enter the circulation is determined by the intensity of the stimulus. If exercise has been for a prolonged duration and/or of very high intensity, the total concentration of lymphocytes declines. The mechanisms for this probably include the lack of mature cells which can be recruited, as well as the redistribution of lymphocytes from the circulation to organs. In animal models [114], there is some information available about the organs to which these lymphocytes are redistributed after exercise, although the proportion of lymphocyte subsets varies as a function of lymphoid compartments. A recent animal study indicated that redistribution to skeletal muscles did not occur after exercise [115]. Whether or not post-exercise lymphopenia occurs is therefore dependent on a combination of intensity and duration.

3.2. NK cells

Exercise of various types, durations and intensities induces recruitment to the blood of cells expressing characteristic NK cell markers [116,117]. Using in vitro assays, NK cell activity (lysis per fixed number of BMNC) increases consequent to the increased proportions of cells mediating non-MHC-restricted cytotoxicity. During exercise the NK cell activity on a per NK cell basis is unchanged [118,119] or reduced [120] depending on exercise intensity. In an early publication [121], it was shown that NK cells with a high IL-2 response capacity were recruited to the blood during bicycle exercise. When BMNC were preincubated with cytokines, IFN-α or IL-2, or with the cyclooxygenase inhibitor, indomethacin, a significant increase in the NK cell activity was registered at all the time points studied. During exercise the IL-2-enhanced NK cell activity increased significantly more than the IFN-α-enhanced NK cell activity. When BMNC were incubated with IL-2 for more than three days, the LAK cell activity of cells from blood sampled at the end of the exercise period was significantly increased [122]. These data support the early findings [121] that during exercise NK cells with a high IL-2 response capacity are recruited to the blood. Following intense exercise of long duration, the concentration of NK cells and NK cytolytic activity declines below exercise values. Maximal reduction in NK cell concentrations, and hence the lower NK cell activity, occurs 2 to 4 hours after exercise.

The percentage of NK cells was suppressed below prevalues [123] or unchanged compared to prevalues [116]. In accordance with these controversial findings, the post-exercise suppression of the NK cell activity has been ascribed to a decreased proportion of NK cells among BMNC. However, it has also been reported that NK cell activity was not lower on a per NK cell basis following moderate exercise; in fact NK cell activity on a "per cell" basis was elevated post-exercise [118]. Increases in NK cell activity were accompanied by a corresponding increase in serine-esterase activity [124]. Other investigators suggest that reductions in NK cell activity were due to down-regulation of the NK cell activity by prostaglandins (PG) [123]. This hypothesis is based on the observation that indomethacin partly restored post-exercise impairment of NK cell function [123] and that the NK cell activity was partly reduced by PGE1, PGE2 and PGD2 [125].

Generally, NK cell activity is increased when measured immediately after or during both moderate and intense exercise of a few minutes. The intensity, more than the duration of exercise, is responsible for the degree of increment in the number of NK cells. If the exercise has lasted for a long period and has been very intense (e.g., a triathlon race), only a modest increase in NK cells is found post-exercise [126]. NK cell count and the NK cell activity are markedly lower only following intense exercise of at least one hour duration. The definitive study to map the time-course in terms of post-exercise NK cell immune impairment has not been done. Initial fitness level or sex, do not appear to influence the magnitude of exercise-induced changes in NK cells [127,128].

3.3. Mucosal immunity

Gleeson and Pyne recently reviewed the literature [129]. They report that while habitual exercise at an intense level can cause suppression of mucosal immune parameters, moderate exercise may have positive effects. Lower concentrations of the salivary IgA have been reported in cross-country skiers after a race [130]. This finding was confirmed by a 70% decrease in salivary IgA which persisted for several hours after completion of intense, long duration ergometer cycling [131]. Decreased salivary IgA was found after intense swimming [132,133], after running [134], and after incremental treadmill running to exhaustion [135]. Submaximal exercise had no effect on salivary IgA [135,136]. Salivary IgA and IgM concentrations decline immediately after a bout of intense exercise, but usually recover within 24 h. Training at an intense level over many years can result in a chronic suppression of salivary immunoglobulin levels. The degree of immune suppression and the recovery rates after exercise are associated with the intensity of exercise and the duration or volume of the training [129].

3.4. Cellular activation

Increased plasma concentrations of soluble intercellular adhesion molecule 1 (ICAM1), CD23 and neopterin were recorded in 18 individuals during or after long-duration exercise [137]. Exercise has been found to render mouse splenocytes more resistant to the blockade effect of antibodies to LFA-1 (the intercellular adhesion molecule ICAM) [138]. These results suggest that there is some immune system activation during intense exercise of long duration. However, in another study the levels of colony-stimulating factor and neopterin remained unchanged after concentric exercise [139]. Prolonged severe physical exercise has been associated with an initial increase and delayed decrease in circulating immune complexes [140,141]. However, the changes were, although statistically significant, quantitatively small, and the values were only occasionally above the upper limit. Other studies did not indicate these changes [142,143]. The lack of increased concentrations of immune complexes and also the lack of occurrence of C3c and C3d indicate that immune complex-induced complement activation does not occur during concentric exercise [142]. Furthermore, the levels of complement receptor type one (CR1) on erythrocytes do not change in relation to concentric exercise, neither in healthy subjects nor in patients with rheumatoid arthritis [142]. A similar time course of changes in myeloperoxidase and C5a, and the highly significant relationship between these two variables lend some support to the hypothesis that complement activation contributes to post-exercise neutrocytosis in eccentric exercise [144]. The disparity between the studies [140–144] may be explained by the fact that only exercise of long duration or exercise involving an eccentric component cause activation of the complement cascade. In support of this hypothesis downhill running, but not uphill walking, induced increased plasma levels of myeloperoxidase and elastase [145].

4. REPETITIVE BOUTS OF EXERCISE

In contrast to a vast number of investigations on immune cell responses to a single bout of exercise, there is limited information on how repeated bouts of exercise on the same day affect the immune system. The few studies that have measured changes in concentration and function of leukocytes associated with repeated bouts of exercise have all used different exercise and recovery protocols, as well as subjects with varying training status [43,146,147]. A methodological limitation that applies to all of the previous investigations is the lack of control for diurnal variations in various blood constituents, as the response to a first bout of exercise in the morning has been compared with a second or third bout later on the same day. Besides, the exercise and recovery protocols used in the aforementioned studies hardly reflect the daily exercise and recovery regime practised by most elite endurance athletes. A recent study used a study design that eliminated the effect of diurnal variations. This study [148] compared leukocyte counts and lymphocyte responsiveness during and after a second bout of high-intensity endurance exercise on the same day with the response to a similar but single bout of exercise. Athletes participated in three 24-h trials: 1) rest in bed (Rest); 2) one bout of exercise (One); and 3) two bouts of exercise (Two). All bouts consisted of 75 min at approximately 75% of maximal O_2 uptake on a cycle ergometer. The second bout of exercise in the Two trial was associated with significantly increased concentrations of total leukocytes, neutrophils and $CD56^+$ NK cells. These differences suggest a "carry-over" effect in the immune system from a first to a second bout of exercise on the same day, whereas immune changes in response to five repetitive bouts of cycling over five days (each separated by a rest of 24 hours) were not different from those elicited by the first bout [146]. Ronsen et al. [149] further described enhanced plasma IL-6 and IL-1ra responses to repeated versus single bouts of cycling in athletes. The response was more pronounced if the recovery between the two exercise episodes was 3 hours versus 6 hours.

5. EXERCISE AND HYPOXIA

The effect of acute hypoxia on lymphocyte subpopulations resembles the effect of exercise [150]. Thus, when subjects were placed in a decompression chamber (380 Torr) for 20 min with or without supplemental oxygen, the lymphocyte concentration increased during the exposure and declined below prevalues in the post-hypoxic period. All lymphocyte subpopulations were influenced by the hypoxia, but the NK cells were more sensitive to the stress induced by hypoxia [151]. Also, the NK cell function demonstrated the same pattern as with exercise. The NK cell activity did not decline following the 20 min of hypoxia, which is in accordance with the short term exercise induced recruitment of NK cells to the circulation, but not post-stress immune impairment. Meehan et al. [152] demonstrated that there was no change in NK cells after 4 weeks, indicating that the effect of hypoxia on NK cells is transient. Hypoxia induced a small increase in neutrophil number [151]. However, a marked increase in the chemiluminescence response of neutrophils was found 2 h after hypoxia [151]. Thus, hypoxia and exercise induce the same effects on neutrophil number and function. When exercise is performed during hypoxic conditions, the exercise-induced effects on lymphocyte subpopulations are in general pronounced [153]. This was especially so regarding the combined effect of exercise and hypoxia on NK cells and NK cell function [153]. Interestingly, this effect was not abolished by blocking the nerve impulses from active muscles and was not mediated by beta-endorphins [153].

6. MECHANISMS OF ACTION

Acute, intense muscular exercise increases the concentrations of a number of stress hormones in the blood, including adrenaline, noradrenaline, growth hormone, beta-endorphins, and cortisol, whereas the concentration of insulin slightly decreases [154–156]. In this section the evidence for exercise induced changes in neuro-immune interactions is discussed.

6.1. Catecholamines

During exercise adrenaline is released from the adrenal medulla and noradrenaline is released from the sympathetic nerve terminals. Arterial plasma concentrations of adrenaline and noradrenaline increase almost linearly with duration of dynamic exercise and exponentially with intensity, when it is expressed relative to the individuals maximal oxygen uptake [154]. The expression of beta-adrenoceptors on T, B and NK cells, macrophages and neutrophils in numerous species provide the molecular basis for these cells to be targets for catecholamine signalling [157]. The numbers of adrenergic receptors on the individual lymphocyte subpopulations may determine the degree to which the cells are mobilised in response to catecholamines. In accordance with this hypothesis, it has been shown that different subpopulations of BMNC have different numbers of beta-adrenergic receptors [158–161]. NK cells contain the highest number of beta-adrenergic receptors with CD4+ lymphocytes having the lowest number. B lymphocytes and CD8+ lymphocytes are intermediate between NK cells and CD4+ lymphocytes [158]. Dynamic exercise upregulates the beta-adrenergic density, but only on NK cells [158]. Interestingly, NK cells are more responsive to exercise and other stressors than any other subpopulation. CD4+ cells are less sensitive and CD8+ cells and B cells are intermediate [1]. Thus, a correlation exists between numbers of beta-adrenergic receptors on lymphocyte subpopulations and their responsiveness to exercise. Selective administration of adrenaline to obtain plasma-concentrations comparable to those obtained during concentric cycling for 1 hour at 75% of VO_2max, mimicked the exercise-induced effect on BMNC subsets, NK cell activity, LAK cell activity and the lymphocyte proliferative response [42,162–164]. However, adrenaline infusion caused either a very small or no increase in neutrophil concentrations compared to levels observed following exercise [162,163]. Thus, adrenaline seems to be responsible for the recruitment of lymphocytes, and in particular NK cells, to the blood during physical exercise.

6.2. Growth hormone

Plasma levels of pituitary hormones increase in response to exercise both with duration and intensity. Growth hormone responses are more related to the peak exercise intensity rather than to duration of exercise or total work output [154]. An intravenous bolus injection of growth hormone at blood concentrations comparable to those observed during exercise, had no effect on BMNC subsets, NK cell activity, cytokine production, or lymphocyte function, but induced a highly significant neutrocytosis [165].

6.3. Cortisol

The plasma concentrations of cortisol increases only in relation to exercise of long duration [155]. Thus, short term exercise does not increase the cortisol concentration in plasma, and only minor changes in the concentrations of plasma cortisol were described in relation to acute time-limited exercise stress of one hour [155]. It is well documented that corticosteroids given intravenously to humans cause lymphocytopenia, monocytopenia, eosinopenia and neutrophilia which reach their maximum 4 hours after administration [159]. The increase in cortisol during exercise is mediated by IL-6 [91]. Linking exercise-induced lymphocyte changes to an effect of IL-6 on cortisol production is further supported by several studies demonstrating that carbohydrate loading during exercise attenuates both the exercise-induced increase in circulating IL-6 as well as the exercise effect on lymphocyte number and function [34,92,93].

To summarise, adrenaline, and to a lesser extent, noradrenaline contribute to the acute effects on NK cells. The increase in growth hormone mediates the acute effects on neutrophils. The exercise-induced increase in cortisol is mediated by IL-6. Cortisol exerts its effects within a time lag of at least two hours and contributes to the maintenance of low NK cell activity and neutrophilia after prolonged exercise.

7. DIETARY INTERVENTION

Given that the mechanisms underlying exercise-induced immune changes are multifactorial and include altered metabolism during exercise as well as a pronounced neuroendocrinological response, many theories have been put forward. Free oxygen radicals and prostaglandins (PG) released by the elevated number of neutrophils and monocytes may influence the function of lymphocytes and contribute to the impaired function of the later cells. Thus, nutritional supplementation with carbohydrate, glutamine, antioxidant and PG inhibitors may in principle influence exercise-associated immune function. However, with regard to effect on exercise-related changes in natural immunity, it is possible only to make firm conclusions about carbohydrate and glutamine, whereas the available information is sparse regarding other interventions.

7.1. Carbohydrate, NK and neutrophil function

As described above, carbohydrate ingestion attenuates elevations in plasma IL-6 during both running and cycling [34,45]. Post-exercise decline in NK cell function and post-exercise neutrophilia are mediated by cortisol. The increase in cortisol is mediated by IL-6 [91]. Thus, in theory if IL-6 is inhibited, post-exercise immune impairment will be less pronounced. Earlier research had established that a reduction in blood glucose levels is linked to hypothalamic-pituitary-adrenal activation, an increased release of adrenocorticotrophic hormone and cortisol, increased plasma growth hormone, decreased insulin, and a variable effect on blood epinephrine level [166]. Given the link between stress hormones and immune responses to prolonged and intensive exercise [167], carbohydrate compared to placebo ingestion should maintain plasma glucose concentrations, attenuate increases in stress hormones, and thereby diminish changes in immunity. The new observation is that IL-6 is linking the effect of low blood glucose and low glycogen concentration in the muscle to the effect on cortisol, which thereby may influence the effect of exercise on the immune system. The hypothesis that carbohydrate may influence exercise-induced immune changes has been tested in a number of studies by Nieman et al. [34,92,93] using double-blind, placebo-controlled randomised designs. Carbohydrate beverage ingestion before, during (about 1 litre/hour), and after 2.5 hours of exercise was associated with higher plasma glucose levels, an attenuated cortisol and growth hormone response, fewer perturbations in blood immune cell counts, lower granulocyte and monocyte phagocytosis and oxidative burst activity.

7.2. Glutamine, NK cell and neutrophil function

Skeletal muscle is the major tissue involved in glutamine production and known to release glutamine into the blood stream at a high rate. Therefore, skeletal muscle may play a vital role in maintenance of the key process of glutamine utilisation in the immune cells. Consequently, the activity of the skeletal muscle may directly influence the immune system. It has been hypothesised (the so called "glutamine-hypothesis") that under intense physical exercise, or in relation to surgery, trauma, burn and sepsis, the demands on muscle and other organs for glutamine are such that the lymphoid system may be forced into a glutamine debt, which temporarily affects its function. Thus, factors that directly or indirectly influence glutamine synthesis or release, could theoretically influence the function of lymphocytes and monocytes [168,169]. Following intense long-term exercise and other physical stress disorders, the glutamine concentration in plasma declines [170–173]. In four placebo-controlled glutamine intervention studies [174–177], it was found that glutamine abolished the post-exercise decline in plasma glutamine without influencing post-exercise impairment of NK and LAK cell function, or mitogen-induced proliferative responses or salivary IgA. Thus, contrary to the glutamine-hypothesis, the latter studies did not support the idea that post-exercise decline in immune function is caused by a decrease in the plasma glutamine concentration [178].

8. CHRONIC EXERCISE

In contrast to the large number of studies on the immune response to acute exercise, much less is known concerning the effect of physical conditioning or training on immune function. This is largely due to the difficulties in separating fitness effects from the actual physical exercise, and the long duration studies that need to be performed. Thus, the changes induced by intense physical exercise may last at least 24 hours, and even moderate acute exercise induces significant immune changes for several hours. In brief, a number of human studies report that the NK cell activity as measured at rest is elevated in trained versus untrained humans [179–181] and animals [182–186], whereas the lymphocyte proliferative responses have been described as decreased [187], elevated [188,189] or unchanged [179–181,190,191] when comparing athletes and non-athletes. Neutrophil function is either suppressed [192,193] or not significantly influenced by exercise training [194,195]. Neutrophil function was unchanged in athletes during a low training period, but decreased during periods of high intensity training [189,196].

9. EXERCISE AND INFECTIONS

Without doubt exercise and training influence natural immunity. An important question is, however, to what degree are these cellular changes of clinical significance, especially with respect to resistance to infectious diseases. From animal studies [197–199] it is clear that effects of exercise on disease lethality vary with the type and time that it is performed. In general, exercise or training before infection has either no effect or decreases morbidity and mortality. Exercise during the incubation period of the infection appears to have either no effect or to increase severity of infection. In contrast to the limited experimental evidence, there are several epidemiological studies on exercise and upper respiratory tract infections (URTI). These studies are based on self-reported symptoms rather than clinical verification. In general, increased numbers of URTI symptoms have been reported in the days following strenuous exercise (e.g., a marathon race) [127,200–202] whereas moderate training has been claimed to reduce the number of symptoms [188,203]. However, in neither strenuous nor moderate exercise have these symptoms been causally linked to exercise-induced changes in immune function.

10. CONCLUSION

Natural immunity is highly influenced by muscular exercise. Highly consistent changes are found in the production of IL-6 as well as in the number and function of NK cells and neutrophils. During exercise and other physical stress reactions (trauma, surgery, burn) as well as environmental stimuli (hyperthermia and hypoxia), increased catecholamine levels in the circulation induce recruitment of NK cells to the circulation. In response to muscle contractions, IL-6 is produced and released from working skeletal muscles. IL-6 induces increased levels of other anti-inflammatory cytokines such as IL-1ra and IL-10 and induces cortisol production and hence suppression of natural killer cell cytotoxicity and neutrophilia. IL-6 also works as an energy sensor. Thus, the production of IL-6 from working muscles is further enhanced if muscle glycogen content is low. In addition, carbohydrate intake during the exercise attenuates the IL-6 production and consequently exercise-induced cortisol production and fluctuations in NK cells and neutrophils. The major new finding is that exercise-induced immune changes are not a secondary phenomenon to exercise-induced hormonal changes. Rather, muscle contractions per se induce the release of a cytokine, IL-6, which is produced by muscle fibres. By producing IL-6, muscle fibres are directly involved in exercise-induced immune changes, and exercise-induced cortisol changes can be viewed as a secondary phenomenon, which in turn leads to altered leukocyte subset composition. As IL-6 works as an energy sensor, it is also clear that dietary factors such as carbohydrate may influence the immune response to exercise. It is a hallmark that a cytokine, previously known as a component of the natural immune defence, should now also be viewed as an important player in metabolism.

REFERENCES

1. Hoffman-Goetz L, Pedersen BK. Exercise and the immune system: a model of the stress response? Immunol Today 1994;15(8):382–7.
2. Pedersen BK, Hoffman- Goetz L. Exercise and the immune system: regulation, integration and adaption. Physiol Rev 2000;80(3):1055–81.
3. Pedersen BK, Kappel M, Klokker M, Nielsen HB, Secher NH. The immune system during exposure to extreme physiologic conditions. Int J Sports Med 1994;15 Suppl 3:S116–21.
4. Febbraio MA, Pedersen BK. Muscle-derived interleukin-6: mechanisms for activation and possible biological roles. FASEB J 2002;16(11):1335–47.
5. Pedersen BK, Steensberg A, Keller P, Keller C, Fischer C, Hiscock N, et al. Muscle derived interleukin-6-lipolytic, antiinflammatory and immune regulatory effects. Eur J Physiol 2003;446:9–16.
6. Ostrowski K, Rohde T, Zacho M, Asp S, Pedersen BK. Evidence that interleukin-6 is produced in human skeletal muscle during prolonged running. J Physiol 1998;508 (pt 3): 949–53.
7. Ostrowski K, Hermann C, Bangash A, Schjerling P, Nielsen JN, Pedersen BK. A trauma-

like elevation of plasma cytokines in humans in response to treadmill running. J Physiol 1998; 513(Pt3):889–94.
8. Ostrowski K, Rohde T, Asp S, Schjerling P, Pedersen BK. Pro- and anti-inflammatory cytokine balance in strenuous exercise in humans. J Physiol 1999; 515(Pt1):287–91.
9. Pedersen BK, Ostrowski K, Rohde T, Bruunsgaard H. The cytokine response to strenuous exercise. Can J Physiol Pharmacol 1998;76(5):505–11.
10. Starkie RL, Rolland J, Angus DJ, Anderson MJ, Febbraio MA. Circulating monocytes are not the source of elevations in plasma IL-6 and TNF-alpha levels after prolonged running. Am J Physiol Cell Physiol 2001;280(4):C769–74.
11. Toft AD, Thorn M, Ostrowski K, Asp S, Møller K, Iversen S, et al. N-3 polyunsaturated fatty acids do not affect cytokine response to strenuous execise. J Appl Physiol 2000;89(6): 2401–6.
12. Suzuki K, Yamada M, Kurakake S, Okamura N, Yamaya K, Liu Q, et al. Circulating cytokines and hormones with immunosuppressive but neutrophil-priming potentials rise after endurance exercise in humans. Eur J Appl Physiol 2000;81:281–7.
13. Ostrowski K, Rohde T, Asp S, Schjerling P, Pedersen BK. Chemokines are elevated in plasma after strenuous exercise in humans. Eur J Appl Physiol 2001;84(3):244–5.
14. Niess AM, Sommer M, Schlotz E, Northoff H, Dickhuth HH, Fehrenbach E. Expression of the inducible nitric oxide synthase (iNOS) in human leukocytes: responses to running exercise. Med Sci Sports Exerc 2000;32(7):1220–5.
15. van Eeden SF, Terashima T. Interleukin 8 (IL-8) and the release of leukocytes from the bone marrow. Leuk Lymphoma 2000;37(3–4):259–71.
16. Drenth JP, Van Uum SH, Van Deuren M, Pesman GJ, Van der Ven Jongekrijg J, Van der Meer JW. Endurance run increases circulating IL-6 and IL-1ra but downregulates ex vivo TNF-alpha and IL-1beta production. J Appl Physiol 1995;79(5):1497–503.
17. Weinstock C, Konig D, Harnischmacher R, Keul J, Berg A, Northoff H. Effect of exhaustive exercise stress on the cytokine response. Med Sci Sports Exerc 1997; 29(3):345–54.
18. Haahr PM, Pedersen BK, Fomsgaard A, Tvede N, Diamant M, Klarlund K, et al. Effect of physical exercise on in vitro production of interleukin 1, interleukin 6, tumor necrosis factor-alpha, interleukin 2 and interferon- gamma. Int J Sports Med 1991;12(2):223–7.
19. Pannen BH, Robotham JL. The acute-phase response. New Horiz 1995;3(2):183–97.
20. Gleeson M, Almey J, Brooks S, Cave R, Lewis A, Griffiths H. Haematological and acute-phase responses associated with delayed- onset muscle soreness in humans. Eur J Appl Physiol Occup Physiol 1995;71(2-3):137–42.
21. Ray A, Ray BK. Serum amyloid A gene expression level in liver in response to different inflammatory agents is dependent upon the nature of activated transcription factors. DNA Cell Biol 1997;16(1):1–7.
22. Rojanasakul Y, Shi X, Deshpande D, Liang WW, Wang LY. Protection against oxidative injury and permeability alteration in cultured alveolar epithelium by transferrin-catalase conjugate. Biochim Biophys Acta 1996;1315(1):21–8.
23. Kargotich S, Goodman C, Keast D, Fry RW, Garcia-Webb P, Crawford PM, et al. Influence of exercise-induced plasma volume changes on the interpretation of biochemical data following high-intensity exercise. Clin J Sport Med 1997;7(3):185–91.
24. Hubinger L, Mackinnon LT, Barber L, McCosker J, Howard A, Lepre F. Acute effects of treadmill running on lipoprotein(a) levels in males and females. Med Sci Sports Exerc 1997;29(4):436–42.
25. Bourque SP, Pate RR, Branch JD. Twelve weeks of endurance exercise training does not

affect iron status measures in women. J Am Diet Assoc 1997;97(10):1116–21.
26. Nindl BC, Friedl KE, Frykman PN, Marchitelli LJ, Shippee RL, Patton JF. Physical performance and metabolic recovery among lean, healthy men following a prolonged energy deficit. Int J Sports Med 1997;18(5):317–24.
27. Gunga HC, Wittels P, Gunther T, Kanduth B, Vormann J, Rocker L, et al. Erythropoietin in 29 men during and after prolonged physical stress combined with food and fluid deprivation. Eur J Appl Physiol Occup Physiol 1996;73(1–2):11–6.
28. Pyne DB, Baker MS, Telford RD, Weidermann MJ. A treadmill protocol to investigate independently the metabolic and mechanical stress of exercise. Aust J Sci Med Sport 1997;29(3):77–82.
29. Schuit AJ, Schouten EG, Kluft C, de Maat M, Menheere PP, Kok FJ. Effect of strenuous exercise on fibrinogen and fibrinolysis in healthy elderly men and women. Thromb Haemost 1997;78(2):845–51.
30. Akira S, Taga T, Kishimoto T. Interleukin-6 in biology and medicine. Adv Immunol 1993;54:1–78.
31. Nagaraju K, Raben N, Merritt G, Loeffler L, Kirk K, Plotz P. A variety of cytokines and immunologically relevant surface molecules are expressed by normal human skeletal muscle cells under proinflammatory stimuli. Clin Exp Immunol 1998;113(3);407–14.
32. Pedersen BK, Steensberg A, Schjerling P. Muscle-derived interleukin-6: possible biological effects. J Physiol 2001;536(Pt2):329–37.
33. Northoff H, Berg A. Immunologic mediators as parameters of the reaction to strenuous exercise. Int J Sports Med 1991;12 Suppl 1:S9–15.
34. Gadient RA, Patterson PH. Leukemia inhibitory factor, Interleukin 6, and other cytokines using the GP130 transducing receptor: roles in inflammation and injury. Stem Cells 1999;17(3):127–37.
35. Nehlsen-Cannarella SL, Fagoaga OR, Nieman DC, Henson DA, Butterworth DE, Schmitt RL, et al. Carbohydrate and the cytokine response to 2.5 hours of running. J Appl Physiol 1997;82(5):1662–7.
36. Castell LM, Poortmans JR, Leclercq R, Brasseur M, Duchateau J, Newsholme EA. Some aspects of the acute phase response after a marathon race, and the effects of glutamine supplementation. Eur J Appl Physiol Occup Physiol 1997;75(1):47–53.
37. Rohde T, MacLean DA, Richter EA, Kiens B, Pedersen BK. Prolonged submaximal eccentric exercise is associated with increased levels of plasma IL-6. Am J Physiol 1997; 273(1Pt1):E85–91.
38. Hellsten Y, Frandsen U, Orthenblad N, Sjodin B, Richter EA. Xanthine oxidase in human skeletal muscle following eccentric exercise: a role in inflammation. J Physiol 1997;498 (Pt1):239–48.
39. Nieman DC, Nehlsen-Cannarella SL, Fagoaga OR, Henson DA, Utter A, Davis JM, et al. Effects of mode and carbohydrate on the granulocyte and monocyte response to intensive, prolonged exercise. J Appl Physiol 1998;84(4):1252–9.
40. Starkie RL, Arkinstall MJ, Koukoulas I, Hawley JA, Febbraio MA. Carbohydrate ingestion attenuates the increase in plasma interleukin-6, but not skeletal muscle interleukin-6 mRNA, during exercise in humans. J Physiol 2001;533(Pt 2):585–91.
41. Steensberg A, van Hall G, Osada T, Sacchetti M, Saltin B, Klarlund Pedersen B. Production of interleukin-6 in contracting human skeletal muscles can account for the exercise-induced increase in plasma interleukin-6. J Physiol 2000;529 Pt1:237–42.
42. Steensberg A, Febbraio MA, Osada T, Schjerling P, van Hall G, Saltin B, et al. Interleukin-

6 production in contracting human skeletal muscle is influenced by pre-exercise muscle glycogen content. J Physiol 2001;537 (Pt 2):633–9.
43. Steensberg A., Toft A.D, Schjerling P, Halkjaer-Kristensen J., Pedersen B.K. Plasma interleukin-6 during strenuous exercise: role of epinephrine. Am J Physiol Cell Physiol 2001; 281(3):C1001–4.
44. Nielsen HB, Secher NH, Christensen NJ, Pedersen BK. Lymphocytes and NK cell activity during repeated bouts of maximal exercise. Am J Physiol 1996;271(1Pt2):R222–7.
45. Ostrowski K, Schjerling P, Pedersen BK. Physical activity and plasma interleukin-6 in humans - effect of intensity of exercise. Eur J Appl Physiol 2000;83(6):512–5.
46. Nieman DC, Nehlsen-Cannarella SL, Fagoaga OR, Henson DA, Utter A, Davis JM, et al. Influence of mode and carbohydrate on the cytokine response to heavy exertion. Med Sci Sports Exerc 1998;30(5):671–8.
47. Northoff H, Weinstock C, Berg A. The cytokine response to strenuous exercise. Int J Sports Med 1994;15 Suppl 3:S167–71.
48. Sprenger H, Jacobs C, Nain M, Gressner AM, Prinz H, Wesemann W, et al. Enhanced release of cytokines, interleukin-2 receptors, and neopterin after long-distance running. Clin Immunol Immunopathol 1992;63(2):188–95.
49. Ullum H, Haahr PM, Diamant M, Palmo J, Halkjaer-Kristensen J, Pedersen BK. Bicycle exercise enhances plasma IL-6 but does not change IL-1alpha, IL-1beta, IL-6, or TNF-alpha pre-mRNA in BMNC. J Appl Physiol 1994;77(1):93–7.
50. Nehlsen Cannarella SL, Fagoaga OR, Nieman DC, Henson DA, Butterworth DE, Schmitt RL, et al. Carbohydrate and the cytokine response to 2.5 h of running. J Appl Physiol 1997; 82(5):1662–67.
51. Bruunsgaard H, Galbo H, Halkjaer-Kristensen J, Johansen TL, MacLean DA, Pedersen BK. Exercise-induced increase in serum interleukin-6 in humans is related to muscle damage. J Physiol 1997;499(Pt3):833–41.
52. Croisier JL, Camus G, Venneman I, Deby-Dupont G, Juchmes-Ferir A, Lamy M, et al. Effects of training on exercise-induced muscle damage and interleukin 6 production. Muscle Nerve 1999;22(2):208–12.
53. Toft AD, Jensen LB, Bruunsgaard H, Ibfelt T, Halkjaer-Kristensen J, Febbraio M, et al. Cytokine response to eccentric exercise in young and elderly humans. Am J Physiol Cell Physiol 2002;283(1):C289–95.
54. Rhind SG, Castellani JW, Brenner IK, Shephard RJ, Zamecnik J, Montain SJ, et al. Intracellular monocyte and serum cytokine expression is modulated by exhausting exercise and cold exposure. Am J Physiol Regul Integr Comp Physiol 2001;281(1):R66–75.
55. DeRijk RH, Boelen A, Tilders FJ, Berkenbosch F. Induction of plasma interleukin-6 by circulating adrenaline in the rat. Psychoneuroendocrinology 1994;19(2):155–63.
56. Moldoveanu AI, Shephard RJ, Shek PN. Exercise elevates plasma levels but not gene expression of IL-1beta, IL- 6, and TNF-alpha in blood mononuclear cells. J Appl Physiol 2000;89(4):1499–504.
57. Starkie RL, Angus DJ, Rolland J, Hargreaves M, Febbraio MA. Effect of prolonged submaximal exercise and carbohydrate ingestion on monocyte intracellular cytokine production in humans. J Physiol 2000;528(Pt3):647–55.
58. Jonsdottir IH, Schjerling P, Ostrowski K, Asp S, Richter EA, Pedersen BK. Muscle contractions induce interleukin-6 mRNA production in rat skeletal muscles. J Physiol 2000;528 Pt1:157–63.
59. Febbraio MA, Steensberg A, Starkie RL, McConell GK, Kingwell BA. Skeletal muscle

interleukin-6 and tumor necrosis factor-alpha release in healthy subjects and patients with type 2 diabetes at rest and during exercise. Metabolism 2003;52(7):939–44.

60. Bartoccioni E, Michaelis D, Hohlfeld R. Constitutive and cytokine-induced production of interleukin-6 by human myoblasts. Immunol Lett 1994;42(3):135–8.
61. De Rossi M, Bernasconi P, Baggi F, de Waal Malefyt R, Mantegazza R. Cytokines and chemokines are both expressed by human myoblasts: possible relevance for the immune pathogenesis of muscle inflammation. Int Immunol 2000;12(9):1329–35.
62. Yan SF, Tritto I, Pinsky D, Liao H, Huang J, Fuller G, et al. Induction of interleukin 6 (IL-6) by hypoxia in vascular cells. Central role of the binding site for nuclear factor-IL-6. J Biol Chem 1995;270(19):11463–71.
63. Klouche M, Bhakdi S, Hemmes M, Rose-John S. Novel path to activation of vascular smooth muscle cells: up-regulation of gp130 creates an autocrine activation loop by IL-6 and its soluble receptor. J Immunol 1999;163(8):4583–9.
64. Keller C, Steensberg A, Pilegaard H, Osada T, Saltin B, Pedersen BK, et al. Transcriptional activation of the IL-6 gene in human contracting skeletal muscle: influence of muscle glycogen content. Faseb J 2001;15(14):2748–50.
65. Nybo L, Nielsen B, Pedersen BK, Moller K, Secher NH. Interleukin-6 release from the human brain during prolonged exercise. J Physiol 2002;542(Pt 3):991–5.
66. Langberg H, Olesen JL, Gemmer C, Kjaer M. Substantial elevation of interleukin-6 concentration in peritendinous tissue, in contrast to muscle, following prolonged exercise in humans. J Physiol 2002;542(Pt 3):985–90.
67. Keller C, Keller P, Marshall-Gradisnik SM, Pedersen BK. IL-6 gene expression in human adipose tissue in response to exercise - effect of carbohydrate ingestion. J Physiol 2003;550(3):927–31.
68. Penkowa M, Keller C, Keller P, Jauffred S, Pedersen BK. Immunohistochemical detection of interleukin-6 in human skeletal muscle fibers following exercise. FASEB J 2003;17(14): 2166–8.
69. Gleeson M, Bishop NC. Special feature for the Olympics: effects of exercise on the immune system: modification of immune responses to exercise by carbohydrate, glutamine and anti-oxidant supplements. Immunol Cell Biol 2000;78(5):554–61.
70. Stouthard JM, Romijn JA, Van der Poll T, Endert E, Klein S, Bakker PJ et al. Endocrinologic and metabolic effects of interleukin-6 in humans. Am J Physiol 1995;268(5 Pt 1):E813–9.
71. Stouthard JM, Oude Elferink RP, Sauerwein HP. Interleukin-6 enhances glucose transport in 3T3-L1 adipocytes. Biochem Biophys Res Commun 1996;220(2):241–5.
72. Hardin J, Kroeker K, Chung B, Gall DG. Effect of proinflammatory interleukins on jejunal nutrient transport. Gut 2000;47(2):184–91.
73. Nonogaki K, Fuller GM, Fuentes NL, Moser AH, Staprans I, Grunfeld C, et al. Interleukin-6 stimulates hepatic triglyceride secretion in rats. Endocrinology 1995;136(5):2143–9.
74. Wallenius V, Wallenius K, Ahren B, Rudling M, Carlsten H, Dickson SL, et al. Interleukin-6-deficient mice develop mature-onset obesity. Nat Med 2002;8(1):75–9.
75. Yudkin JS, Kumari M, Humphries SE, Mohammed-Ali V. Inflammation, obesity, stress and coronary heart disease: is interleukin-6 the link? Atherosclerosis 2000;148(2):209–14.
76. Bruunsgaard H, Andersen-Ranberg K, Jeune B, Pedersen AN, Skinhoj P, Pedersen BK. A high plasma concentration of TNFalpha is associated with dementia in centenarians. J Gerontol A Biol Sci Med Sci 1999;54(7):M357–64.

77. Bastard JP, Jardel C, Bruckert E, Blondy P, Capeau J, Laville M, et al. Elevated levels of interleukin 6 are reduced in serum and subcutaneous adipose tissue of obese women after weight loss. J Clin Endocrinol Metab 2000;85(9):3338–42.
78. Pickup JC, Chusney GD, Thomas SM, Burt D. Plasma interleukin-6, tumour necrosis factor alpha and blood cytokine production in type 2 diabetes. Life Sci 2000;67(3):291–300.
79. Katsuki A, Sumida Y, Murashima S, Murata K, Takarada Y, Ito K, et al. Serum levels of tumor necrosis factor-alpha are increased in obese patients with noninsulin-dependent diabetes mellitus. J Clin Endocrinol Metab 1998;83(3):859–62.
80. Mishima Y, Kuyama A, Tada A, Takahashi K, Ishioka T, Kibata M. Relationship between serum tumor necrosis factor-alpha and insulin resistance in obese men with Type 2 diabetes mellitus. Diabetes Res Clin Pract 2001;52(2):119–23.
81. Vozarova B, Weyer C, Hanson K, Tataranni PA, Bogardus C, Pratley RE. Circulating interleukin-6 in relation to adiposity, insulin action, and insulin secretion. Obes Res 2001;9(7):414–7.
82. Ridker PM, Rifai N, Stampfer MJ, Hennekens CH. Plasma concentration of interleukin-6 and the risk of future myocardial infarction among apparently healthy men. Circulation 2000;101(15):1767–72.
83. Fried SK, Bunkin DA, Greenberg AS. Omental and subcutaneous adipose tissues of obese subjects release interleukin-6: depot difference and regulation by glucocorticoid. J Clin Endocrinol Metab 1998;83(3):847–50.
84. Hotamisligil GS, Shargill NS, Spiegelman BM. Adipose expression of tumor necrosis factor-alpha: direct role in obesity-linked insulin resistance. Science 1993;259(5091): 87–91.
85. Qi C, Pekala PH. Tumor necrosis factor-alpha-induced insulin resistance in adipocytes. Proc Soc Exp Biol Med 2000;223(2):128–35.
86. Hauner H, Petruschke T, Russ M, Rohrig K, Eckel J. Effects of tumour necrosis factor alpha (TNF alpha) on glucose transport and lipid metabolism of newly-differentiated human fat cells in cell culture. Diabetologia 1995;38(7):764–71.
87. Hotamisligil GS. Mechanisms of TNF-alpha-induced insulin resistance. Exp Clin Endocrinol Diabetes 1999;107(2):119–25.
88. Hotamisligil GS, Budavari A, Murray D, Spiegelman BM. Reduced tyrosine kinase activity of the insulin receptor in obesity-diabetes. Central role of tumor necrosis factor-alpha. J Clin Invest 1994;94(4):1543–9.
89. Patton JS, Shepard HM, Wilking H, Lewis G, Aggarwal BB, Eessalu TE et al. Interferons and tumor necrosis factors have similar catabolic effects on 3T3 L1 cells. Proc Natl Acad Sci U S A 1986;83(21):8313–7.
90. Boden G. Role of fatty acids in the pathogenesis of insulin resistance and NIDDM. Diabetes 1997;46(1):3–10.
91. Fiers W. Tumor necrosis factor. Characterization at the molecular, cellular and in vivo level. FEBS Lett 1991;285(2):199–212.
92. Matthys P, Mitera T, Heremans H, Van Damme J, Billiau A. Anti-gamma interferon and anti-interleukin-6 antibodies affect staphylococcal enterotoxin B-induced weight loss, hypoglycemia, and cytokine release in D-galactosamine-sensitized and unsensitized mice. Infect Immun 1995;63(4):1158–64.
93. Mizuhara H, O'Neill E, Seki N, Ogawa T, Kusunoki C, Otsuka K, et al. T cell activation-associated hepatic injury: mediation by tumor necrosis factors and protection by interleukin

6. J Exp Med 1994;179(5):1529–37.

94. McCarthy DA, Dale MM. The leucocytosis of exercise. A review and model. Sports Med 1988;6(6):333–63.
95. Steensberg A, Toft AD, Bruunsgaard H, Sandmand M, Halkjaer-Kristensen J, Pedersen BK. Strenuous exercise decreases the percentage of type 1 T cells in the circulation. J Appl Physiol 2001;91(4):1708–12.
96. Nieman DC, Henson DA, Garner EB, Butterworth DE, Warren BJ, Utter A, et al. Carbohydrate affects natural killer cell redistribution but not activity after running. Med Sci Sports Exerc 1997;29(10):1318–24.
97. Nieman DC, Fagoaga OR, Butterworth DE, Warren BJ, Utter A, Davis JM, et al. Carbohydrate supplementation affects blood granulocyte and monocyte trafficking but not function after 2.5 h of running. Am J Clin Nutr 1997;66(1):153–9.
98. Pedersen BK. In: Pedersen BK, editor. Exercise Immunology. Austin,Texas, U.S.A.: R.G.Landes Bioscience, 1997;1–206.
99. Keast D, Morton AR. Long-term exercise and immune functions. In: Watson RR, Eisinger M, editors. Exercise and Disease. Florida, Boca Raton: CRC Press, 1992;89–120.
100. Mackinnon LT. Current challenges and future expectations in exercise immunology: back to the future. Med Sci Sports Exerc 1994;26(2):191–4.
101. Pedersen BK, Ostrowski K, Rohde T, Bruunsgaard H. Nutrition, exercise and the immune system. Proc Nutr Soc 1998;57(1):43–7.
102. Pedersen BK, Nieman DC. Exercise immunology: integration and regulation. Immunol Today 1998;19(5):204–6.
103. Keast D, Cameron K, Morton AR. Exercise and the immune response. Sports Med 1988;5(4):248–67.
104. Nieman DC. Exercise, upper respiratory tract infection, and the immune system. Med Sci Sports Exerc 1994;26(2):128–39.
105. Brines R, Hoffman-Goetz L, Pedersen BK. Can you exercise to make your immune system fitter? Immunol Today 1996;17(6):252–4.
106. Hoffman-Goetz L. Exercise, Immunity, and colon cancer. In: Hoffman- Goetz L, Husted J, editors. Exercise and immune function. Boca Raton, FL: CRC Press; 1996. p. 179–98.
107. Kurokawa Y, Shinkai S, Torii J, Hino S, Shek PN. Exercise-induced changes in the expression of surface adhesion molecules on circulating granulocytes and lymphocytes subpopulations. Eur J Appl Physiol Occup Physiol 1995;71(2–3):245–52.
108. Smith JA, Gray AB, Pyne DB, Baker MS, Telford RD, Weidemann MJ. Moderate exercise triggers both priming and activation of neutrophil subpopulations. Am J Physiol 1996;270(4 Pt 2):R838–45.
109. Smith JA, Telford RD, Mason IB, Weidemann MJ. Exercise, training and neutrophil microbicidal activity. Int J Sports Med 1990;11(3):179–87.
110. Ortega E, Collazos ME, Maynar M, Barriga C, De la Fuente M. Stimulation of the phagocytic function of neutrophils in sedentary men after acute moderate exercise. Eur J Appl Physiol Occup Physiol 1993;66(1):60–4.
111. Smith JA, McKenzie SJ, Telford RD, Weidemann MJ. Why does moderate exercise enhance, but intense training depress, immunity? In: Husband AJ, editor. Behavior and Immunity. Boca Raton, FL: CRC Press;1992. p.155–68.
112. Peters AM, Allsop P, Stuttle AW, Arnot RN, Gwilliam M, Hall GM. Granulocyte margination in the human lung and its response to strenuous exercise. Clin Sci (Lond) 1992;82(2):237–44.

113. Pabst R. The spleen in lymphocyte migration. Immunol Today 1988;9(2):43–5.
114. Katafuchi T, Ichijo T, Take S, Hori T. Hypothalamic modulation of splenic natural killer cell activity in rats. J Physiol 1993;471:209–21.
115. Steel CM, French EB, Aitchison WR. Studies on adrenaline-induced leucocytosis in normal man. I. The role of the spleen and of the thoracic duct. Br J Haematol 1971;21(4): 413–21.
116. Nielsen HB, Secher NH, Kristensen JH, Christensen NJ, Espersen K, Pedersen BK. Splenectomy impairs lymphocytosis during maximal exercise. Am J Physiol 1997; 272(6 Pt 2):R1847-R52.
117. Iversen PO, Arvesen BL, Benestad HB. No mandatory role for the spleen in the exercise-induced leucocytosis in man. Clin Sci (Lond) 1994;86(5):505–10.
118. Randall Simpson JA, Hoffman-Goetz L, Thorne R, Arumugam Y. Exercise stress alters the percentage of splenic lymphocyte subsets in response to mitogen but not in response to interleukin-1. Brain Behav Immun 1989;3(2):119–28.
119. Espersen GT, Stamp I, Lidang Jensen M, Elbaek A, Ernst E, Kahr O, et al. Lymphocyte redistribution in connection with physical activity in the rat. Acta Physiol Scand 1995;155(3):313–21.
120. Mackinnon LT. Exercise and natural killer cells. What is the relationship? Sports Med 1989;7(3):141–9.
121. Pedersen BK, Ullum H. NK cell response to physical activity: possible mechanisms of action. Med Sci Sports Exerc 1994;26(2):140–6.
122. Nieman DC, Miller AR, Henson DA, Warren BJ, Gusewitch G, Johnson RL, et al. Effects of high- vs moderate-intensity exercise on natural killer cell activity. Med Sci Sports Exerc 1993;25(10):1126–34.
123. Palmø J, Asp S, Daugaard JR, Richter EA, Klokker M, Pedersen BK. Effect of eccentric exercise on natural killer cell activity. J Appl Physiol 1995;78(4):1442–6.
124. Nielsen HB, Secher NH, Kappel M, Hanel B, Pedersen BK. Lymphocyte, NK and LAK cell responses to maximal exercise. Int J Sports Med 1996;17(1):60–5.
125. Pedersen BK, Tvede N, Hansen FR, Andersen V, Bendix T, Bendixen G, et al. Modulation of natural killer cell activity in peripheral blood by physical exercise. Scand J Immunol 1988;27(6):673–8.
126. Tvede N, Kappel M, Halkjaer-Kristensen J, Galbo H, Pedersen BK. The effect of light, moderate and severe bicycle exercise on lymphocyte subsets, natural and lymphokine activated killer cells, lymphocyte proliferative response and interleukin 2 production. Int J Sports Med 1993;14(5):275–82.
127. Pedersen BK, Tvede N, Klarlund K, Christensen LD, Hansen FR, Galbo H, et al. Indomethacin in vitro and in vivo abolishes post-exercise suppression of natural killer cell activity in peripheral blood. Int J Sports Med 1990;11(2):127–31.
128. Hoffman-Goetz I. Serine esterase (BLT-esterase) activity in murine splenocytes is increased with exercise but not training. Int J Sports Med 1995;16(2):94–8.
129. Droller MJ, Perlmann P, Schneider MU. Enhancement of natural and antibody-dependent lymphocyte cytotoxicity by drugs which inhibit prostaglandin production by tumor target cells. Cell Immunol 1978;39(1):154–64.
130. Rohde T, MacLean DA, Hartkopp A, Pedersen BK. The immune system and serum glutamine during a triathlon. Eur J Appl Physiol Occup Physiol 1996;74(5):428–34.
131. Kendall A, Hoffman-Goetz L, Houston M, MacNeil B, Arumugam Y. Exercise and blood lymphocyte subset responses: intensity, duration, and subject fitness effects. J Appl Physiol

1990;69(1):251–60.

132. Brahmi Z, Thomas JE, Park M, Dowdeswell IR. The effect of acute exercise on natural killer-cell activity of trained and sedentary human subjects. J Clin Immunol 1985;5(5): 321–8.
133. Gleeson M, Pyne DB, McDonald WA, Clancy RL, Cripps AW, Horn PL, et al. Pneumococcal antibody responses in elite swimmers. Clin Exp Immunol 1996;105(2): 238–44.
134. Tomasi TB, Trudeau FB, Czerwinski D, Erredge S. Immune parameters in athletes before and after strenuous exercise. J Clin Immunol 1982;2(3):173–8.
135. Mackinnon LT, Chick TW, van As A, Tomasi TB. The effect of exercise on secretory and natural immunity. Adv Exp Med Biol 1987;216A:869–76.
136. Tharp GD, Barnes MW. Reduction of saliva immunoglobulin levels by swim training. Eur J Appl Physiol Occup Physiol 1990;60(1):61–4.
137. Gleeson M, McDonald WA, Cripps AW, Pyne DB, Clancy RL, Fricker PA. The effect on immunity of long-term intensive training in elite swimmers. Clin Exp Immunol 1995;102(1):210–6.
138. Steerenberg PA, van Asperen IA, van Nieuw Amerongen A, Biewenga A, Mol D, Medema GJ. Salivary levels of immunoglobulin A in triathletes. Eur J Oral Sci 1997;105(4):305–9.
139. McDowell SL, Hughes RA, Hughes RJ, Housh DJ, Housh TJ, Johnson GO. The effect of exhaustive exercise on salivary immunoglobulin A. J Sports Med Phys Fitness 1992;32(4): 412–5.
140. Housh TJ, Johnson GO, Housh DJ, Evans SL, Tharp GD. The effect of exercise at various temperatures on salivary levels of immunoglobulin A. Int J Sports Med 1991;12(5):498–500.
141. Tilz GP, Domej W, Diez-Ruiz A, Weiss G, Brezinschek R, Brezinschek HP, et al. Increased immune activation during and after physical exercise. Immunobiology 1993;188(1–2): 194–202.
142. Hoffman-Goetz L. Effect of acute treadmill exercise on LFA-1 antigen expression in murine splenocytes. Anticancer Res 1995;15(5B):1981–4.
143. Smith JA, Telford RD, Baker MS, Hapel AJ, Weidemann MJ. Cytokine immunoreactivity in plasma does not change after moderate endurance exercise. J Appl Physiol 1992;73(4): 1396–401.
144. Dufaux B, Order U. Complement activation after prolonged exercise. Clin Chim Acta 1989;179(1):45–9.
145. Dufaux B, Muller R, Hollmann W. Assessment of circulating immune complexes by a solid-phase C1q- binding assay during the first hours and days after prolonged exercise. Clin Chim Acta 1985;145(3):313–7.
146. Thomsen BS, Rodgaard A, Tvede N, Hansen FR, Steensberg J, Halkjaer Kristensen J, et al. Levels of complement receptor type one (CR1, CD35) on erythrocytes, circulating immune complexes and complement C3 split products C3d and C3c are not changed by short-term physical exercise or training. Int J Sports Med 1992;13(2):172–5.
147. Simpson IJ, Myles MJ, Smith GW. Immune complexes in normal subjects. J Clin Lab Immunol 1983;11(3):119–22.
148. Camus G, Duchateau J, Deby-Dupont G, Pincemail J, Deby C, Juchmes-Ferir A, et al. Anaphylatoxin C5a production during short-term submaximal dynamic exercise in man. Int J Sports Med 1994;15(1):32–5.

149. Camus G, Pincemail J, Ledent M, Juchmes-Ferir A, Lamy M, Deby-Dupont G, et al. Plasma levels of polymorphonuclear elastase and myeloperoxidase after uphill walking and downhill running at similar energy cost. Int J Sports Med 1992;13(6):443–6.
150. Hoffman-Goetz L, Simpson JR, Cipp N, Arumugam Y, Houston ME. Lymphocyte subset responses to repeated submaximal exercise in men. J Appl Physiol 1990;68(3):1069–74.
151. Field CJ, Gougeon R, Marliss EB. Circulating mononuclear cell numbers and function during intense exercise and recovery. J Appl Physiol 1991;71(3):1089–97.
152. Ronsen O, Pedersen BK, Oritsland TR, Bahr R, Kjeldsen-Kragh J. Leukocyte counts and lymphocyte responsiveness associated with repeated bouts of strenuous endurance exercise. J Appl Physiol 2001;91(1):425–34.
153. Ronsen O, Lea T, Bahr R, Pedersen BK. Enhanced plasma IL-6 and IL-1ra responses to repeated vs. single bouts of prolonged cycling in elite athletes. J Appl Physiol 2002;92(6): 2547–53.
154. Pedersen BK, Steensberg A. Exercise and hypoxia: effects on leukocytes and interleukin-6-shared mechanisms? Med Sci Sports Exerc 2002;34(12):2004–13.
155. Klokker M, Kharazmi A, Galbo H, Bygbjerg I, Pedersen BK. Influence of in vivo hypobaric hypoxia on function of lymphocytes, neutrocytes, natural killer cells, and cytokines. J Appl Physiol 1993;74(3):1100–6.
156. Meehan R, Duncan U, Neale L, Taylor G, Muchmore H, Scott N, et al. Operation Everest II: alterations in the immune system at high altitudes. J Clin Immunol 1988;8(5):397–406.
157. Klokker M, Kjaer M, Secher NH, Hanel B, Worm L, Kappel M, et al. Natural killer cell response to exercise in humans: effect of hypoxia and epidural anesthesia. J Appl Physiol 1995;78(2):709–16.
158. Kjaer M, Dela F. Endocrine responses to Exercise. In: Hoffman-Goetz L, editor. Exercise and immune function. Boca Raton, FL: CRC Press; 1996. p. 1–20.
159. Galbo H. Hormonal and metabolic adaption to exercise. New York: Thieme Verlag;1983.
160. Volek JS, Kraemer WJ, Bush JA, Incledon T, Boetes M. Testosterone and cortisol in relationship to dietary nutrients and resistance exercise. J Appl Physiol 1997;82(1): 49–54.
161. Madden KS, Felten DL. Experimental basis for neural-immune interactions. Physiol Rev 1995;75(1):77–106.
162. Maisel AS, Harris T, Rearden CA, Michel MC. Beta-adrenergic receptors in lymphocyte subsets after exercise. Alterations in normal individuals and patients with congestive heart failure. Circulation 1990;82(6):2003–10.
163. Rabin BS, Moyna MN, Kusnecov A, Zhou D, Shurin MR. Neuroendocrine effects of immunity. In: Hoffman- Goetz L, editor. Exercise and Immune Function. Boca Raton, FL: CRC; 1996. p. 21–38.
164. Khan MM, Sansoni P, Silverman ED, Engleman EG, Melmon KL. Beta-adrenergic receptors on human suppressor, helper, and cytolytic lymphocytes. Biochem Pharmacol 1986;35(7):1137–42.
165. van Tits LJ, Graafsma SJ. Stress influences CD4+ lymphocyte counts. Immunol Lett 1991;30(1):141–2.
166. Kappel M, Tvede N, Galbo H, Haahr PM, Kjaer M, Linstow M, et al. Evidence that the effect of physical exercise on NK cell activity is mediated by epinephrine. J Appl Physiol 1991;70(6):2530–4.
167. Tvede N, Kappel M, Klarlund K, Duhn S, Halkjaer-Kristensen J, Kjaer M, et al. Evidence

that the effect of bicycle exercise on blood mononuclear cell proliferative responses and subsets is mediated by epinephrine. Int J Sports Med 1994;15(2):100–4.
168. Tonnesen E, Christensen NJ, Brinklov MM. Natural killer cell activity during cortisol and adrenaline infusion in healthy volunteers. Eur J Clin Invest 1987;17(6):497–503.
169. Kappel M, Hansen MB, Diamant M, Jorgensen JO, Gyhrs A, Pedersen BK. Effects of an acute bolus growth hormone infusion on the human immune system. Horm Metab Res 1993;25(11):579–85.
170. Nieman DC, Pedersen BK. Exercise and immune function: Recent developments. Sports Med 1999;27(2):73–80.
171. Pedersen BK, Bruunsgaard H, Klokker M, Kappel M, MacLean DA, Nielsen HB, et al. Exercise-induced immunomodulation - possible roles of neuroendocrine and metabolic factors. Int J Sports Med 1997;18 Suppl 1:S2–7.
172. Newsholme EA. Biochemical mechanisms to explain immunosuppression in well- trained and overtrained athletes. Int J Sports Med 1994;15 Suppl 3:S142–7.
173. Newsholme EA. Psychoimmunology and cellular nutrition: an alternative hypothesis. Biol Psychiatry 1990;27(1):1–3.
174. Parry-Billings M, Budgett R, Koutedakis Y, Blomstrand E, Brooks S, Williams C, et al. Plasma amino acid concentrations in the overtraining syndrome: possible effects on the immune system. Med Sci Sports Exerc 1992;24(12):1353–8.
175. Keast D, Arstein D, Harper W, Fry RW, Morton AR. Depression of plasma glutamine concentration after exercise stress and its possible influence on the immune system. Med J Aust 1995;162(1):15–8.
176. Essen P, Wernerman J, Sonnenfeld T, Thunell S, Vinnars E. Free amino acids in plasma and muscle during 24 hours post- operatively-a descriptive study. Clin Physiol 1992;12(2): 163–77.
177. Lehmann M, Huonker M, Dimeo F, Heinz N, Gastmann U, Treis N, et al. Serum amino acid concentrations in nine athletes before and after the 1993 Colmar ultra triathlon. Int J Sports Med 1995;16(3):155–9.
178. Rohde T, MacLean DA, Pedersen BK. Effect of glutamine supplementation on changes in the immune system induced by repeated exercise. Med Sci Sports Exerc 1998;30(6): 856–62.
179. Rohde T, Asp S, MacLean DA, Pedersen BK. Competitive sustained exercise in humans, lymphokine activated killer cell activity, and glutamine - an intervention study. Eur J Appl Physiol Occup Physiol 1998;78(5):448–53.
180. Krzywkowski K, Petersen EW, Ostrowski K, Link-Amster H, Boza J, Halkjaer-Kristensen J, et al. Effect of glutamine and protein supplementation on exercise-induced decreases in salivary IgA. J Appl Physiol 2001;91(2):832–8.
181. Krzywkowski K, Petersen EW, Ostrowski K, Kristensen JH, Boza J, Pedersen BK. Effect of glutamine supplementation on exercise-induced changes in lymphocyte function. Am J Physiol Cell Physiol 2001;281(4):C1259–65.
182. Hiscock N, Pedersen BK. Exercise-induced immunodepression- plasma glutamine is not the link. J Appl Physiol 2002;93(3):813–22.
183. Tvede N, Steensberg J, Baslund B, Halkjaer Kristensen J, Pedersen BK. Cellular immunity in highly trained elite racing cyclists during periods of training with high and low intensity. Scand J Med Sci Sports 1991; 1:163–6.
184. Pedersen BK, Tvede N, Christensen LD, Klarlund K, Kragbak S, Halkjr-Kristensen J. Natural killer cell activity in peripheral blood of highly trained and untrained persons. Int

J Sports Med 1989;10(2):129–31.
185. Nieman DC, Buckley KS, Henson DA, Warren BJ, Suttles J, Ahle JC, et al. Immune function in marathon runners versus sedentary controls. Med Sci Sports Exerc 1995;27(7): 986–92.
186. Hoffman-Goetz L, Arumugam Y, Sweeny L. Lymphokine activated killer cell activity following voluntary physical activity in mice. J Sports Med Phys Fitness 1994;34(1): 83–90.
187. Hoffman-Goetz L, MacNeil B, Arumugam Y, Randall Simpson J. Differential effects of exercise and housing condition on murine natural killer cell activity and tumor growth. Int J Sports Med 1992;13(2):167–71.
188. MacNeil B, Hoffman-Goetz L. Effect of exercise on natural cytotoxicity and pulmonary tumor metastases in mice. Med Sci Sports Exerc 1993;25(8):922–8.
189. MacNeil B, Hoffman-Goetz L. Exercise training and tumour metastasis in mice: influence of time of exercise onset. Anticancer Res 1993;13(6A):2085–8.
190. Jonsdottir IH, Hoffmann P, Thoren P. Physical exercise, endogenous opioids and immune function. Acta Physiol Scand Suppl 1997;640:47–50.
191. Papa S, Vitale M, Mazzotti G, Neri LM, Monti G, Manzoli FA. Impaired lymphocyte stimulation induced by long-term training. Immunol Lett 1989;22(1):29–33.
192. Nieman DC, Henson DA, Gusewitch G, Warren BJ, Dotson RC, Butterworth DE, et al. Physical activity and immune function in elderly women. Med Sci Sports Exerc 1993;25(7):823–31.
193. Baj Z, Kantorski J, Majewska E, Zeman K, Pokoca L, Fornalczyk E, et al. Immunological status of competitive cyclists before and after the training season. Int J Sports Med 1994;15(6):319–24.
194. Nieman DC, Brendle D, Henson DA, Suttles J, Cook VD, Warren BJ, et al. Immune function in athletes versus nonathletes. Int J Sports Med 1995;16(5):329–33.
195. Oshida Y, Yamanouchi K, Hayamizu S, Sato Y. Effect of acute physical exercise on lymphocyte subpopulations in trained and untrained subjects. Int J Sports Med 1988;9(2): 137–40.
196. Lewicki R, Tchorzewski H, Majewska E, Nowak Z, Baj Z. Effect of maximal physical exercise on T-lymphocyte subpopulations and on interleukin 1 (IL 1) and interleukin 2 (IL2) production in vitro. Int J Sports Med 1988;9:114–7.
197. Pyne DB. Regulation of neutrophil function during exercise. Sports Med 1994;17(4): 245–58.
198. Hack V, Strobel G, Rau JP, Weicker H. The effect of maximal exercise on the activity of neutrophil granulocytes in highly trained athletes in a moderate training period. Eur J Appl Physiol Occup Physiol 1992;65(6):520–4.
199. Green RL, Kaplan SS, Rabin BS, Stanitski CL, Zdziarski U. Immune function in marathon runners. Ann Allergy 1981;47(2):73–5.
200. Hack V, Strobel G, Weiss M, Weicker H. PMN cell counts and phagocytic activity of highly trained athletes depend on training period. J Appl Physiol 1994;77(4):1731–5.
201. Nicholls EE, Spaeth RA. The relation between fatigue and the susceptibility of guinea pigs to infections of type I pneumococcus. Am J Hygiene 1922;2:527–35.
202. Cannon JG, Kluger MJ. Exercise enhances survival rate in mice infected with Salmonella typhimurium. Proc Soc Exp Biol Med 1984;175(4):518–21.
203. Ilback NG, Friman G, Crawford DJ, Neufeld HA. Effects of training on metabolic responses and performance capacity in Streptococcus pneumoniae infected rats. Med Sci

Sports Exerc 1991;23(4):422–7.
204. Nieman DC, Johanssen LM, Lee JW. Infectious episodes in runners before and after a roadrace. J Sports Med Phys Fitness 1989;29(3):289–96.
205. Nieman DC, Johanssen LM, Lee JW, Arabatzis K. Infectious episodes in runners before and after the Los Angeles Marathon. J Sports Med Phys Fitness 1990;30(3):316–28.
206. Heath GW, Ford ES, Craven TE, Macera CA, Jackson KL, Pate RR. Exercise and the incidence of upper respiratory tract infections. Med Sci Sports Exerc 1991;23(2):152–7.
207. Nieman DC, Nehlsen-Cannarella SL, Markoff PA, Balk-Lamberton AJ, Yang H, Chritton DB, et al. The effects of moderate exercise training on natural killer cells and acute upper respiratory tract infections. Int J Sports Med 1990;11(6):467–73.

Natural Immunity
Edited by L. Bertók and D.A. Chow

© 2005 Elsevier B.V. All rights reserved

New Prospect for the Enhancement of Natural Immunity.

LÓRÁND BERTÓK

"Fodor József" National Center of Public Health, "Frédéric Joliot-Curie" National Research Institute for Radiobiology and Radiohygiene ,H-1221 Anna u. 5, Budapest, Hungary

ABSTRACT

It is well demonstrated that serial endotoxin injections produce endotoxin tolerance and elevate natural resistance. However, such injections may also have harmful effects such as high fever, hypotension and abortion. For this reason LPS injections are not suitable to enhance nonspecific resistance in endotoxin-sensitive mammalian species including man. Various techniques have been designed (physical, chemical, etc.) for the detoxification of endotoxins while the beneficial effects were maintained. Perhaps one of the best detoxification techniques is treatment with ionizing radiation. The irradiation of LPS with ^{60}Co (100–200 kGy) decreased its toxicity in a dose-dependent manner. Such radiodetoxified endotoxin (RD-LPS) preparations showed decreased toxicity whereas the beneficial effects were preserved (150 kGy:TOLERIN®). These findings have been confirmed in other laboratories. Irradiation causes marked chemical alteration in LPS, such as the decrease of glucosamine, KDO and fatty acids. A single parenteral injection of TOLERIN® is capable of preventing the various forms of shock in experimental animals. This preparation has a membrane-stabilizing effect and thereby can prevent the membrane-damaging effect of LPS and of some cytostatic agents. Unlike endotoxin, TOLERIN has barely any hypotensive effect and pretreatment with this preparation can prevent practically all the haemodynamic changes induced by LPS. LPS plays an important role in the pathogenesis of the intestinal syndrome of radiation disease, which may be prevented by up to 70% in rats with RD-LPS pretreatment. TOLERIN retains the adjuvant activity of LPS and it is a good adjuvant for inactivated virus vaccines. TOLERIN can also evoke the regeneration of the immune system in irradiated animals. The decrease of nonspecific resistance in immunodeficient or immunosuppressed patients is the most important cause of opportunistic infections that may lead to sepsis, endotoxaemia, pneumonia and so on. Organ transplant recipients commonly die of septicaemia. Antilymphocyte serum (ALS) is used in such patients as an immunosuppressant. The augmentation of natural resistance and the induction of endotoxin tolerance are of major significance in such patients. We found that in ALS-treated rats RD-LPS induced tolerance against the lethal dose of LPS. This experiment demonstrated that in spite of the suppressive effect of ALS on T lymphocytes the induction of LPS tolerance (the enhancement of natural resistance) was normal. Facultative pathogenic organisms may flourish and cause disease when specific and nonspecific resistance is impaired. RD-LPS could produce significant proliferation of lymphoid cells in germ-free animals which are immunodeficient. Many other beneficial effects are preserved by RD-LPS preparations, such as the activation of macrophages and of the reticuloendothelial system, antitumour activity, etc. On the basis of these favourable experimental results, TOLERIN was tested on 350 surgical patients suffering from gastrointestinal tumours, on other patients suffering from AIDS and on cancer patients treated with CYSPLATIN[c]. TOLERIN treatment prevented sepsis and activated bone marrow function in these patients.

1. INTRODUCTION

At the beginning of the last century Wright [1] first studied natural resistance (NR). He observed that after vaccination with killed bacteria a 'negative' phase occurred which was followed by increased natural resistance tied to the production of specific antibodies. Landy [2] and Rowley [3] made similar observations later independently, and demonstrated that this preimmune resistance was due to the LPS content of the vaccines used. It was also observed that changes in immune status were closely related to the production of natural antibodies [4]. The properdin system, which was originally discovered by Pillemer et al. [5], was also stimulated by LPS. Beeson [6] discovered that low doses of toxic LPS given repeatedly led to the induction of endotoxin tolerance and prevented the pyrogenic effect of LPS (pyrogen tolerance). It was also observed that small LPS doses could decrease the severity of various forms of experimental shock and of the lethal effect of radiation. Later it was demonstrated that LPS functions as an immunological adjuvant, capable of inducing tumour necrosis: it stimulated bone marrow activity and increased the production of interferon. Moreover, it was possible to prevent the development of infectious diseases by small endotoxin doses, which increased natural resistance significantly. These observations evoked great interest in the phenomenon of endotoxin tolerance [7].

The question was posed whether or not endotoxin tolerance could be used for the prevention of endotoxin shock and of shock due to other causes. It was clear that during endotoxin tolerance no lysosomal membrane damage occurred even if LPS was given repeatedly [8], and the animals survived the endotoxin challenge [9]. However, the use of endotoxin for preventive treatment was limited by the excessive sensitivity of man and of higher animals to LPS. For this reason, numerous attempts were made using physical, chemical and immunological approaches to produce LPS preparations that would maintain its ability to induce tolerance, increase natural resistance, act as an adjuvant and exert a necrotic effect on tumours while decreasing or entirely eliminating its toxicity. Methylation [10] and the modification of the structure of LPS molecule of the so-called monophosphoryl lipid A [11–13] were successful in detoxifying LPS but the capacity to induce natural resistance was best preserved when ionizing radiation (^{60}Co-gamma) was used for detoxification [14–17].

2. THE PRODUCTION AND BIOLOGICAL EFFECTS OF RADIODETOXIFIED LPS

In our laboratory E. coli bacteria are produced in bulk by fermentation and extracted by the phenol-water method of Westphal with some modifications [14]. The LPS is further purified by ultracentrifugation and dissolved in water by ^{60}Co-gamma radiation using 50, 100, 150 or 200 kGy doses. The toxicity of LPS is decreased as shown in Fig. 1.

The biological effects of radiation-treated LPS are presented in Table I. The harmful effects of LPS are decreased after radiation, whereas its capacity to induce tolerance, to function as an immunoadjuvant and immunomodulator, to protect against shock and radiation and to stimulate natural resistance are preserved to a large extent. The lethal effect of such preparations (LD_{50}

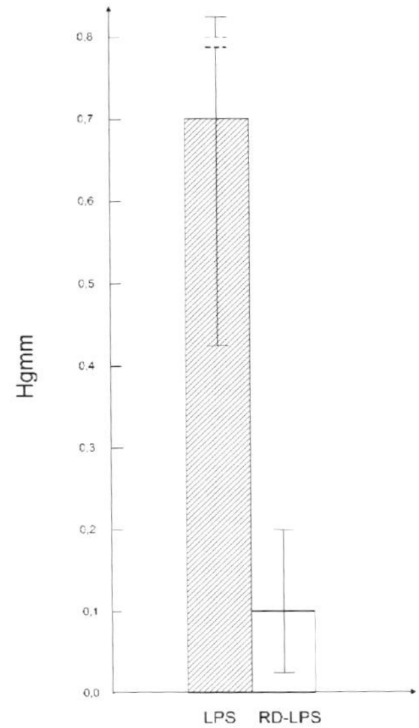

Figure 1. Blood pressure decreasing effect of endotoxin (LPS) and radiodetoxified endotoxin (RD-LPS: 200 kGy) in dogs 4–6 minutes after the treatment. (mean ±SEM for LPS:61±24 Hgmm; RD-LPS: 9.8±8.8 Hgmm; with n=14; P<0.01).

Table I Comparison of various biological effects of intact endotoxin (LPS) and radiodetoxified (5 Mrads) E.coli endotoxin (radiodetoxified endotoxin) preparations.

Effects	LPS	RD-LPS
LD50 [rat, mg/kg, n=50]	20	50
Hypotension [dog, Hgmm, n=10]	<60	>10
Leukocyte decrease [rabbit, % , n=10]	66	45
Platelet decrease [rabbit, %]	80	50
Fibrinogen decrease [rabbit, %. n=10]	40	17
Reptilase time increase [rabbit, /%]	90	10
Pyrogenecity [rabbit, ° C, n=10]	2.4	1.2
Sanarelli-Shwartzman local [rabbit, mm^2 , n=5]	1200	600
Hyperlipidemic effect [mouse, n=20]	+	–
Fetopathy [rat, % , n=50]	100	2
Complement depletion in vivo [rabbit, %]	35	10
Spermatozoon agglutination in vitro [swine, n=50]	+	–
Anticomplement activity in vitro [μg]	30	174
Adjuvant effect [rat, %, n=100]	508	470
Interferon induction [mouse, n=40]	+	+
Stem cell mobilization [CFUS /mouse, n=25]	521	247
Endotoxin tolerance {rat, pig, n=200, 10, protection, %]	100	100
Shock preventing [rat, dog, n=250; 10, protection, %]	80	80
Radioprotective effect [rat, n=300, protection, %]	70	70

and LDM) is dependent on the amount of radiation applied [14,16,17]. It was shown that the anti-complement and platelet-aggregating effect (indicating membrane damage) of detoxified endotoxin was partly maintained [18], which was dependent on the radiation dose used (Fig. 2). The decrease of membrane perturbation by radiated LPS was proven in these studies by the measurement of ^{3}H-concanavalin binding [19]. Table I shows the comparison of major effects

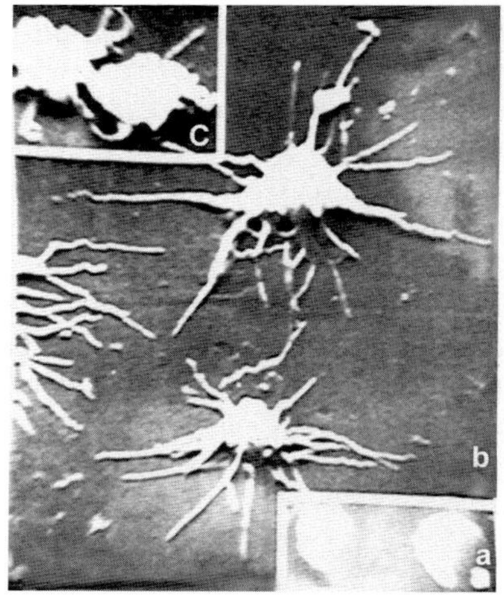

Figure 2. Effect of endotoxin (LPS) and radiodetoxified endotoxin (RD-LPS: 150 kGy) on human thrombocytes (in vitro). Scanning electronmicroscopic studies (15000X) (n=5). (a) untreated, (b) LPS-treated, (c) RD-LPS-treated [18].

of LPS and RD-LPS.

It was demonstrated in mice that toxic LPS increased the blood level of very low density lipoprotein (VLDL) whereas the RD-LPS did not, indicating that hyperlipidaemia is a marker of LPS toxicity [20]. We also found that RD-LPS inhibited membrane-bound adenylate cyclase (AC) less than its toxic counterpart [21].

Depending on the radiation dose used, RD-LPS preparations do not release or show a decreased release of lysosomal enzymes (beta-glucuronidase, cathepsin D). The capacity to induce the Sanarelli-Shwartzman reaction was decreased by half, as was pro-coagulant activity as measured with rabbit leukocytes [8,22,23].

We found that radiation treatment of mice (10 Gy; ^{60}Co-gamma) significantly increased their LPS sensitivity and 300 μg doses led to 100% mortality on days 3 and 7 after treatment, whereas identical doses of RD-LPS induced no ill effects. It was also observed that animals bearing Lewis lung carcinomas showed increased sensitivity to LPS but RD-LPS had no ill effects in such animals [24].

It is long recognized that bacterial endotoxins have significant metabolic effects. In the liver microsomal monooxygenase enzyme systems are sensitive to endotoxin [25]. Because of the potential anti-shock effect of RD-LPS, we examined its effect on the microsomal monooxygenase system. The metabolic inactivation of narcotic agents is dependent on microsomal enzyme activity. We demonstrated that RD-LPS, in contrast with toxic LPS, exerts a significantly decreased inhibitory effect on liver microsomal mono-oxygenase enzymes. In LPS-treated animals phenobarbital was unable to induce these enzymes, whereas in RD-LPS (150 kGy) treated animals enzyme induction was present. The mechanism of enzyme inhibition by LPS is unknown. It is possible that LPS damages the cytochrome P-450 enzyme [25].

We studied the mechanism of endotoxin detoxification by radiation. It was indicated that a dose-dependent induction of free radicals in the water phase induced or led to the induction of structural changes in endotoxin. This led to the decrease of glucosamine, keto-deoxy-octonic acid and fatty acids [26,27]. Ionizing radiation has been used in several other laboratories for the detoxification of endotoxin and confirmed our observations [17,28–32].

3. THE INTERACTION OF RD-LPS WITH THE COMPLEMENT SYSTEM

The complement system is fundamental to host defence, and LPS is capable of activating this system. Therefore, it was important to examine RD-LPS from this point of view and to compare it with toxic LPS. Ionizing radiation decreased, in a dose-dependent manner, the hypotensive (in dogs) and shock-inducing capacity (in dogs and rats) and complement-activating capacity of LPS. Thus, both the lethal and anti-complement effect of LPS was decreased by ionizing radiation. We observed that LPS is capable to activate complement by both the 'classical' and 'alternative' pathways. Although RD-LPS showed a dose-dependent decrease in the activation of both pathways, the activation of the alternative pathway was less affected. This observation confirms our earlier findings that the two pathways are activated by different parts of the LPS molecule [33]. Our results clearly demonstrated that there is a close correlation between LPS toxicity and its complement-activating capacity. It was concluded that complement activation may be used for the measurement of detoxification.

4. THE EFFECT OF RD-LPS ON THE ENDOCRINE SYSTEM

4.1. Thyroid gland

LPS affects the membrane and TSH receptor of follicular cells in the thyroid [34,35]. We demonstrated in rats that RD-LPS, although it decreases T4 (thyroxin) level in the serum, has no significant effect on the membrane and TSH receptor of follicular cells, and TSH was found to be effective in the stimulation of T4 production. This indicates that RD-LPS is not capable of inducing membrane alterations, which would damage membrane receptors, yet it affects membranes as indicated by the induction of endotoxin tolerance [36,37]. Similar results were found in irradiated animals or in various animal models of experimental shock [35,38,39].

4.2. Pituitary-adrenal axis

It is known from experiments in rats that LPS, either by direct effect or via cytokines – increases the circulating level of stress hormones (ACTH, corticosteroid, beta-endorphin) and activates the pituitary-adrenal axis. Such activation is present in the absence of the paraventricular nucleus, which secretes releasing neuropeptides towards the hypophysis [40,41]. In contrast, RD-LPS does not increase significantly ACTH, corticosteroid or beta-endorphin levels. These results indicate that ionizing radiation destroys the capacity of LPS to induce cytokines and to activate the pituitary-adrenal axis [37,42].

5. THE EFFECT OF RD-LPS ON ARACHIDONIC ACID METABOLISM IN MACROPHAGES.

Endotoxin tolerance is so far the best model to study natural resistance. For this reason it is imperative that we understand its mechanisms. During the mediator production of macrophages is altered, which is considered to be of significance for the induction of natural resistance. Therefore, it was warranted to study in rats the effect of RD-LPS on macrophages in comparison with unaltered LPS. Our results indicate that RD-LPS is capable of inducing macrophage activation

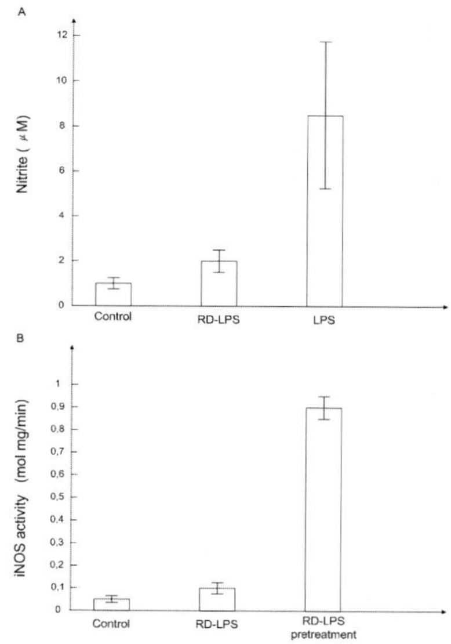

Figure 3. Nitrite production (A) and iNOS activity (B) by J774 macrophages exposed to DMEM only (control), RD-LPS or native LPS (10 ng/ml) for 24 h. Each value represents the mean ± SEM of N=18 wells from three independent experiments. Pc 0.01 versus control.

A. NO formation	control:	1 ± 0.8 μM	B. iNOS activity	control:	0.1 ± 0 $pM(mg/min)^{-1}$
	RD-LPS:	2.3 ± 2.0 μM		RD-LPS:	0.3 ± 0.01 $pM(mg/min)^{-1}$
	LPS:	8.3 ± 3.8 μM		LPS:	0.9 ± 0.02 $pM(mg/min)^{-1}$

similar to toxic LPS, and LPS tolerance is also induced. Its capacity to induce arachidonic acid production persisted significantly longer than its capacity to inhibit endotoxin shock [43].

6. THE PROTECTION OF RES BY RD-LPS AGAINST RADIATION AND ALCOHOL-INDUCED INJURY

The reticuloendothelial system (RES) plays an important role in host defence by the removal of foreign material. For this reason we have examined the effect of RD-LPS on RES activity. A method of isotope (^{99m}Tc-labelled nanoalbumon microcolloid) removal from the blood was established. This method is very sensitive and is suitable for the detection of granulopetic activity and efficiency. The clearance curve that described RES activity was of exponential nature and it was well characterized by the granulopectic index. The liver, spleen and bone marrow cells took up the ^{99m}Tc-labelled nanoalbumon microcolloid. The extent of RES damage was measured by colloid clearance and organ distribution. The effect of radiation and chronic alcohol consumption has been investigated. Under these conditions colloid clearance was decreased, as was phagocytic activity in the liver, spleen and bone marrow. It was shown that large doses of LPS damaged the RES system, whereas identical doses of RD-LPS were actually stimulatory on phagocytosis. Moreover, the harmful effects of damaging agents on RES activity could be decreased or fully prevented by treatment with RD-LPS. It is likely that the increase in RES activity plays a role in the stimulation of natural resistance [44,45].

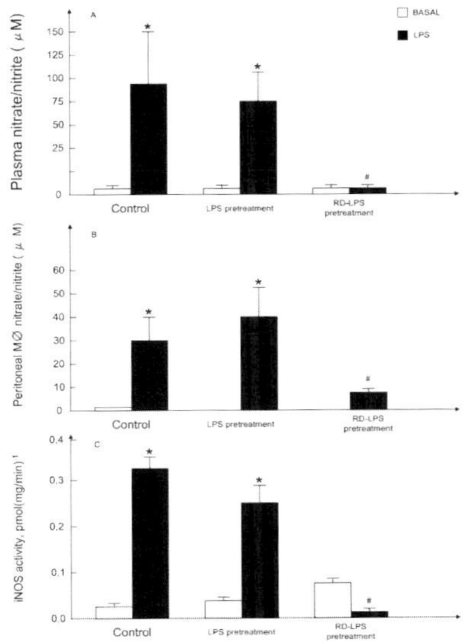

Figure 4. Effect of RD-LPS or LPS pretreatment in rats on plasma nitrate/nitrite levels (A), peritoneal macrophage (Mř) nitrate/nitrite levels (B) and lung iNOS activity (C) after subsequent endotoxin challenge. Rats, given sublethal doses of RD-LPS, LPS (1 mg/kg i.p.) or saline solution only (control) for four days, were challenged with a high dose of LPS (15 mg/kg i.p.) on the fifth day. Open columns represent basal values before lethal LPS challenge; filled columns represent values obtained 6 h after high-dose LPS challenge. Each value represents the mean ± SEM of five rats for each group. *P < 0.01 versus control. # P < 0.01 versus LPS pretreatment.

7. THE EFFECT OF RD-LPS ON NITRIC OXIDE (NO) PRODUCTION

During the study of pro-inflammatory mediators the importance of nitric oxide (NO) has been recognised. NO plays an important role in endotoxin-induced circulatory and metabolic alterations. LPS stimulates the production of the inductive NO synthase enzyme (iNOS) in various cell types. This mechanism contributes to LPS toxicity. For this reason we have examined the effect of LPS and RD-LPS on the NO system. LPS-treated (10 ng/ml) macrophages (J774 cell line) produced iNOS, which resulted in increased NO production. If, however, the cells were pretreated 24 hours earlier with RD-LPS (10 ng/ml), no NO response was detected after the subsequent LPS treatment. In contrast, when the cells were pretreated with LPS, no change was observed in the NO response to subsequent LPS challenge. The treatment of rats with repeated LPS injections (1 mg/kg/day ip. for 4 days) prevented the rise of nitrate/nitrite levels in the blood. These results indicate that RD-LPS induced tolerance towards NO induction by toxic LPS [46] (Figs. 3 and 4).

8. RD-LPS INCREASES NATURAL RESISTANCE, PROTECTS AGAINST VARIOUS FORMS OF SHOCK, AND EXERTS ADJUVANT AND ANTITUMOUR EFFECTS. POSSIBLE MECHANISMS OF ACTION.

8.1. Endotoxin shock

It is well known that an adequate dose of endotoxin is capable of inducing severe shock [47,48]. This phenomenon is readily induced in sensitive animals simply by LPS injection into the bloodstream or into the peritoneal cavity. We demonstrated that RD-LPS pretreatment of rats, mice, hamsters, guinea pigs, dogs, piglets, horses and monkeys was capable of inducing full endotoxin tolerance. Tolerance will develop within 24 hours and will disappear between 1 and 4 weeks. The protective effect of RD-LPS was further supported by the measurement of circulatory parameters. LPS caused major alterations in blood pressure and cardiac output. Pretreatment with RD-LPS moderated, or fully protected against, the haemodynamic effects of toxic LPS [49].

8.2. Peritonitis caused by intestinal bacteria and septic shock

The prevention of peritonitis due to faecal bacteria and of sepsis is important in clinical practice. Therefore, we studied the effect of RD-LPS in experimental models of these conditions. It was shown that pre-treatment with RD-LPS protected 90% of the animals against lethal peritonitis or septic shock [9,47,50]. Other investigators confirmed these results [51]. It is indicated that RD-LPS may be used prior to abdominal surgery for the elevation of natural resistance [7,9,52].

8.3. Haemorrhagic shock

Haemorrhagic shock is a significant problem in surgery. Fine and co-workers [53] presumed several years ago that endotoxaemia plays a role in the pathology of this condition. For this reason we studied the effect of RD-LPS on haemorrhagic shock and demonstrated that the pretreatment of dogs resulted in survival of the majority (70%) of the animals affected by lethal shock [47,49,54].

8.4. Intestinal ischaemic shock

The occlusion of the superior mesenteric artery (arteria mesenterica superior or cranialis) leads to severe intestinal ischaemia in man, which frequently results in death even when the occlusion is successfully removed by surgery. In animals the experimental intestinal ischaemia induced by temporary closure of the superior mesenteric artery is an excellent model for the examination of that injury. It has been demonstrated earlier that LPS absorbed from the gut during reperfusion plays an important role in the pathogenesis of this condition [48,53,55–57]. We studied the effect of RD-LPS in experimental intestinal ischaemia and showed that the majority of rats (70%) were saved from lethal intestinal ischaemic injury by our preparation [9,48].

8.5. Pulmonary shock

This condition is of clinical importance and bacterial endotoxins play an important role in its pathogenesis. In animal model systems LPS is used for induction, which evokes a characteris-

Table II Protection by radiodetoxified endotoxin (RD-LPS) against various forms of experimental shock, radiation disease and infections.

Experimental intervention /[species]	Protective value [%]
Endotoxin shock [LPS, rat, pig]	100
Radiation disease [X ray or 60Co-γ, rat]	70
Septic shock [fecal peritonitis, rat]	90
Tourniquet shock [limb ischemia, rat]	60
Intestinal ischemic shock [AMSO, rat]	74
Haemorrhagic shock [hypotension, dog]	70
Abortion [LPS, rat]	50
Pasteurella infection [X ray + infection, rat]	100
Klebsiella infection [rat]	90
Aujeszky virus infection [rat]	70
Immunosuppression [ALS, rat]	100

tic neutrophilic granulocyte infiltration into the lungs. This condition can only be moderately induced by RD-LPS, and pretreatment with radiodetoxified LPS (endotoxin tolerance) protects against the LPS-induced lung infiltration [58].

8.6. Tourniquet shock

Bacterial endotoxins may play a significant role in the pathogenesis of this condition as well. Pre-treatment with RD-LPS prevented endotoxin shock induced by ischaemia of the hind leg in 60% of the rats tested [9,59,60].

8.7. Foetal death and abortion induced by LPS

Bacterial endotoxins play a role in the pathogenesis of these conditions during urogenital infections [61]. It is not possible to protect against LPS-induced abortion by pharmaceutical means [62,63]. Therefore, we studied whether or not RD-LPS would prevent LPS-induced foetal death and abortion. We found that RD-LPS hardly exerts any toxic effect on the foetus, yet it protects 90% of the animals against LPS-induced foetal death and abortion [62].

8.8. Radiation-induced disease

It has been known for some time that the toxic form of LPS in small doses protects against radiation, but such treatment was not practical because of the imminent danger of toxicity. We showed earlier that bacterial endotoxins play an important role in the intestinal syndrome of radiation disease [9,64–66]. It is also known that ionizing radiation damages the bone marrow, which results in deficient haematopoiesis. For these reasons, it was warranted to study the effect of RD-LPS on radiation-induced disease. Our experiments revealed that RD-LPS protected 70% of rats from a lethal radiation dose [9]. This result prooves the effectiveness of this preparation.

8.9. Immunosuppression

It is well known that sub-lethal radiation significantly decreases natural resistance and adaptive immunity, increases the susceptibility to infection, may lead to the activation of dormant infection, and could lead to further sepsis induced by facultative pathogenic organisms. Thus, sub-lethal radiation damages all forms of immune function and leads to general immunosuppression [4,67]. Early observations in radiation biology revealed the atrophy of immune organs (e.g., spleen, thymus, lymph nodes) and the hypertrophy of the adrenal gland. The lymphoid organs represent the anatomical basis of host defence and for this reason it is understandable that radiation damage to these organs leads to a profound or complete immunosuppression. It is imperative that after radiation the regeneration of the immune system be accelerated as much as possible. Such situations occur daily during radiation treatment of cancer patients. We have examined the effect of RD-LPS on immune regeneration after non-lethal irradiation in rats. RD-LPS given 21 days after radiation damage (at this point no adaptive immune response was present) produced significant improvements in immune function and accelerated immune regeneration [67]. Radioresistant T-helper cells seem to be important in the mediation of the immunostimulatory effect of RD-LPS [19].

8.10. Immunosuppression due to antilymphocyte serum

RD-LPS induces endotoxin tolerance and elevates natural resistance. It is well known that transplant patients die because of infectious disease rather than inadequate surgical procedures. In most cases sepsis or endotoxaemia is the cause of death. These patients receive strong immunosuppressive agents in order to prevent graft rejections. It is common knowledge that immunosuppressive drugs decrease natural resistance to a large extent and for this reason the patients become susceptible even to bacteria that have moderate pathogenicity. Antilymphocyte serum is also used in these patients as an immunosuppressive agent. We examined whether or not RD-LPS is capable of inducing endotoxin tolerance and enhanced natural resistance in antilymphocyte serum treated animals. It was found in rats immunized with sheep red blood cells that antilymphocyte serum treatment, that led to complete immunosuppression, did not prevent the induction of endotoxin tolerance in response to RD-LPS. Therefore, endotoxin tolerance and indeed the increase of natural resistance was independent of the suppression of adaptive immunity by antilymphocyte serum. A possible reason for this is that endotoxin tolerance is primarily related to B-cell function. On the basis of these experiments it is possible that RD-LPS would protect transplant patients from septicaemia and endotoxaemia [9,68]. The results of these experiments are summarized in Table II.

8.11. RD-LPS as an immunological adjuvant

It has long been known that bacterial endotoxins are excellent immunological adjuvants [67,69]. However, the use of endotoxins in vaccine production was limited due to the undesirable side effects (fever, local inflammation). Nevertheless, the efficacy of some combination vaccines is improved by the small amount of LPS present. We observed in rats that RD-LPS maintains its adjuvant potential [67,69,70]. The adjuvant effect of RD-LPS could also be demonstrated by thymidine incorporation in human white blood cells treated with phytohaemagglutinin [19]. For this reason it is possible that RD-LPS would be useful also for the potentiation of viral antigens. Inactivated viral vaccines are often used in order to avoid the danger of reversion of attenuated viruses to pathogenic strains. However, inactivated viruses are less immunogenic, which requires the use of adjuvants for the production of acceptable vaccines. Good adjuvants are in short supply. This warranted the trial of RD-LPS for the potentiation of viral vaccines. We produced a vaccine against foot and mouth disease with RD-LPS, which was superior to the vaccine in use when tested in mice and pigs. We also succeeded in the production of vaccines against equine and human influenza viruses, which were significantly better than the ones in use (these findings are the subject of several patents) [71–73].

It should be noted that the RD-LPS adjuvant also increased natural resistance in the vaccinated animals that lasted for 1 to 3 weeks. Therefore, it provides natural protection prior to the induction of adaptive immunity [52].

Newborn mice become more susceptible to the lymphocytic choriomeningitis virus if treated with LPS or RD-LPS. This is related to the immunoadjuvant effect of LPS/RD-LPS [74]. Ionizing radiation does not affect the stimulation of the lymphoid system by LPS [74–76]. Similar results were obtained in experiments with Haemophilus influenzae [77,78].

In other experiments we treated newborn germ-free miniature piglets aged a few days with a single dose of RD-LPS and examined the effect on the lymphoid system. In contrast with untreated germ-free animals that had an underdeveloped immune system, the animals treated with RD-LPS showed a fully developed lymphoid system in a short period (10–14 days), which was comparable histologically to the immune system of conventional animals of similar age [52].

It is likely that natural resistance, or rather its decrease, plays an important role in tumour progression. It is known that killed bacterial cultures [79] and bacterial endotoxins exert antitumour activity [11,80]. It is unfortunate that the use of LPS is limited again in this situation by the harmful effects it may have. One of the most important cytokines induced by LPS is tumour necrosis factor (TNF), which has been tested for tumour therapy with great expectations. Unfortunately, the expected results did not materialize. It became clear that TNF is responsible in part for LPS toxicity. Thus, the toxic effect is related to the antitumour activity. This assumption is supported by the observation that it is possible to inhibit most of the harmful effects of LPS by anti-TNF monoclonal antibodies. One should note, however, that a chemically detoxified toxin preparation, monophosphoryl lipid A, exerts some anti-tumour effect [11].

It is very important that LPS preparations enhance natural resistance [2,3,5]. It is common knowledge that radiation treatment, chemotherapeutic agents, radiation sensitizing agents, steroids, local heat treatment and even surgical procedures induce a profound decrease in natural resistance. For this reason the patients become sensitive to infectious agents and a significant proportion fall victim to sepsis caused by Gram-negative bacteria, become endotoxaemic or develop pneumonia. Anticancer agents as well as ionizing radiation are harmful not only to tumour cells but also to normal cells, especially to the membranes. For instance, formyl-leurosine (Kőbányai Gyógyszerárugyár, Budapest), which was effective in animal experiments, could not be used on patients because of cardiotoxicity. It causes hypotonia and membrane damage of cardiac muscle [81]. For this reason we tested the effect of RD-LPS pretreatment on formyl-leurosine cardiotoxicity. It was observed in dogs that RD-LPS pretreatment had a minimal effect on the hypotensive effect of formyl leurosin; however, after 30 minutes blood pressure and cardiac function returned to normal. Examination of the cardiac muscle of RD-LPS treated dogs did not show the pathological changes of membrane injury, which were present in formyl-leurosine treated animals [82]. This experiment indicates that treatment with RD-LPS may protect against the side effects of chemotherapeutic agents and radiation treatment.

It is possible that the mechanism of protection by RD-LPS is mediated by the so-called lysosomal membrane 'concentration'. In RD-LPS tolerant animals no lysosomal membrane damage occurs after LPS challenge and consequently lysosomal enzymes are not released (beta-glucuronidase, cathepsin D, etc.) [8].

Most of the desirable effects of LPS are preserved with RD-LPS treatment. These are RES activation, stimulation of phagocytosis and macrophage activity, elevation of natural antibody and properdin levels, and so on. RD-LPS is capable of activating the entire immune system, which includes both humoral and cellular immunity. This is the reason for the effectiveness of RD-LPS against diverse noxious agents [9]. It is possible that RD-LPS will gain application in complex therapeutic approaches to neoplasia.

8.12. Hepato-protection by RD-LPS in experimental myocardial infarction.

We examined in dogs whether or not RD-LPS would protect against liver damage caused by myocardial infarction elicited by the occlusion of the left coronary artery. It was observed that in RD-LPS treated dogs there was moderate or no disturbance of permeability, and liver function, including detoxification, remained normal [47,83]. These results indicate that RD-LPS may be useful in several clinical situations.

8.13. The effect of RD-LPS on haematopoiesis

It has long been known that endotoxin affects bone marrow function [84]. Numerous drugs (such as chemotherapeutic agents) and medical procedures (radiation therapy) impair the host defence system. Damage to the bone marrow and lymphatic system leads to the decrease of natural resistance. The number of stem cells will decrease in the bone marrow, which leads to a decreased production of white blood cells (especially granulocytes) and agranulocytosis will develop.

For these reasons we examined whether or not RD-LPS treatment could improve or restore bone marrow function under these conditions. Rabbits were used for these experiments. The animals were given immunosuppressive agents (Imuran, hydrocortisone) in order to suppress and damage the bone marrow. Comparative blood count was performed after RD-LPS treatment. RD-LPS increased significantly the production of white blood cells in healthy animals and restored almost completely bone marrow function in Imuran- and hydrocortisone-treated rabbits [52].

8.14. The effect of RD-LPS on apoptosis

It is known that HIV-infected lymphocytes show increased apoptosis. We studied the effect of RD-LPS on this phenomenon. Lymphocytes were isolated from healthy HIV-infected individuals (CD4 < 500/μl) and treated in vitro with interleukin-2 (hrIL-2). Twenty-four hours later the cells were treated with HIV peptides or with RD-LPS. It was observed that the HIV peptides increased apoptosis in all experiments, whereas RD-LPS inhibited this reaction in over 60 percent of the experiments. These experiments suggest the use of RD-LPS for the prevention of apoptosis in HIV-infected individuals [52].

8.15. The effect of RD-LPS on the stimulation of HIV-infected lymphocytes

In man there is an asymptomatic phase after HIV injection, while the virus proliferates in infected lymphocytes and macrophages. The loss of CD4+ T lymphocytes is central to the development of acquired immunodeficiency syndrome (AIDS). It is possible that the augmentation of immune function would delay the development of AIDS. Therefore, we examined lymphocytes from patients with different stages of HIV infection for the reaction to RD-LPS and to some other agents. These studies indicated that during the initial stage of AIDS RD-LPS stimulated immature T-lymphocytes [85].

9. THE EVALUATION OF RD-LPS (TOLERIN®) FOR HUMAN USE ON VOLUNTEERS

These experiments have been performed with the permission of the Hungarian Ministry of Health, using human volunteers. The first experiment included five subjects (4 male and 1 female). It was observed that TOLERIN given at the dose of 7 μg/kg subcutaneously (1000 μg/ml solution was used) caused no adverse effects (circulatory, respiratory, urinary tract, cardiac function, nausea, vomiting, diarrhoea) within the 24-hour observation period. A moderate febrile reaction, increase in blood pressure and some swelling at the injection site have been observed. These symptoms significantly diminished or disappeared completely within the 24-hour observation period. Repeated laboratory testing revealed no changes in blood coagulation, liver and kidney function. In contrast, the C3 complement component was elevated in the blood and at 24 hours so was the leukocyte count. On this basis it may be concluded that the dose applied does not elicit a greater reaction than vaccines do, and may be considered harmless and suitable for further clinical studies.

For the second experiment 40 volunteers were recruited from university students. We observed that TOLERIN administered subcutaneously at a dose of 4 μg/kg did not produce clinical symptoms (circulatory, respiratory, urinary, cardiac damage, nausea, diarrhoea) at all. At various times after application there was a moderate elevation in body temperature with a maximum of 37.9 °C in one individual. There was a moderate swelling at the site of application. These changes disappeared within 24 hours after application. The laboratory tests performed at 24 hours did not show any alteration in blood coagulation, liver and kidney function. In the serum of treated individuals, taken at 24 hours, TNF was detected. There was also a moderate elevation of serum T_4 (thyroxin) in most individuals. The leukocyte count and the C3 complement fraction in the serum were also increased. The treated individuals were followed for three weeks, and two individuals developed a mild form of cold syndrome during that period. It may be concluded on the basis of both experiments that TOLERIN is essentially harmless and it causes only a very mild clinical reaction and therefore it is suitable for further clinical trials.

9.1. Clinical trials with RD-LPS (TOLERIN®)

After our initial clinical trials had been completed, the Hungarian National Agency of Public Health and Infectious Diseases gave permission for the trial of TOLERIN in 9 health institutions in both open and double-blind experiments. During these studies 110 surgical patients were treated with TOLERIN and 241 patients receiving similar medical treatment served as control. The majority of patients had been operated on for colon carcinoma. TOLERIN was given to patients 24–48 hours prior to surgery. It has been observed so far that in the treated individuals there was a decrease of infections and complications and natural resistance was increased on the basis of laboratory tests (increase in white blood cell count and C3 complement levels).

We also studied testicular carcinoma patients treated with Cysplatin for the correction of granulocytopenia. The experiment performed on five patients is presented in Fig. 5 [52]. TOLERIN treatment stimulated bone marrow function, and leukocyte and granulocyte counts were increased significantly. This experiment indicates that TOLERIN may be used for the correction of bone marrow suppression caused by chemotherapeutic agents.

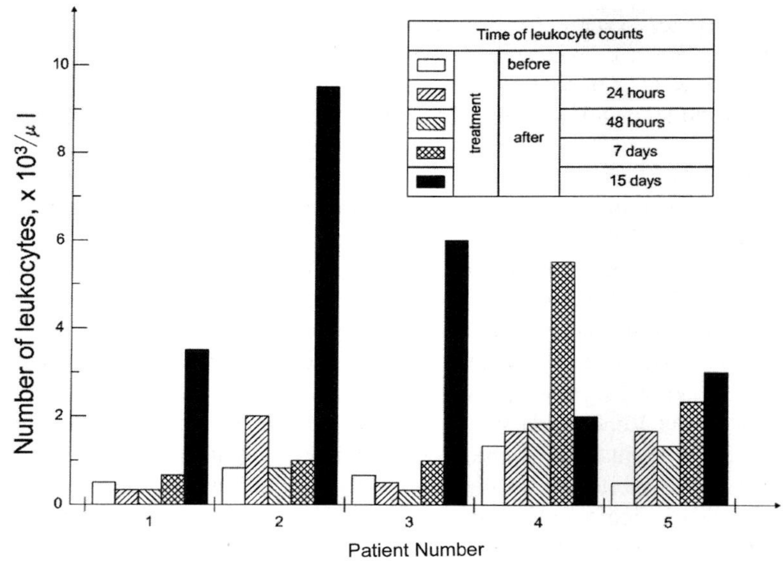

Figure 5. Effect of radiodetoxified endotoxin (RD-LPS: TOLERIN) on the number of leucocytes in CYSPLATIN treated patients bearing testis tumours.

We also treated five individuals suffering from immunodeficiency in addition to the usual treatment regimes given to these patients. Although TOLERIN increased CD4 number in patients with full-blown AIDS, no clinical improvement was obvious in the treated individuals. This observation correlates with our in vitro studies performed earlier. However, in one patient aged 28 years there was a significant clinical improvement after TOLERIN treatment. This patient suffered from severe meningitis and encephalitis of unknown origin, Candida sepsis and mixed bacterial infections. The CD4+ and CD8+ T-cell count was 250 and 261, respectively. TOLERIN was given two times at 280 μg subcutaneously (the second treatment was given 60 days after the first), and it increased significantly the CD4+ and CD8+ lymphocyte count. There was improvement already after the first treatment and after the second treatment the CD4+/CD8+ ratio was 1.05. One year later the CD4+/CD8+ ratio increased to 2.0, which is slightly over normal. Bone marrow function was normalized by this treatment [86].

REFERENCES

1. Wright AE. A short treatise on anti-typhoid inoculation, containing an exhibition of the principle of the method and summary of the results achieved by its application. Westminster: Constable;1904.
2. Landy M, Pillemer L. Elevation of properdin levels in mice following administration of bacterial lipopolysaccharides. J Exp Med 1956;103:823–830.
3. Rowley D. Stimulation of natural immunity to Escherichia coli infections. Lancet 1965;1: 232–240.
4. Merétey K. Changes of immunological balance in the mirror of the production of natural antibody (Hungarian) [PhD Thesis Hung Acad Sci]. Budapest: 1972.

5. Pillemer L, Blum L, Lepow IH, Ross OA, Todd EW, Wardlaw AC. The properdin system and immunity. Science 1954;120:279–284.
6. Beeson RB. Tolerance of bacterial pyrogens. J Exp Med 1947;86:29–35.
7. Bertók L. Bacterial endotoxins and nonspecific resistance. Acta Microbiol Immunol Hung 1997;44:361–365.
8. Szilagyi T, Csernyanszky H, Gazdy E, Bertok L. Studies on lysosomal enzyme liberating and endotoxin tolerance inducing capacity of radio-detoxified endotoxin. Acta Microbiol Acad Sci Hung 1982;29:155–159.
9. Bertók L. Radiodetoxified endotoxin as a potent stimulator of nonspecific resistance. Persp Biol Med 1980;24:61–66.
10. Nowotny A. Endotoxin preparations. Nature 1963;197:221–230.
11. Ribi E, Amano K, Cantrell J, Shwartzman S, Parker R, Takayama K. Preparation and antitumour activity of nontoxic lipid A. Canc Chemother Pharmacol 1982;12:91–96.
12. Toyoda T, Kassell NF, Lee KS. Induction of tolerance against ischemia/reperfusion injury in the rat brain by precondititoning with the endotoxin analog diphosphoryl lipid A. J Neurosurg 2000;92:435–441.
13. Xi L. Nitric oxide-dependent mechanism of anti-ischemic myocardial protection induced by monophosphoryl lipid A. Zhongguo Yao Li Xue Bao 1999;20:865–871.
14. Bertók L, Kocsár L, Várterész V, et al. inventors; Method for the production of ionizing radiation induced detoxified bacterial endotoxin preparation. (Hungarian). Budapest: Hungarian Patent;(No: 162,973/-61-k-27/02,23/00)1973.
15. Previte JJ, Chang Y, El-Bisi HM. Detoxification of Salmonella typhimurium lipopolysaccharide by ionizing radiation. J Bacteriol 1967;93:1607–1612.
16. Naidu MD, Chander R. Immunomodulation of macrophages by radio-detoxified lipopolysaccharide of Salmonella typhimurium. Indian J Exp Biol 1999;37:283–289.
17. Nerkar DP, Bandekar JR. Stimulation of macrophages and antitumour activity of radiodetoxified endotoxin. Microbiol Immunol 1986;30:893–897.
18. Kubasova T, Somosy Z, Bertók L, Köteleski J. Effect of endotoxin and radio-detoxified endotoxin on cell membranes in vitro. Acta Microbiol Acad Sci Hung 1982;29:235–243.
19. Temesi A, Bertók L, Pellet S. Stimulation of human peripheral lymphocytes with endotoxin and radiodetoxified endotoxin. Acta Microbiol Acad Sci Hung 1983;30:13–17.
20. Gaàl D, Kremmer T, Bàlint Z, Holczinger L, Bertók L, Nowotny A. Effects of bacterial endotoxins and their detoxified derivatives on serum and liver lipids in mice. Toxic Appl Pharmacol 1984;75:437–443.
21. Takáts A, Borsos B, Bertók L. A possible mechanism of the inhibitory effect of endotoxin on adenylate cyclase. Acta Biochim Biophy Hung 1989;23:191–202.
22. Szilágyi T, Csernyánszky H, Gazdy E, Bertók L. Haematologic effect and Shwartzman reactivity of radiodetoxified endotoxin. Acta Microbiol Acad Sci Hung 1978;25:159–164.
23. Szilágyi T, Csernyánszky H, Gazdy E, Bertók L. The procoagulant activity of leukocytes pretreated with radiodetoxified endotoxin. Acta Microbiol Acad Sci Hung 1980;27:191–194.
24. Walker RI, Ledney GD, Bertók L. Reduced toxicity of irradiated endotoxin in mice compromised by irradiation, tumours or infections. J Trauma 1983;23:225–230.
25. Bertók L, Szeberényi S. Effect of radio-detoxified endotoxin on the liver microsomal drug metabolizing enzyme system in rats. Immunopharmacol 1983;6:1–5.
26. Elekes E, Lüderitz O, Galanos C, Bertók L. Alterations in the chemical composition and

antigenicity of Escherichia coli O89 lipopolysaccharide and lipid A after 60Co gamma irradiation. Acta Microbiol Acad Sci Hung 1988;35:301–305.
27. El Sabbagh M, Galanos C, Bertók L, Füst G, Lüderitz O. Effect of ionizing radiation on chemical and biological properties of Salmonella minnesota R595 lipopolysaccharide. Acta Microbiol Acad Sci Hung 1982;29:255–261.
28. Csákó G, Tsai CM, Slomiany BL, Hep A, Elin RJ. Modification of the chemical composition and structure of the US reference standard endotoxin (RSE) by 60Co radiation. Radiat Res 1986;105:283–288.
29. Csákó G, Elin RJ, Hochstein HD, Tsai CM. Physical and biological properties of US standard endotoxin EC after exposure to ionizing radiation. Infect Immun 1983;41(1): 190–194.
30. Csákó G, Tsai CM, Hochstein HD, Elin RJ. The concentration, physical state, and purity of bacterial endotoxin affect its detoxification by ionizing radiation. Radiat Res 1986;108: 158–163.
31. Csákó G, Suba EA, Tsai CM, Mocca LF, Elin RJ. Dose-dependent changes in the antigenicity of bacterial endotoxin exposed to ionizing radiation. J Clin Lab Immunol 1987;24:193–198.
32. Elin RJ, Csákó G. Response of humans to gamma-irradiated reference Escherichia coli endotoxin. J Clin Lab Immunol 1989;29:17–23.
33. Füst G, Bertók L, Juhász-Nagy S. Interactions of the radio-detoxified E.coli endotoxin preparation with the complement system. Infect Immun 1977;16:26–31.
34. Nagy SU, Csaba G, Bertók L. Effect of thyrotropin (TSH) treatment on the responsiveness of the thyroid gland during endotoxin shock in adult rats. Acta Physiol Hung 1983;62: 187–190.
35. Nagy SU, Bertók L. Influence of experimentally induced endotoxemias on the thyroid function of rats. Acta Physiol Hung 1990;76:137–144.
36. Bertók L, Nagy SU. The effect of endotoxin and radio-detoxified endotoxin on the serum T4 level of rats and response of their thyroid gland to exogenous TSH. Immunopharmacology 1984;8:143–146.
37. Bertók L. Endotoxins and endocrine system. Domest Anim Endocrinol 1998;15:305–308.
38. Bertók L, Nagy SU. Effect of irradiation on serum T_4 level and response of thyroid gland to exogenous TSH in rats. J Radiat Res (Tokyo)1986;27:225–229.
39. Nagy SU, Bertók L. Effect of experimental shock conditions on the serum T_4 level of rats and response of their thyroid gland to exogenous TSH. Z Exp Chir Transplant Kunstliche Organe 1987;20:113–116.
40. Elenkov IJ, Kovács K, Kiss J, Bertók L, Vizi ES. Lipopolysaccharide is able to bypass corticoetrophin-releasing factor in affecting plasma ACTH and corticosterone levels: evidence from rats with lesions of the paraventricular nucleus. J Endocrinol 1992;133: 231–236.
41. Herzyk DJ, Ruggieri EV, Cunningham L, Polsky R, Herold C, Klinkner AM, et al. Single-organism model of host defense against infection: a novel immunotoxicologic approach to evaluate immunomodulatory drugs. Toxicol Phathol 1997;25:351–362.
42. Barna I, Bertók L, Koenig JI, Makara GB. Radiodetoxified lipopolysaccharide fails to activate the hypophyseal-pituitary-adrenal axis in the rat. Neuro Immunomodulation 2000;8:128–131.
43. Bertók L, Takáts A, Chen H, Cook J. Radiodetoxified endotoxin-induced tolerance, effect

on endotoxin lethality and macrophage arachidonic acid metabolism. Acta Microbiol Immunol Hung 1995;42:409–417.
44. Gál K, Bertók L. The effect of X-radiation on reticuloendothelial system and its treatment with radiodetoxified-endotoxin and trace elements in rats. Acta Microbiol Immunol Hung 1994;41:457–463.
45. Gál K, Bertók L. Effect of radiodetoxified endotoxin and trace elements on reticulo-endothelial system damaged by ethanol in rats. Acta Microbiol Immunol Hung 1994;41: 465–471.
46. Gilad E, Zingarelli B, O'Connor M, Salzman AL, Bertók L, Szabó C. Effects of radiodetoxified endotoxin on nitric oxide production in J774 macrophages and in endotoxin shock. J Endotoxin Res 1996;3:513–519.
47. Balogh Á. Inhibition of the irreversible surgical shock by radiodetoxified endotoxin pretreatment (Hungarian) [PhD Thesis Hung Acad Sci]. Budapest: 1981.
48. Kisida E. Experimental study of the phathophysiology of the vascular ileus (Hungarian) [PhD Thesis Hung Acad Sci]. Budapest: 1975.
49. Balogh Á, Bertók L, Nemes A, Juhász-Nagy S. Effect of radiodetoxified endotoxin (TOLERIN) on the blood circulation in the endotoxin-shock of dogs (Hungarian). Orv Hetil 1974;115:2055–2056.
50. Balogh Á, Bertók L. Experimentelle Abwehr des septischen und hämorrhagischen Schocks durch Vorbehandlung mit detoxifiziertem Endotoxin. Acta Chir Acad Sci Hung 1974;15: 21–27.
51. Conall TP, Zhang J, Vaziri ND, Schwartz RJ, Kaupke CJ, Oveisi F, et al. Radiodetoxified endotoxin-induced tolerance alters monocyte but not neutrophil CD11b and CD18 expression in response to lipopolysaccharide. Arch Surg 1994;129:1152–1156.
52. Bertók L. Nonspecific resistance: The role of bile acids and bacterial endotoxins (Hungarian). Studia Physiologica (Monographic Serie) 12 (2nd edit.). Budapest: Scientia;2002.
53. Fine J. Shock. In: Hamilton WF, Dow P, editors. Handbook of Physiology. Washington: American Physiology Society, 1965;2031–2046.
54. Balogh Á, Bertók L, Juhász-Nagy S. Wirkung der Vorbehandlung mit strahlendetoxifiziertem Endotoxin auf den Endotoxinschock bei Hunden. Acta Chir Acad Sci Hung 1981;22: 23–29.
55. Cuevas P, Fine J. Demonstration of a lethal endotoxemia in experimental occlusion of the superior mesenteric artery. Surg Gynecol Obstet 1971;33:81–87.
56. Cuevas P, Ischimayania M, Koizumi S, Woodruff PWH, Kaufmann A, Fine J. Role of endotoxemia of intestinal origin in early death from large burns. Surg Gynecol Obstet 1974;138:725–732.
57. Fine J, Frank ED, Ravin HA, Rutenburg JH, Schweinburg FB. The bacterial factor in traumatic shock. New England J Med 1959;260:214–220.
58. Szabó LG, Tóth TB, Benedek G, Bertók L. Prevention of endotoxin-induced leukocytic infiltration of lung with radio-detoxified endotoxin (TOLERIN) pretreatment. Acta Chir Hung 1987;28:309–313.
59. Orbán I. About prognosis and complications of acute limb-ischaemias: Experimental studies (Hungarian) [PhD Thesis Hung Acad Sci]. Budapest: 1977.
60. Orbán I, Bertók L, Regős J, Gazsó L. Die Rolle der bakteriellen Endotoxin beim Tourniquet Schock der Ratte. Acta Chir Acad Sci Hung 1978;19:399–404.
61. Skarnes RC, Harper MJ. Relationship between endotoxin induced abortion and the

synthesis of prostaglandin F. Prostaglandins 1972;1:191–203.
62. Csordás T, Bertók L, Csapó Z. Experiments on prevention of the endotoxin-abortifacient effect by radiodetoxified endotoxin pretreatment in rats. Gynecol Obstet Invest 1978;9: 57–64.
63. Szőcs G, Csordás T, Bertók L. Study of the endotoxin sensitivity of pregnant rats and their fetuses. Acta Chir Hung 1990;31:263–269.
64. Bertók L, Kocsár L. Die Rolle des Endotoxins beim intestinalen Syndrom der StrahlenkrankheitWiss. Z K Marx-Univ Leipzig (Math-Naturwiss) 1974;23:65–66.
65. Bertók L, Jr., Sztanyik LB, Bertók L. Possible role of bile deficiency in the development of intestinal syndrome of acute radiation disease. Acta Physiol Hung 1992;79:29–32.
66. Bertók L, Jr., Sztanyik LB, Bertók L. The effect of kanamycin treatment of rats on the development of gastro-intestinal syndrome of radiation disease. Acta Microbiol Hung 1992;39:155–158.
67. Elekes E. Nonspecific stimulation of antibody production in intact and immuno-depressed animals (Hungarian) [PhD Thesis Hung Acad Sci]. Budapest: 1978.
68. Bertók L, Elekes E, Merétey K. Endotoxin tolerance in rats treated with antilymphocyte serum. Acta Microbiol Acad Sci Hung 1979;26:135–137.
69. Merétey K, Elekes E, Bertók L. Antibody production in rats treated with endotoxin. Ann Immunol Hung 1973;17:63–66.
70. Elekes E, Bertók L, Merétey K. Adjuvant activity of endotoxin preparations in normal and irradiated rats. Acta Microbiol Acad Sci Hung 1978;25:17–21.
71. Sólyom F, Bertók L. Application of radio-detoxified endotoxin as adjuvant for experimental foot and mouth disease vaccine. Acta Microbiol. Acad Sci Hung 1985; 32:233–239.
72. Bertók L, Tanyi J, Nemesi M, Sólyom F. Production of a new, potent horse influenza vaccine. (Hungarian). Budapest: Hungarian Patent;2001.
73. Bertók L, Jankovics I. Production of a new, potent human influenza vaccine. (Hungarian). Budapest: Hungarian Patent;2001.
74. Bános Z, Szeri I, Anderlik P, Wessely M, Bertók L. Effect of endotoxin preparations on the course of lymphocytic choriomeningitis virus infection in suckling mice. Acta Microbiol Acad Sci Hung 1982;29:99–103.
75. Anderlik P, Szeri I, Bános Z, Wessely M, Bertók L, Radnai B. Effect of an irradiated Escherichia coli endotoxin preparation on the sensitivity to a lymphotropic cytostatic agent in germfree and conventional mice. Acta Microbiol Hung 1983;30:239–245.
76. Bános Z, Anderlik P, Szeri I, Wessely M, Bertók L. Bacterial modulation of the cellular immune response in mice. II. Stimulation by endotoxin of the reduced cellular immune response to LCM virus infection in aged mice. Acta Microbiol Hung 1983;30:233–237.
77. Csukás Z, Horváth J, Slowik F, Bertók L. Respiratory effect of Haemophilus influenzae endotoxin in mice. Acta Microbiol Hung 1983;30:139–146.
78. Csukás Z, Horváth J, Slowik F, Bertók L. Effect of irradiated Haemophilus influenzae endotoxin preparations in mice. Acta Microbiol Hung 1983;30:247–253.
79. Coley WB. The treatment of malignant tumors by repeated inoculation of erysipelas. Am J Med Sci 1883;105:487–492.
80. Fukushi K, Asano H, Sasaki J. Bacterial endotoxin as an antitumor agent. Jap J Med Sci Biol 1982;35:105–109.
81. Juhász-Nagy S, Sótonyi P, Bertók L. Haemodynamic pattern of formyl-leurosine induced acute cardiovascular depression in the dog. Acta Chir Acad Sci Hung 1985;26:35–49.
82. Bertók L, Juhász-Nagy S, Sótonyi P. Prevention of cardiac damages induced by formyl-

leurosine, a potent cytostatic agent, by radio-detoxified endotoxin (TOLERIN) in dogs. Immunopharmacol 1984;8:13–17.
83. Balogh Á, Furka I, Sótonyi P, Dalmy L, Bertók L. Leberprotektive Wirkung der Vorbehandlung mit strahlendetoxifiziertem Endotoxin (Tolerin)[R] beim akuten Myokardifarkt des Hundes. Z Exper Chirurg 1981;14:156–164.
84. Bán A. Studies of the bone-marrow function by bacterial lipopolysaccharides (Hungarian) [PhD Thesis Hung Acad Sci]. Budapest: 1968.
85. Ongrádi J, Hadden JW, Bertók L, Specter S, Nelson R, Friedman H. Human herpesvirus 6 variant A enchances in vitro HIV-1 replication by soluble mediators, which effect is diminished by endotoxin. (Hungarian). Orv Hetil 1995;136:653–659.
86. Bánhegyi D, Várnai F, Horváth A, Bertók L. Treatment of severe immune deficiency with radio-detoxified endotoxin. J Med 1992;23:154–156.

V. PHYSIOLOGICAL, PATHOLOGICAL AND BEHAVIORAL SIGNIFICANCE

Natural Immunity
Edited by L. Bertók and D.A. Chow
© 2005 Elsevier B.V. All rights reserved

Physiological Activities of the Natural Immune System

DONNA A. CHOW

Department of Immunology, University of Manitoba, Winnipeg, MB, Canada, R3E 0W3

ABSTRACT

Our understanding of the extent of the role of the innate immune response against pathogens has expanded enormously with the knowledge of an increasing number of mediators, an increasing variety and complexity of function, and central roles in the initiation and mediation/resolution of the adaptive immune response. However, this search for understanding has also revealed the extensive underlying physiological role of the innate immune system in the development and homeostasis of the organism. The impact on development is evident during embryogenesis and also during normal cyclical changes in reproductive tissues in the adult. Mediators of the innate immune system are essential for normal tissue renewal and healing. This chapter explores, as examples of its physiological role, the critical contributions of the innate immune system in wound healing, reproduction and normal tissue homeostasis including, regeneration, air breathing, cell signalling and cancer control. Natural immunity contributes to the normal physiology of the organism in many and diverse ways arguing for an evolutionary selection centred on self-organization for survival.

1. HOMEOSTASIS

1.1. Tissue homeostasis

Normal physiological cell renewal is considered to be a balance between proliferation, differentiation and death. Epidermal structure depends on cutaneous (or epidermal) homeostasis which is based on a balance of continual proliferation of basal cells, nuclear breakdown in the granular layer and termination of cell death in the stratus corneum [reviewed in 1,2]. Basal keratinocytes appeared resistant to apoptosis while upward migration was associated with increasing susceptibility possibly due to a shorter half-life of apoptosis inhibitors than death proteins which were demonstrated in basal cells. Two modes of cell death are thought to contribute to keratinocyte termination. Passive (or intrinsic) cell death initiated by loss of survival stimuli including, nerve growth factor (NGF), epidermal growth factor (EGF) and integrins, likely leads to apoptosis which is inhibited by bcl-2 in basal keratinocytes and by bcl-XL in upper level keratinocytes. Activation-induced (or extrinsic) cell death occurs via two pathways, the TNF-α pathway and the Fas-mediated pathway, both important in lymphocytes. However, keratinocytes appear relatively resistant to the TNF-α pathway probably due to protection from the constitutive NF-κB activity in normal skin. NF-κB , an important transcription factor for inflammatory and innate immune responses, is thought to promote keratinocyte viability during their upward migration and differentiation, contributing to spacial control and maintenance of tissue architecture. Keratinocytes except those in the granular layer express Fas constitutively, and all appear relatively resistant to the Fas pathway which is dominant in lymphocytes [reviewed in 1]. The regulation of keratinocyte survival and death is considered a complex, redundant and highly coordinated process, with stem cell proliferation in the basal layer and terminal differentiation and apoptosis limited to the upper layers of the epidermis [reviewed in 1,2]. Apoptotic keratinocytes shrink and are phagocytosed by nearby keratinocytes acting as "non-professional" phagocytes, while terminally differentiated keratinocytes flatten, form the stratum corneum and eventually are sloughed off [reviewed in 1].

1.2. Regeneration

The identification of DMBT1 (deleted in malignant brain tumour 1), a large mucin-like scavenger receptor cysteine rich (SRCR) B protein which is broadly expressed in epithelia particularly the respiratory and alimentary systems, revealed a link in a single molecule between defence and regeneration functions [reviewed in 3,4]. The participation of two products of alternative splicing, gp340 and salivary gland agglutinin in mucosal innate immunity suggested that DMBT1 was a pattern recognition receptor, probably acting through one or more of its SRCR domains. However, DMBT1 participation in an epithelial proliferation to differentiation switch and its upregulation during inflammation, suggested a role as a local regulator of epithelial homeostasis probably associated with the CUB (C1r/C1s Uegf Bmpl)and ZP (zona pellucida) domains on its C-terminus interacting with growth factors or cell surface molecules [reviewed in 4]. The dual functions exhibited by this molecule, consistent with the multifunctionality of mucins, demonstrate an interesting strategy for a tight, evolutionarily conserved, multifunctional molecular link between innate defence and regeneration functions exerted through distinct motifs [4].

1.3. Cytoprotective chaperones

Heat shock proteins (HSPs) are highly conserved, and constitute the most abundant and ubiquitously expressed soluble intracellular proteins from single-cell organisms to vertebrates [reviewed in 5,6]. While HSP60 is a ligand for TLR4 [reviewed in 7] an activating receptor of the innate immune system, HSPs act as internal chaperones and provide multiple cytoprotective housekeeping services in normal cells through their constitutive expression which is multiplied through induction under stress conditions. HSPs provide functions essential for maintaining protein homeostasis, protein folding and unfolding, transport, translocation, degradation and assembly of multiple subunit complexes. They protect against thermal insult and the pathological expression of transforming mutations [reviewed in 5]. Interactions between HSPs, their co-chaperones and molecules of signalling pathways suggest their regulation of cell growth and death [reviewed in 8]. More recently the observed release of HSPs from viable cells, their presence in the circulation of normal individuals and evidence that exposure to self-HSP60 or self-HSP70 is associated with Th2 rather than Th1 responses, has led to the proposal that they act as anti-inflammatory regulators of the immune response [reviewed in 6].

1.4. Air-breathing

Surfactant-specific proteins include SP-A, SP-B, SP-C and SP-D. While SP-B and SP-C are hydrophobic and limited to the lung, SP-A and SP-D are hydrophobic, found also in extrapulmonary tissues and are members of the collectin family of lectins which contribute to pathogen recognition in the innate immune response [reviewed in 9]. SP-B and SP-C participate in the classical role of surfactants, reducing the surface tension at the alveolar lining of the lung by facilitating lipid insertion. Sp-B forms essential tubular myelin structures and both SP-B and SP-C contribute to the molecular organization of the phospholipid monolayer. SP-A is thought to contribute to the regulation of the structural formation of the surface film through the provision of a lattice framework for tubular myelin formation. Experiments in SP-D knock-out mice suggested that SP-D may contribute to surfactant lipid homeostasis [reviewed in 9].

1.5. Cell signalling

C5b-C9, termed the complement membrane attack complex is responsible for the cytolytic function of complement, a potent mechanism contributing to innate defence against pathogens. However, terminal complement sequences, C5b-7, C5b-8 and C5b-C9 can induce non-lethal cell signals which are associated with an influx of Ca^{++}, in addition to other second messengers dependent upon the cell type [10]. C5b-9 insertion into cell membranes can activate guanine-nucleotide-binding (G) proteins without the need for a specific membrane receptor [11]. Phylogenetic analysis of their amino acid sequences supporting the emergence of C6 and C7 followed by C8 and C9 was interpreted as an evolutionary drive to improve the C5b-7 cell signalling through Ca^{++} flux [12]. Activation of the signal transducer and activator of transcription (STAT) transcription factors have been implicated in programming gene expression for many biological processes including innate immunity, cell growth regulation, embryonic development, organogenesis cell growth regulation and programmed cell death [reviewed in 13]. The STATs are activated by Janus kinases (JAKs) associated with transmembrane receptors, and by other receptors with intrinsic tyrosine kinases. The signalling of TLRs has been shown to be interconnected with the JAK/STAT signalling pathway [reviewed in 14].

The nuclear factor (NF)-κB/Rel transcription factor family participates in signalling for diverse biological processes linked with the innate immune system including embryo development, hematopoiesis and apoptosis [15]. Signals are initiated through TLRs and cytokine receptors such as those for IL-1and INF-γ.

1.6. Cancer control

Impaired cellular homeostasis is the hallmark of cancer. The concept of immune surveillance has gained new credence with evidence from mice genetically manipulated to make them immune deficient [reviewed in 16]. Support has increased for the idea that the innate immune response contributes to tumour surveillance with the increasing identification of mediators which recognize tumour cells including NK cells, NKT cells, γδ T cells, macrophages and natural antibodies. Down regulation of MHC class I in many tumours, including breast, prostate and lung cancer [reviewed in 16], which would reduce their susceptibility to MHC-dependent cytotoxic αβ T cells, increases their susceptibility to NK cells by reducing expression of the targets of NK cell inhibiting receptors [reviewed in 17].

The stimulatory receptor NKG2D is expressed in humans by circulating NK cells, $CD8^+$ T cells, stimulated macrophages and γδ T cells including intestinal intraepithelial (IEL) Vδ1 γδ T cells where it is particularly well expressed, and in mice by NK cells, activated $CD8^+$ cells and activated macrophages, some NKT cells, some splenic and epidermal γδ T cells but not those of the intestinal epithelium [reviewed in 17]. NKG2D recognizes ligands distantly related to MHC including human MHC class I related molecules MICA and MICB found on normal colonic epithelium, murine retanoic early inducible (RAE 1) protein and H60 described as a minor histocompatibility antigen and human UL16 binding proteins (ULBPs ALCAN or human RAE1 proteins), all of which are upregulated on tumour cells [reviewed in 17]. Thus, recognition of induced self-antigens is critical for innate immune control of aberrant cell development. Considering that the epithelial lining of many organs is the most common site of tumours which develop later in life, Vδ1 γδ T cells of the intraepithelial lymphocytes (IELs) which express somewhat organ-specific TCR V region repertoires, are well placed for tumour surveillance in the tissue [reviewed in 18], while NK cells would provide protection against systemic tumours [reviewed in 16] and while a minor population in the circulation, human γδ T cells of the Vγ9 and Vδ2 subset are considered to defend against haematological cancer [reviewed in 18]. Vδ2 T cells also recognize non-peptide antigens found on microbes and on mammalian cells [reviewed in 18]. Receptors specific to NK cells, NKp46 and NKp30 expressed on all NK cells and NKp44 of activated NK cells have been implicated in recognition of tumour cells [reviewed in 19]. NKT cells have demonstrated antitumor activity in experimental models after α-galactosylceramide or low dose IL-12 administration, and in the prevention of primary tumours initiated by the potent carcinogen methylcholanthrene [reviewed in 20,21].

Macrophages are considered to play essential roles in normal tissue homeostasis by removing transformed and dying cells [reviewed in 22]. Activated macrophages, stimulated by for example INF-γ or LPS are tumoricidal, directly by the release of toxic materials into the tumour targets, TNFα, serine proteases and reactive nitrogen intermediates, or through antibody-dependent cell-mediated cytotoxicity, or indirectly through the secretion of factors which induce anti-tumour activity in other cell types or lead to tumour death indirectly as through the macrophage metalloproteinase-12 generation of angiostatin [reviewed in 23]. While local proliferation of tissue macrophages contributes to tumour-associated macrophages (TAM), recruitment from the blood provides the majority of the cells with monocyte chemotactic protein-1 (MCP-1) produced in the main by tumour cells and also endothelial cells, fibroblasts and TAMs, considered a major macrophage chemotactic and activating factor [reviewed in 23]. Macrophage migration inhibitory factor (MIF) is produced by macrophages and tumour cells and stimulates macrophage phagocytosis, tumoricidal activity and release of TNFα and IL-1β in addition to inhibiting their random migration [23]. Furthermore, tumour release of granulocyte/macrophage-colony stimulating factor (G/M-CSF) likely enhances direct tumour killing by TAMs [23]. IL-12 and IL-18 produced by macrophages would be expected to activate NK cells augmenting their proliferation, cytotoxicity and production of INF-γ and IL-2. Similar activation of T cells would occur leading to a Th1-type anti-tumour response. However, the high complexity of TAM-tumour interaction has been revealed by evidence that TAMs also promote tumour growth and progression [reviewed in 22–24]. The ancestral role of mononuclear phagocytes in tissue remodelling and repair during ontogenesis and adult life is evident in pro-tumour action of TAMs [23,24]. TAMs produce growth factors, EGF and FGF which increase tumour proliferation, VEGF which promotes angiogenesis and enzymes, MMPs, plasmin, urokinase-type plasminogen activator, which contribute to the digestion of extracellular matrix in tumours [reviewed in 23,24]. In a non-tumourigenic melanoma model, CCL2-induced 'physiological' accumulation of TAMs promoted tumour formation, while massive macrophage infiltration lead to tumour destruction [reviewed in 24].

Dendritic cells (DCs) are considered the most important antigen presenting cells for activating T cells in the adaptive immune response. However monocyte-derived, immature human DCs exhibited tumoricidal activity in vitro, inducing tumour-specific apoptosis, through TNF family ligands TNF, lymphotoxin-$\alpha_1\beta_2$, Fas ligand and TNF-related apoptosis inducing ligand on DCs acting against tumour cells which express the corresponding death receptors [reviewed in 25,26]. Thus, DCs may contribute to an early response against tumours. While more mature DCs accumulated in the tumour periphery, tumour associated DCs (TADCs) within the tumour showed an immature phenotype which may contribute to maintenance of tolerance to tumour antigens, so that both TAMs and TADCs may contribute to tumour progression and metastasis, [reviewed in 24].

Neutrophils play an important role in inflammatory responses and neutrophil-dependent resistance against tumours has been demonstrated in experimental systems where they may be critical for initiating and maintaining an inflammatory response [reviewed in 24,27]. The Fas/FasL system is considered one of the major cytotoxic mechanisms used by neutrophils and has been shown to play a role in neutrophil-induced apoptosis of tumours [27]. Eosinophils, key inflammatory cells of responses against helminthic infections, have been detected as tumour infiltrating cells in a variety of cancers and reports have tended to link tumour-associated tissue infiltration by eosinophils with a good prognosis [reviewed in 28,29]. The spectrum of eosinophil activities have been proposed to contribute to resistance against tumours including release of TNF-α [reviewed in 28,29]. Mast cells are also known to play key roles in inflammation and increased numbers have often been associated with many human tumours [reviewed in 30,31]. While high counts of infiltrating mast cells were associated with a good prognosis for some tumours possibly due to TNF-α release from mast cells, they have also been associated with promotion of tumour growth and dissemination, with release of angiogenic EGF considered to be a contributing factor [reviewed in 30,31].

Clearance of dead and no-longer-needed autologous cells is a necessary function of the phagocytic system contributing to developmental and homeostatic processes essential for life as a complex organism. Recent investigations summarized in an excellent review [32] have provided a better understanding of phagocytosis of apoptotic cells. Macrophage interactions with apoptotic cells have been shown to suppress inflammatory responses [reviewed in 32]. Many phagocyte receptors, their targets and bridging molecules participate in this complex process. Macrophage clearance of apoptotic cells occurs mainly through recognition by the integrin $\alpha_v\beta_3$, CD36 (and thrombospondin), a phosphatidylserine receptor and CD14 [reviewed in 22]. Recognition of apoptotic cells by innate immune receptors including collectins, complement and CD14 which induce inflammatory responses against microbial pathogens, reveal a blurring between PAMPs and ACAMPs (apoptotic-cell-associated molecular patterns). Phagocyte recognition of altered-self, oxidized or desialylated molecules or phosphatidylserine exposed on apoptotic cells which also contributed to clearance, exhibited some interactions which suggested a close relationship with innate recognition of nonself. The failure of apoptotic cells to disengage from intercellular adhesion molecules on probing phagocytes may also contribute to their elimination. Phagocytosis of apoptotic cells by macrophages stimulated by LPS or necrotic cells suppressed their release of pro-inflammatory cytokines including TNF and increased the release of TGF-β1which exhibited anti-inflammatory activity. CD36, the $\alpha_v\beta_3$ integrin (vitronectin receptor) and the phosphatidylserine receptor have been implicated in the release of TGF-β1 and the apoptotic cells themselves may also release immunosuppressive cytokines including, IL-10 and TGF-β1[reviewed in 32,33]. Investigation of the kinetics of the cytokine response revealed that macrophages doubly stimulated by apoptotic cells and LPS, secreted increased TNF-α before the secretion of TGF-β1began and inhibited TNF-α release, suggesting that elimination of apoptotic cells may augment an initial inflammatory response but assist in the later resolution [34].

Preparations of antigen-negative heat shock/chaperone protein including gp96, have demonstrated antigen-independent activation of the innate immune system and peptide antigen-independent gp96-mediated tumour suppression obtained with gp96 preparations from normal tissue argue for a role for HSPs in innate anti-tumour responses [reviewed in 35].

While natural antibody (NAb), those antibodies in normal individuals which are produced in the absence of intentional immunization, has long been considered an important contributor to the early defence against pathogenic microbes and the clearance of metabolic waste and effete cells, they have also been implicated in the downregulation of inflammatory and autoimmune responses, surveillance against tumours and internalization of antigen for presentation to cells [reviewed in 36].

Our investigations with syngeneic murine models using immortalized and tumorigenic cells suggested that NAb 1) bound to activated cells including activated T cells and 2) reduced the growth of these cells in vitro and in vivo. Every approach taken consistently revealed an inverse relationship between the ability of a cell to bind polyclonal NAb with its survival in vivo. Correlative studies using different tumours [37], genetically B cell deficient mice [38,39] and the natural defence-resistant phenotype of tumours which grew out from threshold SC inocula of T-lymphomas [40–42] all supported an inverse relationship between tumour NAb binding capacity and tumourigenicity or metastatic potential in vivo. NAb reduced the cloning efficiency of the L5178Y-F9 in sloppy agar [43]. Oncogenic ras transformation of 10T½ fibroblasts increased their protein kinase C (PKC) activity and NAb binding [44,45], and reduced their tumourigenicity [46] and in vitro growth in NAb [43]. Preneoplastic, rat PKC-β1 overexpressing 10T½ cells also exhibited higher NAb binding and a more rapid elimination in vivo of ^{131}I-dUrd-labelled cells [47]. Thus, constitutive increases in the basal activity of PKC argued for PKC upregulation of NAb binding structures and for NAb binding to activated cells. In a direct assay, preincubation of tumour cells in serum NAb versus tumour-absorbed NAb reduced their tumourigenicity [37]. Furthermore, IV pretreatment of mice with syngeneic serum NAb, ammonium sulfate precipitated fractions of NAb, or human IVIG reduced the incidence and/or increased the latency of syngeneic tumours injected SC [45,48] and reduced the metastasis of tumours injected IV [49].

Repeated in vitro treatment of the L5178Y-F9 T lymphoma with the tumour promoters' 12-O-tetradecanoylphorbol-13-acetate (TPA) to generate variants followed by selection for high NAb binding through fluorescence-activated cell-sorting (FACS) yielded the LYNAb$^+$ which exhibited an inversely correlating reduction in SC tumourigenicity [50]. Increases in binding of anti-CD45RA monoclonal antibody and expression of higher molecular weight CD45 isoforms suggested that CD45 was an NAb target [51]. Reversal of the phenotype upon growth in vivo was consistent with a CD45-directed NAb-dependent surveillance mechanism and increased NAb binding to neuraminidase treated tumours suggested that the NAb targets were in the asialo form. Furthermore, the demonstration that CD45RA was increased transiently after T cell activation [52] suggests that NAb can regulate neoplastic and normal activated cells. Confirmatory data has been obtained using a similar approach with selection for high human serum IgG plus IgM and high IVIg binding Jurkat cells [manuscript in prep].

Polyclonal intravenous immunoglobulin inhibited proliferation of Schwann cells and fibroblasts in vitro [53] and IVIg treatment has been implicated in the prevention of metastatic spread of cancer in murine systems [54,55]. An immunoregulatory role for NAb has been demonstrated primarily through investigations with human immunoglobulin for intravenous use (IVIg) [reviewed in 56]. IVIg has been shown to recognize numerous molecules which are essential for immune system function, cytokines including INF-γ, cell surface receptors of lymphocytes including CD4, CD5, TCR, Fas, arguing that IVIg is a key factor in homeostasis of the immune system including the inflammatory response and healing [36,57].

Together the data argue for a pivotal role of the innate immune system in the defence against tumours.

2. WOUND HEALING

The response to tissue injury comprises the action of a complex but highly organized, sequence of interacting mediators, many of which are familiar to us from the innate immune response to carry out the processes necessary for healing. The sequence in dermal wound repair is in principle analogous to repair in other sites. After hemostasis is achieved, an initial inflammatory response is critical not only for a defence against pathogens and to clear debris, but also to stimulate reepithelialization with tissue remodelling, cell proliferation and angiogenesis [reviewed in 58–60]. The ability to heal well depends on the immune status of the host. The inflammatory stage of wound healing is the clearest demonstration of the action of the innate immune system cells, however, they are also important to the proliferative/reepithelialization/wound repair stage and the tissue remodelling/granulation phases [59].

2.1. Inflammatory phase

In the inflammatory phase, platelet degranulation, complement activation and extravasation of blood constituents into the damaged tissues leads to the release of chemokines, cytokines and growth factors which lead to the sequential recruitment of inflammatory cells in addition to the direct stimulation of the repair process in local keratinocytes and fibroblasts. Immediate entrance of some neutrophils into the wound is thought to occur passively, facilitated by their large number in the circulation [61]. One day after injury in humans, maximal expression of IL-8 and growth-related oncogene α (GROα) was spatially and temporally associated with infiltration of numerous neutrophils and on day 2 monocyte/macrophage recruitment into the injury site peaked and monocyte chemoattractant protein-1 (MCP-1) mRNA and MCP-1 were detected [61,62]. The major function of neutrophils is phagocytosis, providing a first line of defence against pathogens [60]. Macrophages are phagocytic in the wound bed removing debris, dead and senescing cells, particularly dying neutrophils [reviewed in 63], and both macrophages and neutrophils produce cytokines which augment the inflammatory response by stimulating the lymphocytes of the innate and the adaptive immune responses. Wound macrophages are considered a pivotal cell, stimulated by many agents within wounds [reviewed in 60], and transforming the response from an inflammatory phase to a proliferation and repair stage with the release of angiogenic, fibrogenic, matrix and proteolytic proteins and their inhibitors which contribute to tissue remodelling.

2.2. Reepitheliazation

Reepitheliazation is primarily the function of fibroblasts/keratinocytes and epidermal cells with growth factors from tissue fibroblasts and inflammatory cells including epidermal growth factor (EGF) and fibroblast growth factor (FGF) stimulating keratinocyte proliferation, contributing to their migration into the wound. In an in vitro scrape-wound model, EGF receptors and NF-κB were activated in epithelial cells at the wound-edge [64]. Intraepithelial (IEL) γδT cells have been shown to produce epithelial growth factor [reviewed in 65]. Cytokines are considered important for coordinating wound healing [reviewed in 58] and IL-8 and growth-related oncogene α profiles also corresponded to keratinocyte migration [62]. Macrophages regulate deposition of stromal components through release of cytokines such as TGF-β, which activates fibroblasts to secrete collagen. A tumour necrosis factor -α (TNF-α) released from macrophages after exposure to bacteria or matrix fragments stimulates other macrophages and contributes to the increased expression of adhesion molecules, which support keratinocyte migration [reviewed in 58]. Interleukin-1 (IL-1) produced by monocytes/macrophages and by keratinocytes increases expression of adhesion molecules which increase keratinocyte migration and collagen synthesis [58]. IL-6 released by inflammatory cells and fibroblasts stimulates fibroblast proliferation while INF-γ produced by T cells and also NK cells has been shown to have a negative regulatory effect on reepithelialization [reviewed in 58]. Perhaps INF-γ control is critical to successful wound healing? TGF-β secreted in wounds by platelets, fibroblasts and macrophages enhances reepithelialization by augmenting fibroblast migration and maturation [reviewed in 59]. Macrophages would contribute to altering the extracellular matrix (ECM) by the production of proteases such as metalloproteinases which in addition to proteinases secreted by keratinocytes would degrade the ECM and by the production of ECM components including fibronectin and proteoglycans [reviewed in 60]. The small gaseous molecule, nitric oxide, is important for wound healing, participating in collagen deposition, cell proliferation, the formation of new blood vessels and wound closure [reviewed in 58,66,67]. A major component of the inducible nitric oxide (NO) synthase (iNOS) in the inflammatory stage is produced by macrophages in the wound and increasingly by fibroblasts, keratinocytes and epithelial cells during the proliferative and regenerative phases [reviewed in 58,66]. Recently "alternatively activated macrophages" generated in response to IL-4 or glucocorticoids have been implicated in immunosuppression and tissue repair [reviewed in 68].

In experimental wound healing, there is an early disappearance of mast cells from the wound edge, followed in rapid sequence by mast cell recovery, hyperplasia and normalization [reviewed in 69]. Degranulation is the immediate response of tissue mast cells to wounding, releasing preformed mediators into the local connective tissue which results in the recruitment of cellular and soluble effectors [reviewed in 70]. Histamine causes vasodilation and increased vascular permeability and heparin with anticoagulant properties maintains perfusion of the connective tissue adjacent to the wound needed for cell influx and nutritional supply [60]. Synthesis and release of leukotriene B_4 after mast cell activation facilitates the recruitment of PMNs [reviewed in 70]. Evidence supported a direct relationship between mast cell activation and the initiation of fibrosis, and/or fibroblast activation and proliferation and mast cells enhanced their migration and proliferation in wound healing in vitro [reviewed in 69]. Histamine has also been implicated in fibroblast growth and collagen synthesis in vitro and in vivo.

2.3. Angiogenesis

Angiogenesis, the growth of new blood vessels from already existing ones is essential for normal physiological processes including growth, development, reproduction and wound healing. Angiogenesis provides for the delivery of nutrients, inflammatory cells and oxygen to the remodelling tissue or wound site and for the removal of debris. Macrophages are phagocytic and cytotoxic and secrete over 100 different bioactive substances [reviewed in 71]. They contribute to angiogenesis by secreting factors which directly stimulate growth of new blood vessels, degrade tissue matrix or stimulate other cell types to produce angiogenic factors [reviewed in 71]. Vascular endothelial cell growth factor (EGF), a major factor for sustaining the induction of blood vessel growth is produced by macrophages, keratinocytes, fibroblasts and endothelial cells in wounds providing for a massive and redundant source of this key angiogenic factor [reviewed in 71]. In parallel, proteolytic enzymes are released to degrade the extracellular matrix and make room for the outgrowth of new blood vessels [reviewed in 63]. Chemokines, particularly the CXC family, which contain an ELR (Glu-Leu-Arg) motif adjacent to their first cysteine amino acid in the NH_2 terminus, have been implicated in direct regulation of angiogenesis [reviewed in 61]. The expression profile of IL-8 and GRO-α in human wounds increasing from 1–4 days after injury and decreasing thereafter correlated with the rate of appearance of new blood vessels [reviewed in 63]. Neutrophils may contribute to early angiogenesis by producing TNF-α and IL-1 in addition to EGF [reviewed in 71]. Chemokines, including IL-8, have been shown to elicit expression of metalloproteinases from different leukocyte types contributing to tissue remodelling [reviewed in 61]. Mast cells have been proposed as a central modulator of angiogenesis [reviewed in 70]. Angiogenic factors including EGF, bFGF and PDGF attract mast cells to sites of neovascularization [reviewed in 72], and MCP-1 attracts mast cells at later time points so that increases in mast cells are likely due to recruitment rather than proliferation [61]. Mast cells accumulate in areas undergoing angiogenesis including wound healing and ovulation and some mast cell mediators including histamine, chymase, EGF and basic fibroblast growth factor (bFGF) are angiogenic regulating endothelial cell proliferation and function while others degrade connective tissue [reviewed in 72]. Angiogenesis is a fine balance between angiogenic and angiostatic factors [reviewed in 73].

Support has been obtained for a role for mast cells in the generation of new blood vessels, an essential process in angiogenesis [reviewed in 69]. Connective tissue mast cells are located around small vessels and upon activation they induced angiogenesis. Mast cell mediators modulate endothelial growth, function and role in angiogenesis. Histamine through both H_1 and H_2 receptors, heparin and TNF-α, a mast cell-derived cytokine, were all able to stimulate angiogenesis. While TNF-α has been implicated in the regulation of several endothelial cell functions, the long duration of the impact of mast cell degranulation on angiogenesis suggested that rapidly released mast cell mediators, such as histamine or heparin, may be stimulating other cells known to promote angiogenesis. Thus, fibroblasts and macrophages may in turn be induced to release angiogenic proteases and cytokines. TGF-β increased fibroblast and endothelial cell expression of vascular endothelial cell growth factor (EGF). EGF induced proliferation and migration of endothelial cells and increased vascular permeability leading to extravascular deposition of fibrin, which promotes growth of new blood vessels. Mast cells further provide products which degrade the connective tissue matrix opening space for the new blood vessels.

2.4. Resolution

During the resolution phase the growth of cellular and connective tissue slows and the abundant new capillary bed regresses. Resolution/downregulation of an ongoing inflammatory response occurring in wound healing likely involves the innate immune system in several mechanisms including: active suppression via anti-inflammatory mediator release, including IL-1ra, IL-4, IL-10, IL-13, TGF-β, and NO; suppressor cell activity by possibly macrophages and in some sites NKT or γδT cells; apoptotic cell death; passive dissipation of the activating/inflammatory stimuli [reviewed in 59]. Chemokines also exhibit angiostatic activity, particularly ELR-negative CXC chemokines such as IP-10 which is present in the late phase of normal wound healing after day four and inhibits EGF-induced fibroblast motility [reviewed in 63]. Macrophages also secrete factors which contribute to new capillary regression, for example thrombospondin, as the nutritive demand within the tissue recedes during wound resolution [reviewed in 71].

3. REPRODUCTION

3.1. Cycling uterus and menstruation

While T and B cells have been detected in human endometrium, any roles in implantation and pregnancy maintenance remain questions [reviewed in 74,75]. $CD3^-/CD16^-/CD56^+$ uterine NK (uNK) cells (endometrial granulocytes, eGL, in humans) which exhibit a different phenotype from peripheral NK cells, macrophages, mast cells and eosinophils are present in human and mouse/rat endometria [reviewed in 74,75]. Estrogens promote migration increasing uNK, macrophage and eosinophil densities [74]. Progesterone reduces proliferation and supports cell-specific differentiation preparing the endometrium for pregnancy [reviewed in 76]. Increases in eGL cytotoxicity and expression of activation markers in the late proliferative phase may contribute to resistance against infection, however, the toxic contents of their granules could contribute to tissue destruction [75]. Since macrophages are rich sources of growth factors, cytokines and proteases, they likely contribute to cycle-associated cell proliferation and destruction, in addition to phagocytic removal of cells and debris during menstruation [74]. While increases in macrophages, uNK cells and eosinophils are considered to contribute to successful implantation, mast cells present throughout the menstrual cycle and markedly activated just prior to menstruation, release TNF-α and IL-1 which induces stromal cell production of matrix metalloproteinases (MMP-3 and MMp1) probably a key to the initiation of tissue destruction in menstruation [reviewed in 74]. Neutrophils, closely associate with tissue damage in an inflammatory response, are barely detectable except when they increase during the perimenstrual period [reviewed in 75]. Many contain MMPs and INF-γ [75], the latter the main activator of macrophages. Together with the observations that eosinophils, important for late-type inflammatory reactions, increase markedly just prior to menstruation with some positive for MMP, the evidence supports the idea that menstruation occurs as a result of an inflammatory process [reviewed in 75] initiated by the withdrawal of progesterone and based on complex interactions between migratory cells and endometrial stromal and epithelial cells [reviewed in 77]. The MMP system is considered to contribute to the remodelling of the ovarian and uterine extracellular architecture throughout each reproductive cycle, necessary for growth of the follicle, follicle rupture during ovulation, generation and regression of the corpus luteum [reviewed in 78–80]. Cell adhesion molecules ICAM-1 and VCAM-1 as well as E-selectin induced by cytokines in inflammatory responses are also detected in the ovary and uterus, peaking during maximal leukocyte density, during ovulation and/or luteal regression in the ovary and for ICAM-1 and E-selectin during menstruation or parturition [reviewed in 81].

Complement components and membrane regulators have been detected in epithelial and vascular tissues lining the female reproductive tract [reviewed in 82]. Evidence for functions for complement beyond the inflammatory response against pathogens has been suggested by the demonstration of hormone dependent, tissue-specific or differentiation stage-specific expression patterns of various complement components during the menstrual cycle [reviewed in 82]. Thus, regulated production for example of C3, factor B, decay accelerating factor (DAF) and various complement membrane regulators suggests roles in normal reproduction including endometrium function, gamete maturation, follicular development, ovulation and fertilization [reviewed in 82].

3.2. Oocyte, ovary, ovulation

Leukocyte subsets of the innate immune system including, macrophage/monocytes, neutrophils, lymphocytes, eosiniphils and mast cells have been implicated in ovary function [reviewed in 83]. Ovulation has been compared to an inflammatory reaction with repeated rupture of healthy tissue resulting from cyclic fluxes of leukocytes, all coordinated with changes in lymphatic and blood flow. Macrophages contribute to folliculogenesis. Neutrophils and macrophages have been implicated in ovulation. Cytokines from endothelial cells and resident leukocytes attract more leukocytes, upregulate their integrin expression and adhesion. As ovulation approaches, the leukocytes release proteolytic enzymes, which are essential for follicular rupture. Progressive infiltration of both macrophages and neutrophils and their production of reactive oxygen species is associated with regression of the corpus luteum. Hormone regulation of IL-8, which is chemotactic for and activates neutrophils, and is also angiogenic, is thought to be important for neutrophil action in follicle development and atresia (resolution). IL-1 and TNFα, together with lutenizing hormone promote ovulation. IL-1 induces production of IL-6 which promotes angiogenesis essential for growing follicles. TNFα, a cytotoxic agent secreted by macrophages is thought to contribute to luteolysis, and T lymphocytes and INF-γ were associated with the final stages of luteal regression [83,84]. Granulocyte-macrophage colony stimulating factor has been implicated in the augmentation of IL-1β-induced histamine-release from mast cells during ovulation [85]. Oocytes were shown to both produce TNFα and express TNF receptors and TNF stimulation of oocyte apoptosis was proposed to restrict the size of the primordial follicle pool [86].

3.3. Pregnancy

3.3.1. Innate system activity in the circulation (systemic)

The traditional view of the immunological paradox of pregnancy is that a state of immunosuppression must exist to allow the foetus, a semi-allogeneic graft, to implant and develop. The suggestion has been that while type 1 cytokines are harmful, a type 2 response at the foetal-maternal interface allows the foetus to survive [reviewed in 87–90]. However, recent flow cytometry studies of cell surface markers and extracellular and intracellular cytokines aimed at investigating the impact of pregnancy on the mother's immune system have suggested that the innate immune system is activated [87–89,91,92]. During pregnancy, circulating granulocytes and monocytes increased in number with the proportions of granulocytes increasing, monocytes remaining constant and lymphocytes decreasing [88, reviewed in 89,91]. Increases in monocyte surface expression of activation-associated adhesion molecules, CD11a, CD54 and CD64 [93], and upon stimulation, higher production of the type I cytokine IL-12 [86,87] and IL-1β, peaking in late gestation, suggested that monocytes are progressively activated during pregnancy [88, rev in 91]. An increase in CD11b with the onset of labour suggested that monocytes were further activated at this stage [88]. Granulocytes showed a similar increase in IL-8 synthesis while T cells were less able to produce IL-6 [88]. Peripheral NK cells and their production of INF-γ were decreased [reviewed in 90]. During pregnancy CD14 was increased on granulocytes

[92] and monocytes [reviewed in 89]. Increases in baseline intracellular reactive oxygen species, oxidative burst and stimulation index demonstrated that the metabolic activity of granulocytes and monocytes was increased during pregnancy [92]. Collectively, pregnancy was considered a proinflammatory state similar to patients with sepsis [87–92], with the innate response activated and in contrast, the adaptive response thought to be suppressed [88]. Pregnancy hormones and the placenta have been suggested as the activators of the innate response [reviewed in 90]. Sacks et al [89] have argued that material of foetal origin including whole cells or membrane vesicles could stimulate a signal 2 (adjuvant-type) response through phagocytosis or monocyte activation via their lipid receptors CD14 and CD11b, which in the absence of specific antigen presentation, signal 1, generates a response particular to pregnancy, leading to their speculation that viviparous reproduction may have influenced the evolution of the immune system in addition to the need to defend against infection. While the dominant γδ T cells in human peripheral blood are Vγ9Vδ2 receptor-positive, the number of γδ T cells and the ratio of Vγ1Vδ1 to Vγ9Vδ2 expression associated with Th2 versus Th1 cytokine production respectively, are increased in the peripheral blood of pregnant women. Most express progesterone receptors suggesting they are already activated and decidua has been proposed as a transient site of extrathymic maturation and the origin of these cells [reviewed in 94], extending the support for the idea that pregnancy is a proinflammatory state.

3.3.2. Innate system activity in utero and at the materno/foetal interface

Following implantation, the maternal component of the placenta, the decidua develops providing for close contact between maternal and foetal cells. Although the maternal uterine leukocytes would be expected to recognize the trophoblast cells as foreign, they appear to be programmed to protect the foetus and to facilitate processes essential to a successful pregnancy [reviewed in 74,90]. uNK cells and macrophages increase markedly in the decidua in early pregnancy, while mast cells and eosinophils become difficult to find [reviewed in 90]. Foetal trophoblast expression of classical MHC class I HLA-C and non-classical MHC class I HLA-E and HLA-G is thought to prevent attack from uNK which bear inhibitory receptors CD94/NKG2 which bind HLA-E and unidentified NK receptors for HLA-C, while HLA-G is a target for the inhibitory receptor ILT-4 on macrophages [reviewed in 74,90]. The high number of uNK in the uterus during early pregnancy are well placed for protection against infection but comparisons of normal and complex pregnancies suggest that they provide a negative regulation of implantation and placentation [reviewed in 90]. Some cytokines produced by uNK including colony stimulating factors (CSFs) promoted implantation and trophoblast growth while TGF-β inhibits trophoblast proliferation and differentiation and type I cytokines including TNF-α and INF-γ also likely have negative effects on implantation and trophoblast invasion [reviewed in 90]. Decidual macrophages are considered to contribute to local resistance against infection. However, as phagocytes they likely remove debris generated by trophoblast invasion, they produce cytokines, CSFs, TNF-α and TGF-β, which affect pregnancy and they also produce prostaglandins, which are immunosuppressive for T cells and uNK cells [reviewed in 90]. T cells detected in human decidua decrease during pregnancy, however, they can produce a variety of cytokines, which may affect acceptance of the foetus; type 2, which generally stimulate trophoblast outgrowth and invasion, and type I, which are helpful for pregnancy [reviewed in 90]. Thus, it is clear that a balance in cytokine production from the various immune cells at the maternal-foetal interface is of major importance for a successful pregnancy [reviewed in 90]. γδ T cells are found in endometrium and are significantly increased in the decidua, particularly in allogeneic rather than syngeneic pregnancy, suggesting their recognition of foetal antigens [reviewed in 94]. Trophoblast recognition was TCR-dependent and activation by trophoblast from other species argued for targeting of a conserved mammalian sequence [reviewed in 94], a homologue. Activated γδ T cells in decidua preferentially use the Vδ1 chain, which has been associated with the Th2 cytokine profile. However, two γδ populations have been identified in murine decidua, one appears early, produces Th1 cytokines and is abortogenic, the later appearing, Th2/3 subtype protects the pregnancy.

The presence of TLR1-TLR10 mRNA has been documented in the human placenta [reviewed in 95] and analysis of the cellular distribution showed that TLR2 and TLR4 were present and likely in an upregulated state on the villous and intermediate trophoblasts arguing for a role in an in utero defence against infection [95]. However, costimulation of TLR2 and TLR4 appears to be needed to generate a reliable signal for a proinflammatory response, providing a safety mechanism against inappropriate stimulation [reviewed in 95]. Questions remain regarding possible roles in development analogous to the action of Toll in the *Drosophila* embryo and regarding the impact of uncoordinated signalling. TLR2 and TLR4 mRNA detected in foetal tissue could participate in a defence against pathogens, however, the organ-specific and differentiation stage-dependence of expression in murine foetal lung, liver and placenta [96] and the sterility of the environment, argue for a role in development.

The accumulation of $CD16^{+}$NK cells in decidua at the end of pregnancy suggests that innate immunity may play a major role near parturition [97]. Defensin transcripts were identified in the placenta [reviewed in 95]. Proinflammatory cytokines IL-1β, IL-6 and TNF-α are important for labour at full term pregnancy [reviewed in 98]. At the beginning of term, high quantities of IL-1β and IL-6 are produced by placental endothelial cells. Together with TNF-α produced by macrophages and increased after the membranes are broken, these cytokines activate the acute phase response which in conjunction with IL-8 lead to parturition [reviewed in 98]. Parturition at term is associated with increases in neutrophil defensin HNP 1–3 in amniotic fluid [99].

3.3.3. Abortion/miscarriage

Recent studies have revealed a major role for the innate immune system in spontaneous abortions [100]. Th evidence suggests that just before or during abortion, localized non-adaptive events including inflammation and haemorrhaging occur with activation of complement or infiltration of leukocytes but not lymphocytes. These responses may be initiated by local necrosis due to stress or infection in the placenta. Endothelial cells have been reported to synthesize in vitro and in vivo all of the components of the complement cascade and nearly all of the complement regulators [reviewed in 101]. Complement regulatory proteins prevent attack of self tissue by complement and the importance of complement in a successful pregnancy was demonstrated in mice deficient for complement receptor 1-related gene/protein y, which was associated with spontaneous deposition of complement in the placenta at the foetal/maternal interface, PMN invasion of the embryos and ultimately foetal loss [reviewed in 100].

3.3.4. Innate system activity in foetus/neonate (development)

Foetal tissues and placental trophoblast produce cytokines, either constitutively as for IL-8 from thymic epithelium or induced as for TNF-α and IL-6 from foetal Kupffer cells [98]. They play essential roles during foetal life. Hematopoietic growth factors regulate proliferation and differentiation of all stages of hematopoiesis which shifts from the yolk sac at 4–8 weeks of gestation to the foetal liver for macrophage production and erythropoiesis. IL-1, IL-6 and IL-3 are general stimulators of hematopoiesis with stem cell factor (SCF) and IL-6 stimulating multipotent self-replicating stem cells and CSFs and IL-6 among other cytokines stimulating noncommitted progenitors and lineage specific colony forming units. Early macrophages are phagocytic and play a role in developmentally regulated tissue remodelling and in foetal defence against infection. Proinflammatory cytokines including IL-1, IL-6, IL-8 and TNF-α are powerful augmentors of phagocytosis. Both foetal and placental cytokines contribute to foetal defence against pathogens and placental IL-4, IL-10 and INF-α promote a humoral maternal response and suppress the cell-mediated response, which could lead to rejection of the foetus [reviewed in 98].

4. CONCLUSIONS

Clearly the mediators of the innate immune response are essential for normal tissue remodelling typified in the continuous homeostasis of the epidermis, wound healing and the cyclical changes associated with mammalian reproduction. Embryonic development depends upon the components of the innate immune system and the evidence is extended by the discovery that Toll receptors which are essential for fly development are major signalling receptors of the innate immune response. The evidence supports physiologic roles beyond defence for the natural immune system. The questions regarding the evolutionary pressure responsible for the development of the innate immune system can not be denied and this is completely entangled in the issue regarding self-nonself discrimination, suggesting a self-centred organizational strategy for survival.

REFERENCES

1. Weisfelner ME, Gottlieb AB. The role of apoptosis in human epidermal keratinocytes. J Drugs Dermatol 2003;2(4):385–91.
2. Nickoloff BJ, Qin JZ, Chaturvedi V, Bacon P, Panella J, Denning MF. Life and death signalling pathways contributing to skin cancer. J Investig Dermatol Symp Proc 2002;7(1):27–35.
3. Mollenhauer J, Herbertz S, Helmke B, Kollender G, Krebs I, Madsen J, et al. Deleted in Malignant Brain Tumors 1 is a versatile mucin-like molecule likely to play a differential role in digestive tract cancer. Cancer Res 2001;61(24):8880–6.
4. Kang W, Reid KB. DMBT1, a regulator of mucosal homeostasis through the linking of mucosal defence and regeneration? FEBS Lett 2003;540(1–3):21–5.
5. Srivastava P. Roles of heat-shock proteins in innate and adaptive immunity. Nat Rev Immunol 2002;2(3):185–94.
6. Pockley AG. Heat shock proteins as regulators of the immune response. Lancet 2003;362(9382):469–76.
7. Underhill DM, Ozinsky A. Toll-like receptors: key mediators of microbe detection. Curr Opin Immunol 2002;14(1):103–10.
8. Nollen EA, Morimoto RI. Chaperoning signaling pathways: molecular chaperones as stress-sensing 'heat shock' proteins. J Cell Sci 2002;115(Pt 14):2809–16.
9. Haagsman HP, Diemel RV. Surfactant-associated proteins: functions and structural variation. Comp Biochem Physiol A Mol Integr Physiol 2001;129(1):91–108.
10. Nicholson-Weller A, Halperin JA. Membrane signaling by complement C5b-9, the

membrane attack complex. Immunol Res 1993;12(3):244–57.
11. Niculescu F, Rus H, Shin ML. Receptor-independent activation of guanine nucleotide-binding regulatory proteins by terminal complement complexes. J Biol Chem 1994;269(6):4417–23.
12. Mondragon-Palomino M, Pinero D, Nicholson-Weller A, Laclette JP. Phylogenetic analysis of the homologous proteins of the terminal complement complex supports the emergence of C6 and C7 followed by C8 and C9. J Mol Evol 1999;49(2):282–9.
13. Horvath CM. STAT proteins and transcriptional responses to extracellular signals. Trends Biochem Sci 2000;25(10):496–502.
14. Dalpke A, Heeg K. Signal integration following Toll-like receptor triggering. Crit Rev Immunol 2002;22(3):217–50.
15. Liou HC. Regulation of the immune system by NF-kappaB and IkappaB. J Biochem Mol Biol 2002;35(6):537–46.
16. Pardoll D. Does the immune system see tumors as foreign or self? Annu Rev Immunol 2003;21:807–39.
17. Diefenbach A, Raulet DH. The innate immune response to tumors and its role in the induction of T-cell immunity. Immunol Rev 2002;188:9–21.
18. Ferrarini M, Ferrero E, Dagna L, Poggi A, Zocchi MR. Human gammadelta T cells: a nonredundant system in the immune-surveillance against cancer. Trends Immunol 2002;23(1):14–8.
19. Soloski MJ. Recognition of tumor cells by the innate immune system. Curr Opin Immunol 2001;13(2):154–62.
20. Smyth MJ, Crowe NY, Hayakawa Y, Takeda K, Yagita H, Godfrey DI. NKT cells - conductors of tumor immunity? Curr Opin Immunol 2002;14(2):165–71.
21. Taniguchi M, Harada M, Kojo S, Nakayama T, Wakao H. The regulatory role of Valpha14 NKT cells in innate and acquired immune response. Annu Rev Immunol 2003;21:483–513.
22. Reiter I, Krammer B, Schwamberger G. Cutting edge: differential effect of apoptotic versus necrotic tumor cells on macrophage antitumor activities. J Immunol 1999;163(4):1730–2.
23. Bingle L, Brown NJ, Lewis CE. The role of tumour-associated macrophages in tumour progression: implications for new anticancer therapies. J Pathol 2002;196(3):254–65.
24. Mantovani A, Sozzani S, Locati M, Allavena P, Sica A. Macrophage polarization: tumor-associated macrophages as a paradigm for polarized M2 mononuclear phagocytes. Trends Immunol 2002;23(11):549–55.
25. Lu G, Janjic BM, Janjic J, Whiteside TL, Storkus WJ, Vujanovic NL. Innate direct anticancer effector function of human immature dendritic cells. II. Role of TNF, lymphotoxin-alpha(1)beta(2), Fas ligand, and TNF-related apoptosis-inducing ligand. J Immunol 2002;168(4):1831–9.
26. Joo HG, Fleming TP, Tanaka Y, Dunn TJ, Linehan DC, Goedegebuure PS, et al. Human dendritic cells induce tumor-specific apoptosis by soluble factors. Int J Cancer 2002;102(1):20–8.
27. Chen YL, Chen SH, Wang JY, Yang BC. Fas ligand on tumor cells mediates inactivation of neutrophils. J Immunol 2003;171(3):1183–91.
28. Furbert-Harris P, Parish-Gause D, Laniyan I, Hunter KA, Okomo-Awich J, Vaughn TR, et al. Inhibition of prostate cancer cell growth by activated eosinophils. Prostate 2003;57(2):165–75.

29. Dorta RG, Landman G, Kowalski LP, Lauris JR, Latorre MR, Oliveira DT. Tumour-associated tissue eosinophilia as a prognostic factor in oral squamous cell carcinomas. Histopathology 2002;41(2):152–7.
30. Gallagher SJ, Marshall JS, Hoskin DW. Human mast cells induce caspase-independent DNA fragmentation in leukemic T cells. Oncol Rep 2003;10(4):1019–23.
31. Fischer M, Juremalm M, Olsson N, Backlin C, Sundstrom C, Nilsson K, et al. Expression of CCL5/RANTES by Hodgkin and Reed-Sternberg cells and its possible role in the recruitment of mast cells into lymphomatous tissue. Int J Cancer 2003;107(2):197–201.
32. Savill J, Dransfield I, Gregory C, Haslett C. A blast from the past: clearance of apoptotic cells regulates immune responses. Nat Rev Immunol 2002;2(12):965–75.
33. Huynh ML, Fadok VA, Henson PM. Phosphatidylserine-dependent ingestion of apoptotic cells promotes TGF-beta1 secretion and the resolution of inflammation. J Clin Invest 2002;109(1):41–50.
34. Lucas M, Stuart LM, Savill J, Lacy-Hulbert A. Apoptotic cells and innate immune stimuli combine to regulate macrophage cytokine secretion. J Immunol 2003;171(5):2610–5.
35. Baker-LePain JC, Reed RC, Nicchitta CV. ISO: a critical evaluation of the role of peptides in heat shock/chaperone protein-mediated tumor rejection. Curr Opin Immunol 2003;15(1):89–94.
36. Lacroix-Desmazes S, Kaveri SV, Mouthon L, Ayouba A, Malanchere E, Coutinho A, et al. Self-reactive antibodies (natural autoantibodies) in healthy individuals. J Immunol Methods 1998;216(1–2):117–37.
37. Chow DA, Wolosin LB, Greenberg AH. Murine natural antitumor antibodies II. The contribution of natural antibodies to tumor surveillance. Int J Cancer 1981;27:459–69.
38. Chow DA, Bennet RD. Low natural antibody and low in vivo tumor resistance in xid-bearing deficient mice. J Immunol 1989;142:3702–6.
39. Bennet RD, Chow DA. Inverse correlation between natural anti-tumor antibodies and tumor susceptibility in individual xid-bearing mice. Nat Immun & Cell Growth Regul 1991;10:45–55.
40. Chow DA. Tumor selection in vivo for reduced sensitivity to natural resistance and natural antibodies. J Natl Cancer Inst 1984;72:339–46.
41. Brown GW, Lesiuk T, Chow DA. Phenotypic alterations in tumors that develop from threshold subcutaneous inocula. I Reduced binding of natural antibodies and sensitivity to hypotonic lysis. J Immunol 1986;136:3116–23.
42. Reese MR, Chow DA. Tumor progression in vivo: Increased SBA lectin binding, N-acetylgalactosamine-specific lectin expression and liver metastasis potential. Cancer Res 1992;52:5235–43.
43. Wang H, Chow, DA. Natural antibody-induced intracellular signaling and growth control in C3H 10T½ fibroblast variants. Immunol 2000;101:458–67.
44. Tough DF, Chow DA. Natural antibody recognition of v-H-ras induced 10T½ transformation. Natural Immun Cell Growth Regul 1991;10:83–93.
45. Tough DF, Haliotis T, Chow DA. Regulation of natural antibody binding and susceptibility to natural killer cells through Zn^{++}-inducible ras oncogene expression. Int J Cancer 1992;50:423–30.
46. Tough DF, Feng X, Chow DA. $p21^{ras}$ independent down-regulation of ras-induced increases in natural antibody binding during tumor progression. Nat Immun 1995;14:20–34.
47. Wang H, Chow DA. PKC expression in 10T½ cells associated increased acquisition of natural antibodies with surveillance of preneoplasia and homeostasis of the organism.

Scand J Immunol 1999;49:381–90.
48. Chow DA. Reduced tumorigenicity of threshold tumor inocula in xid-bearing mice treated with natural antibodies. Int J Cancer 1995;60:848–53.
49. Chow DA, Yuan X-y, Tough DF. Polyclonal natural antitumor antibody binding dynamics: Preferential release of surface membrane molecules and increased metastasis. Inv & Met 1992;12:218–32.
50. Tough DF and Chow DA. Tumorigenicity of murine lymphomas selected through fluorescence-detected natural antibody binding. Cancer Res 1988;48:270–75.
51. Zhang Z, Chow DA. Differential CD45 isoform expression accompanies reduced natural antibody binding in L5178Y-F9 tumor progression. J Immunol 1997;159(1):44–50.
52. Deans JP, Serra HM, Shaw J, Shen YJ, Torres RM, Pilarski LM. Transient accumulation and subsequent rapid loss of messenger RNA encoding high molecular mass CD45 isoforms after T cell activation. J Immunol 1992;148:1898–1905.
53. Van Schaik IN, Vermeulen M, Brand A. Immunomodulation and remyelination: two aspects of human polyclonal immunoglobulin treatment in immune mediated neuropathies ? Mult. Scler. 1997;3:98–104.
54. Fishman P, Bar-Yehuda S, Shoenfeld Y. IVIg to prevent tumor metastases (Review). Int J Oncol 2002;21(4):875–80.
55. Merimsky O, Meller I, Inbar M, Bar-Yehuda S, Shoenfeld Y, Fishman P. A possible role for IVIg in the treatment of soft tissue sarcoma: a clinical case and an experimental model. Int J Oncol 2002;20(4):839–43.
56. Bayry J, Misra N, Latry V, Prost F, Delignat S, Lacroix-Desmazes S, et al. Mechanisms of action of intravenous immunoglobulin in autoimmune and inflammatory diseases. Transfus Clin Biol 2003;10(3):165–9.
57. Amital H, Rewald E, Levy Y, Bar-Dayan Y, Manthorpe R, Engervall P, et al. Fibrosis regression induced by intravenous gammaglobulin treatment. Ann Rheum Dis 2003;62(2): 175–7.
58. Hackam DJ, Ford HR. Cellular, biochemical, and clinical aspects of wound healing. Surg Infect (Larchmt) 2002;3 Suppl 1:S23–35.
59. Ayala A, Chung CS, Grutkoski PS, Song GY. Mechanisms of immune resolution. Crit Care Med 2003;31(8 Suppl):S558–71.
60. DiPietro LA. Wound healing: the role of the macrophage and other immune cells. Shock 1995;4(4):233–40.
61. Gillitzer R, Goebeler M. Chemokines in cutaneous wound healing. J Leukoc Biol 2001;69(4):513–21.
62. Engelhardt E, Toksoy A, Goebeler M, Debus S, Brocker EB, Gillitzer R. Chemokines IL-8, GROalpha, MCP-1, IP-10, and Mig are sequentially and differentially expressed during phase-specific infiltration of leukocyte subsets in human wound healing. Am J Pathol 1998;153(6):1849–60.
63. Sylvia CJ. The role of neutrophil apoptosis in influencing tissue repair. J Wound Care 2003;12(1):13–6.
64. Egan LJ, De Lecea A, Lehrman ED, Myhre GM, Eckmann L, Kagnoff MF. Nuclear factor-{kappa}B activation promotes restitution of wounded intestinal epithelial monolayers. Am J Physiol Cell Physiol 2003;285(5):C1028-C1035.
65. Chen ZW. Comparative biology of gamma delta T cells. Sci Prog 2002;85(Pt 4):347–58.
66. Witte MB, Barbul A. Role of nitric oxide in wound repair. Am J Surg 2002;183(4):406–12.

67. Frank S, Kampfer H, Wetzler C, Pfeilschifter J. Nitric oxide drives skin repair: novel functions of an established mediator. Kidney Int 2002;61(3):882–8.
68. Mosser DM. The many faces of macrophage activation. J Leukoc Biol 2003;73(2):209–12.
69. Metcalfe DD, Baram D, Mekori YA. Mast cells. Physiol Rev 1997;77(4):1033–79.
70. Gottwald T, Coerper S, Schaffer M, Koveker G, Stead RH. The mast cell-nerve axis in wound healing: a hypothesis. Wound Repair Regen 1998;6(1):8–20.
71. Lingen MW. Role of leukocytes and endothelial cells in the development of angiogenesis in inflammation and wound healing. Arch Pathol Lab Med 2001;125(1):67–71.
72. Hiromatsu Y, Toda S. Mast cells and angiogenesis. Microsc Res Tech 2003;60(1):64–9.
73. Distler J, Hirth A, Kurowska-Stolarska M, Gay RE, Gay S, Distler O. Angiogenic and angiostatic factors in the molecular control of angiogenesis. Q J Nucl Med 2003;47(3): 149–61.
74. Hunt JS, Petroff MG, Burnett TG. Uterine leukocytes: key players in pregnancy. Semin Cell Dev Biol 2000;11(2):127–37.
75. Salamonsen LA, Lathbury LJ. Endometrial leukocytes and menstruation. Hum Reprod Update 2000;6(1):16–27.
76. Osteen KG, Bruner-Tran KL, Keller NR, Eisenberg E. Progesterone-mediated endometrial maturation limits matrix metalloproteinase (MMP) expression in an inflammatory-like environment: a regulatory system altered in endometriosis. Ann N Y Acad Sci 2002;955: 37–47; discussion 86–8, 396–406.
77. Salamonsen LA, Woolley DE. Menstruation: induction by matrix metalloproteinases and inflammatory cells. J Reprod Immunol 1999;44(1–2):1–27.
78. Curry TE, Jr., Osteen KG. The matrix metalloproteinase system: changes, regulation, and impact throughout the ovarian and uterine reproductive cycle. Endocr Rev 2003;24(4): 428–65.
79. Smith MF, Ricke WA, Bakke LJ, Dow MP, Smith GW. Ovarian tissue remodeling: role of matrix metalloproteinases and their inhibitors. Mol Cell Endocrinol 2002;191(1):45–56.
80. Ny T, Wahlberg P, Brandstrom IJ. Matrix remodeling in the ovary: regulation and functional role of the plasminogen activator and matrix metalloproteinase systems. Mol Cell Endocrinol 2002;187(1–2):29–38.
81. Bonello N, Norman RJ. Soluble adhesion molecules in serum throughout the menstrual cycle. Hum Reprod 2002;17(9):2272–8.
82. Mastellos D, Lambris JD. Complement: more than a 'guard' against invading pathogens? Trends Immunol 2002;23(10):485–91.
83. Bukulmez O, Arici A. Leukocytes in ovarian function. Hum Reprod Update 2000;6(1): 1–15.
84. Komatsu K, Manabe N, Kiso M, Shimabe M, Miyamoto H. Changes in localization of immune cells and cytokines in corpora lutea during luteolysis in murine ovaries. J Exp Zoolog Part A Comp Exp Biol 2003;296(2):152–9.
85. Tamura K, Kogo H. Granulocyte-macrophage colony-stimulating factor enhances interleukin-1beta stimulated histamine release in the preovulatory rat ovary. Eur J Pharmacol 1999;373(2–3):207–13.
86. Marcinkiewicz JL, Balchak SK, Morrison LJ. The involvement of tumor necrosis factor-alpha (TNF) as an intraovarian regulator of oocyte apoptosis in the neonatal rat. Front Biosci 2002;7:d1997–2005.
87. Sacks GP, Redman CW, Sargent IL. Monocytes are primed to produce the Th1 type

cytokine IL-12 in normal human pregnancy: an intracellular flow cytometric analysis of peripheral blood mononuclear cells. Clin Exp Immunol 2003;131(3):490–7.
88. Luppi P, Haluszczak C, Betters D, Richard CA, Trucco M, DeLoia JA. Monocytes are progressively activated in the circulation of pregnant women. J Leukoc Biol 2002;72(5): 874–84.
89. Sacks G, Sargent I, Redman C. An innate view of human pregnancy. Immunol Today 1999;20(3):114–8.
90. Veenstra van Nieuwenhoven AL, Heineman MJ, Faas MM. The immunology of successful pregnancy. Hum Reprod Update 2003;9(4):347–57.
91. Luppi P. How immune mechanisms are affected by pregnancy. Vaccine 2003;21(24): 3352–7.
92. Naccasha N, Gervasi MT, Chaiworapongsa T, Berman S, Yoon BH, Maymon E, et al. Phenotypic and metabolic characteristics of monocytes and granulocytes in normal pregnancy and maternal infection. Am J Obstet Gynecol 2001;185(5):1118–23.
93. Sacks GP, Studena K, Sargent K, Redman CW. Normal pregnancy and preeclampsia both produce inflammatory changes in peripheral blood leukocytes akin to those of sepsis. Am J Obstet Gynecol 1998;179(1):80–6.
94. Szekeres-Bartho J, Barakonyi A, Miko E, Polgar B, Palkovics T. The role of gamma/delta T cells in the feto-maternal relationship. Semin Immunol 2001;13(4):229–33.
95. Holmlund U, Cebers G, Dahlfors AR, Sandstedt B, Bremme K, Ekstrom ES, et al. Expression and regulation of the pattern recognition receptors Toll-like receptor-2 and Toll-like receptor-4 in the human placenta. Immunology 2002;107(1):145–51.
96. Harju K, Glumoff V, Hallman M. Ontogeny of Toll-like receptors Tlr2 and Tlr4 in mice. Pediatr Res 2001;49(1):81–3.
97. Hayano C, Koi H, Ogawa K, Nagata K, Matsumoto Y, Nakamura M, et al. Accumulation of CD16+ cells with secretion of Ksp37 in decidua at the end of pregnancy. Am J Reprod Immunol 2002;48(1):57–62.
98. Nesin M, Cunningham-Rundles S. Cytokines and neonates. Am J Perinatol 2000;17(8): 393–404.
99. Espinoza J, Chaiworapongsa T, Romero R, Edwin S, Rathnasabapathy C, Gomez R, et al. Antimicrobial peptides in amniotic fluid: defensins, calprotectin and bacterial/ permeability-increasing protein in patients with microbial invasion of the amniotic cavity, intra-amniotic inflammation, preterm labor and premature rupture of membranes. J Matern Fetal Neonatal Med 2003;13(1):2–21.
100. Caucheteux SM, Kanellopoulos-Langevin C, Ojcius DM. At the innate frontiers between mother and fetus: linking abortion with complement activation. Immunity 2003;18(2): 169–72.
101. Monsinjon T, Gasque P, Chan P, Ischenko A, Brady JJ, Fontaine MC. Regulation by complement C3a and C5a anaphylatoxins of cytokine production in human umbilical vein endothelial cells. Faseb J 2003;17(9):1003–14.

Natural Immunity
Edited by L. Bertók and D.A. Chow
© 2005 Elsevier B.V. All rights reserved

Pathological Relevance of the Natural Immune System

STEFANO SALVIOLI, MIRIAM CAPRI, CRISTIANA FUMELLI, FRANCESCO LESCAI, DANIELA MONTI[1] and CLAUDIO FRANCESCHI

Department of Experimental Pathology, University of Bologna, via S. Giacomo 12, Bologna, 40126 Italy, [1]Department of Experimental Pathology and Oncology, University of Florence, via Morgagni 50, Florence, 50139 Italy

ABSTRACT

The natural immune response is a pre-programmed, non specific first line of defence that is primarily responsible for eliminating or containing pathogens at the site of entrance into the host. This evolutionary conserved function was primarily described in cells of the immune system, but it is now known to exist in various tissues, where its activation plays a significant role in host defence, autoimmunity, inflammatory disease and pathogenesis of sepsis-induced multiorgan dysfunction. It is also emerging in the last years as a possible role for natural immunity in the aging process, and its role in tumour immunosurveillance is undergoing a great revival. This Chapter will briefly summarise the importance of natural immunity in all of these phenomena.

1. ROLE IN HOST DEFENCE AGAINST INFECTION

In contrast to adaptive immunity, natural immunity is highly conserved from invertebrates to vertebrates. It is able to provide the organisms with an efficient and satisfactory level of protection against infectious challenges, indeed even invertebrates harbouring only natural immunity have effective host defence systems. Nevertheless, the role of natural immunity in host defence in higher mammals and in humans has long been underestimated, mostly because of the fact that the mechanisms of nonself recognition remained largely unclear. In the last years, with the discovery of Toll-like receptors (TLR, described elsewhere in this Volume), it became clear that, unlike the adaptive immunity, where subtle molecular structures are recognised, the natural immunity can recognise highly conserved patterns common to entire classes of pathogens, the so called pathogen-associated molecular patterns, PAMPs [1]. Examples of PAMPs are lipopolysaccharide (LPS), an outer membrane component of Gram-negative bacteria, teichoic acids of Gram-positive organisms, and glycolipids of mycobacteria. Recognition of PAMPs results in the activation of different intracellular cascades, leading to the expression of effector molecules such as cytokines, chemokines, and adhesion molecules that are involved in inflammation. This feature enables, for example, TLR4 to detect Gram-negative bacteria through the recognition of the lipid A moiety of LPS, or TLR2 to recognise lipoproteins of Gram-positive bacteria, etc. [reviewed in 2]. The importance of TLR function is demonstrated by extensive experimental evidence. Among others are: the resistance to LPS toxicity of mice lacking TLR4 [3], the increased resistance to sepsis of mice lacking MyD88, a protein that initiates the signalling cascade of TLR [4], and the fact that an LPS antagonist for TLR4 is able to suppress endotoxin toxicity [5].

The activation *via* TLR of immature dendritic cells occurs in response to microbial components. Mature dendritic cells then migrate to the nearest lymph node where they can interact with naive T cells to initiate the adaptive immune response [6]. In particular, the stimulation of dendritic cells mediated by TLR steers the course of an adaptive response towards an inflammatory Th1 response [7], *via* the up-regulation of MHC class II and B7 molecules, which can in turn interact with naive T cells supporting their differentiation into Th1 cells [8]. Because of the ability of TLR stimulation to activate natural immunity and the Th1 response, microbial components able to trigger this pathway, such as CpG oligonucleotides, are now under investigation for possible clinical usage as adjuvants for vaccinations [8]. CpG motifs are rare in vertebrate genomic DNA and highly methylated. On the contrary, hypomethylated CpG motifs are quite frequent in bacterial DNA and can thus be recognised as a PAMP, in particular by TLR9. Moreover, the administration of CpG oligonucleotides completely protected mice against challenges with *Plasmodium yoelii, Listeria monocytogenes, Leishmania major*, and *Francisella tularensis* [reviewed in 8]. This suggests that a therapy based on CpG oligonucleotides could potentially be used to increase the readiness of natural immunity, thus providing a general, short-lived protection against various bacterial infections, as a sort of universal vaccine [9]. Nevertheless, an excessive and continuing cytokine production in response to bacterial LPS or superantigens is a hallmark of the systemic inflammatory response, which can be life-threatening. Dissemination of these bacterial products induces the TLR-mediated production of proinflammatory cytokines that cause vascular injury and multiple organ dysfunction. This will be further discussed on section 6.

Recently, the production of natural antibiotic peptides has emerged as an important mechanism of natural immunity in plants and animals. Defensins are diverse members of a large family of antimicrobial peptides, contributing to the antimicrobial action of granulocytes, mucosal host defence in the small intestine and epithelial host defence in the skin and elsewhere (see also Chapter 4 and 10). It has been proposed that a defensin deficiency may play a pivotal role in the aetiopathogenesis of Crohn's disease [11]. Moreover, defensins and other antimicrobial peptides such as cathelicidins, are found to be increased in patients with psoriasis and decreased in patients with atopic dermatitis. A deficiency in the expression of these antimicrobial peptides may account for the susceptibility of patients with atopic dermatitis to skin infection [12]. It has also been reported that pathologies characterised by severe neutropenia and frequent bacterial infections such as morbus Kostmann [13] and Specific Granule Deficiency [14], display a significant deficiency in defensins. All these observations clearly indicate the great importance of these antimicrobial peptides in the defence of the host against possible opportunistic infections.

2. HOST DEFENCE AGAINST CANCER

There is no doubt that the immune system can recognise and eliminate malignant tumour cells *in vivo*, even though the immunosurveillance against tumour clones has likely not been the main purpose that drove the evolution of the immune system. Consequently, it is believed that tumours, which emerge in cancer patients, have been previously selected to escape immune elimination. There is compelling evidence that both natural and adaptive immune responses are involved in tumour clearance. In particular, as far as natural immunity is concerned, it is known that nude athymic mice have comparable rates of cancer incidence relative to normal mice, this fact being mostly due to their maintained NK activity [15]. In contrast, knockout mice lacking the gene for perforin [16], IFN-γ [17] or IFNR-γ [18] have been shown to have a higher incidence of carcinogen-induced tumours and in some cases spontaneous carcinomas. From a clinical perspective, since the end of the XIX century, experimental observations on cancer patients indicated that spontaneous remission was often accompanied by an inflammatory response against a concomitant bacterial infection [19]. On the whole, both historical clinical experience and modern experimental data converge in indicating an important role for natural immunity in cancer clearance. In this regard, it has long been recognised that NK cells spontaneously kill MHC-deficient tumour cells *in vivo* [20]. More recently, it has been observed that cancer cells can be recognised by NK, NKT, CD8+ T cells and γδ T cells through the binding of stress-induced molecules that structurally resemble MHC class I molecules. These molecules are called MICA, MICB and the ULBP family, the ortholog of the murine RAE-1 family [21,22]. These molecules are normally expressed on gut epithelium and can be induced by viral infection or other stress, such as heat shock, and bind to the NKG2D receptor expressed on the surface of NK, NKT, CD8+ T cells and γδ TCR cells [23]. This receptor is associated with DAP10, a transmembrane-anchored adapter protein that can activate the PI3-kinase pathway [24], and thus is able to trigger cell-mediated cytotoxicity [23].

Dendritic cells (DC), the major antigen presenting cells, play an important role in immunosurveillance against cancer. These cells have to be activated in order to induce fully effective T cell immunity. There is a series of studies indicating that DC, when appropriately activated and induced to present tumour-derived peptides, can very effectively elicit tumour-specific T cell immunity [25]. Tumour associated antigens (TAA), such as MAGE1 and MART1 melanoma antigens, can be captured by immature DC which in turn can mature and migrate to the draining lymph node, where they can stimulate both specific CD8+ and CD4+ T cells upon expression of costimulatory molecules such as CD28 and CD40 [26]. Activated CD8+ CTL and T helper CD4+ cells can then migrate into tissues and mount an attack against the developing melanoma. Based on this, different clinical trials on vaccines against melanoma are now underway. Unfortunately, most of the tumours are not targeted by the immune system for a series of rational reasons (among others, lack of specific TAAs or adequate co-stimulation, or the production of inhibitory cytokines). One of these handicaps can be overridden by inducing a localised inflammatory reaction. The production of Th1 cytokines can in fact activate and orientate macrophages and T cells not only against the inflammatory agents, but also against tumour cells. This is the rationale for the most effective immune therapy that has been established up to now, i.e., Coley's toxin (a toxin from *S. pyogenes*, that was used for over 40 years by William Coley in the first half of the past century, with a cure rate of 10% in inoperable sarcomas [19]), and the Bacillus Calmette-Guérin (BCG), used not only to vaccinate against TBC, but also against superficial bladder cancer [27]. At present, local generation of an *immune milieu* by agents of the imidazoquinoline family leading to a Th1-dominance and cell-mediated immunity has been used clinically to treat viral infections such as human papillomavirus (HPV), herpes simplex virus (HSV), and cancerous lesions including initial squamous cell and basal cell carcinoma in immunocompetent and immunosuppressed patients [28].

3. NATURAL IMMUNITY AND AGING

Human aging can be considered as a dynamic process that leads to a continuous adaptation of the body to the deteriorative changes occurring lifelong. This picture is conceptualised in the remodelling theory of aging [29,30], based on experimental evidence obtained from studies on human immunosenescence and on healthy very old people (centenarians) as a model of successful aging. Specifically, these results show that the aging process affects immune responses differently; some of them decline while others remain unchanged or increase [31–33]. Accordingly, a variety of immune responses and parameters are well conserved in centenarians [34–40].

Data from the literature seem to indicate that natural immunity remains preserved or less affected by aging than clonotypic and adaptive immunity. Indeed, the absolute number of cells belonging to the natural immunity compartment, such as dendritic cells (DCs), monocytes/macrophages and granulocytes is not affected by age, while their ability to function, responsiveness, or number of precursors can change, as described in detail below.

Rapid progress in the characterisation of DCs, the most important antigen-presenting cells with a central role in initiating and modulating immune responses, has been made in recent years. DC activity appears to be well preserved during aging [41], even if some alterations seem to occur. For instance, one type of DC precursor, i.e., plasmacytoid DC, a rare circulating population of blood cells, seems to be decreased together with its capacity to produce IFN-α [42]. As far as migratory capacity is concerned, it is not yet clear whether it is impaired in aged DC [43,44], while DC responsiveness to some pathogens and vaccines has been found to be unimpaired [41].

Monocytes and macrophages appear to be mostly activated in aged subjects, based on the observed immunophenotype as well as on biological activity assays [45]. Specifically, their production of cytokines, such as IL-1β, IL-6, IL-10, and chemokines, such as RANTES and MIP-1α, is up-regulated during aging [45–48]. These results are very important and the central role of monocytes in the pro-inflammatory status, which can contribute to the onset of major age-related diseases such as cardiovascular diseases, neurodegenerative disorders and diabetes, will be discussed in the paragraph dedicated to the inflammatory diseases. The number of circulating neutrophil cells in the peripheral blood is not altered with age, though the proliferative response of neutrophil progenitors to G-CSF appears to be reduced [49,50]. It is well known that during bacterial infection neutrophil growth is massively up-regulated by the action of pro-inflammatory cytokines, leading to neutrophilia. Reduced responsiveness of neutrophil progenitors to G-CSF can therefore potentially affect the ability of the elderly to increase the number of neutrophil cells during infection, leading to a higher susceptibility to infectious diseases. This fact has been observed in elderly people affected by chronic infection [50], and suggest that neutrophil production is modified under conditions of persistent infection. Moreover, a reduced neutrophil phagocytic capacity is found in elderly donors, together with a decreased expression of CD16, one of the key receptors inducing phagocytosis of bacteria [51]. This loss of membrane receptors could be a major factor contributing to reduced neutrophil function and increased susceptibility to bacterial infections in the oldest old. Nevertheless, when healthy centenarians are considered, the number of granulocytes (mainly neutrophils) has been found to be increased. Moreover, phagocytic function and production of cytokines such as IL-1β and TNF-α in granulocytes from centenarians, seem to be increased, whereas the production of superoxides is decreased in comparison with that measured in middle-age subjects [52].

An increased number and percentage of NK cells (CD16+, CD56+, CD57+) has been found in the elderly and even more in centenarians [36,52,53]. It has been proposed that the increased number of NK cells can be a compensatory mechanism that counteracts their decreased functionality. Such a functionality is correlated with a preserved metabolism of thyroid hormones and vitamin D [53,54]. These findings are very important, since multiple interactions are known to exist between the endocrine and immune system, and thus alterations in hormone metabolism and responsiveness occurring with age can be the cause of impairment in the NK compartment. Moreover, NK cells from healthy aged subjects and centenarians seem to have a peculiar impairment of some activation pathways such as that involving Protein Kinase C, while others such as the antibody-dependent pathway, seem to be preserved [52,53]. A decreased level of chemokine production in isolated and stimulated NK cells from nonagenarian subjects has been demonstrated [55]. Other authors have found an increased production of IFN-γ by NK cells both in middle-age subjects and centenarians [52].

During ageing, an increase in the proportion of T cells expressing NK markers (CD16, CD56, CD57) has also been reported particularly in centenarians [36,52,53]. Studies on human NKT cells and aging are limited. Nevertheless, some authors have found a decreased percentage of cells bearing CD3 and Valpha24, a membrane marker for a subpopulation of human NKT cells, together with an increase of Valpha24+CD8+ cells in peripheral blood from the elderly, indicating a redistribution of this subset according to the CD4/CD8 phenotype [56]. Moreover, unhealthy centenarians have a high level of Valpha24+ cells that produce high amounts of IFN-γ [52]. It also has been speculated that in humans an age-related shift in lymphocyte populations from canonic T and NK cells to NKT cells would be responsible for a progressive difficulty in discriminating NK from T cells of aged individuals on the basis of phenotypic markers [57–59].

The number of circulating γδ T cells is found to be reduced in old people and centenarians together with an altered pattern of cytokine production, particularly evident at the level of TNF-α production. In spite of these alterations, the level of γδ T cell cytotoxicity appears to be well preserved [60,61]

As far as the complement system is concerned, it appears well preserved in elderly subjects and centenarians. Indeed, the immunochemical levels of C3 and C4 together with serum functional haemolytic activity for classical (CH50) and alternative pathways (AP50) are found to be in the normal range [62].

On the whole, natural immunity seems to be affected by age to a lesser degree than clonotypical immunity. Actually, it is emerging that different cells, such as monocytes, granulocytes, NK and NKT cells can up-regulate their production of cytokines and chemokines thus inducing a pro-inflammatory status. These findings suggest that the reshaping of the organism occurring with age can be, at least in part, orchestrated by a shift in cytokine production toward a pro-inflammatory profile, together with other endocrine and metabolic alterations [63]. Moreover, the progressive accumulation of clones of memory cells, together with the age-related decrease of thymic output of new T cells, leads to a progressive filling of the available immunological space with antigen-experienced, low-responder cells and to a correspondent decline in the number of virgin T cells [64]. This renders the subjects likely more prone to a variety of infectious and non-infectious diseases, where immunity and inflammation play a major role [64].

4. AUTOIMMUNE DISEASES

The term autoimmunity refers to a wide variety of diseases with different aetiologies. A characteristic feature of autoimmune diseases is the selective targeting of a single cell type, tissue or organ by a certain population of autoreactive B or T cells that escaped negative selection during development. Nevertheless, it is now widely accepted that also cellular and soluble components of the natural immunity also play a crucial role in the pathogenesis and maintenance of many autoimmune disorders. As discussed elsewhere in this Volume, natural immunity plays a crucial role in the early response to infections and injuries by eliciting an inflammatory response, and indeed it has been observed that the onset and the recrudescence of many clinical and experimental autoimmune diseases are sustained by infection-driven inflammatory responses [65,66]. Because most autoreactive responses are self-limiting, several criteria must be met for the self-reactive lymphocytes to be pathologic. In particular, the antigen must be presented in a persistent fashion, and co-stimulatory signals that allow full activation of reactive T cells must be present. Both criteria can be achieved by cells and cytokines belonging to the natural branch of the immune system.

Frequent associations between infections and autoimmune diseases have been reported in humans and mice, and an infection often exacerbates an ongoing autoimmune response [67–69]. Some mechanisms have been proposed to explain how infections break self-tolerance, including bystander damage, unveiling of hidden epitopes, molecular mimicry and determinant spreading [70]. Nevertheless, the most convincing evidence on the role of infections in triggering autoimmunity comes from the observation that microorganisms can induce inflammatory events. Inflammation can in turn activate one or more cellular subsets of natural immunity such as NK, NKT, γδ T cells, interferon producing cells (IPC) and mast cells, which can provide co-stimulatory signals for both adaptive immune response and autoimmunity. Cells of the natural immune system can activate autoreactive B and T cells by direct interaction or indirectly with cytokines that can drive a Th1 or Th2 response, as it is summarised below.

It has long been recognised that mast cells play a direct role in the inflammatory process associated with allergic diseases [71]. A brand-new role for mast cells is now emerging also in autoimmune pathogenesis. It has been reported that mast cells infiltrate the salivary glands of Sjögren syndrome patients [72] and the synovial fluid of patients with rheumatoid arthritis and systemic lupus erythematosus (SLE) [73] In both human and rodents mast cells are associated with sites of demyelinisation in multiple sclerosis (MS), or experimental autoimmune encephalomyelitis (EAE) [74]. It has been proposed that mast cells, activated through a variety of mechanisms can initiate and sustain both Th1- and Th2-type responses [75] and thus modulate autoimmune B and T cell clones. In agreement with this hypothesis, it has been reported that two strains of mice deficient in mast cells, W/Wv and Sl/Sld, were resistant to the development of erosive arthritis and that susceptibility was restored in the W/Wv strain by mast cell engraftment [76]. Alternatively, it has also been proposed that mast cells, which are the major producers of histamine and vasoactive amines, can have a role in altering the blood barrier, and thus facilitating the entry of T cells into tissues, especially in the brain of MS patients [77].

NK cells are frequently present in many target organs in autoimmunity, including rheumatoid synovial tissue, muscle, pancreas, brain, and are considered a pathognomonic sign of GVHD. Their role in the control of immune responses to autoantigens remains quite elusive, since at present it has been impossible to determine whether an alteration in NK activity is primary or secondary to the pathological condition. Moreover, in different diseases NK cell activity is either enhanced or decreased. Indeed, in murine EAE [78] and in T-cell transfer induced colitis [79], the depletion of NK cells enhanced the diseases, suggesting that NK cells may play an inhibitory role in such diseases. On the contrary, in cyclophosphamide-induced diabetes [80], in experimental autoimmune myasthenia gravis (EAMG) and in eosinophilic airway inflammation [81], the depletion of NK cells dramatically reduced the clinical disease. This apparent paradox may be due to the wide variety of cytokines produced by NK cells. Indeed, following stimulation, NK cells can rapidly produce IFN-γ and many other immunoregulatory mediators including TGF-β, TNF-α/β, GM-CSF, macrophage inflammatory protein 1α (MIP 1α), IL-1, IL-3, IL-5, IL-8 and IL-10 [81]. IFN-γ can direct naive T cells to differentiate into Th1 proinflammatory phenotype [82], while TGF-β can synergise with cytokines produced by Th2 cells in generating suppressive activity [83]. Thus, it is possible that the opposite roles played by NK cells in different autoimmune diseases would depend upon the particular microenvironmental conditions and on the prevalent production of pro- or anti-inflammatory cytokines.

It is also possible that NK cells can contribute to the development of autoimmunity by directly interacting with antigen presenting cells, such as macrophages and dendritic cells [84], or with antigen specific T and B cells [85]. Direct lysis of dendritic cells by NK cells would be expected to impact negatively on the generation of antigen-specific T cell responses.

As far as NKT cells are concerned, it has been reported that they can produce both IFN-γ and IL-4 after stimulation [86], even though their *in vivo* function is still a subject of debate. Also in this case as for NK cells, contrasting reports are suggesting different roles for NKT cells in autoimmunity. Indeed, patients with myasthenia gravis can have significant increases of Valpha24 NKT cells [87], while patients with MS, systemic sclerosis and type I diabetes show reduced numbers of Valpha24-JalphaQT cells [88]. It has been reported that, upon activation, NKT cells can interact with and activate NK, T and B cells [89,90]. Thus, it has been hypothesised that the collaboration of NKT cells and other cell types, such as NK, B and T cells, might contribute to the genesis of autoimmunity [70].

Some observations have led to the speculation that γδ T cells also might be involved in the induction of autoimmunity. Indeed, they express functional NK inhibitory receptors [91], and are increased in number in Guillian-Barré syndrome patients [92]. Moreover, the depletion of such cells ameliorates the severity of some experimental autoimmune conditions, such as adjuvant arthritis, diabetes in NOD mice and EAE in SJL mice [93–95]. Although the mechanisms are still unproven, the possibility that γδ T cells can interact with other cells of the natural immune system has been suggested.

Interferon-producing cells constitute a small population of leukocytes that secrete high levels of type I interferons (e.g., IFN-α, β, ω) in response to viruses. Evidence has been reported that chronic production of type I IFN by IPC may contribute to autoimmune diseases such as SLE [96]. The mechanisms by which type I IFN induces autoimmunity are under investigation. It has been reported that type I IFNs induce differentiation of monocytes into activated dendritic cells, which may present self-epitopes to autoreactive T cells [97].

On the basis of the data outlined above, a role of primary importance clearly emerges for cytokines that can mediate the communication between the cellular components of natural and adaptive immunity. A wide range of cytokines and chemokines is produced by macrophages, dendritic cells and non-immune cells, such as IFN-α/β, IL-1, TNF-α, IL-12, IL-18, RANTES, MIP-1α and monocyte chemotactic protein (MCP) [98]. These inflammatory mediators are designated as innate cytokines, and there are several lines of evidence suggesting that they can participate in the development of autoimmune responses [70]. Indeed, treatment of mice with some of these cytokines exacerbates the diseases, while on the contrary, mice deficient in IL-1β, IL-12, IL-18 and TNF-α are relatively resistant to the induction of autoimmune diseases [70]. The involvement of such mediators in other pathological conditions will be described later in this Chapter.

Another component of the natural immune system is the pool of IgM natural antibodies, i.e., antibodies that are present prior to antigen stimulation. Antibodies that recognise the red blood cell ABO antigens belong to this class. A high proportion of natural IgM is self-reactive [99], they can thus form immune complexes that may enhance an autoantibody response. Consistent with this notion, rheumatoid diseases are often associated with elevated levels of autoantibodies [100]. The onset of the diseases correlates with a switch from production of IgM to IgG antibodies. Nevertheless, the exact role of autoreactive IgM in the autoantibody response and the switch to other isotypes is not known [101]. Moreover, it has to be mentioned that IgM autoantibodies can have a role in protecting from autoimmunity, either by facilitating the removal of apoptotic cells, which expose many self antigens, or by increasing the tolerance of B cells to self antigen. The timing of exposure, the level of affinity of the autoreactive IgM and its local concentration may determine which scenario applies, i.e., autoimmunity or tolerance.

A very important soluble component of natural immunity is complement. It has been reported that some complement components, namely C1q and C4, have a protective effect against autoimmunity. Indeed, it can be expected that the formation of an immune complex between a self antigen and an autoantibody would lead to the activation of complement, and this would lead to the appropriate clearance of the immune complex. This is in agreement with the fact that in both mice [102] and humans [101], a deficiency in C1q or C4 leads to the development of glomerulonephritis, SLE, antinuclear and anti-DNA autoantibodies. Also in the case of complement, as for the other components of natural immunity, an opposite role has been reported in different autoimmune disorders. In particular, it has been shown that higher levels of the terminal complement complex in the intrathechal space of MS patients correlated significantly with neurological disability [103]. It is known that myelin can indeed bind complement, and activated complement can either act as a bridge between myelin and scavenger cells such as microglia [104], or disrupt the myelin lamellae [105].

On the whole, most of the components of natural immunity are reported to be in some way involved in autoimmune disorders. Some of them act mainly in the pathogenesis of the diseases (early stages), while others can have a role in the development of chronic disease or in some of its clinical features. The complex role played by natural immunity in autoimmune phenomena is underlined by the fact that the same component, just like a two-faced Janus, can have a protective or a triggering role according to the micro-environmental, genetic and anatomic conditions that apply.

5. INFLAMMATORY DISEASE

As inflammation is the first response of the organism to a variety of stimuli, including infection, tissue damage and stress, it has to be expected that a consistent number of pathologies have a heavy inflammatory background [106,107]. Indeed, as already mentioned in this Chapter, inflammation can be in some cases an important cause of damage, by itself or by the interaction of inflammatory molecules with pathological molecular mechanisms, thus contributing to the acceleration of the disease [108]. The close association between inflammation and disease can be more clearly highlighted during ageing, when a progressive pro-inflammatory state is going to be established, thus resulting in a higher risk to develop age-associated disorders, as most of them show a strong inflammatory component [109,110]. During inflammation, among the great number of cells and mediators involved, cytokines represent the central architectural communication network, thus being of primary importance in the modulation and outcome of the inflammatory response. In this sense, the individual variation in the intensity of the inflammatory response can be traced back to a number of genetic differences accounting for differences in the capacity to produce high or low levels of these mediators, thus conferring upon them the ability to develop a higher or a lower inflammatory response involved in the disease evolution [47,111]

One of the primary causes of mortality, which is cardiovascular disease, is strictly associated with inflammatory phenomena mediated by different molecules, such as leukocyte adhesion molecules, chemoattractans, TNF-α and interferons. All stages of initiation, growth and complication of the atherosclerotic plaque can be considered to be an inflammatory response to initial injury at the endothelial level [112]. Thus, these mediators can be identified as potential targets for therapies against acute coronary syndrome (ACS). In particular IL-1β, TNF-α, IL-6, or products of the hepatic activation (C-reactive protein, CRP or serum amyloid, SAA) have been proposed as good candidates for inhibitor therapies [113–116]. Elevated values of CRP, SAA, IL-6 and IL-1 receptor antagonist (IL-1RA) commonly accompany ACS: such an elevation correlates with an adverse prognosis and may reflect not only an effect of the ACS itself, but also the presence of a pre-existing inflammatory status able to trigger coronary instability [117–119].

Given this framework, the importance of individual capability to mount an inflammatory response, due to underlying genetic variation, is particularly relevant. In particular, a polymorphism in the promoter of the IL-6 gene, referred to as -174 C/G polymorphism, has been widely studied. The two possible alleles were differently associated with risk of coronary hearth disease and systolic blood pressure in healthy men [119]. The same single nucleotide polymorphism (SNP) seems to interact with another SNP in the gene encoding for an adhesion molecule (ICAM-1) important in leukocyte migration during inflammatory responses in patients with a history of ischaemic stroke [120].

Another relevant pathology such as diabetes is characterised by the presence of increased inflammatory markers. It is possible to consider diabetes as a trigger for vascular inflammation (production of advanced glycation end-products), but there is also substantial evidence that low-grade inflammation is an important pathogenetic determinant for type-2 diabetes. CRP level is a predictive parameter for the risk of developing this form of diabetes, independent from other determinants such as body mass index or glucose levels [121]. Many cytokines, in particular IL-1β, TNF-α and IL-6 act ultimately on the hypothalamic pituitary-adrenal axis, whose activation is associated with hypertension and insulin resistence [122]. Cytokines released by both T lymphocytes and activated macrophages, and in particular IL-1β, have been implicated as effectors that both inhibit insulin release and induce beta-cell destruction [122–127]. Even in this case genetic polymorphisms play a fundamental role in shaping the background upon which the disease develops, since high levels of cytokines such as IL-6 and TNF-α are risk factors for type 2 diabetes [128–130]. The TNF-α gene accounts for another A/G SNP in the promoter (-308 A/G): both IL-6 and TNF-α SNPs have been associated with different risks and an interaction between them has been proposed [131–133].

In a completely different context such as the central nervous system, a peculiar inflammatory process called neuroinflammation is present in patients affected by age-related disorders like Alzheimer's Disease (AD). The interlinked pathways connecting inflammatory response and disease progression can be traced through all stages of the disease and can better explain how the innate response can also accelerate the pathological evolution: molecules like α-1-antichymotrypsin can act as a chaperone for the insoluble amyloid peptides, binding the fragment without displaying its proteolytic activities and thus preventing its degradation. This results in a faster deposition of fibrillary forms and in the reduction of the scavenging activities on pro-inflammatory mediators [134–137]. The inflammatory process appears to be chronic and it is clearly able to activate a response that has the potential to injure and even kill neurons, through the release of highly toxic products (reactive oxygen species, nitric oxide, cytokines and complement components). Thus, it is clear that inflammation significantly contributes to AD pathogenesis [138,139].

Two main actors in regulating this process (IL-1β and IL-6) have been studied to answer the question whether it is possible to find in the population pro-inflammatory genotypes more disadvantaged and with a higher risk to develop AD. The results of the studies concluded that IL-1β genotypes (base substitutions at -511 and -889 positions) may actually confer different risks for AD through IL-1β over-expression and IL-1β-driven neurodegenerative cascades [139–142], while polymorphisms of the IL-6 gene play a complex role, due to the possible interaction of alleles at different loci in the sequence [138,143–145].

On the whole, these findings suggest that inflammation plays a central role in this neurological pathology, and that the genetic background of individual patients affects the regulation of brain responses, which in turn may contribute to neurodegeneration.

6. SEPTIC AND TRAUMATIC SHOCK

In the initial response to a localised infection, the release of endotoxins or exotoxins by a bacterial infection induces tissue macrophages, as well as other cells, to generate inflammatory cytokines. Although these early-response cytokines play an important role in host defence (see above) by attracting activated neutrophils to the site of infection, the entry of these cytokines and bacterial products into the systemic circulation can induce widespread microvascular injury. Systemic alterations observed in patients affected by disseminated sepsis are identified as systemic inflammatory response syndrome. All the clinical features of this syndrome are due to the effects of cytokines expressed in response to PAMPs. They may include fever and haematic increase of neutrophils and acute phase-proteins in patients with a moderate clinical expression. In contrast, a massive septic process induces a marked systemic inflammatory response syndrome caused by high levels of circulating cytokines induced by large quantities of PAMPs released by pathogens, resulting in disseminated intravascular coagulation (DIC). Thrombosis and inflammation are responsible for the damage to tissues and organs and lead to functional collapse and septic shock. Additional damage is caused by neutrophil activation before their migration out of the vascular system, with consequent endothelial damage and slowing of the haematic flux, that affect particularly lungs and liver, leading to an inadequate hepatic gluconeogenesis and respiratory distress syndrome due to plasma outflow into interstitial pulmonary space. Kidney and gut are also damaged by reduced perfusion. Excessive amounts of nitric oxide (NO) produced by myocardial cells and vasal muscular cells upon cytokine stimulation lead to cardiac decompensation, pressure collapse and cardiovascular shock. TNF-α, IL-1β and NO seem to play an important role in sepsis-induced myocardial dysfunction [146]. Disseminated intravascular coagulation, hypoglycaemia and cardiovascular decompensation are the clinical expression of septic shock that is mostly lethal.

TNF-α, produced by LPS-activated macrophages, is the main mediator responsible for this syndrome. In fact TNF-α plasma levels are elevated during experimental and clinical sepsis and increasing concentrations of TNF-α during sepsis are associated with increasing mortality [147,148]; exogenous TNF-α administration in humans and animals leads to multiorgan failure simulating sepsis and LPS effects, moreover TNF-α neutralization often leads to amelioration of sepsis syndrome and improves survival [149,150].

Also traumatic shock, such as acute hypovolemic hemorragic shock, initiates a similar inflammatory response characterized by the up-regulation of cytokine expression [151] and accumulation of neutrophils in various tissues [152] with consequent multiple organ failure. The mechanism by which this type of shock triggers the inflammatory response still remains to be elucidated. Elevated adrenergic activity [153] and systemic release of proinflammatory agents from the gut [154], have been hypothesized to contribute to organ injury. In addition, reactive oxygen species are implicated in various signal transduction pathways [155]. Acute hemorragic shock is characterized by severe hypotension, increased levels of TNF-α and vascular failure due to the loss of vascular activity after stimulation with vasoconstrictive stimuli. The early activation of NFκB in the liver induced by blood loss in turn activates an inflammatory cascade, leading to the expression of TNF-α, finally culminating in the fatal outcome for the host [156].

The possible therapeutic use of inhibitors of TLR or complement components to abrogate or minimize the effects of uncontrolled inflammatory response and sepsis is at present under investigation. Basing on the experimental and clinical evidence reported in this Chapter, a number of studies on molecules able to inhibit the function of complement components C1q and MBL [157] or the signaling of TLR4 [158] or CD14 [159] are ongoing to exploit this possibility.

REFERENCES

1. Medzhitov R, Janeway C Jr. Innate Immunity. N Engl J Med 2000;343:338–44.
2. Takeda K, Akira S. Roles of Toll-like receptors in innate immune responses. Genes Cells 2001 Sep;6(9):733–42.
3. Hoshino K, Takeuchi O, Kawai T, Sanjo H, Ogawa T, Takeda Y, et al. Cutting edge: Toll-like receptor 4 (TLR4)-deficient mice are hyporesponsive to lipopolysaccharide; evidence for TLR4 as the Lps gene product. J Immunol 1999;162:3749–52.
4. Weighardt H, Kaiser-Moore S, Vabulas RM, Kirschning CJ, Wagner H, Holzmann B. Cutting edge: myeloid differentiation factor 88 deficiency improves resistance against sepsis caused by polymicrobial infection. J Immunol 2002;Sep 15;169(6):2823–7.
5. Mullarkey M, Rose JR, Bristol J, Kawata T, Kimura A, Kobayashi S, et al. Inhibition of endotoxin response by e5564, a novel Toll-like receptor 4-directed endotoxin antagonist. J Pharmacol Exp Ther 2003 Mar;304(3):1093–102.
6. Banchereau J, Steinman RM. Dendritic cells and the control of immunity. Nature 1998 Mar 19;392(6673):245–52.
7. Schnare M, Barton GM, Holt AC, Takeda K, Akira S, Medzhitov R. Toll-like receptors control activation of adaptive immune responses. Nat Immunol 2001 Oct;2(10):947–50.
8. Lawton JA, Ghosh P. Novel therapeutic strategies based on toll-like receptor signaling. Curr Opin Chem Biol 2003 Aug;7(4):446–51.
9. Mutwiri G, Pontarollo R, Babiuk S, Griebel P, van Drunen Littel-van den Hurk S, Mena A, et al. Biological activity of immunostimulatory CpG DNA motifs in domestic animals. Vet Immunol Immunopathol 2003 Jan 30;91(2):89–103.
10. Ganz T. Defensins: antimicrobial peptides of innate immunity. Nat Rev Immunol 2003 Sep;3(9):710–20.
11. Fellermann K, Wehkamp J, Herrlinger KR, Stange EF. Crohn's disease: a defensin deficiency syndrome? Eur J Gastroenterol Hepatol 2003 Jun;15(6):627–34.
12. Ong PY, Ohtake T, Brandt C, Strickland I, Boguniewicz M, Ganz T, et al. Endogenous antimicrobial peptides and skin infections in atopic dermatitis. N Engl J Med 2002 Oct 10;347(15):1151–60.

13. Putsep K, Carlsson G, Boman HG, Andersson M. Deficiency of antibacterial peptides in patients with morbus Kostmann: an observation study. Lancet 2002 Oct 12;360(9340): 1144–9.
14. Ganz T, Metcalf JA, Gallin JI, Boxer LA, Lehrer RI. Microbicidal/cytotoxic proteins of neutrophils are deficient in two disorders: Chediak-Higashi syndrome and "specific" granule deficiency. J Clin Invest 1988 Aug;82(2):552–6.
15. Lanier LL. A renaissance for the tumor immunosurveillance hypothesis. Nat Med 2001 Nov;7(11):1178–80.
16. van den Broek ME, Kagi D, Ossendorp F, Toes R, Vamvakas S, Lutz WK, et al. Decreased tumor surveillance in perforin-deficient mice. J Exp Med 1996 Nov 1;184(5):1781–90.
17. Kaplan DH, Shankaran V, Dighe AS, Stockert E, Aguet M, Old LJ, et al. Demonstration of an interferon gamma-dependent tumor surveillance system in immunocompetent mice. Proc Natl Acad Sci U S A 1998 Jun 23;95(13):7556–61.
18. Shankaran V, Ikeda H, Bruce AT, White JM, Swanson PE, Old LJ, et al. IFN gamma and lymphocytes prevent primary tumour development and shape tumour immunogenicity. Nature 2001 Apr 26;410(6832):1107–11.
19. Parish CR. Cancer immunotherapy: The past, the present and the future. Immunol Cell Biol 2003 Apr;81(2):106–13.
20. Whiteside TL, Herberman RB. The role of natural killer cells in immune surveillance of cancer. Curr Opin Immunol 1995 Oct;7(5):704–10.
21. Groh V, Bahram S, Bauer S, Herman A, Beauchamp M, Spies T. Cell stress-regulated human major histocompatibility complex class I gene expressed in gastrointestinal epithelium. Proc Natl Acad Sci U S A. 1996 Oct 29;93(22):12445–50.
22. Cosman D, Mullberg J, Sutherland CL, Chin W, Armitage R, Fanslow W, et al. ULBPs, novel MHC class I-related molecules, bind to CMV glycoprotein UL16 and stimulate NK cytotoxicity through the NKG2D receptor. Immunity 2001 Feb;14(2):123–33.
23. Diefenbach A, Jensen ER, Jamieson AM, Raulet DH. Rae1 and H60 ligands of the NKG2D receptor stimulate tumour immunity. Nature 2001 Sep 13;413(6852):165–71.
24. Wu J, Song Y, Bakker AB, Bauer S, Spies T, Lanier LL, et al. An activating immunoreceptor complex formed by NKG2D and DAP10. Science 1999 Jul 30;285(5428):730–2.
25. Mayordomo JI, Zorina T, Storkus WJ, Zitvogel L, Celluzzi C, Falo LD, et al. Bone marrow-derived dendritic cells pulsed with synthetic tumour peptides elicit protective and therapeutic antitumour immunity. Nat Med 1995 Dec;1(12):1297–302.
26. Smyth MJ, Godfrey DI, Trapani JA. A fresh look at tumor immunosurveillance and immunotherapy. Nat Immunol 2001 Apr;2(4):293–9.
27. Bassi P. BCG (Bacillus of Calmette Guerin) therapy of high-risk superficial bladder cancer. Surg Oncol 2002 Jun;11(1–2):77–83.
28. Hengge UR, Benninghoff B, Ruzicka T, Goos M. Topical immunomodulators-progress towards treating inflammation, infection, and cancer. Lancet Infect Dis 2001 Oct;1(3): 189–98.
29. Franceschi C, Monti D, Sansoni P, Cossarizza A. The immunology of exceptional individuals: the lesson of centenarians. Immunol Today 1995 Jan;16(1):12–6.
30. Franceschi C, Cossarizza A. Introduction: the reshaping of the immune system with age. Int Rev Immunol 1995;12(1):1–4.
31. Fagnoni FF, Vescovini R, Mazzola M, Bologna G, Nigro E, Lavagetto G, et al. Expansion of cytotoxic CD8+ CD28- T cells in healthy ageing people, including centenarians. Immunology 1996 Aug;88(4):501–7.

32. Fagnoni FF, Vescovini R, Passeri G, Bologna G, Pedrazzoni M, Lavagetto G, et al. Shortage of circulating naive CD8(+) T cells provides new insights on immunodeficiency in aging. Blood 2000 May 1;95(9):2860–8.
33. Wack A, Cossarizza A, Heltai S, Barbieri D, D'Addato S, Fransceschi C, et al. Age-related modifications of the human alphabeta T cell repertoire due to different clonal expansions in the CD4+ and CD8+ subsets. Int Immunol 1998 Sep;10(9):1281–8.
34. Paganelli R, Quinti I, Fagiolo U, Cossarizza A, Ortolani C, Guerra E, et al. Changes in circulating B cells and immunoglobulin classes and subclasses in a healthy aged population. Clin Exp Immunol 1992 Nov;90(2):351–4.
35. Mariotti S, Sansoni P, Barbesino G, Caturegli P, Monti D, Cossarizza A, et al. Thyroid and other organ-specific autoantibodies in healthy centenarians. Lancet 1992 Jun 20;339(8808): 1506–8.
36. Sansoni P, Cossarizza A, Brianti V, Fagnoni F, Snelli G, Monti D, et al. Lymphocyte subsets and natural killer cell activity in healthy old people and centenarians. Blood 1993 Nov 1;82(9):2767–73.
37. Sansoni P, Fagnoni F, Vescovini R, Mazzola M, Brianti V, Bologna G, et al. T lymphocyte proliferative capability to defined stimuli and costimulatory CD28 pathway is not impaired in healthy centenarians. Mech Ageing Dev 1997 Jun;96(1–3):127–36.
38. Fagiolo U, Cossarizza A, Scala E, Fanales-Belasio E, Ortolani C, Cozzi E, et al. Increased cytokine production in mononuclear cells of healthy elderly people. Eur J Immunol 1993 Sep;23(9):2375–8.
39. Cossarizza A, Ortolani C, Paganelli R, Barbieri D, Monti D, Sansoni P, et al. CD45 isoforms expression on CD4+ and CD8+ T cells throughout life, from newborns to centenarians: implications for T cell memory. Mech Ageing Dev 1996 Mar 29;86(3):173–95.
40. Bagnara GP, Bonsi L, Strippoli P, Bonifazi F, Tonelli R, D'Addato S, et al. Hemopoiesis in healthy old people and centenarians: well-maintained responsiveness of CD34+ cells to hemopoietic growth factors and remodeling of cytokine network. J Gerontol A Biol Sci Med Sci 2000 Feb;55(2):B61–6.
41. Lung TL, Saurwein-Teissl M, Parson W, Schonitzer D, Grubeck-Loebenstein B. Unimpaired dendritic cells can be derived from monocytes in old age and can mobilize residual function in senescent T cells. Vaccine 2000 Feb 25;18(16):1606–12.
42. Shodell M, Siegal FP Circulating, interferon-producing plasmacytoid dendritic cells decline during human ageing. Scand J Immunol 2002 Nov;56(5):518–21.
43. Steger MM, Maczek C, Grubeck-Loebenstein B. Morphologically and functionally intact dendritic cells can be derived from the peripheral blood of aged individuals. Clin Exp Immunol 1996 Sep;105(3):544–50.
44. Pietschmann P, Hahn P, Kudlacek S, Thomas R, Peterlik M. Surface markers and transendothelial migration of dendritic cells from elderly subjects. Exp Gerontol 2000 Mar;35(2):213–24.
45. Sadeghi HM, Schnelle JF, Thoma JK, Nishanian P, Fahey JL. Phenotypic and functional characteristics of circulating monocytes of elderly persons. Exp Gerontol 1999 Dec;34(8): 959–70.
46. Bonafe M, Olivieri F, Cavallone L, Giovagnetti S, Mayegiani F, Cardelli M, et al. A gender--dependent genetic predisposition to produce high levels of IL-6 is detrimental for longevity. Eur J Immunol 2001 Aug;31(8):2357–61.
47. Olivieri F, Bonafe M, Cavallone L, Giovagnetti S, Marchegiani F, Cardelli M, et al. The -174 C/G locus affects in vitro/in vivo IL-6 production during aging. Exp Gerontol 2002

Jan-Mar;37(2–3):309–14.
48. Mariani E, Pulsatelli L, Neri S, Dolzani P, Meneghetti A, Silvestri T, et al. RANTES and MIP-1alpha production by T lymphocytes, monocytes and NK cells from nonagenarian subjects. Exp Gerontol 2002 Jan-Mar;37(2–3):219–26.
49 Chatta GS, Andrews RG, Rodger E, Schrag M, Hammond WP, Dale DC. Hematopoietic progenitors and aging: alterations in granulocytic precursors and responsiveness to recombinant human G-CSF, GM-CSF, and IL-3.J Gerontol 1993 Sep;48(5):M207–12.
50. Born J, Uthgenannt D, Dodt C, Nunninghoff D, Ringvolt E, Wagner T, et al. Cytokine production and lymphocyte subpopulations in aged humans. An assessment during nocturnal sleep. Mech Ageing Dev 1995 Oct 13;84(2):113–26.
51. Butcher SK, Chahal H, Nayak L, Sinclair A, Henriquez NV, Sapey E, et al. Senescence in innate immune responses: reduced neutrophil phagocytic capacity and CD16 expression in elderly humans. J Leukoc Biol 2001 Dec;70(6):881–6.
52. Miyaji C, Watanabe H, Toma H, Akisaka M, Tomiyama K, Sato Y, Abo T. Functional alteration of granulocytes, NK cells, and natural killer T cells in centenarians. Hum Immunol 2000 Sep;61(9):908–16.
53. Mariani E, Ravaglia G, Forti P, Meneghetti A, Tarozzi A, Maioli F, et al. Vitamin D, thyroid hormones and muscle mass influence natural killer (NK) innate immunity in healthy nonagenarians and centenarians. Clin Exp Immunol 1999 Apr;116(1):19–27.
54. Kmiec Z, Mysliwska J, Rachon D, Kotlarz G, Sworczak K, Mysliwski A. Natural killer activity and thyroid hormone levels in young and elderly persons. Gerontology 2001 Sep-Oct;47(5):282–8.
55. Mariani E, Meneghetti A, Neri S, Ravaglia G, Forti P, Cattini L, et al. Chemokine production by natural killer cells from nonagenarians. Eur J Immunol 2002 Jun;32(6): 1524–9.
56. DelaRosa O, Tarazona R, Casado JG, Alonso C, Ostos B, Pena J, et al. Valpha24+ NKT cells are decreased in elderly humans. Exp Gerontol 2002 Jan-Mar;37(2–3):213–7.
57. Globerson A, Effros RB. Ageing of lymphocytes and lymphocytes in the aged. Immunol Today 2000 Oct;21(10):515–21.
58. Solana R, Mariani E. NK and NK/T cells in human senescence. Vaccine 2000 Feb 25;18(16):1613–20.
59. Tarazona R, DelaRosa O, Alonso C, Ostos B, Espejo J, Pena J, et al. Increased expression of NK cell markers on T lymphocytes in aging and chronic activation of the immune system reflects the accumulation of effector/senescent T cells. Mech Ageing Dev 2000 Dec 20;121(1–3):77–88.
60. Argentati K, Re F, Donnini A, Tucci MG, Franceschi C, Bartozzi B, et al. Numerical and functional alterations of circulating gammadelta T lymphocytes in aged people and centenarians. J Leukoc Biol 2002 Jul;72(1):65–71.
61. Colonna-Romano G, Potestio M, Aquino A, Candore G, Lio D, Caruso C. Gamma/delta T lymphocytes are affected in the elderly. Exp Gerontol 2002 Jan-Mar;37(2–3):205–11.
62. Bellavia D, Frada G, Di Franco P, Feo S, Franceschi C, Sansoni P, et al. C4, BF, C3 allele distribution and complement activity in healthy aged people and centenarians. J Gerontol A Biol Sci Med Sci 1999 Apr;54(4):B150–3.
63. Paolisso G, Barbieri M, Bonafe M, Franceschi C. Metabolic age modelling: the lesson from centenarians. Eur J Clin Invest 2000 Oct;30(10):888–94.
64. Franceschi C, Bonafe M, Valensin S. Human immunosenescence: the prevailing of innate immunity, the failing of clonotypic immunity, and the filling of immunological space.

Vaccine 2000 Feb 25;18(16):1717–20.
65. Regner M, Lambert PH. Autoimmunity through infection or immunization? Nat Immunol 2001; 2(3):185–8.
66. Wucherpfennig KW. Mechanisms for the induction of autoimmunity by infectious agents. J Clin Invest 2001;108(8):1097–104.
67. Horwitz MS, Sarvetnick N. Viruses, host responses, and autoimmunity. Immunol Rev 1999; 169:241–53.
68. Di Rosa F, Barnaba V. Persisting viruses and chronic inflammation: understanding their relation to autoimmunity. Immunol Rev 1998;164:17–27.
69. Aichele P, Bachmann MF, Hengartner H, Zinkernagel RM. Immunopathology or organ-specific autoimmunity as a consequence of virus infection. Immunol Rev 1996;152: 21–45.
70. Shi F, Ljunggren HG, Sarvetnick N. Innate immunity and autoimmunity: from self-protection to self-destruction. Trends Immunol 2001;22(2):97–101.
71. Williams CM, Galli SJ. The diverse potential effector and immunoregulatory roles of mast cells in allergic disease. J Allergy Clin Immunol 2000;105(5):847–59.
72. Skopouli FN, Li L, Boumba D, Stefanaki S, Hanel K, Moutsopoulos HM, et al. Association of mast cells with fibrosis and fatty infiltration in the minor salivary glands of patients with Sjogren's syndrome. Clin Exp Rheumatol 1998;16(1):63–5.
73. Woolley DE, Tetlow LC. Mast cell activation and its relation to proinflammatory cytokine production in the rheumatoid lesion. Arthritis Res 2000;2(1):65–74.
74. Ibrahim MZ, Reder AT, Lawand R, Takash W, Sallouh-Khatib S. The mast cells of the multiple sclerosis brain. J Neuroimmunol 1996;70(2):131–8.
75. Robbie-Ryan M, Brown M. The role of mast cells in allergy and autoimmunity. Curr Opin Immunol 2002;14(6):728–33.
76. Lee DM, Friend DS, Gurish MF, Benoist C, Mathis D, Brenner MB. Mast cells: a cellular link between autoantibodies and inflammatory arthritis. Science 2002;97(5587):1689–92.
77. Bebo BF Jr, Yong T, Orr EL, Linthicum DS. Hypothesis: a possible role for mast cells and their inflammatory mediators in the pathogenesis of autoimmune encephalomyelitis. J Neurosci Res 1996;5(4):340–8.
78. Zhang B, Yamamura T, Kondo T, Fujiwara M, Tabira T. Regulation of experimental autoimmune encephalomyelitis by natural killer (NK) cells. J Exp Med 1997;86(10): 1677–87.
79. Fort MM, Leach MW, Rennick DM. A role for NK cells as regulators of CD4+ T cells in a transfer model of colitis. J Immunol 1998;61(7):3256–61.
80. Maruyama T, Watanabe K, Takei I, Kasuga A, Shimada A, Yanagawa T, et al. Anti-asialo GM1 antibody suppression of cyclophosphamide-induced diabetes in NOD mice. Diabetes Res 1991;7(1):37–41.
81. Korsgren M, Persson CG, Sundler F, Bjerke T, Hansson T, Chambers BJ, et al. Natural killer cells determine development of allergen-induced eosinophilic airway inflammation in mice. J Exp Med 1999;89(3):553–62.
82. Shi FD, Takeda K, Akira S, Sarvetnick N, Ljunggren HG. IL-18 directs autoreactive T cells and promotes autodestruction in the central nervous system via induction of IFN-gamma by NK cells. J Immunol 2000;65(6):3099–104.
83. Gray JD, Hirokawa M, Horwitz DA. The role of transforming growth factor beta in the generation of suppression: an interaction between CD8+ T and NK cells. J Exp Med 1994;80(5):1937–42.

84. Fernandez NC, Lozier A, Flament C, Ricciardi-Castagnoli P, Bellet D, Suter M, et al. Dendritic cells directly trigger NK cell functions: cross-talk relevant in innate anti-tumor immune responses in vivo. Nat Med 1999;(4):405–11.
85. Yuan D, Koh CY, Wilder JA. Interactions between B lymphocytes and NK cells. FASEB J 1994; 8(13):1012–8.
86. Park SH, Bendelac A. CD1-restricted T-cell responses and microbial infection. Nature 2000; 406(6797):788–92.
87. Reinhardt C, Melms A. Elevated frequencies of natural killer T lymphocytes in myasthenia gravis. Neurology 1999;2(7):1485–7.
88. Illes Z, Kondo T, Newcombe J, Oka N, Tabira T, Yamamura T. Differential expression of NK T cell V alpha 24J alpha Q invariant TCR chain in the lesions of multiple sclerosis and chronic inflammatory demyelinating polyneuropathy. J Immunol 2000;64(8):4375–81.
89. Carnaud C, Lee D, Donnars O, Park SH, Beavis A, Koezuka Y, et al. Cutting edge: Cross-talk between cells of the innate immune system: NKT cells rapidly activate NK cells. J Immunol 1999;63(9):4647–50.
90. Eberl G, MacDonald HR. Selective induction of NK cell proliferation and cytotoxicity by activated NKT cells. Eur J Immunol 2000;0(4):985–92.
91. Fisch P, Moris A, Rammensee HG, Handgretinger R. Inhibitory MHC class I receptors on gammadelta T cells in tumour immunity and autoimmunity. Immunol Today 2000;1(4): 187–91.
92. Borsellino G, Poccia F, Placido R, Tramonti D, Mancino G, Luchetti S, et al. Phenotypic and functional properties of gamma delta T cells from patients with Guillain Barre syndrome. J Neuroimmunol 2000;02(2):199–207.
93. Peterman GM, Spencer C, Sperling AI, Bluestone JA. Role of gamma delta T cells in murine collagen-induced arthritis. J Immunol 1993;51(11):6546–58.
94. Usami J, Hiromatsu K, Matsumoto Y, Maeda K, Inagaki H, Suzuki T, et al. A protective role of gamma delta T cells in primary infection with Listeria monocytogenes in autoimmune non-obese diabetic mice. Immunology 1995;6(2):199–205.
95. Rajan AJ, Gao YL, Raine CS, Brosnan CF. A pathogenic role for gamma delta T cells in relapsing-remitting experimental allergic encephalomyelitis in the SJL mouse. J Immunol 1996;57(2):941–9.
96. Ronnblom L, Alm GV. An etiopathogenic role for the type I IFN system in SLE. Trends Immunol 2001;2(8):427–31.
97. Blanco P, Palucka AK, Gill M, Pascual V, Banchereau J. Induction of dendritic cell differentiation by IFN-alpha in systemic lupus erythematosus. Science 2001;94(5546): 1540–3.
98. Biron CA, Nguyen KB, Pien GC, Cousens LP, Salazar-Mather TP. Natural killer cells in antiviral defence: function and regulation by innate cytokines. Annu Rev Immunol 1999;1189–220.
99. Casali P, Notkins AL. CD5+ B lymphocytes, polyreactive antibodies and the human B-cell repertoire. Immunol Today 1989;0(11):364–8.
100. Naparstek Y, Plotz PH. The role of autoantibodies in autoimmune disease. Annu Rev Immunol 1993;1:79–104.
101. Boes M. Role of natural and immune IgM antibodies in immune responses. Mol Immunol 2000; 37(18):1141–9.
102. Mitchell DA, Taylor PR, Cook HT, Moss J, Bygrave AE, Walport MJ, et al. Cutting edge: C1q protects against the development of glomerulonephritis independently of C3

activation. J Immunol 1999;62(10):5676–9.

103. Sellebjerg F, Jaliashvili I, Christiansen M, Garred P. Intrathecal activation of the complement system and disability in multiple sclerosis. J Neurol Sci 1998;57(2):168–74.
104. Smith ME. Phagocytic properties of microglia in vitro: implications for a role in multiple sclerosis and EAE. Microsc Res Tech 2001;4(2):81–94.
105. Vanguri P, Koski CL, Silverman B, Shin ML. Complement activation by isolated myelin: activation of the classical pathway in the absence of myelin-specific antibodies. Proc Natl Acad Sci USA 1982;9(10):3290–4.
106. Volpato S, Guralnik JM, Ferrucci L, Balfour J, Chaves P, Fried LP, et al. Cardiovascular disease, interleukin-6, and risk of mortality in older women: the women's health and aging study. Circulation 2001 Feb 20;103(7):947–53.
107. Reuben DB, Ferrucci L, Wallace R, Tracy RP, Corti MC, Heimovitz H, et al. The prognostic value of serum albumin in healthy older persons with low and high serum interleukin-6 (IL-6) levels. J Am Geriatr Soc 2000 Nov;48(11):1404–7.
108. Gruol DL, Nelson TE. Physiological and pathological roles of interleukin-6 in the central nervous system. Mol Neurobiol 1997 Dec;15(3):307–39.
109. Franceschi C, Bonafe M, Valensin S, Olivieri F, De Luca M, Ottaviani E, et al. Inflamm-aging. An evolutionary perspective on immunosenescence. Ann N Y Acad Sci 2000 Jun;908:244–54.
110. Ershler WB, Keller ET. Age-associated increased interleukin-6 gene expression, late-life diseases, and frailty. Annu Rev Med 2000;51:245–70.
111. Lio D, Scola L, Crivello A, Colonna-Romano G, Candore G, Bonafe M, et al. Inflammation, genetics, and longevity: further studies on the protective effects in men of IL-10 -1082 promoter SNP and its interaction with TNF-alpha -308 promoter SNP. J Med Genet 2003 Apr;40(4):296–9.
112. Libby P. Inflammation in atherosclerosis. Nature 2002;420:868–74.
113. Maseri A., Biasucci LM. Liuzzo G. Inflamrnation in ischaemic heart disease. BMJ 1996;312: 1049–50.
114. Paulus WJ. Cytokines and heart failure. Heart Fail Monit 2000;1:50–6.
115. Robbie L, Libby P. Inflamation and atherothrombosis. Ann NY Acad Sci 2001;947: 167–79; discussion 179–80.
116. Ross R. Atherosclerosis: an inflammatory disease. N Engl J Med 1999;340:115–26.
117. Biasucci LM, Liuzzo G, Cobizzi C, Rizzelbo V. Clinical use of C-reactive protein for the prognostic stratification of patients with ischemic heart disease. Ital Heart J 2001;2: 164–71.
118. Febdman AM, Kadokami T, Higuichi Y, Ramani R, McTiernan CF. The role of anticytokine therapy in heart failure: recent lessons from preclinical and clinical trials? Med Clin North Am 2003;87:419–40.
119. Humphries SE, Luong LA, Ogg MS, Hawe E, Miller GJ. The interleukin-6 -174 G/C promoter polymorphism is associated with risk of coronary heart disease and systolic blood pressure in healthy men. Eur Heart J 2001 Dec;22(24):2243–52.
120. Pola R, Flex A, Gaetani E, Flore R, Serricchio M, Pola P. Synergistic effect of -174 G/C polymorphism of the interleukin-6 gene promoter and 469 E/K polymorphism of the intercellular adhesion molecule-1 gene in Italian patients with history of ischemic stroke. Stroke 2003 Apr;34(4):881–5.
121. Freeman DJ, Norrie J, Caslake MJ, Gaw A, Ford I,.Lowe GD, et al. C-reactive protein is an independent predictor of risk for the development of diabetes in the West of Scotland

Coronary Prevention Study. Diabetes 2002;51:1596–600.
122. Yudkin JS, Kumari M,Humphries SE, Mohamed-Ali V. Inflammation, obesity, stress and coronary heart disease: is interleukin-6 the link? Atherosclerosis 2000;148:209–14.
123. Biondi-Zoccai GG, Abbate A, Liuzzo G, Biasucci LM. Atherothrombosis, inflammation, and diabetes. JAm Coll Cardiol 2003;41:1071–7.
124. Brownlee M. Negative consequences of glycation. Metabollsm 2000;49:9–13.
125. McCarty MF. Interleukin-6 as a central mediator of cardiovascular risk associated with chronic inflammation, smoking, diabetes, and visceral obesity: down-regulation with essential fatty acids, ethanol and pentoxifylline. Med Hypotheses 1999;52:465–77.
126. McDaniel ML, Kwon G, Hill JR, Marshall CA, Corbett JA. Cytokines and nitric oxide in is inflammation and diabetes. PMC Soc Exp Bio Mad 1996;211:24–32.
127. Pickup JS, Mattock MB, Chutney GD, Burt D. NIDDM as a disease of the innate immune system: association of acute-phase reactants and interleukin-6 with metabolic syndrome X. Diabetologia 1997;40:1286–92.
128. Nilsson J, Jovinge S, Niemann A, Reneland R, Lithell H. Relation between plasma tumour necrosis factor-alpha and insulin sensitivity in elderly men with non-insulin-dependent diabetes mellitus. Arterioscler Thromb Vasc Biol 1998;18 :1199–202.
129. Pradhan AD, Manson JE, Rifai N, Buring JE, Ridker PM. C-reactive protein, interleukin 6, and risk of developing type 2 diabetes mellitus. JAMA 2001;286:327–34.
130. Kubaszek A, Pihlajamaki J, Komarovski V, Lindi V, Lindstrom J, Eriksson J, et al. Finnish Diabetes Prevention Study. Promoter polymorphisms of the TNF-alpha (G-308A) and IL-6 (C-174G) genes predict the conversion from impaired glucose tolerance to type 2 diabetes: the Finnish Diabetes Prevention Study. Diabetes 2003 Jul;52(7):1872–6.
131. Vozarova B, Fernandez-Real JM, Knowler WC, Gallart L, Hanson RL, Gruber JD, et al. The interleukin-6 (-174) G/C promoter polymorphism is associated with type-2 diabetes mellitus in Native Americans and Caucasians. Hum Genet 2003 Apr;112(4):409–13.
132. Costa A, Fernandez-Real JM, Vendrell J, Broch M, Casamitjana R, Ricart W, et al. Lower rate of tumour necrosis factor-alpha -863A allele and higher concentration of tumour necrosis factor-alpha receptor 2 in first-degree relatives of subjects with type 2 diabetes. Metabolism 2003 Aug;52(8):1068–71.
133. Janciauskiene S, Wright HT. Inflammation, antichymotrypsin, and lipid metabolism: autogenic etiology of Alzheimer's disease. Bioassays 1998 Dec;20(12):1039–46.
134. Styren SD, Kamboh MI, DeKosky ST. Expression of differential immune factors in temporal cortex and cerebellum: the role of alpha-1-antichymotrypsin, apolipoprotein E, and reactive glia in the progression of Alzheimer's disease. J Comp Neurol 1998 Jul 13;396(4):511–20.
135. Wang X, DeKosky ST, Luedecking-Zimmer E, Ganguli M, Kamboh IM. Genetic variation in alpha(1)-antichymotrypsin and its association with Alzheimer's disease. Hum Genet 2002 Apr;110(4):356–65. Epub 2002;Mar 19.
136. Morgan K, Licastro F, Tilley L, Ritchie A, Morgan L, Pedrini S, et al. Polymorphism in the alpha(1)-antichymotrypsin (ACT) gene promoter: effect on expression in transfected glial and liver cell lines and plasma ACT concentrations. Hum Genet 2001 Sep;109(3): 303–10.
137. Franceschi, CS, Valensin F, Lescai, F Olivieri, F Licastro, Grimaldi LM, et al. Neuroinflammation and the genetics of Alzheimer's disease: the search for a pro-inflammatory phenotype. Aging (Milano) 2001;13:163–70.
138. Akiyama H., Barger S. Barnum B. Bradt J, Bauer GM, Cole, NR, et al. Inflammation and

Alzheimer's disease. NeumbiolAging 2000;21:383–421.
139. Ehl C, Kolsch H, Ptok U, Jessen F, Schmitz S, Frahnert C, et al. Association of an interleukin-1beta gene polymorphism at position -511 with Alzheimer's disease. Int J Mol Med 2003 Feb;11(2):235–8.
140. Pirskanen M, Hiltunen M, Mannermaa A, Iivonen S, Helisalmi S, Lehtovirta M, et al. Interleukin 1 alpha gene polymorphism as a susceptibility factor in Alzheimer's disease and its influence on the extent of histopathological hallmark lesions of Alzheimer's disease. Dement Geriatr Cogn Disord 2002;14(3):123–7.
141. Griffin WS, Mrak RE. Interleukin-1 in the genesis and progression of and risk for development of neuronal degeneration in Alzheimer's disease. J Leukoc Biol 2002 Aug;72(2):233–8.
142. Mrak RE, Griffin WS. Interleukin-1, neuroinflammation, and Alzheimer's disease. Neurobiol Aging 2001 Nov-Dec;22(6):903–8.
143. Bagli M, Papassotiropoulos A, Knapp M, Jessen F, Luise Rao M, Maier W, et al. Association between an interleukin-6 promoter and 3' flanking region haplotype and reduced Alzheimer disease risk in a German population. Neurosci Lett 2000;283:109–12.
144. Du Y, Dodel RC, Eastwood AJ, Bales KR, Gao, F, Lohmuller F, et al. Association of an interleukin 1 alpha polymorphism with Alzheimer's disease. Neurology 2000;55: 480–3.
145. Licastro F, Pedrini S, Ferri C, Casadei V, Govoni M, Pession A, et al. Gene polymorphism affecting alphal-antichymotrypsin and interleukin-1 plasma levels increases Alzheimer's disease risk. Ann Neurol 2000;48:388–91.
146. Knuefermann P, Nemoto S, Baumgarten G, et al. Cardiac inflammation and innate immunity in septic shock. Is there a role for Toll-like receptors? Chest 2002;121:1329–36.
147. Casey LC, Balk RA, Bone RC. Plasma cytokine and endotoxin levels correlate with survival in patients with the sepsis syndrome. Ann Int Med 1993;119:771–8.
148 Debets JM, Kampmeijer R, van der Linden MP, et al. Plasma tumour necrosis factor and mortality in critically ill septic patients. Crit Care Med 1989;17:489–494.
149. Beutler B, Milsark IW, Cerami AC. Passive immunization against cathectin/tumour necrosis factor protects mice from lethal effects of endotoxin. Science 1985;229:869–71.
150. Tracey KJ, Fong Y, Hesse DG, et al. Anti-cathectin /TNF monoclonal antibodies prevent septic shock during lethal bacteraemia. Nature 1987;330:662–4.
151. Chaudry IH, Ertel W, Ayala A. Alterations in inflammatory cytokine production following haemorrhage and resuscitation. In: Schlag G., Redl H, Traber DL. Editors. Shock. Sepsis and organ failure, Third Wiggers Bernard Conference, Springer, Berlin 1993; 73–127.
152. Abraham E, Bursten S, Shenkar R, Allbee J, Tuder R, Woodson P, et al. Phosphatidic acid signaling mediates lung cytokine expression and lung inflammatory injury after haemorrhage in mice. J Exp Med 1995;181:569–75.
153. Le Tulzo Y, Shenkar R, Kaneko D, Moine P, Fantuzzi G, Dinarello CA, et al. Haemorrhage increases cytokine expression in lung mononuclear cells in mice: involvement of catecholamines in nuclear factor-kB regulation and cytokine expression. J Clin Invest 1997;18:529–36.
154. Deitch EA, Morrison J, Berg R, Specian RD. Effect of hemorragic shock on bacterial translocation, intestinal morphology, and intestinal permeability in conventional and antibiotic-decontaminated rats. Crit Care Med 1990;18:529–36.
155. Lander HM. An essential role for free radicals and derived species in signal transduction. FASEB J 1997;11:118–24.

156. Altavilla D, Saitta A, Guarini S, Galeano M, Squadrito G, Santamaria LB, et al. Nuclear factor kB as a target of cyclosporin in acute hypovolemic hemorragic shock. Cardiovasc Res 2001;52:143–52.
157. Roos A, Ramwadhdoebe TH, Nauta AJ, Hack CE, Daha MR. Therapeutic inhibition of the early phase of complement activation. Immunobiology 2002 Sep;205(4–5):595–609.
158. Lynn M, Rossignol DP, Wheeler JL, Kao RJ, Perdomo CA, Noveck R, et al. Blocking of responses to endotoxin by E5564 in healthy volunteers with experimental endotoxemia. J Infect Dis 2003 Feb 15;187(4):631–9.
159. Axtelle T, Pribble J. IC14, a CD14 specific monoclonal antibody, is a potential treatment for patients with severe sepsis. J Endotoxin Res 2001;7(4):310–4.

Natural Immunity
Edited by L. Bertók and D.A. Chow
© 2005 Elsevier B.V. All rights reserved

Behavioural Mechanisms for Defence Against Pathogens

SUSAN J. LARSON[1] and ADRIAN J. DUNN[2]

[1]*Department of Psychology, Concordia College, Moorhead MN, 56562, USA;* [2]*Department of Pharmacology and Therapeutics, Louisiana State University Health Sciences Center, Shreveport, LA 71130, USA*

ABSTRACT

Behavioural strategies can assist organisms to defend themselves against pathogens. Both reflexive and learned behaviours can play important roles in pathogen defence. Reflexive behaviours, like coughing and vomiting, can be instrumental in expelling pathogens from the body, and avoidance of excrement is an important strategy for minimizing contact with pathogens. Learned food aversions and the avoidance of stimuli previous associated with illness minimize contact with pathogens. Considerable evidence has shown that behavioural changes can be induced by immune activation, and it has been argued that this "sickness behaviour" may assist the organism to recover from infection. Immune activation is associated with the production of cytokines, some of which (most notably, interleukin-1, IL-1) have potent behavioural activities. IL-1 decreases several behavioural activities, such as food intake, and sexual activity in females. These changes in behaviour can facilitate the return to health. Thus sickness behaviour can be an important mechanism for defence against pathogens. It is significant that sickness behaviour is not stereotyped and can be adapted to the nature of the threat and the immediate needs of the organism. Certain kinds of behavioural experiences, most notably stressful ones, may induce immune activation and cytokine production. Environmental stressors and immune activation produce some similar physiological responses: increased body temperature, and activation of the sympathetic nervous system, the adrenal medulla, and the hypothalamo-pituitary-adrenal axis, as well as brain catecholamines and indoleamines. These observations have led to the concept that pathogen invasion induces "immune stress". The physiological responses induced can assist the defence of the organism against infections, at least in part by changing behaviour. It is argued that learned and reflexive behavioural strategies, and physiological and behavioural responses to illness, are all important components of host defence against pathogens.

1. INTRODUCTION

The behaviour of animals typically changes when they become sick. Although sickness is often deduced from physical symptoms, such as coughing, vomiting, and obvious injuries, behavioural symptoms are also important, and sickness is often inferred from behavioural symptoms alone. For example, when people are sick, they often do not feel like eating and may avoid many other kinds of activities. Changes in sleep patterns are also common. Such changes were recog-

Table I Behavioural changes associated with infection and injury. Arrows reflect direction of change typically observed (↓: decreased; ↑: increased).

Behaviour	Typical Change
Food intake	↓
Slow-wave sleep	↑
Environmental exploration	↓
Social exploration	↓
Sexual activity	↓ females
Cognitive function	Impaired
Anhedonia (lack of interest in pleasurable stimuli)	↑

nized many years ago by Hans Selye who identified a state he called the "syndrome of just being sick". He noted that sick people displayed many common features that were independent of the nature of their diseases. "They are all indisposed, they look tired, have no appetite, gradually lose weight, they do not feel like going to work, they prefer to lie down rather than to stand up" [1]. Substantial changes in behaviour, resembling those reported by humans, are also noted in sick pets, livestock and research animals. Experimental investigations have shown that infected mammals undergo behavioural changes such as decreased motor activity, decreased ingestive behaviour, decreased exploratory behaviour, impaired cognitive functioning, altered sexual behaviour, increased sleep, and changes in affective states (e.g., [2–5]; see Table I).

Such changes are induced not only by infections and other pathologies, but can be induced by compounds that stimulate the immune system, such as lipopolysaccharide (LPS, also known as endotoxin), a component of the cell walls of Gram-negative bacteria. This suggests that being sick is not a direct consequence of the infection or the tissue damage, but may be related to the activation of the immune system associated with the pathology. The suggestion is reinforced by the observation that similar patterns of behaviour can be induced by administration of certain cytokines, soluble factors (proteins or glycoproteins) released by immune cells during immune activation [4,5]. Thus it is not the pathogens themselves that induce the sickness, but the response of the host's immune system, most likely involving cytokines.

Cytokines known to be behaviourally active include tumour necrosis factor-α (TNFα), interleukin-1α (IL-1α), interleukin-1β (IL-1β), interleukin-6, (IL-6), and the interferons (IFNα, IFNβ, and IFNγ). These cytokines are largely pro-inflammatory; they can activate the acute phase response, and are activated during various disease states. Cytokines are released after LPS administration as well as after the administration of pathogens and antigens. It is well documented that the pro-inflammatory cytokine, IL-1β, administered both peripherally and centrally, has behavioural effects and induces a profile of behavioural changes similar to LPS and many pathogens (see [4,5] for reviews of cytokine effects on behaviour). In addition to IL-1, other cytokines, notably IL-2, TNFα, IL-6, IFNα and IFNγ may induce behavioural effects, although these cytokines are generally less potent than IL-1, and may induce different behavioural effects. Thus laboratory research has confirmed anecdotal observations of changes of behaviour induced by immune activation, and has suggested cytokines as mediators of these effects.

Medical professionals have long been aware that illness involves changes in behaviour (see the reference to Selye above [1]). Nevertheless, until recently scientists and practitioners have paid little attention to these sickness-induced changes in behaviour. The changes associated with illness were assumed to reflect debilitation of little or no benefit to the organism, and were rarely studied. In retrospect, the lack of attention given to the behavioural changes associated with ill-

Table II Components of Behavioural Defense.

Aspects of behavioral defense	Role in Health
Avoidance behaviours: Reflexive	Avoiding materials likely to be pathogen-infected
Avoidance behaviours: Learned	Avoid stimuli associated with past illness
	Learn to avoid (or indulge in) activities by observing other animals
Sickness behaviours	Reduce energy expenditure
	Avoid activities that expose animals to risk (food gathering, exploration)
	Facilitate fever
	Minimize contact with pathogens
Immune responses induced by behaviour	Conditioned immune-enhancing responses
	Priming of behavioral defense by stress-induced increase in cytokines

ness is surprising. Changes in behaviour in sick animals are well conserved evolutionarily. They are expressed in many species and may result from many different diseases and activators of the immune system [2,3]. It is unlikely that such changes would be so well conserved evolutionarily if they were not in some way beneficial to the organism. In a seminal review paper, Benjamin Hart argued that such behavioural changes were adaptive and discussed what he saw as their value [2]. Since this paper was published, scientists and practitioners have looked more closely at what has come to be known as 'sickness behaviour' [3], and have investigated it systematically. Most agree with Hart that sickness behaviour is a defensive strategy for the organism facilitating its return to health.

The purpose of this chapter is to assess these assertions by describing the adaptive value of behavioural changes during sickness and evaluating these changes as defensive behaviour. Before so doing, we will describe behaviours other than sickness behaviour that may be important for defence against pathogens. As indicated above, Hart argued that the behavioural changes that occur during illness are defensive and can facilitate recovery [2]. However, these are not the only behaviours that fulfil a defensive function. Animals adapt their behaviour in order to minimize contact with pathogens. Such adaptations can involve reflexively avoiding pathogens or learning to avoid stimuli previously associated with pathogens. In this chapter, we will consider some examples of each of these forms of behavioural defence (Table II).

2. REFLEXIVE AND LEARNED RESPONSES TO PATHOGENS

Animals must adapt to their environment or suffer the consequences. Obvious examples of environmental adaptation include appropriate food-seeking and storage, as well as behaviours that facilitate thermoregulation and avoid predators [6]. Other behavioural adaptations may involve avoiding pathogens and responding in ways that minimize the effects of pathogens.

The best defence against an infection is to avoid contact with the pathogen. Thus responding to the environment in a way that minimizes contact with pathogens is an important component of behavioural defence. Avoidance behaviours can result from simple reflexes as well as learning from previous experience, and the spectrum of avoidance-related behaviours can be quite varied (e.g., nest building, foraging strategies, eliminative behaviour, food selection and grooming). We will address only a few examples. One such is the response to faeces. Faecal matter avoidance appears in the behavioural repertoire of many animals [7,8], including cattle [8], horses

[9], monkeys [10], and others [7]. In some cases, the unpleasant aroma associated with faecal matter may elicit a reflexive avoidance response without prior training or exposure, allowing the organism to avoid numerous pathogens in its environment. In addition to simply avoiding faeces, animals defecate and feed in ways suggesting faecal matter avoidance. For example, it has been observed that Howler monkeys defecate less often in areas they use predominantly for foraging than in other less foraged areas [10]. This suggests that this species both avoids faeces and defecates in a manner that will minimize contact with faeces and possible food contamination. Other animals (e.g., horses) avoid consuming foodstuffs contaminated with faeces and are known to defecate preferentially in areas where little grazing occurs [9]. Consistent with this, most humans tend to avoid eating in the bathroom.

For humans, one aspect of avoiding faeces is the disgust it invokes. Curtis and Biran suggested that faecal matter is but one of a number of stimuli that elicit a disgust response [11]. Other stimuli include (but are not limited to) other body excretions, body parts, and decaying and spoiled food. These "elicitors of disgust" were compiled after surveying people from four distinct regions (India, Africa, the Netherlands, and the United Kingdom), and in one international airport. Curtis and Biran noted that the primary stimuli that elicit disgust are potential sources of infection. A prime example is faeces, which are considered disgusting by most people, and are a major source of infections (e.g., *Salmonella, Escherichia coli, Shigella, Giardia*). Other objects of disgust such as vomit and saliva are also potential sources of infection. Curtis and Biran argued that the disgust response elicited by stimuli like faeces is adaptive because it produces avoidance of the potential source of a pathogen [11] (also discussed in [12]).

While faecal matter avoidance can be an effective means of pathogen avoidance it is not a universal phenomenon. Some organisms consume faeces (coprophagia) from their own species (see [7]), and less often, faeces from other species (e.g., [13]). There are a number of explanations for this. One is that faeces (or rather the cecal fluid associated with the faeces [14]) may provide animals with essential nutrients or assist them in maintaining their intestinal flora [15,16]. Also, the young of some species consume the faeces of their mothers and this provides the young with appropriate intestinal microflora, and the deoxycholic acid ingested protects them against endotoxins [17]. Additionally, nursing mothers of some species (including numerous rodent species) wash their young by licking them, especially in the anogenital area. Thus the mother is likely to synthesize antibodies to any pathogens ingested, which can then be transferred to the infant in breast milk [18]. Presumably, in these instances the benefits obtained by the faecal ingestion outweigh the costs associated with pathogen exposure from this material.

As indicated above, it has been shown that certain animals avoid faeces. Others have shown that animals may avoid food that is infected with pathogens. Recently, Pujol and colleagues [19] investigated the role of the toll-like receptor in avoidance of pathogens using *C. elegans*. Toll-like receptors are important in innate immunity because they recognize microbe-derived molecules such as LPS, and the activation of these receptors is important for the synthesis of proinflammatory cytokines [20]. Pujol and colleagues demonstrated that variants of *C. elegans* that express the gene tol-1, which encodes a toll-like receptor (TLR1), respond more effectively to certain bacteria in their food than organisms lacking the gene [19]. In particular, it was found that *C. elegans* mutants lacking tol-1 did not avoid the pathogen *S. marcescens* unlike the wild type. Thus the tol-1 receptor appears to be important for recognizing and avoiding certain pathogens and provides animals a behavioural advantage for avoiding bacteria. Based on this observation in *C. elegans*, it is likely that other animals also have genes (possibly for other toll-like receptors) that affect pathogen avoidance, warranting further investigation.

While we have mainly focused on the reflexive avoidance of a pathogen, other behavioural strategies also serve a defensive role. In organisms unable to avoid contact with pathogens, a second line of behavioural defence is to remove the pathogen from the body. Reflexive behaviours such as coughing, vomiting and diarrhoea expel pathogens from the body, minimizing their effects, and facilitating return to health. Other adaptive, health-promoting behaviours include activities like grooming, stomping or tail flicking to remove external pathogens from the body. For a more complete discussion of these behavioural strategies, see Hart [7].

An animal cannot always reflexively avoid or remove pathogens. Thus learning to avoid stimuli previously associated with pathogen exposure or illness is an important line of defence. An important example of this, conditioned taste aversion, was first studied by Garcia and colleagues [21] and is often referred to as the 'Garcia effect.' In a typical taste aversion experiment, thirsty animals are given the opportunity to drink a novel, highly palatable solution (the conditioned stimulus, CS). Following consumption, animals are exposed to an illness-inducing agent (the unconditioned stimulus, US); early experiments used radiation exposure to induce illness, but numerous other treatments (e.g., lithium chloride) have been used for this purpose. Once the association between the illness and the novel tasting solution has been made, animals avoid the solution. A taste aversion can be produced with a single flavour-illness pairing, and even if there is a lengthy delay (e.g., many hours) between the taste and the illness. More recent work has demonstrated that if animals are exposed to an agent such as LPS that induces an acute phase response, a conditioned taste aversion can be induced [22]. Tumour growth may also induce a taste aversion for novel food consumed [23,24], presumably because the tumour serves as the illness-inducing US and the novel tasting food as the CS. In these and other demonstrations, animals learned to associate a flavour with an illness-inducing event and subsequently avoid that flavour.

Although laboratory work has paired specific flavours with distinct illness-inducing agents, conditioned taste aversions occur naturally where the flavour and the illness-inducing agent are often part of the same stimulus complex. For example, a poisonous mushroom may possess a specific novel taste and also delivers a toxin to the animal that consumes it. The animal will learn to associate the effect of the toxin with the taste of the mushroom and will subsequently avoid it. Such taste aversions are highly adaptive; an animal that does not learn to avoid a flavour associated with sickness is at risk of poisoning and death. Thus avoidance of an illness-inducing flavour is an effective behavioural defence.

Conditioned taste aversions may have efficacy beyond inducing flavour avoidance/aversion; they may also condition the immune system. It has been shown that a taste stimulus that precedes inhibition of the immune system will, upon re-exposure, produce a similar inhibition of the immune system [25]. If the conditioned stimuli (taste or otherwise) were to elicit immune system enhancement, an individual re-exposed to these stimuli would be aided by the activity of the immune system. Some work has shown conditioned immunoenhancing responses. For example, Ramirez-Amaya and Bermudez-Rattoni have recently shown that rats can exhibit increased antibody responses when exposed to a stimulus associated with antigen exposure [26]. They paired either a novel taste or a novel odour with a hen egg lysozyme (HEL) antigen. Re-exposure to the taste or odour was associated with enhanced HEL IgG antibody production in conditioned animals. In humans, Stockhorst and colleagues showed that patients undergoing chemotherapy have higher levels of natural killer cells and IFNγ when tested in the hospital setting than when tested at home [27]. Although they did not manipulate the exposure to chemotherapy, they argued that the hospital was a conditioned environment (CS) because of its association with the immune-enhancing effect of chemotherapy (US), and would be expected to induce immune responses not present in the home.

In a conditioned taste aversion paradigm, taste avoidance results from exposure to pathogens or illness-inducing agents. It is also possible that taste avoidance, and presumably pathogen avoidance, can be learned by observation. Much work by Galef and others (for reviews, see [28,29]) has clearly demonstrated that dietary choice and food preference can be passed from one member of the species to others. In a typical procedure, a "demonstrator" animal, for example a rat, is given access to food with a distinct odour and is then allowed to interact with an "observer" rat. The observer rat, though never having had access to this food, will subsequently demonstrate a preference for the food the demonstrator ate over another, novel food. In humans, food preferences may be dependent upon social learning, so that children acquire taste preferences by observing their parents and peers eating and enjoying particular foods [30,31]. The extent to which dietary preference is related to immunocompetence has not been investigated specifically. However, young animals learn from other members of the species which foods are safe to eat, and this can protect the animal against future illness. If the young learn about dietary selection by observation, they enjoy the benefits of the experience of others and avoid the risks, and possible pathogens, associated with the consumption of novel foods.

As can be seen from the examples listed above, animals have a number of behavioural strategies to facilitate pathogen avoidance: avoiding stimuli that may be infected with pathogens, avoiding stimuli that have previously made you sick, and learning to distinguish healthy from unhealthy foods. We have not described the entirety of reflexes and learned behaviours that animals make in response to pathogens, but have merely emphasized the importance of both reflexive and learned behaviours in avoiding and minimizing the effects of pathogens, as part of behavioural defence [7]. Below we shall consider what happens to organisms when such avoidance is not immediately successful.

3. SICKNESS BEHAVIOUR AS BEHAVIOURAL DEFENCE

Up to this point we have considered ways in which an organism can avoid the deleterious effects of the pathogen, either reflexively or by learning about pathogen-associated stimuli. A remaining question is what happens to behaviour as a result of infection and does this behaviour assist the organism to rid itself of the pathogen and return to a healthy state. As indicated above, there is a well-characterized profile of behavioural change observed in sick animals, called sickness behaviour (Table I). This profile of behavioural change includes decreased general activity (especially locomotor activity), decreased food intake [32–34], increased slow-wave sleep [35,36], altered sexual activity [37], decreased environmental [38] and social exploration [39], impaired cognitive function [40,41], and decreased interest in pleasurable stimuli (so-called "anhedonia") [42]. As mentioned previously, Hart [2] argued that the typical profile of behavioural change experienced by organisms infected with a pathogen is a strategy used by the organism to aid return to health. Thus an important question is whether this sickness behaviour profile is a part of behavioural defence.

In his original analysis, Hart described the behavioural changes induced by pathogens (e.g., reduction in general motor activity, grooming and food intake) as being adaptive by assisting the organism to maintain its "emergency thermoregulatory mode" [2, p. 124]. For example, he argued that decreased mobility facilitates fevers because of the lack of movement. In some animals, the curled up position associated with increased sleep and decreased movement enables the animal to conserve heat. Decreased food intake in animals, specifically hunter-gatherers, minimizes heat loss associated with food seeking and allows the animal to conserve energy needed to facilitate a fever. According to this analysis, illness-induced anorexia will be most prevalent when an individual must work hard to obtain food (e.g., travel long distances from the safety of a home territory), and less prevalent when food is easily accessible. While Hart speculated that there were immediate benefits of decreased food intake in sick organisms, it should be acknowledged that in the long term illness-induced anorexia will become deleterious, because decreased food intake decreases the available energy stores.

According to Hart, these sickness behaviours are adaptive because they enhance illness-induced fever, which may aid the animal to combat pathogens. In fact, Kluger and colleagues have shown that animals not allowed to express the typical febrile response associated with illness have a greater risk of dying. Higher mortality rates were observed in lizards forced to remain in a cold environment after exposure to a bacterial infection than those placed in a warm environment [43]. Moreover, lizards in the warm environment that were treated with an antipyretic (salicylate), experienced higher mortality rates than untreated animals [44]. Likewise in humans, the use of antipyretics (aspirin and acetaminophen) has been shown to extend the duration and symptoms of chicken pox [45] and common colds [46], although we cannot be certain these effects of the drugs are attributable to the absence of a fever. The work of others has shown that a behavioural fever (moving to a warmer environment) increases survival, even if it increases the risk of predation, in animals such as flies, grasshoppers and fish (see [8]). It has been argued that the value of the febrile response derives from its ability to: enhance immune functioning (e.g., enhancing lymphocyte proliferation); make the body of the ill animal inhospitable for the pathogen by increasing body temperature above the optimal temperature for its survival and proliferation; and reduce iron concentrations, inhibiting the growth of many pathogens [2].

Following Hart's analysis, many people have investigated the behavioural changes induced by pathogens and immunologically activate agents. However, very little of this work has addressed Hart's main argument which was that behavioural change facilitates a fever in the sick animal and this facilitates its survival. While there is evidence to support the argument that fever is adaptive [43,44], this concept is quite controversial. Immunologically active agents do not necessarily induce fever, and not all fevers enhance survival, although interpretation of these data is not always straightforward [47,48]. Importantly, sickness behaviour can be dissociated from fever. For example, McCarthy and colleagues have shown that administration of an antipyretic decreased endotoxin-induced fever without diminishing endotoxin-induced anorexia [32].

Whether or not sickness behaviours are always expressed to enhance fever, there is evidence to support Hart's contention that sickness behaviours have survival value. For instance, mice that are not allowed to experience the typical anorexia associated with immune activation are less likely to survive endotoxin treatment. Murray and Murray infected mice with *Listeria monocytogenes* and allowed them to feed ad libitum, or they supplemented their food with gastric intubation [49]. Intubated mice, fed daily to match uninfected controls, had lower survival rates than animals allowed to express *Listeria*-induced anorexia. Similarly, animals food-deprived for 24–72 hours prior to infection with *Listeria monocytogenes* survived at higher rates than animals that were not food-deprived [50]. The deprived animals also had fewer bacteria in their spleen 2–4 days after infection. In a comprehensive analysis, Exton reviewed the evidence that anorexia is associated with enhanced immune functioning via increased activation of natural killer cells and macrophages, and increased T cell proliferation [51]. Thus illness-induced anorexia may in part, facilitate survival because of an enhanced immune system response.

Most researchers that have systematically evaluated sickness behaviour have not measured mortality. Nevertheless, other support for Hart's proposal derives from work demonstrating that sickness behaviour is sensitive to test conditions, and does not necessarily occur in the same way for every animal, or every time an animal is sick. Moreover, immune system activation does not necessarily induce generalized decreases in behaviour. It has been shown that animals do not demonstrate typical sickness-induced behaviours when the consequences of doing so are detrimental [52,53] (see below). Variability in sickness behaviour has been suggested to reflect a differential sensitivity of animals to the perceived importance of a particular behaviour. The underlying assumption is that animals can choose to modify the induced sickness behaviour as a strategy to maximize its adaptive value, and it has been argued that animals are able to mitigate illness-induced behavioural changes so as to minimize the negative effects of sickness. This view assumes that animals evaluate their behaviour based on the possible consequences, which would be difficult to verify for nonhuman animals. Despite this, it does appear that the animals behave in a manner that facilitates their survival. Thus this view retains some appeal because, relying on evolutionary principles, it argues that these behavioural changes are adaptive for the animal.

Indeed, much of the variability in sickness behaviour appears to occur when the typical sickness behaviour profile could be detrimental to the organism's health. An example is a task in which rats or mice are allowed to investigate a multi-compartment chamber. The chamber is divided into nine compartments, each of which contains a loosely coiled ball mounted just below a round hole in the floor. Using this task, it has been shown that administration to mice of LPS, IL-1α or IL-1β all decreased exploration [38,54,55]. However, the effect depended upon the aspect of exploration assessed; compartment entries and nose pokes were much less sensitive to IL-1 and LPS than the times spent in contact with the novel stimuli. In other words, exploration of novel stimuli in the environment was more affected by the treatment than general exploration of the chamber. These diverse effects, decreased investigation of specific stimuli while continuing to investigate the entire chamber, can both be considered adaptive. Environmental investigation is important for an animal to ensure the safety of its environment, and thus, is to be expected during illness. On the other hand, investigation of the coiled ball prevents the animal paying attention to its global environment, and in times of weakness this could be dangerous. Therefore, decreased investigation of the novel stimuli may be adaptive for the animal. Because in this example, general motor activity is not impaired, it seems that motor activity is altered during sickness to the extent that it does not impair the animal's safety.

Another example of the differential effects of immune activation is that food-restricted organisms are less likely to show illness- or cytokine-induced anorexia than non food-restricted organisms. Aubert and colleagues compared the effects of LPS on food hoarding and consumption in rats that received all their sustenance from hoarding with those in rats with supplemental food sources [52]. They found that both groups of animals decreased food intake when they were ill. However, in the animals that obtained all their food from hoarding, LPS had less of an effect on hoarding as compared to animals with supplemental food sources. In other words, although LPS decreased eating at the time of analysis, it produced little disruption of hoarding for animals with no alternative food source [52]. In another study, the effects of IL-1β on sweetened milk intake were compared in food-restricted and free feeding mice [53]. Mice were given the opportunity to consume sweetened milk in their home cage for 30 minutes. Milk intake in food-restricted mice was less affected by IL-1β than intake in free feeding animals. Similarly, food-restricted mice trained to nose poke for milk using an operant paradigm were less affected by IL-1β than a group of free feeding mice also trained on the operant paradigm [53]. Based on these data, it is reasoned that food-restricted animals have less stored energy and illness-induced anorexia and disruption of hoarding would be a greater threat so the reduced anorexia is a behavioural defence.

If illness-induced anorexia is health promoting because it promotes decreased activity and thus, conservation of heat, food intake with little behavioural cost should be less affected by immune system activation. Indeed, decreases in feeding-related behaviours are dependent upon how much energy must be expended to access the food. Using animals trained on operant schedules of food-maintained behaviour, it was shown that response cost modifies the IL-1-induced decreases in nose-poking for sweetened condensed milk [53]. In these studies, mice were maintained on either a fixed ratio (FR) 4 (four responses necessary to obtain one drop of milk) or an FR32 (32 responses per drop) schedule of reinforcement. The behaviour of the animals on the FR32 schedule was affected by IL-1β to a greater extent than animals on the FR4 schedule (i.e., a high response requirement is more readily affected by IL-1β than a low response requirement) [53]. Comparable results were obtained when the effect of LPS on animals maintained under an interval schedule (animals are reinforced with a food pellet for responding after a certain time has elapsed) was compared with those on a ratio schedule (animals are reinforced with a food pellet for responding a specified number of times). Interval schedules produce lower response rates and the cost of food is generally lower than ratio schedules. As expected, LPS had a more substantial effect on ratio than on interval schedules (Larson, unpublished observations). Furthermore, Larson and colleagues showed that IL-1 decreases behaviour maintained under progressive ratio schedules of responding [53]. In these schedules, animals must produce an increasing number of responses in order to obtain the reinforcer (e.g., the first reinforcer may be earned after 10 responses; the second reinforcer after 20, the third after 30, etc.). These schedules require considerable behavioural output and, as expected, are sensitive to the effects of IL-1.

The above examples demonstrate that the profile of behavioural changes induced during illness is not stereotyped. In a healthy, well-fed, well-maintained organism, one might expect to observe all the behavioural responses described earlier. However, in an animal that has other constraints, such as a food-restriction, the profile of sickness behaviour may depend on these circumstances. Demonstrations of different effects of immune activation, depending upon circumstance, have been interpreted to suggest that immune activation affects motivation. Motivated behaviours can be defined as those associated with arousal, persistence and directional activity [56]. Many data have shown that sickness decreases motivated behaviours, such as feeding, certain sexual activities, and behaviours maintained by pleasurable stimuli [e.g., 34,37, and 42]. Thus it can be concluded that motivation to engage in certain behaviours is reduced during sickness, perhaps associated with immune activation. In instances where motivation for a particular behaviour is great (as in the case of food-restricted animals as discussed above), behaviours typically decreased by sickness (e.g., eating) are less affected. Thus as speculated by others [4,57], sickness may typically curtail behaviours that are unimportant in times of illness (e.g., sexual activity in females, social exploration). In cases where a particular behaviour might be important for survival (e.g., food intake in a food-restricted organism), an animal will be highly motivated to engage in the relevant behaviour, and the behaviour will be expressed.

Related to this, Aubert, Dantzer and colleagues [4,57] argued that sickness behaviours represent a motivational state, defining motivation as "a central state that organizes perception and action" [57, p. 1031]. Further, they suggested that other motivational states (e.g., fear, or in the case of the above example, hunger) may compete with sickness, and if other behaviours are more pressing, sickness behaviours may be superseded. Whether or not sickness should be regarded as a "motivational state", the evidence discussed above clearly indicates that sickness can affect motivation.

Illness appears to decrease many positively reinforced motivated behaviours but perhaps does so only to the extent that this is beneficial for the animal. Minimal work has evaluated the effect of illness on negatively reinforced motivated behaviours (i.e., behaviours motivated by the removal of aversive events). Miller reported that endotoxin did not disrupt operant behaviour reinforced by the elimination of a mildly aversive stimulus (a rotating drum) and actually increased it, even though the same dose of endotoxin disrupted food- and water-maintained behaviour [58]. Another example is Gibertini's observations on the performance of rats in a Morris water-maze, which was impaired after *Legionella* administration [59]. Interestingly, the magnitude of the disruption was dependent upon the water temperature in the water-maze; cooler water was associated with less impairment than was warmer water. To explain this, he suggested that the animals were more motivated to escape the cooler water and thus were less impaired by their illness [59]. Taken together, these results suggest that behaviours followed by the removal of aversive stimuli are less likely to be affected by immune activators. Because maintaining behaviour that avoids aversive stimuli can in many cases be beneficial for the organism, these data further support suggestions that sickness behaviour is expressed in a manner that is affected by motivation and facilitates survival.

Another example of the dependence of sickness behaviour on the needs of the animal is evident in the effects of IL-1 on sexual behaviour. As indicated above, IL-1 markedly reduces sexual activity in female rats, but not in males [37]. From a biological perspective, it would be detrimental for a sick female to add the burden of a foetus, the growth of which might also be adversely affected by the disease and its consequences. However, there are no such adverse consequences for the male. Indeed copulation may offer a last opportunity for the male to pass on its genes. These considerations may explain the lack of effect of IL-1 on sexual activity in male rats.

An issue rarely addressed by sickness behaviour researchers is the extent to which specific sickness behaviours might directly enhance survival (for example, if illness-induced anorexia were to facilitate an immune response), as opposed to enhancing survival simply by minimizing the risks associated with engaging in these behaviours. Infections and injuries produce effects that typically decrease most ongoing behaviours. Although this may occur to facilitate fever and to decrease to predators (see above), the decreased activity typically associated with sickness may also be adaptive because it minimizes further contact with additional pathogens, which could increase the animal's burden. Thus the reduction in ongoing activity may be the most important aspect of sickness behaviour. In cases where reduced activity would be deleterious (e.g., in food-restricted animals), sickness behaviour is less evident. Infections and injuries may elicit a nonspecific reduction in behaviour so that animals avoid high risk activities, and only perhaps, as Hart argued, enhance fever responses.

Conceiving of sickness behaviour as a nonspecific, general strategy that serves to minimize the activity of the organism does not imply that this profile occurs in the same way for every organism and/or in every circumstance. As described above, this profile may be affected by other factors (e.g., food restriction) that may attenuate typical sickness behaviours. However, the concept of sickness behaviour as a nonspecific, general defence helps us understand some aspects of sickness behaviour that do not readily appear adaptive, for example, the impaired cognitive function associated with immune activation [40,41]. It is not intuitively obvious why cognitive impairment would facilitate survival of the organism. However, impaired learning and memory may simply be a negative consequence of the global and nonspecific changes that serve to facilitate survival. Like other aspects of sickness behaviour, cognitive impairments are likely to be highly selective. According to this line of reasoning, sickness behaviours represent a general, evolutionarily advantageous defence that is adaptive for organisms facilitating their health. The profile is sensitive to environmental and physiological conditions imposed on the organism and

Table III Physiological responses to environmental and immune stressors. ↑ reflects an increase in activity; ↑↑ reflects a larger increase.

	Environmental Stressor	Immune Stressor
HPA Axis	↑↑	↑↑
Sympathetic Nervous System	↑↑	↑
Adrenal Medulla	↑↑	↑
Brain Noradrenergic Systems	↑↑	↑↑
Brain Dopaminergic Systems	↑↑	↑*
Brain Serotonergic Systems	↑	↑
Brain Tryptophan	↑↑	↑↑

*In some cases only.

not every specific aspect of sickness is necessarily adaptive at any given time.

Considering sickness behaviour as a relatively nonspecific behavioural defence strategy provides a rationale for interpreting the many non-immunological triggers that elicit something closely resembling sickness behaviour. For example, it has been shown that in the young of many species, maternal separation elicits a profile of behavioural change that in the past was considered to reflect despair [60]. This pattern of behaviour closely resembles sickness behaviour, including decreased activity, reduced social behaviour and induction of a crouched posture. Moreover, in common with other stressors, maternal separation activates the hypothalamo-pituitary adrenocortical (HPA) axis. Based on these observations, Hennessy and colleagues suggested that maternal separation induces "stress-induced sickness behaviour" [60].

Others have shown that over-training (i.e., excessive exercise) in athletes is associated with both increases in cytokines and a sickness behaviour profile, possibly because the musculoskeletal stress induces an inflammatory response [61]. Over-training is also associated with activation of the HPA axis, indicative of stress. It has been suggested that this over-training syndrome is a protective state that occurs during stress [61]. Given the various ways in which sickness behaviour can be induced, this profile of behavioural changes may be more than a response to immune activation, and may be a behavioural profile that can be elicited in many circumstances, especially stressful ones.

The presence of sickness-like behavioural profiles in maternal separation and over-training probably applies to other forms of stress. Most humans would consider that being sick is stressful. The behavioural similarities are obvious. Under stress, animals may eat less, be less interested in sexual activity, in exploring their environment, etc. Thus from a behavioural perspective, sickness can be considered a form of stress.

The parallels go beyond behaviour. Dunn et al. showed that infection with influenza virus induced a pattern of physiological responses that closely resembled responses to environmental stressors in activating the HPA axis, and certain neurochemical systems in the brain (noradrenergic and serotonergic) long associated with stress [62] (see Table III). Moreover, the responses to influenza virus resembled very closely those to peripheral (and intracerebral) administration of IL-1 and LPS [63].

The similarities between the physiological responses to IL-1, LPS and viral infection and environmental stressors are extensive [64], so that such agents have sometimes been referred to as "immune stressors". Both induce a profound activation of the HPA axis, elevating secretion of corticotropin-releasing factor (CRF) from the hypothalamus, resulting in secretion of adrenocorticotropin (ACTH) from the pituitary, and glucocorticoids from the adrenal cortex.

Moreover, the sympathoadrenal system is also activated by immune challenges, elevating circulating concentrations of the catecholamines, noradrenaline and adrenaline, although to a lesser extent than most environmental stressors. In addition, the responses within the brain are similar. In all cases, there is a widespread activation of cerebral noradrenergic systems, although the ventral (hypothalamic) system is activated by pathogens, IL-1 and LPS to a greater extent than with environmental stressors. In all cases, there is also an increase in brain tryptophan and serotonin metabolism. Cerebral CRF systems other than those associated with ACTH secretion also appear to be activated. The only major difference between immune challenges and environmental stress is in brain dopaminergic systems, which are activated less frequently during immune challenges (although they are affected by LPS, but minimally by IL-1), and in patterns distinct from those observed with environmental stressors, which tend to affect mesocortical and mesolimbic projections preferentially [64]. Thus an immune challenge can be regarded as a stressor from a physiological as well as a behavioural perspective, and it may be that sickness behaviour is but one example of a broad category of stress-related physiological changes.

A further interesting aspect is the relationship between clinical depression and sickness behaviour. Several authors have noted that the profile of behaviour seen in patients with major depression parallels that of sickness behaviour [65–67]. The cardinal symptoms of depression are depressed mood, and anhedonia (the inability to take pleasure in normally pleasurable activities). In fact, depression has been likened to a chronic state of stress. Behaviourally, depression can be associated with decreases in activity, decreased feeding, decreased sexual activity, decreased interest in a variety of activities and altered sleep patterns, behavioural changes that parallel sickness behaviour. Moreover, there are marked parallels in behaviour during stress and depression [68]. In addition, a majority (about two-thirds) of severely depressed patients exhibit a hyperactive or hyper-responsive HPA axis, and there is important evidence for a hyperactivity of brain noradrenergic systems, which are activated in stress [68,69].

Very specific parallels have been drawn between depression and the actions of LPS and IL-1 [65,66]. This has led to a cytokine hypothesis of depression which postulates that increased cytokine production from a variety of causes can induce the symptoms of depression [66]. Consistent with this, increased circulating concentrations of certain cytokines have been observed in depressed patients. However, the parallels between LPS- and IL-1-induced sickness behaviour are imperfect. Depressed patients often exhibit hyperphagia, rather than hypophagia, and the sleep abnormalities in depressed patients are more commonly the inability to sleep than the increased duration of slow-wave sleep observed with IL-1 and LPS [70]. Moreover, plasma cytokines are not elevated in all depressed patients, just as the HPA axis is not elevated in all depressed patients. It is entirely possible that some chronic diseases induce depression and elevate cytokines, and that in some cases the cytokines contribute to the depression. However, it is clear that cytokines are not the sole cause of depression. Nevertheless, there are clear parallels, both behaviourally and physiologically between stress, sickness and depression.

Clearly there are multiple parallels between immune and environmental stressors. An apparent difference between the stress induced by infection and environmental stressors is that the activation of a cytokine response is part of the immune system's response to an unrecognised antigen. However, over-training also appears to increases circulating concentrations of cytokines [61] and through activation of an acute phase response [60], maternal separation may also do so. This observation is consistent with evidence that restraint and footshock elevate the circulating concentrations of certain cytokines (especially IL-6) [71–74]. Such changes in plasma cytokines do not appear to be responsible for the physiological and behavioural changes [75]. A possible explanation for the plasma cytokine (e.g., IL-6) response induced during stress could be that it primes the immune system for a response that may be needed when individuals are under stress, or that it reflects such a priming. By adopting an appropriate behavioural profile and increasing cytokine secretion, the organism may be better prepared to counter pathogens.

This suggestion is congruent with evidence that meal intake activates the mucosal immune system. Hansen et al. have shown that meal consumption results in increased levels of neutrophils and granulocytes and reduced levels of lymphocytes [76]. These authors suggested that these changes reflect cell migration that supports immune responses in the gut. Based on these findings, one could speculate that because the consumption of a meal puts the organism at risk of pathogen exposure, an immune system response to eating minimizes the threat of pathogens ingested during the meal. Similarly, studies have shown that acute restraint produces both a stress response and immunoenhancement, as measured by increased leukocyte trafficking [77,78]. Thus it can be speculated that behaviours that induce an acute stress response may facilitate immune responding. Indeed, Dhabhar [78] speculated that "a hormonal alarm signal released by the brain upon detecting a stressor, may "prepare" the immune system for potential challenges (wounding or infection) which may arise due to the actions of the stress-inducing agent (e.g., a predatory or attacker)" (p. 789). Perhaps the stress-related increases in certain cytokines are such a signal.

The information reviewed above suggests that it may well be that the behavioural responses induced by pathogens are adaptive responses serving to facilitate survival as originally described by Hart [2]. Given the arguments that events like maternal separation, excessive exercise and depression can induce sickness-like behaviour, we may need to extend our thinking about sickness behaviour beyond Hart's original analysis. Stress elicits a behavioural profile resembling sickness behaviour, and increases the secretion of certain cytokines. Thus it is suggested that the immune system is sensitive to the behaviours of the organism, and perhaps can be activated in a manner that minimizes the possible deleterious effects of these behaviours. For example, it can be speculated that mucosal immune activation after a meal minimizes possible deleterious effects of eating, and "sickness behaviour" during maternal separation might prevent activities that result in an immunological challenge. The behavioural changes induced by immune activation likely facilitate survival and they may do so as part of a general, nonspecific response to stressors, immunological or otherwise, that serves to protect the animal.

4. CONCLUSIONS

Animals exhibit multiple behavioural strategies that serve as a defence against pathogens (Table II). Some of these strategies involve reflex responses, for example, to objects that may harbour pathogens, or to sick individuals. Other strategies involve learning from previous experiences, as well as observing the experiences of others. Thus these reflex responses and learned avoidance behaviours are an important component of behavioural defence, allowing an organism to respond to its environment in a way that minimizes the threat from pathogens.

The immune system may also be involved in behavioural defence against pathogens. The behavioural pattern of sick individuals, which has come to be known as sickness behaviour (Table I), clearly has defensive value and is no longer considered maladaptive. The existing evidence supports the idea that sickness behaviour is induced by the immune system, probably through the actions of certain cytokines, hormone-like factors secreted by cells of the immune system, but other factors may also be involved. Thus the immune system affects behaviour. This may explain why quite similar behavioural patterns are observed in sickness, despite very diverse causes. Sickness behaviour has much in common with behavioural patterns observed in individuals under stress, and in clinical depression. Thus sickness behaviour may be a special case of stress-induced behaviours.

The immune system-induced behavioural changes provide an important component of behavioural defence. The general depression of activity serves to conserve energy and to encourage animals to hide in safety from predators, to avoid additional injuries and infections. The increased sleep time adds to this. The lack of activity also conserves energy at a time when the animal may not be able to gather food. It may also fuel a fever, which in some cases impairs proliferation of pathogens, and may enhance the efficacy of the immune system. The general reduction in activity is bolstered by the relative lack of interest in eating, sexual activities, and exploring novel objects or environments. Thus sickness affects motivation. Nevertheless, it is clear that specific sickness behaviours may be absent if they are inappropriate for the particular circumstances of the organism.

There is limited evidence that behaviour can affect immune function. There may be some conditioning effects on immune function. Also, a general increase in the circulating concentrations of certain cytokines (e.g., IL-6) may prime the immune for action, when the environment threatens or a high-risk behaviour occurs. The net result is that, in the event that animals become infected with pathogens or injured, their behaviour changes in a manner that facilitates their recovery.

ACKNOWLEDGEMENTS

The authors' research described was supported by the National Institute of Mental Health (MH46261) and the National Institute of Neurological Diseases and Stroke (NS25370).

REFERENCES

1. Selye H. The stress of my life. New York: Van Nostrand; 1979 pp. 56–7.
2. Hart BL. Biological basis of the behavior of sick animals. Neurosci Biobehav Rev 1988; 12:123–37.
3. Kent S, Bluthé RM, Kelley KW, Dantzer R. Sickness behavior as a new target for drug development. Trends Pharmacol Sci 1992;13:24–8.
4. Dantzer R, Bluthé RM, Castanon N, Chauvet N, Capuron L, Goodall G, et al. Cytokine effects on behavior. In: Ader R, Felten DL, Cohen N, editors. Psychoneuroimmunology, Third Edition; San Diego: Academic Press, 2001;703–27.
5. Larson SJ, Dunn AJ. Behavioral effects of cytokines. Brain Behav Immun 2001;15: 371–87.
6. Alcock J. Animal Behavior: An Evolutionary Approach, Sixth Edition. Sunderland, MA: Sinauer Associates;1998.
7. Hart BL. Behavioral adaptations to pathogens and parasites: Five strategies. Neurosci Biobehav Rev 1990;14:273–94.
8. Moore J. The behavior of parasitized animals. BioScience 1995;45:89–98.
9. Odberg FO, Francis-Smith K. Studies on the formation of ungrazed eliminative areas in fields used by horses. Appl Anim Ethol 1977;3:27–34.
10. Henry RE, Winkler L. Foraging, feeding and defecation site selection as a parasite

avoidance strategy of Alouatta palliata in a dry tropical forest. Am J Physical Anthropol 2001;79.
11. Curtis V, Biran A. Dirt, disgust, and disease. Is hygiene in our genes? Perspect Biol Med. 2001;44:17–31.
12. Neese G, Williams C. Evolution and healing. London: Weidenfeld & Nicolson;1995.
13. Stake MM, Cavanagh PM. Removal of host nestlings and fecal sacs by Brown-headed Cowbirds. Wilson Bull 2001;113:456–60.
14. Krinke GJ (Ed.) The Laboratory Rat. San Diego: Academic Press;2000.
15. Dell'omo G, Alleva E, Carere C. Parental recycling of nestling faeces in the common swift. Anim Behav 1998;56:631–7.
16. Hornicke H, Bjornhag G. Coprophagy and related strategies for digesta utilisation. In: Ruckebusch Y, Thivend P, editors. Digestive Physiology and Metabolism in Ruminants, Westport: AVT Publishing, 1999;707–30.
17. Moltz H. Of rats and infants and necrotizing enterocolitis. Perspect Biol Med 1984;27: 327–35.
18. Butler JE. Immunologic aspects of breast feeding, antiinfectious activity of breast milk. Semin Perinatol 1979;3:255–70.
19. Pujol N, Link EM, Liu LX, Kurz CL, Alloing G, Tan MW, et al. A reverse genetic analysis of components of the Toll signaling pathway in Caenorhabditis elegans. Curr Biol 2001;11: 809–21.
20. Imler JL, Hoffmann JA. Toll receptors in innate immunity. Trends Cell Biol 2001;11: 304–11.
21. Garcia J, Koelling RA. Relation of cue to consequence in avoidance learning. Psychonom Sci 1966;4:123–4.
22. Exton MS, Bull DF, King MG. Behavioral conditioning of lipopolysaccharide-induced anorexia. Physiol Behav 1995;57:401–5.
23. Bernstein IL, Sigmundi RA. Tumor anorexia: A learned food aversion? Science 1980;209: 416–8.
24. Bernstein IL, Treneer CM, Goehler LE, Murowchick E. Tumor growth in rats: Conditioned suppression of food intake and preference. Behav Neurosci 1985;99:818–30.
25. Ader R, Cohen N. Behaviorally conditioned immunosuppression. Psychosom Med. 1975;37:333–40.
26. Ramirez-Amaya V, Bermudez-Rattoni F. Conditioned enhancement of antibody production is disrupted by insular cortex and amygdala but not hippocampal lesions. Brain Behav Immun 1999;13:46–60.
27. Stockhorst U, Spennes-Saleh S, Kornholz D, Gobel U, Schneider ME, Steingruber HJ, et al. Anticipatory symptoms and anticipatory immune responses in pediatric cancer patients recovering from chemotherapy: Features of a classically conditioned response? Brain Behav Immun 2000;14:198–218.
28. Galef Jr BG. An adaptationist perspective on social learning, social feeding and social foraging in Norway rats. In: Dewsbery DA, editor. Contemporary Issues in Comparative Psychology. Sunderland: Sinauer Associates, 1989;55–79.
29. Galef Jr BG, Giraldeau LA. Social influences on foraging in vertebrates: Casual mechanisms and adaptive functions. Anim Behav 2001;61:3–15.
30. Birch LL. Effects of peer models' food choices and eating behaviors on preschoolers' food preferences. Child Devel 1980;51:489–96.
31. Jansen A, Tenney N. Seeing mum drinking a 'light' product: Is social learning a stronger

determinant of taste preference acquisition than caloric conditioning? Eur J Clin Nutr 2001;55:418–22.
32. McCarthy DO, Kluger MJ, Vander AJ. The role of fever in appetite suppression after endotoxin administration. Amer J Clin Nutr 1984;40:310–6.
33. Plata-Salamán CR. Anorexia during acute and chronic disease. Nutrition 1996;12:69–78.
34. Swiergiel AH, Smagin GN, Dunn AJ. Influenza virus infection of mice induces anorexia: Comparison with endotoxin and interleukin-1 and the effects of indomethacin. Pharmacol Biochem Behav 1997;57:389–96.
35. Krueger JM, Toth LA. Cytokines as regulators of sleep. Ann NY Acad Sci 1994;739: 299–310.
36. Krueger JM, Majde JA. Microbial products and cytokines in sleep and fever regulation. Crit Rev Immunol 1995;14:355–79.
37. Avitsur R, Yirmiya R. The immunobiology of sexual behavior: gender differences in the suppression of sexual activity during illness. Pharmacol Biochem Behav 1999;64: 787–96.
38. Dunn AJ, Chapman Y, Antoon M. Endotoxin-induced behavioral changes of mice in the multicompartment chamber are distinct from those of interleukin-1. Neurosci Res Commun 1992;10:63–9.
39. Bluthé RM, Dantzer R, Kelley KW. Effects of interleukin-1 receptor antagonist on the behavioral effects of lipopolysaccharide in rat. Brain Res 1992;573:318–20.
40. Gibertini M, Newton C, Friedman H, Klein TW. Spatial learning impairment in mice infected with *Legionella pneumophila* or administered exogenous interleukin-1-β. Brain Behav Immun 1995;9:113–28.
41. Pugh CR, Kumagawa K, Fleshner M, Watkins LR, Maier SF, Rudy JW. Selective effects of peripheral lipopolysaccharide administration on contextual and auditory-cue fear conditioning. Brain Behav Immun 1998;12:212–29.
42. Yirmiya R. Endotoxin produces a depressive-like episode in rats. Brain Res 1996;711: 163–74.
43. Kluger MJ, Ringler DH, Anver MR. Fever and survival. Science 1975;188:166–8.
44. Bernheim HA, Kluger MJ. Fever: Effect of drug-induced antipyresis on survival. Science 1976;193:237–9.
45. Doran TF, De Angelis C, Baumgardner RA, Mellits ED. Acetaminophen: more harm than good for chickenpox? J Pediatr 1989;114:1045–8.
46. Graham NM, Burrell CJ, Douglas RM, Debelle P, Davies L. Adverse effects of aspirin, acetaminophen, and ibuprofen on immune function, viral shedding, and clinical status in rhinovirus-infected volunteers. J Infect Dis 1990;162:1277–82.
47. Kluger MJ, Kozak W, Conn CA, Leon LR, Soszynski D. Role of fever in disease. Ann N Y Acad Sci 1998;856:224–33.
48. Blatteis, CM. Fever: pathological or physiological, injurious or beneficial? J Thermal Biol 2003;28:1–13.
49. Murray MJ, Murray AB. Anorexia of infection as a mechanism of host defense. Am J Clini Nutr 1979;32:593–6.
50. Wing EJ, Young JB. Acute starvation protects mice against Listeria Monocytogenes. Infect Immun 1980;28:771–6.
51. Exton MS. Infection-induced anorexia: Active host defence strategy. Appetite 1997;29: 369–83.
52. Aubert A, Kelley KW, Dantzer R. Differential effects of lipopolysaccharide on food

hoarding behaviour and food consumption in rats. Brain Behav Immun 1997;11:229–38.
53. Larson SJ, Romanoff RR, Dunn AJ, Glowa JR. Effects of interleukin-1β on food-maintained behavior in the mouse. Brain Behav Immun 2002;16:398–410.
54. Spadaro F, Dunn AJ. Intracerebroventricular administration of interleukin-1 to mice alters investigation of stimuli in a novel environment. Brain Behav Immun 1990;4:308–22.
55. Dunn A J, Antoon, M, Chapman Y. Reduction of exploratory behavior by intraperitoneal injection of interluekin-1 involves brain corticotropin-releasing factor. Brain Res Bull 1991;26:539–42.
56. Bindra D. Motivation: a systematic reinterpretation. New York: Ronald Press Company; 1959.
57. Aubert A. Sickness and behaviour in animals: A motivational perspective. Neurosci Biobehav Rev 1999;23:1029–36.
58. Miller NE. Some psychophysiological studies of motivation and of the behavioral effects of illness. Bull Brit Psych Soc 1964;17:1–20.
59. Gibertini, M. Cytokines and cognitive behavior. Neuroimmunomodul 1998;5:160–5.
60. Hennessy MB, Deak T, Schiml-Webb PA. Stress-induced sickness behaviors: An alternative hypothesis for responses during maternal separation. Dev Psychobiol 2001;39: 76–83.
61. Smith LL. Cytokine hypothesis of overtraining: A physiological adaptation to excessive stress? Med Sci Sports Exerc 2000;32:317–31.
62. Dunn AJ, Powell ML, Meitin C, Small PA. Virus infection as a stressor: influenza virus elevates plasma concentrations of corticosterone, and brain concentrations of MHPG and tryptophan. Physiol Behav 1989;45:591–4.
63. Dunn AJ. Endotoxin-induced activation of cerebral catecholamine and serotonin metabolism: comparison with interleukin-1. J Pharmacol Exptl Therapeut 1992;261: 964–9.
64. Dunn AJ, Wang J-P, Ando T. Effects of cytokines on central neurotransmission. Comparison with the effects of stress. Adv Expl Med Biol 1999;461:117–27.
65. Yirmiya R. Behavioral and psychological effects of immune activation: Implications for 'depression due to a general medical condition'. Cur Opin Psychiat 1997;10:470–6.
66. Dantzer R, Wollman E, Vitkovic L, Yirmiya R. Cytokines, stress and depression. Adv Expl Med Biol 1999;461:317–29.
67. Charlton BG. The malaise theory of depression: Major depressive disorder is sickness behavior and antidepressants are analgesic. Med Hypotheses 2000;54:126–30.
68. Weiss JM, Simson PG, Ambrose MJ, Webster A, Hoffman, LJ. Neurochemical basis of behavioral depression. Adv Behav Med 1985;1:233–75.
69. Stone EA. Brain noradrenergic mechanisms in models of depression. In: Halbreich U, editor. Hormones and Depression. New York: Raven Press, 1987;263–78.
70. de Beaurepaire R. Questions raised by the cytokine hypothesis of depression. Brain Behav Immun 2002;16:610–7.
71. Zhou D, Kusnecov AW, Shurin MR, DePaoli M, Rabin BS. Exposure to physical and psychological stressors elevates plasma interleukin 6: Relationship to the activation of hypothalamic-pituitary-adrenal axis. Endocrinol 1993;133:2523–30.
72. Takaki A, Huang QH, Somogyvari-Vigh A, Arimura A. Immobilization stress may increase plasma interleukin-6 via central and peripheral catecholamines. Neuroimmunomod 1995;1:335–42.
73. Maes M, Song C, Lin A, De Jongh R, Van Gastel A, Kenis G, et al. The effects of

psychological stress on humans: increased production of pro-inflammatory cytokines and a Th1-like response in stress-induced anxiety. Cytokine 1998;10:313–8.
74. Nukina H, Sudo N, Aiba Y, Oyama N, Koga Y, Kubo C. Restraint stress elevates the plasma interleukin-6 levels in germ-free mice. J Neuroimmunol 2001;115:46–52.
75. Swiergiel AH, Dunn AJ. The roles of IL-1, IL-6 and TNFα in the feeding responses to endotoxin and influenza virus infection in mice. Brain Behav Immun 1999;13:252–65.
76. Hansen K, Sickelmann F, Pietrowsky R, Fehm HL, Born J. Systemic immune changes following meal intake in humans. Am J Physiol 1997;273:R548–53.
77. Dhabhar FS, McEwen BS. Acute stress enhances while chronic stress suppresses cell-medicated immunity *in vivo*: A potential role for leukocyte trafficking. Brain Behav Immun 1997;11:286–306.
78. Dhabhar FS. Stress-induced augmentation of immune function – The role of stress hormones, leukocyte trafficking, and cytokines. Brain Behav Immun 2002;16:785–98.

Keyword Index

Symbols

A

B

C

G

H

I

K

L

O

P

R

S

T

U

V

W